YOU CAN'T SEE THEM, TASTE THEM, OR SMELL THEM—BUT CALORIES COUNT.

"My own diet"—what works best for each individual—is the most successful diet in the United States today. Forget fads. With the sound advice and calorie information found in *The Calorie Counter*, 5th Edition, you can make consistent, small changes in the way you eat that will help you lose weight and keep it off.

- **Understand calories**
- **Understand portions**
- **Determine the calories you need daily**
- **Calculate the calories you burn through exercise and everyday activities**
- **Find out the truth about dieting myths**
- **Manage "mindless eating"**
- **Stop battling your weight**

THE CALORIE COUNTER
5th Edition

If you eat it, you'll find it here!

Books by Karen J. Nolan and Jo-Ann Heslin

The Calorie Counter (*Fifth Edition*)

The Ultimate Carbohydrate Counter (*Third Edition*)

Books by Annette B. Natow, Jo-Ann Heslin, and Karen J. Nolan

The Cholesterol Counter (*Seventh Edition*)

The Complete Food Counter (*Third Edition*)

The Diabetes Carbohydrate and Calorie Counter (*Third Edition*)

The Fat Counter (*Seventh Edition*)

The Healthy Wholefoods Counter

The Most Complete Food Counter (*Second Edition*)

Books by Annette B. Natow and Jo-Ann Heslin

Eating Out Food Counter

The Healthy Heart Food Counter

The Protein Counter (*Second Edition*)

The Vitamin and Mineral Food Counter

Published by POCKET BOOKS

THE
CALORIE
COUNTER

FIFTH EDITION

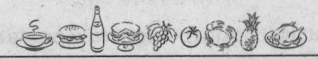

**Karen J. Nolan, Ph.D.
and Jo-Ann Heslin, M.A., R.D.**

POCKET BOOKS
New York   London   Sydney   Toronto

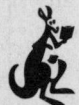 Pocket Books
A Division of Simon & Schuster, Inc.
1230 Avenue of the Americas
New York, NY 10020

This Pocket Books paperback edition January 2010

POCKET and colophon are registered trademarks of Simon & Schuster, Inc.

For information about special discounts for bulk purchases, please contact Simon & Schuster Special Sales at 1-866-506-1949 or business@simonandschuster.com.

The Simon & Schuster Speakers Bureau can bring authors to your live event. For more information or to book an event, contact the Simon & Schuster Speakers Bureau at 1-866-248-3049 or visit our website at www.simonspeakers.com.

Cover photo by Michael Rosenfeld/Getty

Manufactured in the United States of America

10 9 8 7 6 5 4 3 2 1

ISBN 978-1-4165-6667-0
ISBN 978-1-4391-6649-9 (ebook)

For Annette.

We continue to build on the foundation
you helped put in place.

ACKNOWLEDGMENTS

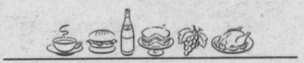

For all her continuous support and help, our agent, Nancy Trichter.

For her suggestions and editing skills, Sara Clemence.

For all her patience, comments, and suggestions—our favorite reviewer, Jean Schwarsin.

Without the tireless cooperation of Stephen Llano and the production department at Pocket Books, *The Calorie Counter, Fifth Edition* would never have been completed.

A special thank-you to our editor, Micki Nuding.

We would also like to thank all of our readers for their suggestions and questions. Your input helps us to provide you with the most useful information.

*Man is to be compared to a clock, going all
the time, rather than to an automobile engine,
working only at intervals. . . .*

*In order to have energy to spend . . . we
must first acquire it . . . protein, fat, and
carbohydrate . . . are the fuels which supply
energy for the human machine.*

Mary Swartz Rose, Ph.D.
Feeding the Family
The MacMillan Company, 1919

CONTENTS

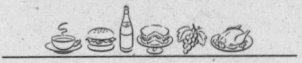

Introduction   1
Understanding Calories   4
Understanding Portions   7
Calories You Need   11
Real Men Can Count Calories   14
The Truth, and Nothing but the Truth   19
Calories You Use   23
Minimize Mindless Eating   30
Tracking Calories   34
Using Your Calorie Counter   38
Definitions   41
Abbreviations   42
Notes   43

PART ONE

Brand Name, Nonbranded (Generic), and Take-Out Foods

45

PART TWO

Restaurant Chains

527

INTRODUCTION

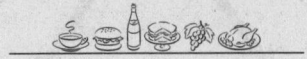

If losing weight were easy, no one would weigh too much.

If you're looking at this book, you are probably trying to lose weight. You aren't alone; *losing weight has become one of the most important health concerns in America.*

Everyone is scrambling to solve the problem of America's expanding waistlines. The federal government, public health and professional organizations, educators, pharmaceutical companies, food manufacturers, and even restaurant chains all want to slow down the nation's weight gain epidemic. But new policies, programs, food formulations, and drug approvals occur slowly. Like most people we talk to every day, you are not willing to wait. *You want to lose weight now!*

So let's get started . . .

Weight gain results from a combination of your genes and your environment. Food is everywhere we turn, all through the day. And most of us live lifestyles that require little physical activity, unless we make an effort to move.

There isn't much you can do about your genetic profile, which was fixed before you were born. But you *can* control your environment, especially your eating environment. And that's what we hope *The Calorie Counter* will help you do.

1

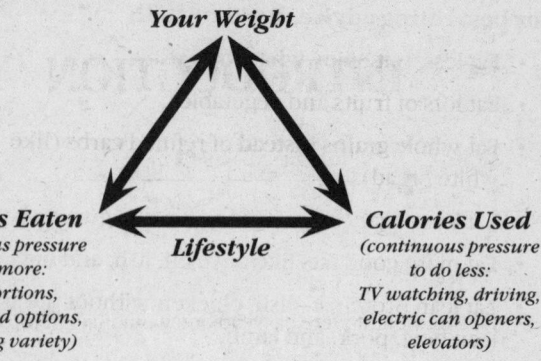

Your Weight

Calories Eaten
*(continuous pressure
to eat more:
large portions,
mobile food options,
increasing variety)*

Lifestyle

Calories Used
*(continuous pressure
to do less:
TV watching, driving,
electric can openers,
elevators)*

Two important things you should know:

***The most successful diet in the U.S. today is what peo-
ple call "my own diet."*** Forget fads. With the sound advice
and the calorie information found in this book, you can de-
sign your own diet—one that works.

Consistent small changes will add up to big results.
When it comes to losing weight and *maintaining* your
weight loss, making many small changes in the way you re-
late to food will result in more success than making a few big
changes, which usually don't last.

Skeptical?

If you eat 100 fewer calories each day for a year, and
change nothing else in your life, you will lose 10 pounds. All
you'd have to do is give up 1 slice of bread or 1 cookie or 1
small soda each day. A small change for a big result. Make a
few more of those small changes and the end result could be
very impressive.

Our best eating advice, in a nutshell:

- Eat less, but enjoy what you eat.
- Eat lots of fruits and vegetables.
- Eat whole grains instead of refined carbs (like white bread).
- Eat less sugar (but you don't have to give it up).
- Eat more good fats like olive oil, fish, and nuts.
- Eat lean proteins—fish, chicken without the skin, lean beef, pork, and lamb.
- Enjoy a glass of wine, but not the whole bottle.
- Move more, and move often—find ways to be active throughout the day.

10%

Losing 10% of your body weight—15 pounds for someone who weighs 150 pounds, 20 pounds for a person weighing 200 pounds, or 30 pounds if the scale says 300 pounds—is all that is needed to significantly improve your health.

Lose 10% of your current body weight and you'll have:

Lower blood pressure
Improved cholesterol levels
Decreased risk for diabetes
Better sex

Reaching your ideal weight is great, but even just a 10% drop in body weight improves both your health and appearance.

UNDERSTANDING CALORIES

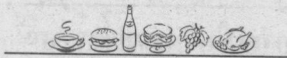

*You can't see them, taste them or smell
them, but calories count!*

Calories are calories, whether they come from apples or chocolate fudge. Every time you eat, you take in calories. All foods except water have some. Your body is a machine that uses food calories as fuel. When the amount of fuel you take in equals the amount of fuel you need to run your body, your weight remains constant. There is no extra fuel to store, and no deficit to make up. Eat too many calories, and your body uses what it needs and stores the leftovers for future use. You see this storage on your thighs, hips, and waist. Eat too few calories, and your body draws on its fuel reserves to meet demands. Your thighs, hips, and waist get slimmer as your fuel surplus is depleted.

You can think of the extra pounds you are carrying around as a warehouse of stored fuel. Empty the warehouse and you lose weight. Fill up the warehouse and you gain weight.

Again and again, studies have shown that if you cut calories, you lose weight. It doesn't matter if those calories come from bread, meat, or salad dressing. When you eat too many calories, even from healthy foods, you gain weight.

The key to long-term weight control is to burn as many calories as you eat. In order to do that effectively, you need to know how many calories you need, and how many calories you burn in activity. Then you can see if the two balance each other.

And the Numbers Are?

On average, we eat 300 more calories a day than we ate 35 years ago and we weigh 24 pounds more.

Women report eating 1,877 calories a day; men 2,618 calories.

The catch—up to 75% of people underreport what they really eat!

Beware of Calories in a Glass (or Bottle . . . or Can . . .)

At most restaurants, drink refills are free. You'll quickly get more soda and coffee without even asking. You get more, so you drink more. You're thinking, It's free, so why shouldn't I drink it? One reason: liquid calories could be helping you pack on extra pounds. It seems our bodies don't process calories from drinks the same way we process calories from food.

Alcoholic drinks and clear liquids like soda, fruit drinks, energy drinks, and sweetened tea are potential diet disasters. Alcoholic drinks can be very calorie dense (see page 303) and they make you eat more. Studies show if you have a glass of wine with dinner, you'll eat more food. Your calorie intake can go up by as much as 40%.

Beverages also have a very low satisfaction level, which means the more you are offered, the more you drink, often without considering the calories. Soda is the single largest source of calories in the American diet. The increased intake of calorie-containing clear drinks parallels our sharp rise in weight gain over the past three decades.

At the same time, the portion sizes of typical beverages have increased. We've gone from an 8-ounce bottle of Coke to unlimited soda refills served in a quart-size glass. A small coffee now averages 10 ounces, in contrast to the old 5-ounce cup. Add cream and sugar and your small coffee equals 100 calories. And few of us ever order "small." Multiply that by 3 or 4 cups a day, and you start to see why it's hard to lose weight.

To keep calories down when you are thirsty:

- Choose low- or no-calorie drinks.

- Drink nonfat milk instead of whole milk.

- Dilute fruit drinks with mineral water.

- Dilute alcohol with low- or no-calorie mixers.

- Drink light beer and not too many.

- Order hot cocoa with skim milk and no whipped topping.

- Order coffee minus the whipped toppings and other add-ons.

- Drink water; it's thirst quenching and calorie free.

UNDERSTANDING PORTIONS

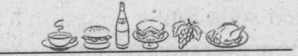

Smaller portions = a smaller you.

With the exception of a slice of bread, the portion sizes of commonly eaten foods have steadily grown over the past 20 years. Even the average restaurant dinner plate is 2 inches larger! We've gotten so used to these exaggerated amounts that we think of them as normal.

What Research Has Shown

Larger portions encourage people to overeat, even foods that they don't like or that don't taste good.

Serving large portions encourages people to eat up to 40% more calories at a meal.

After eating a large portion or a regular portion, people rated their feelings of fullness the same, though they ate more of the large portion.

Twenty years ago, the muffin or bagel you bought with your morning coffee weighed 2 ounces. Today, 4 to 6 ounces is more the norm. When burger shops first opened, an average soda was 8 ounces, regular French fries were 2.5 ounces, and the burger plus bun weighed less than 4 ounces. Today, a medium soda averages 20 ounces, and the French fries and burger have been supersized. They're 2 to 5 times larger than the original, adding up to a 1,000-calorie meal.

PORTION DISTORTION
Today's "normal" portion is actually a supersized serving.

FOOD ITEM	20 YEARS AGO CALORIES (PORTION)	TODAY CALORIES (PORTION)	CALORIE DIFFERENCE
Soda	150 (12 ounces)	400 (32 ounces)	250
Muffin	210 (1.5 ounces)	500 (4 ounces)	290
Pepperoni Pizza	500 (2 slices)	850 (2 slices)	350
Chicken Caesar Salad	390 (1½ cups)	790 (3½ cups)	400
Movie theater popcorn	270 (5 cups)	630 (11 cups)	360
Chicken stir-fry	435 (2 cups)	865 (4½ cups)	430

You may think larger portions are bargains, without appreciating how many extra calories you're eating. According to a government survey, Americans typically eat 2½ times the standard serving of potatoes, 4 times the standard serving of pasta, and 2 times the standard serving of rice. A standard serving for all is ½ cup.

Seeing Is Believing

These visual cues will help you keep portion sizes to a reasonable amount of food, which automatically reduces calories.

computer mouse	=	*4-ounce portion of meat, chicken, seafood*
		or
		1 medium baked potato
yo-yo	=	*a mini bagel or 100 calories (How many yo-yo's fit into your bagel, muffin, or pastry?)*
tennis ball	=	*medium piece of fresh fruit*
ping pong ball	=	*a 2-ounce serving of cheese*
		or
		2 tablespoons of salad dressing, gravy, sour cream, peanut butter
music CD	=	*1 medium-size pancake or small waffle*
quarter	=	*1 pat butter*

We even eat large portions of good-for-you fruits and vegetables. Many people don't realize that larger portions have more calories. They figure a soda is a soda, no matter how big—until you stop and calculate that a 32-ounce soda has 400 calories. Next time you order, think small: soda, coffee, movie theater popcorn, ice cream cones, French fries, even medium-size fruits.

When you snack, pick single-serving packages. How many times have you opened a bag of chips just to have a few, and before you knew it the bag was empty? A 1-ounce snack-size bag of chips allows you to enjoy a favorite treat without sabotaging your weight loss goals. Single-serving pudding, ice cream, pretzels, peanuts, cookies, and snack-size yogurt will help you keep overindulging under control.

CALORIES YOU NEED

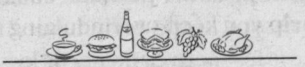

Obesity may soon replace smoking as the country's
leading cause of preventable death.

Most of us eat more than we admit and exercise less than we
should. The consequence is that we weigh more than we
should, and blame it all on our metabolism—even if we're
not quite sure what that is.

Human metabolism is the sum of all the chemical reactions that occur in your body. Your body takes in foods,
burns some to generate power, uses some to produce new
material, and routes the rest into storage for future use. The
chemical reactions that occur either break down large com-
pounds into smaller units (the foods you eat, for example,
are broken down into smaller units of energy), or build com-
plex structures from smaller units (your muscles are made
up of fragments that come from the protein foods you eat,
like eggs). Human metabolism is the sum total of all the energy used to keep your body alive and moving. The energy
required to make all this happen can be translated into the
calories you need each day.

Approximately 60% to 75% of your daily calories are
used just to keep you alive. Energy is needed to maintain
your body's temperature, allow your nerves to work, let you
breathe, keep your heart beating, allow your organs to func-

tion, nourish your body tissues, and repair and replace body fluids and parts. It's a pretty big job that goes on 24 hours a day.

An interesting thing about this basic energy requirement is that different tissues in the body have different levels of activity. Fat tissue is less active and needs less energy. Muscle tissue, even at rest, is more active and uses up more energy. If you exercise and develop more muscle tissue, your body burns more calories every day just keeping your muscles healthy.

The rest of the calories you need each day are used to support your level of activity. You need less if you are relatively inactive, and more if you are very active.

To find out how many calories you need each day, you need to do two things. First, decide how much you want to weigh. What is your target weight? Then, select an activity factor that fits your current activity level.

1. Your target weight is: _____.
2. Your activity factor is: _____.
    20 = Very active men
    15 = Moderately active men or very active women
    13 = Inactive men, moderately active women, and people over 55
    10 = Inactive women, repeat dieters, seriously overweight people
3. Target Weight × Activity Factor = Calories needed each day.

For example, if your target weight is 130 and you are a moderately active woman (factor 13), you need just under 1700 calories a day.

$$130 \text{ pounds} \times 13 = 1690 \text{ calories}$$

Eating this amount of calories each day would guarantee weight loss, because you are getting only enough calories to support your target weight, not your current heavier weight. Couple this calorie intake with some added exercise and the weight will come off even faster.

REAL MEN CAN COUNT CALORIES

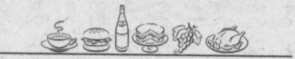

*In contrast to women, if a man cuts calories,
he'll lose more weight and he'll lose it faster.*

Announcing you are on a diet is not manly. Munching on salad, eating yogurt topped with granola, or sipping green tea does not conjure up a macho image. But over half of American men weigh too much, and many are trying to drop pounds.

According to the National Center for Health Statistics, 71% of American men are overweight, while only 62% of women are, based on their Body Mass Index (BMI). Having a BMI of more than 25 tips you into the overweight group. You may be carrying around only a few extra pounds, but as time goes on these "extra" pounds add up as you slide from the overweight category into the much too heavy, obese group. Clearly, losing weight is no longer for women only.

BMI is not a foolproof way to measure overweight. A person with a very muscular, dense body build and a low percentage of body fat could end up with the same BMI as someone who truly is overweight and who has a high percentage of body fat. One way to sort out the difference is to measure waistlines. Experts say that those with a BMI of 25

YOUR BODY MASS INDEX (BMI)

WEIGHT

HEIGHT	100	105	110	115	120	125	130	135	140	145	150	155	160	165	170	175	180	185	190	195	200	205
5'0"	20	21	21	22	23	24	25	26	27	28	29	30	31	32	33	34	35	36	37	38	39	40
5'1"	19	20	21	22	23	24	25	26	26	27	28	29	30	31	32	33	34	35	36	37	38	39
5'2"	18	19	20	21	22	23	24	25	26	27	28	28	29	30	31	32	33	34	35	36	37	37
5'3"	18	18	19	20	21	22	23	24	25	26	27	27	28	29	30	31	32	33	34	35	35	36
5'4"	17	18	19	20	21	21	22	23	24	25	26	27	27	28	29	30	31	32	33	34	34	35
5'5"	17	17	18	19	20	21	22	22	23	24	25	26	27	27	28	29	30	31	32	33	33	34
5'6"	16	17	18	19	19	20	21	22	23	23	24	25	26	27	27	28	29	30	31	31	32	33
5'7"	16	16	17	18	19	20	21	21	22	23	23	24	25	26	27	27	28	29	30	31	31	32
5'8"	15	16	17	18	18	19	20	21	21	22	23	24	24	25	26	26	27	28	29	30	30	31
5'9"	15	16	16	17	18	18	19	20	21	21	22	23	24	24	25	26	27	27	28	29	30	30
5'10"	14	15	16	17	17	18	19	19	20	21	22	22	23	24	24	25	26	27	28	28	29	30
5'11"	14	15	16	16	17	18	18	19	20	20	21	22	22	23	24	24	25	26	27	27	28	29
6'0"	14	14	15	16	16	17	18	18	19	20	20	21	22	22	23	24	24	25	26	26	27	28
6'1"	13	14	15	15	16	17	17	18	18	19	20	20	21	22	22	23	24	24	25	26	26	27
6'2"	13	13	14	15	15	16	17	17	18	19	19	20	21	21	22	22	23	24	24	25	26	26
6'3"	12	13	14	14	15	16	16	17	17	18	19	19	20	21	21	22	23	23	24	24	25	26
6'4"	12	13	13	14	15	15	16	16	17	18	18	19	19	20	21	21	22	23	23	24	24	25

to 35, and with waistlines of 40 inches or more for men and 35 inches or more for women, are considered overweight. They face increased health risks because they are carrying around too many pounds.

Use the BMI scale on page 15 to see where you stand. Find your height on the left of the chart. Find the weight closest to your weight across the top of the chart. Follow the weight column down and the height column across until they meet. Your BMI is the number at the intersection of your weight and height.

Your BMI is _____.

A study with over 50,000 men showed that 3 lifestyle factors predicted weight gain: less time exercising, more time watching TV, and eating between meals. Eating a soup bowl of ice cream while sitting in your recliner, waving the remote at the TV, will not make you trim.

Most weight loss research has been done with women, but the few studies we have on men tell us very good news. Men are very successful at losing weight. They can eat more food and still lose weight; they lose weight faster; and when they trip up, they are less likely to get derailed and feel guilty.

You Should Know

The bigger a man's waistline, the lower his testosterone level, sex drive, sperm count, and likelihood of conceiving a child.

Sadly, many men don't take weight loss seriously until they have a major health problem, like diabetes or a heart attack. What men need to realize is that making lifestyle changes *before* a catastrophe hits could prevent it from ever happening.

You may feel dieting is wimpy, but striving for health and fitness is manly. Aerobic exercise—walking, jogging, and bike riding—helps to lower pounds and reduce fat around your middle. Lowering body weight by as little as 10% can improve your health risks and increase your stamina on the basketball court and in the bedroom.

Watching calories is a simple and easy way for men to lose weight. You don't have to drastically change your eating patterns. You just need to adjust the amount and type of foods you eat, and your buddies will never be the wiser. Swap fried chicken and fries for grilled chicken and a baked potato. Share a bucket of buffalo wings, but eat 3, not 6, and skip the blue cheese dip. Enjoy pizza, but stick with cheese or veggie-topped—just pass on the meat lover's or extra cheese.

You Should Know

Men are more likely to overeat pizza, pasta, hamburger, or casseroles.

Women get tripped up when it comes to sweets and snacks.

Simply downsizing portions will help most men lose weight.

Men, want to be in shape, ripped, trim?

- Drink alcohol, but do it in moderation.

- Go easy on calorie-containing drinks. They add up quickly. Water has zero calories.

- Rev up your metabolism—eat breakfast, lift weights.

- Don't sit around eating chips; go for a run or at least a walk.

- Make smart food choices. Instead of a double burger with bacon and cheese, order a regular burger with lettuce and tomato.

- Cook more at home, where you can control portions and cut calories. Notice all the men cooking on the food channels.

- Don't wait till you've been diagnosed with a problem to start losing weight.

- Count calories. It's a simple strategy to trim down and it works.

A tough guy can count calories and do it successfully; he just doesn't want to announce it to the world.

THE TRUTH, AND NOTHING BUT THE TRUTH

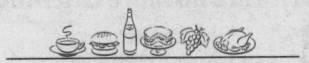

People who wear belts stop eating
sooner than people who don't.

Sugar and fast food do not make you fat.

There is no specific food that causes weight gain. The only thing that makes you fat is eating too many calories. If you eat too much sugar and too many fast foods, you will gain weight. If you eat both in moderation, you won't. People who eat a lot of sugar or fast food also frequently eat larger portions, eat more often, and eat fewer good-for-you foods, like fruits, vegetables, and whole grains.

Smoking is not an effective weight loss strategy.

As a matter of fact, research has shown that smoking encourages the accumulation of belly fat. Smokers, even lean ones, have thicker waists than nonsmokers.

Skipping meals does not help you cut calories.

People who eat many small amounts during the day are slimmer than those who eat fewer but larger meals. Regular breakfast skippers are 450% more likely to be overweight. *Eat when you're hungry, stop when you're full* is a simple rule that is difficult to follow. But those who do, usually eat fewer calories than people who sit down to a big lunch or dinner simply because the clock says it's time to eat.

Nighttime calories are no more fattening than daytime calories.

Time of day doesn't matter; the calorie count does. You can eat all the calories you need for an entire day between midnight and 6 A.M., if you wish. As long as you don't eat any more during the rest of the day, you won't gain weight. The warning against late-night eating *does* have value if the calories eaten watching TV or coping with stress are on top of the calories you've already eaten during the day.

You Should Know

For women, it may be their brains and not their stomachs that lead to overeating.

A recent imaging study showed that a woman's brain drives her to overeat when presented with her favorite foods or when she is under emotional stress.

The same is not true for men.

One package does not always equal one serving.

Read food labels carefully to see if a package—even a small one—contains more than 1 serving. Many foods and snacks are currently packaged as single servings and that's exactly what you are getting: 1 serving. But other smaller-size packages may hold more that 1 serving. For example, a small bag of chips may hold 2½ servings. Eat the whole bag and you've eaten 2½ times the calories listed as a serving.

Fat-free and sugar-free are not calorie free.

Buying fat-free or sugar-free foods seems virtuous and can seduce you into eating larger amounts. But beware: some brands of sugar-free cookies and fat-free crackers have the same number of calories as—and sometimes more than—the regular versions. Few foods are calorie free. If a fat-free salad dressing has half of the calories of the regular version and you use twice as much, or if you eat a whole box of sugar-free cookies, there is no calorie benefit.

You won't burn fat faster if you exercise harder.

The intensity of your exercise makes no difference, as long as you burn more calories than you eat. It doesn't matter how long it takes you to go a distance: the more ground you cover, the more calories you burn. For each pound you weigh, you burn 1 calorie per mile. So whether walking, hiking, jogging, or sprinting, a 100-pound person burns 100 calories per mile on a flat surface, a 200-pound person uses 200 calories, and so on. Keep in mind that the time you exercise is only a small part of the day. A daily active lifestyle may actually burn more calories than a single exercise session. So take the stairs, don't use the drive-thru, play with the kids at the park.

Water is a powerful calorie burner.

Seventy-five percent of people don't drink enough water. When you have too little water in your body, your metabolism slows down and you burn fewer calories. Exercising, running errands, and staying out in the sun can all make you mildly dehydrated. Water, juice, seltzer, mineral water, milk, and even caffeine-containing coffee, tea, and soda all contribute to your fluid intake. If you don't urinate at least every 4 hours when you are awake, you probably need to be drinking more.

Sleep Too Little, Weigh Too Much

People who sleep more weigh less.

Getting too little sleep triggers hormonal changes that lead to increased appetite. Plus, more hours awake means more time to eat, and if you're tired, you're less likely to exercise—all adding up to extra pounds.

Aim for at least 7 hours a night.

CALORIES YOU USE

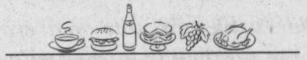

Regular exercise adds years to your life.

Activity burns calories. Activity also builds muscles, which burn calories 70 times faster than fat. Someone who has been relatively inactive will see health benefits from using up just 500 extra calories a week through activity. If you're a true couch potato, this may be the level at which to start, though real weight loss and fitness benefits start to kick in when you use up 1,000 calories a week through activity. Consider 2,000 calories as a great goal to strive for over time.

Everything you do counts, from planned activities to real-life fitness: walking, gardening, golf, tennis, even housework. The more active you are, the more calories you burn. And, the really good news is that research has shown you benefit from exercise whether the activity is continuous or done in small bursts. Being active for as little as 10 minutes at a time not only burns calories but also has a positive impact on your health. The key is to *move* every day.

> ## Walk More, Weigh Less
>
> *A brisk walk burns 100 calories or more per mile, depending on how much you weigh.*
>
> *City dwellers walk more and on average weigh 10 pounds less than their country cousins.*

Real-life Fitness

- Pace while you're talking on the phone.

- Deliver memos and messages in person rather than by email or phone.

- Go window-shopping.

- Clean your house—washing floors, vacuuming carpets, washing windows, and scrubbing bathrooms equal vigorous exercise.

- Garden—weeding, hoeing, cutting the lawn, raking, or trimming bushes burns as many calories as playing a game of tennis.

- Turn your lunch break into an hour-long excursion.

- Carry a basket when shopping for a few items—it's like a free weight that keeps getting heavier and heavier. Switch arms for a maximum workout.

- Sign up for a charity walk, bike, or run.

- Turn off the TV one night a week and plan something active.

- Make exercise a hobby—take golf, tennis, or skating lessons.

- Park your car at the farthest end of the parking lot.

- Take the stairs; you burn 10 calories for every flight

you climb. Over a lifetime, that uses up thousands of calories.

- Dance—salsa, hip-hop, polka, tango, or line dance; square dancers can cover 5 miles in an evening.

- Grocery shop—one hour of pushing, lifting, and bending in the supermarket uses as many calories as a half hour on a treadmill.

- Spend rainy weekend afternoons walking around a museum; when the sun shines, go to the zoo.

- Wash the car.

- Go bowling instead of to the movies.

- Walk the dog.

- Push the baby in a stroller or take the kids to the playground.

- Be an active spectator—walk around the soccer field while the kids are playing.

- Play action games as a family—badminton, volleyball, stickball, croquet.

- Practice yoga.

Don't Sit Your Life Away

Americans average 23 hours a week in front of the TV. That adds up to almost 10 years over a lifetime!

Daily activity helps you reach your target weight faster. Depending on your current level of activity, aim to use up 500 to 1,000 calories a week. Your ultimate goal is to double this amount as you become more fit. In the table "Using Up Calories," pages 26–29, find the activity you've done and the weight column closest to your current weight. Multiply the calories burned in 1 minute by the number of minutes you were active.

For example, if you weigh 150 pounds and you weeded your flower bed for 15 minutes, you used up almost 89 calories.

Gardening (weeding)
5.9 (calories burned in 1 minute) × 15 minutes = 88.5 calories

If your activity goal for the week is to burn 500 calories, you've already burned 89 with one simple chore.

Keep track of the calories you burn each day, and total the amount you burn in a week.

USING UP CALORIES

POUNDS	100	125	150	175	200
ACTIVITY	CALORIES USED PER MINUTE				
Archery	3.1	4.0	4.8	5.6	6.4
Auto repair	2.8	3.5	4.2	4.8	5.5
Badminton	3.6	4.6	5.4	6.4	7.3
Baseball	3.1	4.0	4.7	5.5	6.3
Basketball	4.9	6.2	9.9	11.5	13.2
Bicycling					
5 mph	1.9	2.4	2.9	3.4	3.9
10 mph	4.2	5.3	6.4	7.4	8.5
Bowling	2.7	3.4	4.1	4.5	5.5
Boxing	6.2	7.8	9.3	10.9	12.4
Calisthenics, light	3.4	4.3	5.2	6.1	7.0
Canoeing, 4 mph	4.4	5.5	6.7	7.8	8.9
Card playing	1.0	1.6	1.9	2.2	2.5
Carpentry	2.6	3.2	3.8	4.6	5.3
Chopping wood	4.8	6.0	7.2	8.4	9.6
Croquet	2.7	3.4	4.1	4.7	5.4
Dancing					
Active (square, salsa)	4.5	5.6	6.8	7.9	9.1

POUNDS	100	125	150	175	200
ACTIVITY	**CALORIES USED PER MINUTE**				
Aerobic dance	6.0	7.6	9.1	10.8	12.1
Moderate (waltz)	3.1	4.0	4.8	5.6	6.4
Fencing, moderate	3.3	4.1	5.0	5.8	6.7
Fishing	2.8	3.5	4.2	4.9	5.6
Football, touch	5.5	6.9	8.3	9.7	11.1
Gardening					
Lawn mowing, manual	3.0	3.8	4.6	5.2	5.9
Lawn mowing, power	2.7	3.4	4.1	4.7	5.4
Light gardening	2.4	3.0	3.6	4.2	4.8
Weeding	3.9	4.9	5.9	6.8	7.8
Golf					
Foursome (carry clubs)	2.7	3.4	4.1	4.5	5.4
Twosome (carry clubs)	3.6	4.6	5.4	6.4	7.3
Gymnastics	3.0	3.8	4.5	5.3	6.0
Handball	6.5	6.2	9.9	11.5	13.2
Hiking, 3 mph	4.5	5.5	6.8	7.9	9.1
Hockey, field	5.0	7.6	9.1	10.8	12.1
Hockey, ice	6.6	8.3	10.0	11.7	13.4
Horseback riding					
Gallop	5.7	7.2	8.7	10.1	11.6
Trot	2.7	3.4	4.1	4.8	5.4
Walk	1.9	2.4	2.9	3.4	3.9
Horseshoes	2.5	3.1	3.8	4.4	5.2
House painting	2.3	2.9	3.5	4.0	4.6
Housework					
Dusting	1.8	2.3	2.6	3.1	3.5
Making beds	2.6	3.2	3.8	4.6	5.3
Ice Skating	4.2	5.2	6.4	7.4	8.5
Judo	8.5	10.6	12.8	14.9	17.1
Karate	8.5	10.6	12.8	14.9	17.1
Lacrosse	9.5	11.9	14.3	16.6	19.0
Motorcycling	2.4	3.0	3.6	4.2	4.8
Mountain climbing	6.5	8.2	9.8	11.5	13.1
Paddle ball	5.7	7.2	8.7	10.1	11.6

POUNDS	100	125	150	175	200
ACTIVITY	CALORIES USED PER MINUTE				
Pool (billiards)	1.5	1.9	2.2	2.6	3.0
Racquetball	6.5	8.1	9.8	11.4	13.0
Rollerblading, 9 mph	4.2	5.3	6.4	7.4	8.5
Rowing	3.4	4.2	5.0	5.9	6.7
Rowing machine	9.1	11.4	13.7	16.0	18.2
Running, steady rate					
5 mph	6.0	7.6	9.1	10.8	12.2
7 mph	9.7	12.1	14.6	17.1	19.5
Sailing, small boat	4.2	5.2	6.4	7.4	8.5
Scuba diving, moderate	9.4	11.8	14.1	16.5	18.8
Shoveling snow	5.2	6.5	7.8	8.9	10.2
Skiing, alpine downhill	6.4	8.0	9.6	11.2	12.8
Skiing, cross-country					
2.5 mph	5.0	6.2	7.5	8.8	10.0
4 mph	6.5	8.2	9.9	11.5	13.2
Soccer	5.9	7.4	8.9	10.3	11.8
Squash	6.7	8.4	10.1	11.8	13.5
Swimming					
Backstroke	2.5	3.1	3.8	4.4	5.1
Breaststroke	3.1	4.0	4.8	5.6	6.4
Crawl	4.0	5.0	6.0	7.0	8.0
Table tennis	3.4	4.3	5.2	6.3	7.2
Tennis					
Doubles	3.4	4.3	5.2	6.1	7.0
Singles	5.0	6.2	7.5	6.8	10.0
Typing	1.5	1.9	2.3	2.7	3.1
Volleyball	2.9	3.6	4.4	5.1	5.9
Walking					
1 mph	1.5	1.9	2.3	2.7	3.1
2 mph	2.1	2.6	3.2	3.7	4.3
4 mph	4.2	5.3	6.4	7.4	8.5
Washing floors	3.0	3.8	4.6	5.3	6.1
Washing windows	2.8	3.5	4.2	4.8	5.5
Water skiing	5.0	6.2	7.5	8.8	10.0

POUNDS	100	125	150	175	200
ACTIVITY	**CALORIES USED PER MINUTE**				
Weight training					
Free weights	3.9	4.9	5.9	6.8	7.8
Nautilus	4.2	5.3	6.3	7.4	8.4
Universal	5.3	6.6	8.0	9.3	10.6

Calorie Cost of Love

A kiss = 6 to 12 calories, depending on the intensity.

*Lovemaking = 125 to 300 calories,
depending on the level of passion.*

MINIMIZE
MINDLESS EATING

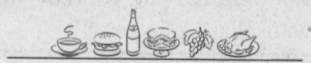

Each of us makes over 112 food decisions a day.

You're thinking, "That's not possible!" But it is. Each morning, you decide to eat or not. Cereal or toast? Toast with butter? Or butter and jelly? One slice or two? Coffee, tea, or Coke? Milk or sugar? One spoonful or two? Fruit or juice? Large or small glass? Seconds?

These choices are considered *low involvement* decisions and often you're not even aware you're making them. They are mindless choices, but over time they can make a significant impact on what and how much you eat.

You Should Know

Eating in response to external signals—food advertisements, food smells, TV commercials, a candy dish on a coworker's desk—is more likely to cause overeating than normal hunger signals. Most of us are rarely hungry.

Your home and office are full of hidden persuaders, but there are a number of things you can do to become a more mindful eater.

Put distance between you and food.

The greater the distance you have to travel to get food, the less you eat. Empty the candy dish on your desk. At home, leave all food in the kitchen cabinets or fridge. Don't stock a mini refrigerator in the family room. Putting distance between you and food gives you enough time to pause and say, "Do I really want that?"

Use small plates, serving spoons, and bowls.

Large serving bowls encourage overeating. People take over 50% more food when they're given a large plate or served from a large bowl. The next time you eat ice cream, use a dessert dish instead of a soup bowl. You generally eat whatever you serve yourself, so if you over-serve, you over-eat. Shapes also affect consumption. You drink less from tall, slim glasses and more out of short, fat ones.

Don't be seduced by the "health halo."

Lowfat, reduced calorie, low carb, sugar free, and *light* are all terms used to make you think a food is good for you. But too much of *any* food equals too many calories. People order more and eat more when they believe the choices are healthy. A restaurant-size salad, drenched in dressing, is more than anyone needs to eat at one sitting. Even healthy foods need to be eaten in moderation.

Buying bulk adds bulk.

Warehouse stores encourage you to buy bigger sizes, which leads to eating more, and eating more frequently. People take larger helpings out of larger packages. Single servings and individual packs are smarter purchases. Or, re-pack larger amounts into smaller sizes to discourage over-eating.

Order small.

Regardless of the choice, go for the smallest option. At a restaurant, order a lunch or half portion, or have an appetizer for your main course. Select the small or regular coffee, even if it's called "tall." Try a "kid's" meal. Eat medium-size apples, oranges, and baked potatoes. Order a one-scoop cone. Remember, *smaller* sizes = *a smaller you*.

Rework your eating environment so it works *for* you, not against you. Now that you are more aware of mindless eating, counteract these choices with mindful solutions. Start small, easy, and doable—success, no matter how small, breeds success.

When Do You Eat Too much?

Asked when they were most likely to overeat, 57% of people said at night, 25% said afternoon, and only 3% noted morning. Simply knowing this can help you cut calories and avoid temptation.

What Do the Experts Recommend?

A group of 23 food and nutrition experts (Jo-Ann Heslin, RD, was invited to be part of the group) were asked to give ideas and suggestions for how Americans could achieve healthy eating and maintain a healthy weight. Here are their recommendations.

- Eating healthy meals and snacks deserves a large slice of our time-stressed lives.

- Give thought to what you eat. Most Americans are totally unaware of the choices they make every day.

- Retrain your taste buds to enjoy the flavor of healthy foods. Eat less sugar, sodium, and fat.

- Eat food for enjoyment and nourishment, not to soothe emotional issues. What are your food triggers?

- Downsize portions.

- Quit the clean plate club.

- Learn more about how many calories are in the foods you regularly eat.

- Learn more about food. It's fun and important to your health.

- Change slowly and the changes are more likely to be permanent.

TRACKING CALORIES

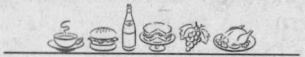

People cut calories by 10% when they simply write
down what they eat; 30% to 50% of those who
keep a food diary change their eating habits.

A large research study done at the Harvard School for Public Health confirmed that the most successful way to lose weight is to keep track of calories. It didn't matter if a person chose a lowfat diet, a low carb diet, a high carb, or a high protein diet. If they counted calories, they lost weight. This proved, once and for all, that calories count!

We know it's a chore to write down everything you eat and keep track of the calories, but it's worth it. After a week of writing down calories, most people have a good idea of how many calories are in 75% of what they usually eat. And people who keep a food diary are more successful at losing weight, even during difficult times like holidays.

"Your Daily Food Diary," on page 37, will tell you a lot about how you eat, why you eat, and what you eat. Research has shown that men are more likely to omit items than women, both sexes are more likely to omit snack items, and meat items are more likely to be underestimated than other foods. No one will ever see what you write down, so be honest.

Why is the day of the week important? Some days, like

on weekends, you may eat more. Some people eat more on Friday, celebrating the end of a work week. Others eat more on Monday in response to the stress of a new week. If you find that some days trigger you to overeat, it will be easier to change the pattern.

We appreciate that many people eat on a crazy schedule, so the day is broken into 3 periods. It will help you figure out when you do the most eating.

A.M. is from midnight till noon. Many people eat in the middle of the night, so A.M. includes middle-of-the-night noshing, breakfast, coffee break, or morning snack.

Midday is from noon until dinner. It includes lunch and any afternoon or pre-dinner snack, like a drink after work.

P.M. is dinnertime through midnight. It includes your evening meal and after-dinner, TV, and bedtime snacks.

After a few days, you'll begin to see patterns in your eating habits. Going too long without food or eating too frequently can both lead to eating too much. Ideally, you want your calories to be spaced evenly throughout the day. But we know that isn't always possible.

By subtotaling your calories 3 times during the day, you can make adjustments for unexpected situations. For example, if a client comes in for lunch, you can skip your afternoon snack and eat a lighter dinner to compensate for the extra calories eaten at lunch.

Why does it matter if you eat alone or with company? Because many of us eat more when we are alone. Most people eat more with family and less with coworkers. Learning this about yourself can help you change habits that may be sabotaging your efforts to lose weight.

And finally, you'll want to note how many calories you burned through activity every day. Some days you may be more active than others, but if you start to fall into an inactive pattern, noting it will help you break the cycle quickly.

One meal or one day does not make a success or failure. But being totally honest with yourself can help keep you on the right track most of the time. Before you realize it, you'll be slimmer and fitter than ever before.

Learning from the Losers

For more than 15 years, the National Weight Control Registry has kept track of people who have lost at least 30 pounds and kept it off. These successful losers used the same general strategies to maintain long-term weight loss:

Eat a low calorie diet.
Eat a lowfat diet and eat less saturated fat.
Eat a moderate amount of carbohydrates.
Go easy on fast food.
Exercise regularly.

It takes knowledge, motivation, action, and time to create change.

DAILY FOOD DIARY

Your Target Calorie Zone _____

Day _____ Date _____

Food	Portion	Calories	Ate Alone	With Company
AM				

AM Calorie Total _____

MIDDAY				

Midday Calorie Total _____

PM				

PM Calorie Total _____

Day's Calorie Total _____

Activity	Minutes Active	Calories Burned

Total Calories Burned _____

USING YOUR
CALORIE COUNTER

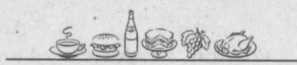

The Calorie Counter lists the calories and portion size for more than 20,000 foods. Now you can compare the values in your favorite foods and, when necessary, choose substitutes when you go out to grocery shop or eat. This will save time and help you decide what to buy.

The counter section of the book is divided into two parts: Part One: Brand Name, Nonbranded (Generic), and Take-Out Foods (page 45); and Part Two: Restaurant Chains (page 527). Each part lists foods or restaurant chains alphabetically.

In Part One, for each category, you will find nonbranded (generic) foods listed first in alphabetical order, followed by an alphabetical listing of brand name foods. The nonbranded listings will help you estimate calorie values when you don't see your favorite brand. They can also help you to evaluate store brands. Large categories are divided into subcategories, such as canned, fresh, frozen, and ready-to-eat, to make it easier to find what you're looking for. Some categories have "see" and "see also" references, to help you find related items.

Because we eat out so often, more than 800 take-out foods are listed in Part One. These are found in the take-out subcategory in many categories throughout this section.

Look there for foods you take out or order in, since they are not nutrition labeled.

Most foods are listed alphabetically. In some cases, though, foods are grouped by category. For example, a tuna sandwich is found in the SANDWICH category. Other group categories include:

ASIAN FOOD (Page 54)
> Includes all types of Asian foods except egg rolls and sushi, which are found in the egg rolls and sushi categories.

DELI MEATS/COLD CUTS (Page 202)
> Includes all sandwich meats except chicken, ham, and turkey, which are found in their own separate categories.

DINNER (Page 204)
> Includes all prepared dinners listed by brand name, except pasta dinners, which are found in the pasta dinner category.

LIQUOR/LIQUEUR (Page 303)
> Includes all alcoholic beverages and mixed drinks except beer, champagne, and wine, which are found in their own separate categories.

NUTRITION SUPPLEMENTS (Page 332)
> Includes all dieting aids, meal replacements, and drinks, except energy bars and energy drinks, which are found in their own separate categories.

SANDWICHES   (Page 422)
Includes popular sandwich, calzone,
and panini choices.

SNACKS   (Page 445)
Includes a variety of snack items such
as pork rinds and cheese puffs.

SPANISH FOOD   (Page 469)
Includes all types of Spanish and
Mexican foods except salsa and
tortillas, which are found in their own
separate categories.

In Part Two, Restaurant Chains, more than 100 national
and regional restaurant, coffee, doughnut, frozen yogurt, ice
cream, pizza, sandwich, soup, and sushi chains are listed.
Brand name foods are required by federal law to have nutrition information on labels, but in most areas of the country,
restaurants only provide this information voluntarily.

With *The Calorie Counter* as your guide, you will never
again wonder how many calories are in the food you eat.

DEFINITIONS

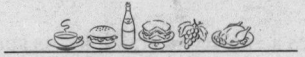

as prep (as prepared): refers to food that has been prepared according to package directions

lean and fat: describes meat with some fat on its edges that is not cut away before cooking, or poultry prepared with skin and fat as purchased

lean only: refers to lean meat that is trimmed of all visible fat, or poultry without skin

not prep (not prepared): refers to food that has not been cooked and may require the addition of other ingredients to prepare

shelf-stable: refers to prepared products found on the supermarket shelf that are not canned or frozen but are packaged and ready-to-eat, or are ready to be heated and do not require refrigeration

take-out: describes prepared dishes that you purchase ready-to-eat; those included serve as a guide to the calories in products you may purchase

ABBREVIATIONS

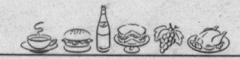

avg	=	average
diam	=	diameter
fl	=	fluid
frzn	=	frozen
g	=	gram
in	=	inch
lb	=	pound
lg	=	large
med	=	medium
mg	=	milligram
oz	=	ounce
pkg	=	package
prep	=	prepared
pt	=	pint
qt	=	quart
reg	=	regular
sec	=	second
serv	=	serving
sm	=	small
sq	=	square
tbsp	=	tablespoon
tsp	=	teaspoon
w/	=	with
w/o	=	without
<	=	less than

NOTES

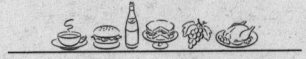

0 (zero) indicates there are no calories in that food.

Discrepancies in figures are due to rounding of values, product reformulation, and reevaluation. The current labeling law allows rounding. Some of the data listed is analysis data, obtained directly from manufacturers, not from labels; therefore, some values may differ slightly from labels because the values have not been rounded.

PART ONE

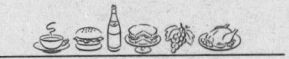

Brand Name, Nonbranded (Generic), and Take-Out Foods

**Eating 100 fewer calories each day
can help you lose 10 pounds in a year!
It can be done with small changes—**

- Use mustard, salsa, or fat-free mayonnaise in place of 1 tablespoon regular mayonnaise
- Eat 1 slice of toast for breakfast instead of 2
- Order a cup of soup instead of a bowl
- Try a plain baked potato with pepper instead of sour cream
- Eat cereal with skim milk instead of whole milk
- Swap breaded and fried chicken fingers for broiled
- Use tuna packed in water rather than oil
- Swap regular soda for diet soda
- Enjoy a glass of wine instead of a martini
- Have a chocolate kiss instead of a chocolate bar

FOOD	PORTION	CALS
ABALONE		
breaded & fried	1 serv (3 oz)	162
steamed	1 serv (3 oz)	127
ACAI JUICE		
Arthur's		
Acai Plus	1 bottle (11 oz)	230
Bossa Nova		
Acai Juice Blueberry	8 oz	89
Acai Juice Mango	8 oz	89
Acai Juice Original	8 oz	94
Acai Juice Passion Fruit	8 oz	89
Acai Juice Raspberry	8 oz	89
O.N.E.		
Amazon Acai	1 bottle (11 oz)	157
Zola		
100% Juice	1 box (11 oz)	170
ACEROLA		
fresh	1 (5 g)	2
ACEROLA JUICE		
juice	1 cup	56
ADZUKI BEANS		
canned sweetened	½ cup	351
dried cooked w/o salt	½ cup	147
Arrowhead Mills		
Organic Dried not prep	¼ cup	130
AKEE		
fresh	3.5 oz	223
ALCOHOL (see BEER AND ALE, CHAMPAGNE, LIQUOR/LIQUEUR, MALT, WINE)		
ALE (see BEER AND ALE)		
ALFALFA		
sprouts	½ cup	40
ALLIGATOR		
cooked	3 oz	126
ALLSPICE		
ground	1 tsp	5

FOOD	PORTION	CALS
ALMONDS		
almond butter w/ salt	2 tbsp	203
almond butter w/o salt	2 tbsp	203
almond extract	1 tsp	38
almond paste	¼ cup	260
chocolate covered	6 (0.6 oz)	102
dry roasted w/ salt	¼ cup	206
dry roasted w/o salt	¼ cup	206
honey roasted	¼ cup	214
jordan almonds	6 (0.7 oz)	99
oil roasted w/ salt	¼ cup	238
oil roasted w/o salt	¼ cup	238
praline	17 (1.4 oz)	210
yogurt covered	6 (0.8 oz)	122
American Almond		
Marzipan	2 tbsp	130
Arrowhead Mills		
Organic Almond Butter Creamy	2 tbsp	200
Blue Diamond		
Almond Roca Buttercrunch	3 (1.3 oz)	210
Honey Roasted	¼ cup	170
Jalapeno Smokehouse	28 (1 oz)	170
Jordon Pastels	15 (1.4 oz)	180
Lime 'N Chili	28 (1 oz)	170
Maui Onion & Garlic	28 (1 oz)	170
Milk Chocolate Covered	9 (1.4 oz)	230
Salted	¼ cup	170
Smokehouse	28 (1.3 oz)	170
Wasabi & Soy Sauce	28 (1 oz)	170
Whole Natural	¼ cup	180
Yogurt Covered	12 (1.4 oz)	210
Brach's		
Chocolate Coated	11	220
Eden		
Tamari	3 tbsp (1 oz)	160
Godiva		
Dark Chocolate Almonds	1 pkg (2 oz)	310
Good Sense		
Hickory Smoked	¼ cup	180
Raw Whole	¼ cup	180

FOOD	PORTION	CALS
Justin's		
Almond Butter Classic	2 tbsp (1.1 oz)	200
Almond Butter Maple	2 tbsp (1.1 oz)	190
Kettle		
Butter Salted	2 tbsp	180
Butter Unsalted	2 tbsp	180
Love'n Bake		
Almond Paste	2 tbsp	140
Almond Schmear	2 tbsp	140
Roasted Butter	2 tbsp	180
Maisie Jane's		
Almond Butter	1 oz	184
Cappuccino	9 (1.4 oz)	220
Chocolate Toffee	9 (1.4 oz)	210
Coffee Glazed	2 tbsp (1 oz)	150
Cowboy BBQ	2 tbsp (1 oz)	140
Mint Chocolate	9 (1.4 oz)	210
Organic Honey Glazed	2 tbsp (1 oz)	160
Tamari	2 tbsp (1 oz)	160
Mrs. May's		
Almond Crunch	1 oz	156
Odense		
Almond Paste	2 tbsp (1.4 oz)	170
Planters		
Chocolate Lovers Dark Chocolate	11 (1.4 oz)	220
Dry Roasted	23 (1 oz)	160
Sunkist		
Accents Italian Parmesan	1 tbsp	40
Accents Original Oven Roasted	1 tbsp	40
AMARANTH		
leaves cooked	½ cup	14
uncooked	½ cup (3.4 oz)	365
Arrowhead Mills		
Organic Whole Grain not prep	¼ cup	180
ANCHOVY		
boneless	1 oz	60
canned in oil drained	1 can (2 oz)	94
fresh	1 (4 g)	8
fresh fillets	3 (0.4 oz)	21

FOOD	PORTION	CALS
Brunswick		
Flat Fillets	1 can (2 oz)	25
Polar		
Rolled Fillets w/ Capers In Olive Oil	7 (0.6 oz)	40
ANGLERFISH		
raw	3.5 oz	72
ANISE		
seed	1 tsp	7
ANTELOPE		
roasted	4 oz	215
APPLE		
CANNED		
sliced sweetened	½ cup	68
Glory		
Fried Apples	½ cup	80
Polar		
Fuji	½ cup	50
DRIED		
chopped	½ cup	104
cooked w/o sugar	½ cup	73
rings	5	78
Bare Fruit		
Chips Cinnamon	1 pkg (0.6 oz)	43
Chukar Cherries		
Cherry Apple Slices	10 (1 oz)	110
Crispy Green		
Crispy Apples	1 pkg (0.36 oz)	35
Fruit Ripples		
Cinnamon Apple	1 pkg	50
Strawberry Apple	1 pkg	50
Mrs. May's		
Fruit Chips	1 pkg	35
Nature's Envy		
Apple Chips Original	1 pkg (0.8 oz)	80
FRESH		
apple	1 sm	55
apple	1 med	72
apple	1 lg	110

FOOD	PORTION	CALS
candied	1 sm (4.9 oz)	179
candied	1 med (6.5 oz)	234
candied	1 lg (9.8 oz)	357
w/ skin sliced	1 cup	57
w/o skin sliced	1 cup	53
Earthbound Farm		
Organic Slices	1 pkg (2 oz)	30
Eastern Select		
Gala	1 (5.5 oz)	80
Mrs. Prindable's		
Caramel Triple Chocolate	¼ apple (1.7 oz)	120
Caramel Walnut	¼ apple (2 oz)	160
Rainier		
Apple	1 med (5.5 oz)	80
Sullivan		
McIntosh	1 (5.4 oz)	80
TreeTop		
Slices Red or Green	1 pkg (2 oz)	35
FROZEN		
sliced w/o sugar	½ cup	42
Roast Works		
Flame Roasted Fuji	1 serv (5 oz)	90
TAKE-OUT		
baked	1 (6 oz)	128
baked no sugar	1 (5.6 oz)	136
fried apple rings	1 serv (2.7 oz)	91
APPLE JUICE		
cider	1 cup	117
juice + vitamin C & calcium	1 cup	117
mulled cider	1 serv	265
unsweetened w/o vitamin C	1 cup	117
After The Fall		
Organic	8 oz	90
Apple & Eve		
100% Juice	8 oz	110
Celestial Seasonings		
Cider Apple Caramel Kiss as prep	1 cup	80
Eden		
Organic Juice	8 oz	90

FOOD	PORTION	CALS
Fizz Ed.		
Green Apple	1 can (8.4 oz)	100
Hansen's		
100% Juice	8 oz	120
Hood		
100% Juice	1 cup	120
Izze		
Sparkling Apple	1 bottle (12 oz)	138
Kedem		
100% Juice	8 oz	110
Land O Lakes		
Juice	1 cup (8 oz)	120
Langers		
Diet Cocktail 50% Juice	8 oz	60
Harvest Apple 100% Juice	8 oz	120
Minute Maid		
100% Juice	8 oz	100
Mott's		
Hot Spiced Cider All Flavors as prep	1 pkg	80
Naked Juice		
Just Apple	8 oz	120
Nantucket Nectars		
100% Juice Pressed Apple	8 oz	120
Organic Cloudy Apple	8 oz	120
Old Orchard		
Cider 100%	8 oz	120
Healthy Balance Apple	8 oz	30
Organic 100% Juice	8 oz	128
Phat Phruit		
Green Apple	8 oz	40
Red Cheek		
100% Juice	8 oz	120
Seneca		
100% Juice	8 oz	110
Snapple		
Diet	8 oz	15
Tree Ripe		
Organic 100% Juice	6 oz	80
TreeTop		
100% Juice	8 oz	120

FOOD	PORTION	CALS
Cider 100% Juice No Sugar Added	8 oz	120
Tropicana		
Orchard Style	1 bottle (14 oz)	200
Walnut Acres		
Organic Juice	8 oz	110
Zeigler's		
Old Fashioned Cider	8 oz	110

APPLESAUCE

sweetened	½ cup	97
unsweetened	½ cup	52
Eden		
Organic	½ cup	60
Organic Apple Cherry	½ cup	70
Organic Apple Strawberry	½ cup	60
Organic Cinnamon	1 pkg (4 oz)	70
Langers		
Unsweetened	½ cup	50
Mott's		
Healthy Harvest Granny Smith No Sugar Added	1 pkg (3.9 oz)	50
Original	½ cup	110
Single-Serve Cinnamon	1 pkg (4 oz)	100
Single-Serve Natural	1 pkg (4 oz)	50
Musselman's		
Lite	1 pkg (4 oz)	50
Unsweetened	1 pkg (4 oz)	50
Revolution Foods		
Organic Unsweetened	1 pkg (4 oz)	50

APRICOT JUICE

nectar	6 oz	106

APRICOTS

canned in heavy syrup	½ cup	91
canned in juice	½ cup	59
canned in water	½ cup	33
canned light syrup	½ cup	80
dried halves	6	51
dried halves cooked w/o sugar	½ cup	106
fresh	1	17
fresh sliced	½ cup	40
frozen sweetened	½ cup	119

FOOD	PORTION	CALS
Crispy Green		
Crispy Dried	1 pkg (0.36 oz)	40
Del Monte		
Halves In Heavy Syrup	½ cup	100
Orchard Select Halves	½ cup	80
Harvest Bay		
Dried	5 (1.4 oz)	60
Mariani		
Ultimate Dried	¼ cup (1.4 oz)	100
Sunsweet		
Dried	6 (1.4 oz)	100
ARROWHEAD		
corm boiled	1 med	9
ARROWROOT		
raw	1 root (1.2 oz)	21
raw root sliced	1 cup	78
Bob's Red Mill		
Starch	¼ cup	110
ARTICHOKE		
CANNED		
hearts in oil	1 serv (3 oz)	100
Cento		
Hearts Quartered Marinated	2	20
Gertie's Finest		
Tapenade	2 tbsp	29
Native Forest		
Organic Hearts Quartered	1 serv (4 oz)	35
Polar		
Hearts	2	18
Hearts Quartered Marinated	1 oz	25
Progresso		
Hearts	2 (4.6 oz)	30
Hearts Marinated	2 (1.1 oz)	60
FRESH		
cooked	1 med	60
hearts cooked	½ cup	42
Ocean Mist		
Lemon	1 (4.2 oz)	60

FOOD	PORTION	CALS
FROZEN		
cooked	1 cup	42
cooked w/o salt	1 pkg (9 oz)	108
C&W		
Hearts	12 (3 oz)	40
TAKE-OUT		
stuffed	1 (8.8 oz)	397

ARUGULA

fresh	1 cup	3

ASIAN FOOD (see also CURRY, DINNER, EGG ROLLS, SAUCE, SOY SAUCE, SUSHI)

FOOD	PORTION	CALS
CANNED		
chow mein chicken w/o noodles	1 cup	194
La Choy		
Chow Mein Beef	1 cup	90
Chow Mein Chicken	1 cup (9.3 oz)	100
Sweet & Sour Noodles	1 cup	150
Teriyaki Chicken	1 cup (8.6 oz)	120
FRESH		
wonton wrappers	1	23
Azumaya		
Round Wraps	10	160
Wrappers Large Square	8	160
Frieda's		
Won Ton Wrappers	4 (1 oz)	80
Nasoya		
Won Ton Wrappers	8	160
FROZEN		
Contessa		
Chow Mein Chicken w/ Sauce not prep	1¾ cups	320
Curry Chicken w/ Sauce not prep	1¾ cups	240
Fried Rice Chicken w/ Sauce not prep	1¾ cups	260
General Tsao Shrimp w/ Sauce not prep	1¾ cups	270
Kung Pao Shrimp w/ Sauce not prep	1¾ cups	200
Lo Mein Shrimp w/ Sauce not prep	1¾ cups	250
Stir-Fry Beef w/ sauce not prep	1¾ cup	190
Stir-Fry Chicken w/ Sauce not prep	1¾ cups	160
Stir-Fry Shrimp w/ Sauce not prep	1¾ cups	120
Sweet & Sour Shrimp w/ Sauce not prep	1½ cups	180
Tandoori Chicken w/ Sauce not prep	1⅓ cups	200

FOOD	PORTION	CALS
Glutino		
Gluten Free Chicken Pad Thai Peach	1 pkg (7 oz)	370
Healthy Choice		
Five Spice Beef & Vegetables	1 pkg (10 oz)	310
General Tso's Spicy Chicken	1 pkg (10.7 oz)	310
Helen's Kitchen		
Thai Yellow Curry w/ Tofu Steaks & Vegetables & Basmati Rice	1 pkg (9 oz)	280
Joy Of Cooking		
Lo Mein Vegetable	1 cup (7.7 oz)	220
Kahiki		
Beef & Broccoli	1 pkg (10.9 oz)	360
Chicken Fried Rice	1 pkg (10.9 oz)	460
General Tso's Chicken	1 pkg (10 oz)	400
Naturals General Tso's Chicken	1 pkg (10 oz)	330
Naturals Mandarin Orange Chicken	1 pkg (10 oz)	340
Naturals Szechuan Peppercorn Beef	1 pkg (10 oz)	350
Naturals Teriyaki Mixed Vegetables	1 pkg (10 oz)	260
Sesame Orange Chicken	1 pkg (10.9 oz)	420
Soothing Lettuce Wraps	4 tbsp (2 oz)	90
Tempura Chicken Nuggets	¾ cup (3.5 oz)	230
Tropical Sweet & Sour Chicken	1 pkg (10.9 oz)	490
Lean Cuisine		
Cafe Classics Asian Style Beef w/ Ginger & Soy	1 pkg (9.25 oz)	210
Cafe Classics Bowl Chicken Fried Rice	1 pkg (10 oz)	310
Cafe Classics Bowl Chicken Teriyaki	1 pkg (11 oz)	320
Cafe Classics Bowl Teriyaki Steak	1 pkg (10.5 oz)	340
Cafe Classics Chicken Teriyaki Stir Fry	1 pkg (10 oz)	300
Cafe Classics Hunan Beef & Broccoli	1 pkg (8.5 oz)	230
Cafe Classics Thai-Style Chicken	1 pkg (9 oz)	230
One Dish Favorites Asian Style Pot Stickers	1 pkg (9 oz)	320
One Dish Favorites Chicken Chow Mein	1 pkg (9 oz)	200
Skillet Asian Style Chicken & Vegetables	1 serv	160
Organic Classics		
Thai Chicken Curry	1 pkg (10 oz)	420
Seeds Of Change		
Asian Stir-Fry Noodles	1 pkg (11 oz)	290
Spicy Peanut Noodles	1 pkg (11 oz)	370
Teriyaki Stir-Fried Rice	1 pkg (11 oz)	340

FOOD	PORTION	CALS
Tyson		
Meal Kit Chicken Fried Rice	2½ cups	440
MIX		
Annie Chun's		
Meal Kit Chow Mein Noodles w/ Garlic Black Bean Sauce	⅓ pkg	230
Meal Kit Chow Mein Noodles w/ Peanut Sesame Sauce	⅓ pkg	270
Meal Kit Chow Mein Noodles w/ Scallion Sauce	⅓ pkg	240
Meal Kit Chow Mein Noodles w/ Teriyaki Sauce	⅓ box	210
Meal Kit Pad Thai Noodles w/ Pad Thai Sauce	⅓ pkg	210
Meal Kit Soba Noodles w/ Soy Ginger Sauce	⅓ pkg	210
Nissin		
Chow Mein Chicken as prep	½ pkg (2 oz)	240
Chow Mein Thai Peanut as prep	½ pkg (2 oz)	270
SHELF-STABLE		
Fantastic		
Pad Thai w/ Rice Noodles	1 pkg (7 oz)	400
Thai Lemon Grass w/ Rice Noodles	1 pkg (7.4 oz)	340
Healthy Choice		
Fresh Mixers Sesame Teriyaki Chicken	1 pkg (7.9 oz)	380
Fresh Mixers Sweet & Sour Chicken	1 pkg (7.9 oz)	390
Fresh Mixers Szechwan Beef w/ Asian Noodles	1 pkg (6.9 oz)	370
TAKE-OUT		
beef & broccoli	1 cup	221
beef w/ black bean sauce	1 serv (7 oz)	288
buddha's delight w/ cellophane noodles fat choi jai	1 serv (7.6 oz)	211
bun baked red bean	1 (1.1 oz)	102
cha siu bao steamed buns w/ chicken filling	1 (2.3 oz)	160
chicken masala	1 serv (8 oz)	430
chicken tandoori	1 serv (4 oz)	156
chicken tikka	1 serv (2.5 oz)	173
chinese garlic chicken	1 cup (5.7 oz)	290
chinese style fried egg noodles w/ seafood & lettuce	1 serv (14 oz)	694
chow mein beef w/o noodles	1 cup	271
chow mein chicken w/ noodles	1 cup (7.7 oz)	273

FOOD	PORTION	CALS
chow mein noodles	1 cup	237
chow mein pork w/o noodles	1 cup	284
chow mein shrimp w/o noodles	1 cup	154
chow mein vegetable w/o noodles	1 cup	224
dim sum deep fried beancurd w/ shrimp	1 (1.1 oz)	77
dim sum deep fried yam	1 (2.4 oz)	201
dim sum meat filled	3 (4 oz)	124
dim sum steamed chives & prawns	1 (1.2 oz)	48
egg foo yung beef	1 patty (6 oz)	243
egg foo yung chicken	1 patty (3 oz)	121
egg foo yung pork	1 patty (3 oz)	125
egg foo yung shrimp	1 patty (3 oz)	153
filipino chicken adobo	1 serv (15 oz)	555
foochow fish ball	1 (1 oz)	36
fried rice	1 cup	333
fried rice beef	1 cup	346
fried rice chicken	1 cup	329
fried rice pork	1 cup	335
fried rice shrimp	1 cup	323
general tsao's chicken	1 cup (5 oz)	296
green beans szechuan style	1 cup	176
indian style fried egg noodles w/ eggs tomato sauce & lime	1 serv (15 oz)	721
korean spicy shredded chicken	1 serv (5 oz)	258
kung pao beef	1 cup	410
kung pao chicken	1 cup (5.7 oz)	434
kung pao pork	1 cup	460
kung pao shrimp	1 cup	345
lemon chicken w/o vegetables	1 serv (6.6 oz)	503
lo mein beef	1 cup	286
lo mein chicken	1 cup (7 oz)	280
lo mein meatless	1 cup	234
lo mein pork	1 cup	314
lo mein shrimp	1 cup	236
moo goo gai pan chicken	1 cup (7.6 oz)	272
moo shu pork w/o pancake	1 cup	512
pakoras	1 (2.5 oz)	163
paneer pakora	1 (2.2 oz)	183
peking duck w/ pancakes & seafood sauce	1 serv (14 oz)	1871
phad thai w/ chicken	1 cup (7 oz)	358

FOOD	PORTION	CALS
pork w/ chinese cabbage	1 serv (4 oz)	120
sesame seed paste bun	1 (2.5 oz)	220
shrimp chips banh phong tom	6 med	214
shrimp w/ lobster sauce	1 cup	298
shu mai chicken & vegetable dumplings	6 (3.6 oz)	160
spring roll deep fried	1 (0.8 oz)	70
sukiyaki beef	1 cup	165
sukiyaki chicken	1 serv (18 oz)	436
sweet & sour chicken w/o rice	1 cup	670
sweet & sour pork w/ rice	1 cup	268
sweet & sour pork w/o rice	1 cup	231
sweet & sour shrimp	1 cup	480
szechuan chicken	1 cup (5.7 oz)	180
szechuan shrimp & vegetables	1 cup	159
tempura vegetable	8 pieces	90
tempura hawaiian fish tofu vegetable	2 cups	285
teriyaki beef	1 cup	454
teriyaki chicken	¾ cup	399
teriyaki chicken w/ rice	1 serv (11 oz)	430
teriyaki shrimp	1 cup	271
thai style pineapple rice w/ ham & pork floss	1 serv (7.7 oz)	408
wonton fried meat filled	1 (0.7 oz)	54
wonton meat & shrimp boiled	1 (0.5 oz)	19

ASPARAGUS
CANNED
spears	1	3
spears	1 cup	46
Del Monte		
Cuts & Tips	½ cup	20
Spears Extra Long	½ cup	20
Tips	½ cup	20
Gertie's Finest		
White	1 oz	15
Green Giant		
Spears Extra Long	5	20
Native Forest		
White	1 serv (4 oz)	20
Tillen Farms		
Crispy Asparagus Pickled	3 spears	10

FOOD	PORTION	CALS
FRESH		
cooked	½ cup	20
cooked	4 spears	13
spears raw	4	10
Apline Fresh		
Fresh Green	5 spears (3.3 oz)	20
Frieda's		
White	⅔ cup	20
Ocean Mist		
Spears	5 (3.3 oz)	25
FROZEN		
cooked	4 spears	11
cooked	1 pkg (10 oz)	53
C&W		
Spears	7 (3 oz)	20
Europe's Best		
Spears	7	15
Joy Of Cooking		
Tender	½ cup (3.3 oz)	70
ATEMOYA		
fresh	½ cup	94
AVOCADO		
california mashed	¼ cup	96
california peeled & pitted	1	289
florida mashed	¼ cup	69
florida peeled & pitted	1	365
Cabilfrut		
Hass fresh	⅕ med (1.1 oz)	55
Calavo		
Fresh	⅕ med (1 oz)	55
Earthbound Farm		
Organic Fresh	⅕ med (1 oz)	55
Frieda's		
Fresh Cocktail	1 (1.4 oz)	60
Simply Avo		
Hass Avocado Pulp	2 tbsp	50
Hass Halves	⅙ pkg (1.1 oz)	50
Wholly Guacamole		
Classic	2 tbsp	50

FOOD	PORTION	CALS
Organic	2 tbsp	50
Pico De Gallo Style	2 tbsp	40
TAKE-OUT		
guacamole	1 serv (2.2 oz)	105

BACON

FOOD	PORTION	CALS
bacon grease	1 tbsp	116
beef breakfast strips cooked	3 strips	153
gammon lean & fat grilled	4.2 oz	274
pan fried	3 strips	109
turkey	2 (0.8 oz)	84
Applegate Farms		
Natural Dry Cured Cooked	2 slices (0.5 oz)	60
Organic Turkey	1 slice (1 oz)	35
Boar's Head		
Fully Cooked Slices	3 (0.5 oz)	70
Butterball		
Turkey Bacon	1 slice (0.5 oz)	25
Hormel		
Real Bits	1 tbsp	25
Jennie-O		
Turkey Bacon	1 slice (0.5 oz)	35
Jimmy Dean		
Lower Sodium	1 slice (0.3 oz)	50
Original	1 slice (0.3 oz)	50
Thick Slice	1 (0.5 oz)	80
Oscar Mayer		
Bacon Bits	1 tbsp (7 g)	25
Center Cut cooked	2 slices (0.4 oz)	50
Hardwood Smoked	2 slices (0.5 oz)	70
Lower Sodium	3 slices (0.5 oz)	70
Ready To Serve	3 slices	70
Uncured	3 slices (0.5 oz)	60
Tyson		
Hickory Thick Cut	2 pieces (0.8 oz)	140
Wellshire		
Beef Uncured	2 oz	114
Panchetta Sliced	1 slice (0.4 oz)	60
Pork Range Sliced Dry Rubbed	2 slices	30
Uncured Turkey	1 slice (1 oz)	20

FOOD	PORTION	CALS
BACON SUBSTITUTES		
bacon bits meatless	1 tbsp	33
meatless	1 strip	16
Bob's Red Mill		
Bac'Ums	4 tsp	25
Lightlife		
Organic Tempeh Smokey Strips	3 (2 oz)	80
Smart Bacon	2 strips (0.8 oz)	45
Worthington		
Stripples	2 strips (0.5 oz)	60
BAGEL		
cinnamon raisin	1 mini	71
cinnamon raisin	1 lg (4 in)	244
egg	1 lg (4.5 in)	364
low carb	1 (4 oz)	216
mini onion	1 (1.4 oz)	100
oat bran	1 lg (4 in)	227
plain	1 sm (3 in)	190
plain	1 med (3.5 in)	289
plain	1 lg (4.5 in)	360
Alvarado Street Bakery		
Sprouted Wheat Cinnamon Raisin	1 (3.3 oz)	280
David's		
Deli Bagels	1 (2.8 oz)	230
Enjoy Life		
Nut Gluten Free Classic Original	1 (3 oz)	270
Natural Ovens		
Blueberry	1 (3 oz)	250
Brainy	1 (3 oz)	230
Whole Wheat	1 (3 oz)	230
New York Style		
Crisps Natural Whole Wheat	6	120
Crisps Plain	7	140
Pepperidge Farm		
100% Whole Wheat	1	250
Everything	1	260
Mini 100% Whole Wheat	1	100
Mini Plain	1	110
Sara Lee		
Apple Cinnamon	1 (4 oz)	310

FOOD	PORTION	CALS
Banana Walnut	1 (4 oz)	350
Blueberry Deluxe	1 (3.3 oz)	260
Blueberry Junior	1 (1 oz)	70
Blueberry Toaster Size	1 (2.1 oz)	160
Cinnamon Raisin Deluxe	1 (3.3 oz)	260
Heart Healthy 100% Whole Wheat	1 (3.3 oz)	220
Heart Healthy Cinnamon Raisin	1 (3.3 oz)	250
Plain	1 (2.1 oz)	160
Sundried Tomato & Basil	1 (4 oz)	300
Whole Grain Plain	1 (3.3 oz)	240
Thomas'		
100% Whole Wheat Mini	1 (1.5 oz)	110
Bagelbread Mini Squares 100% Whole Wheat	1 (2 oz)	150
Carb Consider Plain	1	150
Carb Consider Whole Wheat	1	140
Weight Watchers		
Original	1 (2.8 oz)	190

BAKING POWDER

baking powder	1 tsp	2
low sodium	1 tsp	5
Bob's Red Mills		
Baking Powder	1 tsp	5
Calumet		
Double Acting	⅛ tsp	0
Davis		
Baking Powder	1 tsp	0

BAKING SODA

baking soda	1 tsp	0
Bob's Red Mill		
Baking Soda	¼ tsp	0

BALSAM PEAR (BITTER GOURD)

leafy tips cooked w/o salt	1 cup	20
leafy tips raw	1 cup	14
pods raw sliced	1 cup	16
pods sliced cooked w/ salt	1 cup	24

BAMBOO SHOOTS

canned sliced	½ cup	12
fresh sliced cooked w/ salt	½ cup	7

FOOD	PORTION	CALS
raw sliced	½ cup	20
La Choy		
Bamboo Shoots	½ cup	10
Polar		
Sliced	½ cup	25
BANANA		
baked	1 (4.5 oz)	163
banana chips	1 oz	147
fresh	1 sm (6 in)	90
fresh	1 med (7 in)	105
fresh	1 lg (8 in)	121
fresh baby	1 extra sm (<6 in)	72
fresh mashed	½ cup	100
fresh sliced	1 cup	134
green fried	1 (3.1 oz)	152
green pickled	½ cup	240
green sliced fried	1 cup	323
powder	1 tbsp	21
red ripe	1 (7 in)	93
red ripe sliced	1 cup	134
whole dried	1 piece (1.2 oz)	130
Bob's Red Mill		
Chips	25 (1.4 oz)	210
Brothers-All-Natural		
Crisps	1 pkg (0.58 oz)	66
Frieda's		
Burro	1 (3 oz)	80
Dried	1 piece (1.2 oz)	130
Goodniks		
Nutty Bananas Crunchy Snack	⅔ cup	230
Kopali		
Organic Dark Chocolate Covered	½ pkg (1 oz)	120
Tree Of Life		
Dried Sweetened	½ cup (1.6 oz)	240
TAKE-OUT		
batter dipped fried	1 sm (4 oz)	266
fried dwarf w/ cheese	1 (1.4 oz)	84
fritter	1 (2.3 oz)	197
sliced batter dipped fried	1 cup	335

FOOD	PORTION	CALS
BARBECUE SAUCE		
barbecue	2 tbsp	52
low sodium	2 tbsp	52
Annie's Naturals		
Organic Original	2 tbsp	45
Bear-Man		
Black Bear Boogie	2 tbsp	40
Growlin' Grizzly	2 tbsp	60
Bone Suckin'		
Sauce	2 tbsp	40
Carb Options		
Original	2 tbsp	10
Cattlemen's		
Classic	2 tbsp	60
Honey	2 tbsp	70
Smokehouse	2 tbsp	60
Consorzio		
Organic Original	1 tbsp	50
Organic Spicy	1 tbsp	50
David Burke		
Flavor Spray Memphis BBQ	2 sprays	0
Emeril's		
Original BBQ	2 tbsp	45
Hunt's		
Hickory	2 tbsp	45
Hickory & Brown Sugar	2 tbsp	70
Honey Hickory	2 tbsp	50
Honey Mustard	2 tbsp	50
Hot & Spicy	2 tbsp	45
Mesquite	2 tbsp	40
Original	2 tbsp	50
Original Bold	2 tbsp	45
Nando's		
Barbecue	1 tbsp	7
Naturally Fresh		
BBQ	2 tbsp	40
San-J		
Asian BBQ	2 tbsp	40
Steel's		
Sugar Free	2 tbsp	15

FOOD	PORTION	CALS
Wellshire		
Original	2 tbsp	39
BARLEY		
flour	1 cup	511
pearled cooked	1 cup (5.5 oz)	193
pearled uncooked	¼ cup	176
Arrowhead Mills		
Organic Pearled not prep	¼ cup	160
Robinsons		
Barley Water Lemon as prep	9 oz	48
BARRACUDA		
broiled	4 oz	239
cooked flaked	1 cup	287
poached	4 oz	227
TAKE-OUT		
breaded & fried	4 oz	282
BASIL		
fresh chopped	2 tbsp	1
ground	1 tsp	4
leaves fresh	5	1
Dorot		
Chopped Cube frzn	1 cube (4 g)	5
Eden		
Shiso Leaf Powder	1 tsp	0
BASS		
breaded baked	4 oz	205
pickled mero en escabeche	2 oz	156
striped baked	3 oz	105
striped bass farm raised	4 oz	110
BAY LEAF		
crumbled	1 tsp	2
BEAN SPROUTS (see ALFALFA, SPROUTS)		
BEANS (see also individual names)		
CANNED		
baked beans plain	½ cup	119
baked beans vegetarian	½ cup	119
baked beans w/ franks	½ cup	184

FOOD	PORTION	CALS
baked beans w/ pork	½ cup	134
baked beans w/ pork & tomato sauce	½ cup	119
refried beans	½ cup	134
Allens		
Original Baked	½ cup	150
Refried Black Beans No Fat Added	½ cup	120
B&M		
Baked Original	½ cup (4.6 oz)	180
Barbeque Baked	½ cup (4.6 oz)	190
Country Style	½ cup (4.6 oz)	170
Vegetarian	½ cup (4.6 oz)	160
Bush's		
Barbecue	½ cup	150
Boston Recipe	½ cup	150
Homestyle	½ cup	140
Honey	½ cup	160
Onion 98% Fat Free	½ cup	140
Vegetarian Fat Free	½ cup	130
Campbell's		
Pork & Beans	½ cup	140
Eden		
Organic Baked w/ Sorghum	½ cup	150
Green Giant		
Three Bean Salad	½ cup	80
Heinz		
Vegetarian	1 cup	250
Las Palmas		
Refried	½ cup	150
Old El Paso		
Refried Fat Free	½ cup	100
Refried Fat Free Spicy	½ cup	100
Pace		
Refried Salsa	½ cup	70
Ranch Style		
Original Texas	½ cup	138
Read		
3 Bean Salad	⅓ cup	60
Rosarita		
Refried	½ cup	120
Refried Black Beans No Fat	½ cup	110

FOOD	PORTION	CALS
Refried Fat Free	½ cup	100
Refried Vegetarian	½ cup	120
Van Camp's		
Baked Beans Homestyle	½ cup	170
Beanee Weenee BBQ	1 can	260
Beanee Weenee Original	1 can	240
Beanee Weenee w/ Chili	1 can	240
Pork And Beans	½ cup	110
Wagon Master		
Pork & Beans	½ cup	130
FROZEN		
Lean Cuisine		
Cafe Classics Sante Fe Style Rice & Beans	1 pkg (10.4 oz)	290
MIX		
Fantastic		
Instant Black Beans not prep	⅓ cup	160
Instant Refried Beans not prep	¼ cup	130
TAKE-OUT		
baked beans	½ cup	191
barbecue beans	3.5 oz	120
frijoles a la charra	1 cup	341
w/ pork tomatoes & chili peppers		
refried beans	½ cup	43
three bean salad	1 cup	114
BEAR		
simmered	3 oz	220
BEAVER		
roasted	4 oz	240
BEE POLLEN		
Tree Of Life		
Bee Pollen	1 tsp (7 g)	30
BEECHNUTS		
dried	1 oz	163
BEEF (see also BEEF DISHES, MEATBALLS, VEAL)		
CANNED		
corned beef	1 oz	71
Libby's		
Potted Meat	¼ cup	120

FOOD	PORTION	CALS
FRESH		
arm pot roast trim 0 fat braised	3.5 oz	297
arm pot roast trim ⅛ in fat braised	3.5 oz	302
beef crumbles 70% lean pan browned	3 oz	230
bottom round roast trim 0 fat braised	4 oz	253
bottom round roast trim 0 fat roasted	3.5 oz	187
bottom round roast trim ½ in fat braised	4 oz	337
bottom round roast trim ⅛ in fat braised	4 oz	280
bottom round roast trim ⅛ in fat roasted	4 oz	247
bottom sirloin butt roast trim 0 fat roasted	3.5 oz	182
brisket flat half trim ⅛ in fat braised	3.5 oz	298
brisket flat trim 0 fat braised	3.5 oz	221
brisket point half trim 0 fat braised	3.5 oz	358
brisket point half trim ¼ in fat braised	3.5 oz	404
chuck boston cut roast trim 0 fat roasted	3.5 oz	207
chuck boston cut roast trim ¼ in fat roasted	3.5 oz	242
chuck bottom roast trim 0 fat braised	3.5 oz	334
chuck bottom roast trim ¼ in fat braised	3.5 oz	345
chuck fillet steak trim 0 fat broiled	4 oz	181
chuck top roast trim 0 fat broiled	4 oz	245
club steak trim ½ in fat broiled	4 oz	384
corned beef brisket cooked	3 oz	213
crosscut shank trim ¼ in fat stewed	1 serv (6.8 oz)	510
delmonico steak trim ¼ in fat broiled	4 oz	409
entrecote steak trim ½ in fat broiled	4 oz	413
eye round roast trim 0 fat roasted	4 oz	190
eye round roast trim ¼ in fat roasted	4 oz	283
filet mignon roast trim ¼ in fat roasted	4 oz	376
filet mignon roast trim ⅛ in fat roasted	4 oz	367
filet mignon trim 0 fat broiled	4 oz	247
filet mignon trim ⅛ in fat broiled	4 oz	303
ground 70% lean broiled	3.5 oz	273
ground 75% lean broiled	2.5 oz	195
ground 80% lean broiled	3 oz	234
ground 85% lean pan fried	3 oz	197
ground 90% lean pan fried	3 oz	173
ground 95% lean pan fried	3 oz	139
ground lowfat w/ carrageenan raw	4 oz	160
london broil trim 0 fat broiled	3.5 oz	188
london broil trim ¼ in fat broiled	4 oz	260

FOOD	PORTION	CALS
new york strip steak trim 0 fat broiled	4 oz	219
oxtails cooked	6 pieces (6.3 oz)	472
porterhouse steak trim 0 fat broiled	1 lb	1252
porterhouse steak trim ¼ in fat broiled	1 lb	1492
porterhouse steak trim ⅛ in fat broiled	1 lb	1324
rib eye roast trim ¼ in fat roasted	3.5 oz	365
rib eye steak trim ⅛ in fat broiled	4 oz	221
rib roast trim ¼ in fat roasted	4 oz	406
rib steak trim ¼ in fat broiled	4 oz	388
round tip roast trim 0 fat roasted	4 oz	213
sandwich steaks thinly sliced	1 serv (2 oz)	173
shell steak trim ¼ in fat broiled	4 oz	366
shortribs lean & fat braised	1 serv (7.8 oz)	1060
skirt steak trim 0 fat broiled	4 oz	289
t-bone steak trim 0 fat broiled	4 oz	280
t-bone steak trim ¼ in fat broiled	1 lb	1388
t-bone steak trim ⅛ in fat broiled	1 lb	804
tip round roast trim ⅛ in fat roasted	4 oz	248
top loin steak boneless trim ⅛ in fat broiled	4 oz	299
top round roast trim 0 fat braised	4 oz	237
top round roast trim ¼ in fat braised	4 oz	281
top round roast trim ¼ in fat roasted	4 oz	265
top round steak trim ¼ in fat pan fried	4 oz	314
top sirloin steak trim ⅛ in fat broiled	4 oz	275
top sirloin steak trim ⅛ in fat pan fried	4 oz	355
tri-tip roast trim 0 fat roasted	3.5 oz	218
tri-tip steak trim 0 fat broiled	4 oz	300
Laura's Lean		
Eye Of Round	4 oz	135
Flank Steak	4 oz	140
Ground Beef 92% Lean	4 oz	160
Ground Beef Patties	1 (4 oz)	160
Ground Round 96% Lean	4 oz	140
Ribeye Steak	4 oz	175
Sirloin Steak	4 oz	145
Sirloin Tip	4 oz	130
Strip Steak	4 oz	150
Tenderloin Filet	4 oz	145
Top Round	4 oz	135

FOOD	PORTION	CALS
Organic Prairie		
90% Lean Ground	4 oz	250
Rumba		
Cheekmeat	4 oz	300
Crosscut Hind Shank	4 oz	190
Marrow Bones	4 oz	290
Oxtail	4 oz	260
Short Ribs	4 oz	400
Shady Brook		
Tri-Tip Roast Rosemary Garlic & Chardonnay	4 oz	180
Tri-Tip Roast Sizzling Ginger	4 oz	210
FROZEN		
patty broiled medium	3 oz	240
Organic Prairie		
Rib Eye Steak	1 (6 oz)	470
Soy Lean		
Beef Patty	1 (2.5 oz)	90
READY-TO-EAT		
dried beef smoked chopped	1 oz	37
roast beef spread	¼ cup	127
smoked beef cooked	1 sausage (1.4 oz)	134
Applegate Farms		
Organic Roast Beef	2 oz	80
Boar's Head		
Corned Beef Brisket	2 oz	80
Top Round Deluxe	2 oz	80
Top Round Oven Roasted No Salt Added	2 oz	90
Healthy Ones		
Deli Roast Beef	2 oz	70
Laura's Lean		
Beef Pot Roast Au Jus	3 oz	110
Oscar Mayer		
Slow Roasted Shaved	¼ pkg (1.8 oz)	60
Sara Lee		
Roast Beef Medium or Rare	2 oz	60
Tyson		
Beef Strips Seasoned	1 serv (3 oz)	130
TAKE-OUT		
roast beef rare	2 oz	70

FOOD	PORTION	CALS
BEEF DISHES		
CANNED		
corned beef hash	3 oz	155
Hormel		
Corned Beef Hash 50% Reduced Fat	1 cup	290
Libby's		
Hawaiian Corned Beef	2 oz	120
FROZEN		
Quaker Maid		
Sandwich Steaks Pure Beef	1 serv (1.8 oz)	120
Tyson		
Steak Country Fried	1 (3.2 oz)	310
MIX		
Hamburger Helper		
Beef Pasta as prep	1 cup	270
Cheddar Cheese Melt as prep	1 cup	310
Cheesy Baked Potato as prep	1 cup	310
Chili Cheese as prep	1 cup	340
Double Cheesy Quesadilla as prep	1 cup	350
Italian Sausage as prep	1 cup	290
Microwave Singles Cheesy Lasagna	1 pkg	210
Philly Cheesesteak as prep	1 cup	320
Salisbury as prep	1 cup	260
Tomato Basil Penne as prep	1 cup	300
REFRIGERATED		
Chi Chi's		
For Tacos! Ground Beef	¼ cup	90
Hormel		
Beef Roast Au Jus	1 serv (5 oz)	200
Beef Tips & Gravy	½ cup	170
Huxtable's		
Shepherds Pie Beef	1 pkg (10 oz)	270
Laura's Lean		
Meatloaf w/ Tomato Sauce	1 serv (5 oz)	230
Shredded Beef w/ Barbecue Sauce	1 serv (5 oz)	245
Morton's Of Omaha		
Beef Pot Roast w/ Gravy	1 serv (3 oz)	160
Tyson		
Chuck Roast w/ Vegetables	1 serv (4 oz)	320
Seasoned Meatloaf	1 serv (5 oz)	320

FOOD	PORTION	CALS
Steak Tips In Burbon Sauce	1 serv (5 oz)	180
TAKE-OUT		
beef bourguignonne	1 cup	339
beef satay + peanut sauce	2 skewers	253
bool kogi korean marinated beef ribs	4 oz	190
bracciola	1 roll (4.7 oz)	276
bubble & squeak	5 oz	186
bulgoghi korean grilled beef	1 serv (5.2 oz)	256
chipped beef on toast	1 slice (5 oz)	226
cornish pasty	1 (8 oz)	847
goulash w/ potatoes	1 cup	298
irish stew	1 cup (7 oz)	280
kebab indian	1 (5.4 oz)	553
kheena	6.7 oz	781
koftas	5	280
meatloaf	1 lg slice (5 oz)	294
moussaka	1 serv (8.5 oz)	450
pepper steak	1 cup	317
pot roast w/ gravy	1 serv (6 oz)	320
samosa	2 (4 oz)	652
shepherds pie	1 serv (7 oz)	282
sloppy joes	1 serv (9 oz)	398
steak & kidney pie w/ top crust	1 slice (5 oz)	400
stew w/ potatoes & vegetables	1 cup	199
stroganoff	1 cup	394
swiss steak w/ sauce	1 serv (8 oz)	234
toad in the hole	1 (4.7 oz)	383

BEEFALO

FOOD	PORTION	CALS
roasted	4 oz	213

BEER AND ALE

FOOD	PORTION	CALS
alcohol free beer	7 oz	50
ale brown	10 oz	77
ale pale	10 oz	88
beer cooler	1 (16 oz)	194
beer light	12 oz can	103
beer regular	12 oz can	153
black & tan	1 serv (12 oz)	146
black velvet	1 (10 oz)	160
boilermaker	1 serv	216

FOOD	PORTION	CALS
lager	10 oz	80
lager & black	1 (14 oz)	241
mead	1 serv	250
pilsener lager	7 oz	85
shandy	1 serv	125
stout	10 oz	102
trojan horse	1 (16 oz)	189
Amstel		
Light	1 bottle (12 oz)	95
Beamish		
Stout	12 oz	131
Beck's		
Beer	1 bottle (12 oz)	143
Premium Light	1 bottle	64
Blue Moon		
White	1 bottle (12 oz)	171
Budweiser		
Beer	1 bottle (12 oz)	145
Bud Light	1 bottle (12 oz)	110
Busch		
Light	1 bottle (12 oz)	110
Coors		
Light	1 bottle (12 oz)	102
Corona		
Extra	1 bottle (12 oz)	148
Guinness		
Draft In A Bottle	1 bottle (12 oz)	128
Hamm's		
Light	1 bottle (12 oz)	110
Heineken		
Beer	1 bottle (12 oz)	150
I.C.		
Light	1 bottle (12 oz)	96
Icehouse		
5.0	1 bottle (12 oz)	132
5.5	1 bottle (12 oz)	149
J.W. Dundee		
Honey Brown	1 bottle (12 oz)	150
Keystone		
Light	1 bottle (12 oz)	100

FOOD	PORTION	CALS
LaBatt		
Blue	1 bottle (12 oz)	127
Michelob		
Ultra	1 bottle (12 oz)	95
Miller		
Lite	1 bottle (12 oz)	96
MDG 64	1 bottle (12 oz)	64
Smirnoff		
Ice	1 bottle (12 oz)	241
Weinhard's		
Ale	1 bottle (12 oz)	147
Amber Ale	1 bottle (12 oz)	169
Dark	1 bottle (12 oz)	150
Hefeweizen	1 bottle (12 oz)	128
BEET JUICE		
juice	7 oz	72
BEETS		
CANNED		
harvard	½ cup	90
pickled	½ cup	74
sliced	½ cup	37
Del Monte		
Pickled Sliced	½ cup	35
Sliced	½ cup	35
Freshlike		
Pickled Sliced	4 slices (1 oz)	20
Greenwood		
Harvard	1 serv (4.4 oz)	100
Pickled	1 oz	25
FRESH		
greens cooked w/o salt	½ cup	19
sliced cooked	½ cup	37
whole cooked	2 med (3.5 oz)	44
Frieda's		
Beets	½ cup	35

BEVERAGES (*see* BEER AND ALE, CHAMPAGNE, COFFEE, DRINK MIXERS, ENERGY DRINKS, FRUIT DRINKS, ICED TEA, LIQUOR/LIQUEUR, MALT, MILKSHAKE, SMOOTHIES, SODA, TEA/HERBAL TEA, WATER, WINE, YOGURT DRINKS)

FOOD	PORTION	CALS
BISCUIT		
FROZEN		
Jimmy Dean		
Snack Size Sausage On A Biscuit	2	400
MIX		
plain as prep	1 (2 oz)	190
Bisquick		
Heart Smart	⅓ cup	140
Jiffy		
Buttermilk as prep	1	170
King Arthur		
Whole Grain Buttermilk not prep	¼ cup	100
REFRIGERATED		
plain baked	1 (1 oz)	93
Pillsbury		
Buttermilk	3 (2.2 oz)	150
Flaky Layers	3 (2.2 oz)	160
Grands! Butter Tastin'	1 (2 oz)	190
Grands! Buttermilk Reduced Fat	1 (2 oz)	170
Grands! Golden Wheat Reduced Fat	1 (2.1 oz)	180
Grands! Original	1 (2 oz)	190
Grands! Original Reduced Fat	1 (2 oz)	170
Perfect Portions Butter Tastin'	1 (1.9 oz)	190
TAKE-OUT		
buttermilk	1 lg (2.7 oz)	280
oatcakes	2 (4 oz)	115
plain	1 sm (1.2 oz)	127
tea biscuit	1 (3 oz)	210
w/ egg	1 (4.8 oz)	373
w/ egg & bacon	1 (5.3 oz)	458
w/ egg & ham	1 (6.7 oz)	442
w/ egg & sausage	1 (6.3 oz)	581
w/ egg & steak	1 (5.2 oz)	410
w/ egg cheese & bacon	1 (5.1 oz)	477
w/ ham	1 (4 oz)	386
w/ sausage	1 (4.4 oz)	485
BITTERMELON		
Frieda's		
Foo Qua	1 cup	15

FOOD	PORTION	CALS

BLACK BEANS
dried cooked	1 cup	227
Allens		
Black Beans	½ cup	100
Eden		
Organic Caribbean	½ cup	90
Organic Refried	½ cup	110
Goya		
Black Beans	½ cup (4.3 oz)	90
Tree Of Life		
Organic	½ cup (4.6 oz)	130

BLACKBERRIES
canned in heavy syrup	½ cup	118
fresh	½ cup	31
unsweetened frzn	½ cup	48
Cascadian Farm		
Organic frzn	1 cup	80
Oregon		
In Light Syrup	½ cup	120

BLACKBERRY JUICE
canned	6 oz	65
Izze		
Sparkling Blackberry	8 oz	140

BLACKEYE PEAS
catjang dried cooked	1 cup (2.9 oz)	200
cowpeas canned	1 cup	184
cowpeas frozen cooked	½ cup	112
cowpeas leafy tips chopped cooked	1 cup	12
cowpeas leafy tips raw chopped	1 cup	10
CANNED		
w/pork	½ cup	199
Eden		
Organic	½ cup	90
DRIED		
cooked	1 cup	198
FROZEN		
McKenzie		
Blackeye Peas	1 serv (2.8 oz)	110

FOOD	PORTION	CALS
TAKE-OUT		
blackeye peas & pork	1 cup	236
BLINTZE		
Golden		
Cheese	1 (2.1 oz)	80
Ratner's		
Cheese	1 (2.2 oz)	100
TAKE-OUT		
cheese	1 (2.7 oz)	160
BLUEBERRIES		
canned in heavy syrup	½ cup	113
fresh	½ cup	41
fresh	1 pt	229
frzn unsweetened	½ cup	40
A&L Farms		
Bleuets Fresh	1 pt	80
C&W		
Ulimate	¾ cup	70
Chukar Cherries		
Puget Sound Dried	¼ cup	160
White Chocolate Covered	3 tbsp (1.4 oz)	223
De-Lite		
Dried Sweetened	1 oz	86
Eden		
Organic Dried Wild	¼ cup	150
Emily's		
Dark Chocolate Covered	¼ cup (1.4 oz)	170
Europe's Best		
Woodland frzn	¾ cup	70
Frieda's		
Dried	¼ cup (1.4 oz)	140
Hodgson Mill		
Dried Wild	¼ cup	120
LiteHouse		
Glaze	3 tbsp	70
Marie's		
Glaze	2 tbsp	40
Oregon		
In Light Syrup	½ cup	110

FOOD	PORTION	CALS
Sunsweet		
Dried	¼ cup (1.4 oz)	140
Tree Of Life		
Dried	¼ cup (1.5 oz)	150

BLUEBERRY JUICE
Izze		
Sparkling Blueberry	8 oz	100
Tart Is Smart		
Wild Blueberry Concentrate	0.5 oz	35
Van Dyk's		
100% Juice	6 oz	74
Walnut Acres		
Organic	8 oz	130

BLUEFIN
fillet baked	4.1 oz	186

BLUEFISH
fresh baked	3 oz	135

BOAR
wild roasted	3 oz	136
Natural Frontier Foods		
Wild Boar Steaks	1 (4 oz)	170

BOK CHOY (see CABBAGE)

BONITO
dried	1 oz	50
fresh	3 oz	117

BORAGE
fresh chopped	1 cup	19

BOTTLED WATER (see WATER)

BOYSENBERRIES
frzn unsweetened	½ cup	33
in heavy syrup	½ cup	113

BRAINS
beef pan-fried	3 oz	167
beef simmered	3 oz	123
lamb braised	3 oz	123

FOOD	PORTION	CALS
lamb fried	3 oz	232
pork braised	3 oz	117
veal braised	3 oz	116
veal fried	3 oz	181

BRAN
corn	1 cup (2.7 oz)	170
oat	½ cup (1.6 oz)	116
oat cooked	½ cup (3.8 oz)	44
rice	½ cup (2.1 oz)	187
wheat	½ cup (2 oz)	63
Bob's Red Mill		
Rice Bran	2 tbsp	60
Quaker		
Unprocessed	⅓ cup (0.6 oz)	35
Tree Of Life		
Oat Bran	½ cup (1.6 oz)	120
Organic Wheat Bran	¼ cup (1.1 oz)	190

BRAZIL NUTS
dried unblanched	1 oz	186

BREAD
CANNED
boston brown	1 slice (1.6 oz)	88
B&M		
Raisin Brown Bread	½ in slice (2 oz)	130
FROZEN		
Alexia		
Baguette Garlic	2 pieces (1.6 oz)	130
Cedarlane		
Organic Mediterranean Stuffed Focaccia	1 piece (4 oz)	295
Corbi's		
Chee-Zee Bread Original	½ piece (1.8 oz)	180
Pepperidge Farm		
Garlic	1 slice (2.5 in)	170
Texas Toast Five Cheese	1 slice	150
Whole Grain Texas Toast	1 slice	150
MIX		
cornbread	1 piece (2 oz)	188
Buitoni		
Focaccia Italian Herb & Cheese	1 slice	110

FOOD	PORTION	CALS
Focaccia Rosemary & Garlic	1 piece (1 oz)	110
Carbolite		
Bread Mix as prep	1 slice	45
Keto		
Quick Bread All Flavors as prep	1 slice	55
MiniCarb		
Country White as prep	1 slice	80
READY-TO-EAT		
anadama	1 piece (1.1 oz)	87
baguette whole wheat	2 oz	140
challah	1 slice (1.4 oz)	115
cinnamon	1 slice (0.9 oz)	69
cracked wheat	1 slice (1.1 oz)	78
cuban bread	1 slice (1.1 oz)	83
french	1 slice (1.1 oz)	88
italian	1 loaf (1 lb)	1255
navajo fry	1 piece	281
oat bran	1 slice (1.1 oz)	71
oatmeal	1 slice (0.9 oz)	73
pan criollo	1 piece (0.9 oz)	69
panettone	1 slice (0.9 oz)	86
pita	1 sm (1 oz)	77
pita	1 lg (2 oz)	165
pita whole wheat	1 sm (1 oz)	74
pita whole wheat	1 lg (2.2 oz)	170
pumpernickel	1 slice (0.9 oz)	65
raisin	1 slice (1.1 oz)	88
rye	1 slice (1.1 oz)	83
seven grain	1 slice (1.1 oz)	80
wheat berry	1 slice (0.9 oz)	65
wheat bran	1 slice (1.3 oz)	89
wheat germ	1 slice (1 oz)	73
white cubed	1 cup	93
whole wheat	1 slice (1 oz)	69
Alvarado Street Bakery		
Sprouted Soy Crunch	1 slice (1.2 oz)	90
Sprouted Whole Wheat	1 slice	90
Arnold		
100% Natural Soft Honey Wheat	2 slices (2 oz)	150
Grains & More Double Omega	1 slice	110

FOOD	PORTION	CALS
Jewish Rye	1 slice	90
Sandwich Thins Multi-Grain	1 (1.5 oz)	100
Sandwich Thins Whole Grain White	1 (1.5 oz)	100
Whole Grains 100% Whole Wheat Double Fiber	1 slice	100
Whole Grains 7 Grain	1 slice	110
Whole Grains 12 Grain	1 slice	110
Whole Grains 15 Grain	1 slice	110
Baker's Inn		
9 Grain	1 slice	100
Cracked Wheat	1 slice	100
Honey White Made w/ Whole Grain	1 slice	110
Honey Whole Wheat	1 slice	100
Potato Made w/ Whole Grain	1 slice	100
Comfort Care		
Cabin Hearth Whole Wheat	1 oz	170
Damascus		
Roll-Up Flax	1 (2 oz)	110
Roll-Up Whole Wheat	1 (2 oz)	110
Wraps Honey Wheat	½ wrap (2 oz)	130
Earth Grains		
100% Multi Grain Extra Fiber	1 slice	110
Oat & Nut	1 slice	120
Potato	1 slice	110
Whole Grain Honey	1 slice	110
Whole Wheat Honey	1 slice	110
Ecce Panis		
Classic Ciabatta	⅛ loaf (2 oz)	180
Food For Life		
Brown Rice Bread Yeast Free	1 slice	100
Rice Bread Fruit & Seed Yeast Free	1 slice	140
Rice Bread Multi Seed Yeast Free	1 slice	120
White Rice Bread Yeast Free	1 slice	100
Freihofer's		
100% Whole Wheat	1 slice	90
French Meadow Bakery		
Healthy Hemp	1 slice	110
Organic Men's Bread	1 slice	120
Kangaroo		
Bread Wraps	1 (2.6 oz)	140

FOOD	PORTION	CALS
Greek Pita Flat	1 (2.6 oz)	200
Greek Pita Flat Wheat	1 (2.4 oz)	145
Pita Pockets Onion	½ (1.2 oz)	90
Pita Pockets Wheat N'Honey	½ (1.2 oz)	90
Pita Pockets White	½ (1.2 oz)	90
Salad Pockets	1 (1.2 oz)	90
Sandwich Pockets Whole Grain	1 (1.2 oz)	80
La Tortilla Factory		
Wraps Smart & Delicious Gluten Free Dark Teff	1 (2.3 oz)	180
Wraps Smart & Delicious Gluten Free Ivory Teff	1 (2.3 oz)	180
Matthew's		
All Natural Cinnamon Raisin	1 slice	80
Milton's		
100% Whole Wheat	1 slice	110
Buttermilk	1 slice	90
Gourmet White	1 slice	110
Original Multi-Grain	1 slice	120
Potato	1 slice	90
Whole Grain	1 slice	90
Natural Ovens		
100% Sweet Whole	1 slice	90
Carb Conscious Original	1 slice	80
Healthy Beginnings Better White	1 slice	110
Healthy Beginnings Honey Wheat	1 slice	120
Hunger Filler Whole Grain	1 slice	100
Organic Plus Whole Grain & Flax	1 slice	120
Whole Grain Oat Nut Crunch	1 slice	100
Nature's Own		
100% Whole Wheat	1 slice	50
9 Grain	1 slice	120
Hearty Oatmeal	1 slice	100
Wheat Double Fiber	1 slice	10
Wheat Light	2 slices	80
Wheat N' Fiber	1 slice	60
Whole Wheat w/ Organic Flour	1 slice	100
Nature's Path		
Manna Carrot Raisin	1 slice	130
Manna Millet Rice	1 slice	130
Manna SunSeed	1 slice	160

FOOD	PORTION	CALS
Pepperidge Farm		
100% Natural Whole Grain German Dark Wheat	1 slice	100
Breakfast Apple & Grains	1 slice	90
Canadian White	1 slice	100
Carb Style 7 Grain	1 slice	60
Farmhouse Hearty White	1 slice	120
Farmhouse Honey Wheatberry	1 slice	120
Farmhouse Soft 100% Whole Wheat	1 slice	110
Farmhouse Soft Oatmeal	1 slice	120
Honey Flax Whole Grain	1 slice (1.5 oz)	100
Hot & Crusty Italian	1 slice (2 in thick)	150
Jewish Rye Whole Grain Seeded	1 slice	70
Light Style 7 Grain	1 slice	45
Light Style Oatmeal	3 slices	140
Party Pumpernickel	5 slices	130
Very Thin White	3 slices	120
Whole Grain 100% Soft Whole Wheat Double Fiber	1 slice	100
Whole Grain Honey Oat	1 slice	110
Whole Grain Honey Whole Wheat	1 slice	110
Whole Grain Swirl Cinnamon w/ Raisins	1 slice (1.3 oz)	100
Rudi's Organic Bakery		
100% Whole Wheat	1 slice	100
14 Grain	1 slice	90
Artisan Country French	1 slice	100
Artisan Rosemary Olive Oil	1 slice	100
Low Carb Right Choice	1 slice	45
Spelt Ancient Grain	1 slice	120
Whole Grain Apple N Spice	1 slice	110
S. Rosen's		
Hawaiian	1 slice	110
Rye Black Bavarian	1 slice	100
Sara Lee		
100% Whole Wheat	1 slice	70
Blueberry Crumble	1 slice	180
Cinnamon Raisin	1 slice	190
Classic Wheat	1 slice	70
Delightful Wheat	1 slice	45
Delightful White	1 slice	90

FOOD	PORTION	CALS
Heart Healthy 100% Whole Wheat Essentials	1 slice	80
Heart Healthy Multigrain	1 slice	100
Honey Wheat	1 slice	70
Honey White	1 slice	100
Multigrain	1 slice	100
Soft & Smooth 100% Whole Wheat	1 slice	70
Soft & Smooth Whole Grain White	2 slices	150
Sonoma		
Wraps Organic Multi Grain	1 (2.4 oz)	180
Wraps Organic Wheat	1 (2.4 oz)	190
Wraps Original White Whole Wheat	1 (2.4 oz)	200
Stroehmann		
100% Whole Wheat	1 slice	90
Dutch Country Twelve Grain	1 slice	100
Family Grains Twisted Bread	1 slice	70
Potato	1 slice	100
Soft Rye Seeded	1 slice	90
Super Bakery		
Athlete's Formula	1 slice (1.5 oz)	100
Fitness Formula	1 slice (1.5 oz)	90
Wrap Organic	1 (4 oz)	340
The Baker		
Yoga Bread	1 slice	70
Thomas'		
Breakfast Original	1 slice	90
Corn	1 slice	110
Sahara Pita Pockets Mini Whole Wheat	1 (1 oz)	70
Swirl Cinnamon Raisin	1 slice	120
Tumaro's		
Wraps Chipotle Chili & Peppers	1 (2.3 oz)	170
Wraps Sun Dried Tomato & Basil	1 (2.3 oz)	170
REFRIGERATED		
Pillsbury		
Italian	⅛ pkg (1.6 oz)	110
TAKE-OUT		
banana	1 slice (2 oz)	196
chapati as prep w/ fat	1 (1.6 oz)	95
chapati as prep w/o fat	1 (2.5 oz)	141
cornbread	1 piece (2.3 oz)	183
cornstick	1 (1.4 oz)	118

FOOD	PORTION	CALS
focaccia onion	1 piece (4.6 oz)	282
focaccia rosemary	1 piece (3.5 oz)	251
focaccia tomato olive	1 piece (4.7 oz)	270
garlic bread	1 slice (1 oz)	96
irish soda bread	1 slice (3 oz)	247
italian garlic	1 loaf (11 oz)	990
naan	1 bread (3.5 oz)	286
papadum fried	1 (6 g)	30
paratha plain	1 (1.6 oz)	136
poori indian puffed bread	1 piece (1.3 oz)	112
zucchini	1 slice (1.4 oz)	150

BREAD COATING
Don's Chuck Wagon
Chicken Baking Mix	¼ cup	95
Fish Mix	¼ cup	95
Onion Ring Mix	¼ cup	100

Fryin' Magic
Cornmeal	1 tbsp	30

Hodgson Mill
Vidalia Sweet Onion Mix not prep	¼ cup	100

Zatarain's
Crispy Seasoned Fish-Fri	2 tbsp	50

BREAD MACHINE MIX
Carbsense
Harvest Wheat as prep	1 slice	60

Keto
Cinnamon Raisin as prep	1 slice	79
French Loaf as prep	1 slice	79
Sourdough Rye as prep	1 slice	79

Ketogenics
Low Carb Honey Wheat as prep	1 slice	80
Low Carb Original White as prep	1 slice	62
Low Carb Pumpernickel Rye as prep	1 slice	80

BREADCRUMBS
dry seasoned	¼ cup	115
fresh	¼ cup	30
plain	¼ cup	107

4C
Carb Careful Seasoned	⅓ cup	110

FOOD	PORTION	CALS
Salt Free Seasoned	⅓ cup	110
Edward & Sons		
Organic Lightly Salted	⅓ cup	110
Organic Panko	⅓ cup	110
Ian's		
Panko Italian	¼ cup	70
Panko Original	¼ cup	71
Panko Whole Wheat	¼ cup	70
Krasdale		
Seasoned	¼ cup	120
Progresso		
Garlic & Herb	¼ cup (1 oz)	110
Plain	¼ cup (1 oz)	110
Rienzi		
Italian Style	¼ cup	120
BREADFRUIT		
fresh	1 sm (13.5 oz)	396
fried	1 cup	379
raw	1 cup	227
BREADNUTTREE SEEDS		
dried	1 oz	104
BREADSTICKS		
plain	1 sm	21
plain	1 lg	41
Fattorie & Pandea		
Grissini Sesame	3	70
John Wm Macy's		
CheeseSticks Original Cheddar	3 (1 oz)	130
Pepperidge Farm		
Garlic frzn	1	160
Pillsbury		
Cornbread Twists	1 (1.4 oz)	140
Original Soft	2 (1.8 oz)	140
Stella D'Oro		
Mini Cracked Pepper	4 (0.5 oz)	70
Original	1 (0.3 oz)	40
Roasted Garlic	1	45
Sesame	1 (0.4 oz)	50
Sodium Free	1 (0.3 oz)	40

FOOD	PORTION	CALS

BREAKFAST BARS (see CEREAL BARS, ENERGY BARS)

BREAKFAST DRINKS
Carnation

Instant Breakfast Chocolate Malt as prep w/ fat free milk	1 serv	220
Instant Breakfast Classic French Vanilla as prep w/ fat free milk	1 serv	220
Instant Breakfast Milk Chocolate as prep w/ fat free milk	1 serv	220
Instant Breakfast Ready-To-Drink Carb Conscious French Vanilla	1 pkg	150
Instant Breakfast Ready-To-Drink Carb Conscious Milk Chocolate	1 pkg	150
Instant Breakfast Ready-To-Drink Creamy Milk Chocolate	1 pkg	250
Instant Breakfast Ready-To-Drink French Vanilla	1 pkg	240
Instant Breakfast Ready-To-Drink Strawberry Creme	1 pkg	250
Instant Breakfast Strawberry as prep w/ fat free milk	1 serv	220
Instant Breakfast Junior Vanilla	1 box (8.8 oz)	250
Instant Breakfast No Sugar Added Vanilla as prep w/ fat free milk	1 serv	150

BROCCOFLOWER

fresh raw	½ cup (1.8 oz)	16

BROCCOLI
FRESH

chinese broccoli (gai lan) cooked	½ cup	10
raab cooked	½ cup	28
raw	1 bunch (1.3 lbs)	207
raw flower	1 piece	3
raw flowers	1 cup	20

BroccoSprouts

Broccoli Sprouts	½ cup	16

Mann's

Broccoli Wokly	1 serv (3 oz)	25
Broccolini	8 stalks (3 oz)	35

FOOD	PORTION	CALS
Ocean Mist		
Rapini Broccoli Rabe Chopped Raw	1 cup	9
River Ranch		
Broccoli Slaw	1 cup	25
Florets	1¼ cups	25
FROZEN		
chopped cooked	½ cup	26
spears cooked	1 pkg (10 oz)	70
spears cooked	½ cup	26
Birds Eye		
Broccoli & Cheese Sauce	½ cup	90
Steamfresh Cuts	1 cup (3.1 oz)	30
Steamfresh Florets	1 cup (2.3 oz)	30
C&W		
Broccoli & Cheddar Cheese Sauce	1⅓ cups	70
Florets	1 cup	30
Cascadian Farm		
Organic Florets	⅔ cup	20
Dr. Praeger's		
Broccoli Bites	2 (2 oz)	110
Green Giant		
Broccoli & Cheese Sauce	⅔ cup	60
Butter Sauce Low Fat	3 spears (4 oz)	40
Cuts as prep	⅔ cup	25
Pasta Broccoli & Alfredo Sauce as prep	1 cup	210
TAKE-OUT		
batter dipped & fried	4 pieces	77
w/ cheese sauce	1 cup	242
BROWNIE		
brownie	1 (2 oz)	227
butterscotch	1 (1.2 oz)	151
Arrowhead Mills		
Gluten Free as prep	1	160
Aunt Paula's		
Low Carb Chef Fudge Brownie as prep	1 (2.5 inch)	89
Bob's Red Mill		
Gluten Free as prep	1	140
Foxy's Bake Shop		
Milk Chocolate	½ (1.7 oz)	200
White Chocolate	½ (1.7 oz)	200

FOOD	PORTION	CALS
French Meadow Bakery		
Gluten Free Fudge	1 (1.3 oz)	150
Glenny's		
100 Calorie 75% Organic	1 (1.45 oz)	100
Jiffy		
Fudge as prep	1	160
Joseph's		
Sugar Free	1 (1.5 oz)	150
Keto		
Chocolate Fudge as prep	1	59
Laura's Wholesome Junk Food		
Gluten Free Better Brownie	2	120
Nature's Path		
Organic Double Fudge	1/10 pkg	150
Organic HempPlus	1/10 pkg	140
No Pudge!		
All Flavors as prep	1	100
Pillsbury		
Traditional Chocolate Fudge	1 (1.4 oz)	150
Turtle Supreme Bars	1 (1.4 oz)	180
Sara Lee		
Brownie Bites Chocolate Dipped	1 (0.7 oz)	90
VitaBrownie		
Dark Chocolate Pomegranate	1 (2 oz)	100
Deep Velvety Chocolate	1 (2 oz)	100

BRUSSELS SPROUTS

FOOD	PORTION	CALS
FRESH		
cooked	6 pieces	45
Ocean Mist		
Brussels Sprouts	4 (2 oz)	40
Select Gourmet		
Fresh	½ cup	35
FROZEN		
cooked	1 cup	65
Birds Eye		
Steamfresh Baby	10 (2.9 oz)	45
Steamfresh Singles Baby	1 pkg (3.2 oz)	50
C&W		
Petite	10 (3 oz)	45

FOOD	PORTION	CALS
Green Giant		
Baby & Butter Sauce as prep	½ cup	60
BUCKWHEAT		
groats roasted cooked	½ cup	155
groats roasted uncooked	½ cup	292
Bob's Red Mill		
Organic Kernels	¼ cup	142
BUFFALO (see also JERKY)		
burger	3 oz	202
chuck braised	4 oz	205
top round steak broiled	3 oz	313
water buffalo roasted	3 oz	111
Natural Frontier Foods		
Burgers	1 (5 oz)	170
Ground	4 oz	170
Steaks	1 (4 oz)	160
BULGUR		
cooked	½ cup	76
uncooked	½ cup	239
Bob's Red Mill		
From Soft White Wheat	¼ cup	150
Fantastic		
Tabouli Mix not prep	2 tbsp	70
Near East		
Whole Grain Wheat Pilaf as prep	1 cup	200
Sabra		
Black Bean & Wheat Pilaf	2 oz	45
Cracked Wheat Salad	2 oz	80
Tabouli	2 oz	70
TAKE-OUT		
tabbouleh	1 cup	198
BURBOT (FISH)		
fresh baked	3 oz	98
BURDOCK ROOT		
cooked w/o salt	1 cup	110
cooked w/o salt	1 root (5.8 oz)	146
Frieda's		
Gobo Root	¾ cup	60

FOOD	PORTION	CALS
BUTTER		
clarified butter	¼ cup (1.8 oz)	449
clarified butter	1 tbsp (0.4 oz)	112
ghee cow's milk	1 tbsp	126
ghee vegetable oil	1 tbsp	126
honey butter	¼ cup (2.5 oz)	338
honey butter	1 tbsp (0.6 oz)	85
light butter whipped salted	1 tbsp (0.3 oz)	48
stick salted	1 tbsp (0.5 oz)	102
stick salted	1 stick (4 oz)	810
stick salted	¼ cup (2 oz)	407
stick unsalted	1 tbsp (0.5 oz)	102
stick unsalted	1 (4 oz)	810
stick unsalted	¼ cup (2 oz)	407
whipped salted	¼ cup (1.3 oz)	271
whipped salted	1 tbsp (0.3 oz)	67
Cabot		
Salted	1 tbsp	100
Crystal Farms		
Butter	1 tbsp	100
Whipped	1 tbsp	70
Deerfield		
Creamy	1 tbsp	100
Earth Balance		
Butter Blend Unsalted	1 tbsp	100
Horizon Organic		
European	1 tbsp	100
Land O Lakes		
Light Salted	1 tbsp (0.5 oz)	50
Light Whipped Salted	1 tbsp (0.4 oz)	45
Salted	1 tbsp (0.5 oz)	100
Spreadable w/ Canola Oil	1 tbsp (0.5 oz)	100
Whipped Salted	1 tbsp (0.2 oz)	50
Organic Valley		
European Style	1 tbsp	110
Straus		
Organic European Style Lightly Salted	1 tbsp (0.5 oz)	110
Organic European Style Sweet Butter	1 tbsp (0.5 oz)	110
BUTTER SUBSTITUTES		
stick	1 stick	811

FOOD	PORTION	CALS
Butter Buds		
Granules	1 pkg (2 g)	5
Sunsweet		
Lighter Bake	1 tbsp	35
BUTTERBUR		
canned fuki chopped	1 cup	3
fresh fuki	1 cup	13
BUTTERNUTS		
dried	1 oz	174
BUTTERSCOTCH (see also CANDY)		
E. Guittard		
Baking Chips	33 (0.5 oz)	80
CABBAGE (see also COLESLAW)		
chinese bok choy shredded cooked w/o salt	1 cup	20
chinese pe-tsai shredded cooked w/o salt	1 cup	17
green raw shredded	1 cup	19
green shredded cooked w/o salt	1 cup	34
japanese pickled	½ cup	22
red raw shredded	1 cup	22
red shredded cooked w/o salt	1 cup	44
savoy shredded cooked w/o salt	1 cup	35
Aunt Nellie's		
Sweet & Sour Red	¼ cup	40
Frieda's		
Baby Bok Choy	⅔ cup	10
Bok Choy	1 cup	10
Gai Choy	1 cup (3 oz)	20
Napa	1 cup (3 oz)	15
Salad Savoy	⅔ cup (3 oz)	25
Tuscan	⅔ cup (3 oz)	20
Glory		
Country Cabbage	½ cup	25
Greenwood		
Red	½ cup	100
River Ranch		
Angel Hair	1½ cups	20
TAKE-OUT		
creamed	1 cup	158

FOOD	PORTION	CALS
kimchee	1 cup	32
stuffed cabbage w/ rice & beef	1 (3.6 oz)	117
sweet & sour red cabbage	4 oz	61

CACAO
Kopali
Organic Dark Chocolate Covered Cacao Nibs	½ pkg (1 oz)	140

Navitas Naturals
Butter	1 tbsp	120
Nibs	1 oz	130
Powder	1 oz	120

CACTUS
fresh cooked w/ fat	1 pad (1 oz)	11
fresh cooked w/o fat	1 cup (5.2 oz)	22
pricklypear	1 (3.6 oz)	42
pricklypear fresh	1 cup (5.2 oz)	61

Frieda's
Cactus Pads	¾ cup (3 oz)	20

CAKE (see also CAKE MIX)
battenburg cake	1 slice (2 oz)	204
cream puff shell	1 (2.3 oz)	239
crumpet	1 (2.3 oz)	131
dutch honey cake	1 slice (0.8 oz)	70
eccles cake	1 slice (2 oz)	285
madeira cake	1 slice (1 oz)	98
sponge	1 piece (1.3 oz)	110
sponge cake dessert shell	1 (0.8 oz)	70
treacle tart	1 slice (2.5 oz)	258

Arnold
Date Nut Loaf	1 slice (2 oz)	190

Aunt Trudy's
Organic Baklava Soy Nut	1 (1.8 oz)	190

Balocco
Il Panettone	1 serv (3.5 oz)	380

Bellino
Pandoro	1 (2.8 oz)	330

Boboli
Mini Eclairs Custard Filled	4 (2.3 oz)	224

Chudleigh's
Apple Blossoms	1 (4 oz)	350

FOOD	PORTION	CALS
Drake's		
Coffee Cake Low Fat	2 (2.3 oz)	210
El Monterey		
Cheesecake Bites Caramel	1 (2 oz)	180
Cheesecake Bites Raspberry	1 (2 oz)	200
Entenmann's		
All Butter French Crumb	⅛ cake (1.8 oz)	210
Cheese Cake Deluxe French	⅙ cake (3.8 oz)	390
Coffee Cake Crumb	1 serv (2 oz)	260
Danish Twist Raspberry	⅛ cake	220
Fudge Iced Golden Cake	⅛ cake	290
Loaf All Butter	⅙ cake (2.4 oz)	220
Louisiana Crunch	⅑ cake (2.9 oz)	330
Marble Loaf	⅛ cake	190
Marshmallow Iced Devil's Food	⅛ cake	280
Mini's Carrot Cake	1 (1.4 oz)	160
Strawberry Cheese Buns	1 (3 oz)	320
Fillo Factory		
Organic Apple Strudel	1 (4.4 oz)	290
Organic Apple Turnovers	1 (3 oz)	180
Glenny's		
Blondie 100 Calorie 75% Organic	1 (1.45 oz)	100
Goody Man		
Happy Birthday Cupcake White	1 (1.75 oz)	190
Gourmet Pastries		
Baklava Walnut	1 piece (1.8 oz)	240
Guiltless Gourmet		
Dessert Bowl Bananas Foster Cake	1 pkg (2 oz)	200
Dessert Bowl Black Velvet Cake	1 pkg (2 oz)	200
Hostess		
100 Calorie Pack Mini Carrot Cake	1 pkg (1.2 oz)	100
100 Calorie Pack Mini Chocolate Cupcakes	1 pkg (1.3 oz)	100
100 Calorie Pack Mini Coffee Cake Cinnamon Streusel	1 pkg (1.2 oz)	100
100 Calorie Pack Mini Golden Cupcakes	1 pkg (1.2 oz)	100
Cup Cakes Chocolate	1 (1.8 oz)	170
Ho Ho's	1	120
Twinkies	1 (1.5 oz)	150
Kellogg's		
Pop-Tarts Apple Cinnamon	1 (1.8 oz)	210

FOOD	PORTION	CALS
Pop-Tarts French Toast	1	220
Pop-Tarts Frosted Cookies & Cream	1	200
Pop-Tarts Low Fat Frosted Brown Sugar Cinnamon	1 (1.8 oz)	190
Pop-Tarts Yogurt Blast Strawberry	1 (1.8 oz)	210
Lance		
Honey Bun	1 (3 oz)	320
Mrs. Freshley's		
Golden Cupcakes Creme Filled	1 pkg (1.3 oz)	100
Mrs. Smith's		
Carrot	⅙ cake (2.9 oz)	300
Cobbler Blackberry	1 serv (4 oz)	260
Singles Heavenly 100 New York Cheesecake	1 (0.9 oz)	100
Nature's Path		
Organic Toaster Pastry Apple Cinnamon	1 (2 oz)	210
Organic Toaster Pastry Blueberry	1 (2 oz)	210
Organic Toaster Pastry Frosted Apple Cinnamon	1 (2 oz)	210
Organic Toaster Pastry Frosted Blueberry	1 (2 oz)	200
Organic Toaster Pastry Frosted Strawberry	1 (2 oz)	210
Neuman's		
Date Nut Bread	1 oz	90
Pepperidge Farm		
Chocolate Coconut 3 Layer	⅛ cake	240
Devil's Food 3 Layer	⅛ cake	220
Golden 3 Layer	⅛ cake	230
Lemon 3 Layer	⅛ cake	240
Turnover Apple	1	290
Turnover Peach	1	290
Philadelphia		
Snack Bars Classic Cheesecake	1 (1.5 oz)	190
Snack Bars Strawberry Cheesecake	1 (1.5 oz)	190
Pillsbury		
Caramel Rolls	1 (1.7 oz)	170
Cinnamon Rolls w/ Icing	1 (3.5 oz)	310
Cinnamon Rolls w/ Icing Reduced Fat	1 (1.5 oz)	140
Toaster Strudel	1 (2 oz)	200
Toaster Strudel Blueberry	1 (2 oz)	190
Toaster Strudel Cream Cheese	1 (2 oz)	200
Toaster Strudel Raspberry	1 (2 oz)	190

FOOD	PORTION	CALS
Toaster Strudel Wildberry	1 (2 oz)	190
Turnovers Cherry	1 (2 oz)	180
Sara Lee		
Cheesecake Classic French	1 piece (4.7 oz)	410
Cheesecake French Chocolate	1 piece (4.2 oz)	430
Cheesecake French Strawberry	1 piece (4.3 oz)	320
Cheesecake Strawberry Swirl	1 piece (2.9 oz)	290
Cobbler Anytime Apple	1 (4 oz)	350
Coffee Cake Butter Streusel	1 piece (2 oz)	190
Coffee Cake Crumb	1 serv (2 oz)	190
Layer Cake Coconut	1 slice (2.8 oz)	260
Layer Cake Double Chocolate	1 slice (2.8 oz)	260
Layer Cake Fudge Golden	1 slice (2.8 oz)	260
Layer Cake Vanilla	1 slice (2.8 oz)	260
Pound Cake All Butter	1 slice (0.6 oz)	240
Pound Cake Free & Light	1 slice (2.5 oz)	200
Weight Watchers		
Lemon w/ Lemon Icing	1 (1 oz)	80
TAKE-OUT		
angelfood	1 slice (2 oz)	143
apple crisp	1 serv (8.6 oz)	384
apple turnover	1 (6.6 oz)	661
baklava	1 piece (2.7 oz)	334
basbousa namoura	1 piece (1 oz)	60
bean cake	1 (1.1 oz)	130
black forest chocolate cherry	1 piece (2.5 oz)	187
boston cream pie	1 slice (3.2 oz)	232
cannoli w/ cannoli cream	1	369
carrot w/ icing	1 slice (4.7 oz)	543
cheesecake	1 slice (4.5 oz)	410
cheesecake chocolate	1 slice (4.5 oz)	489
chinese moon cake	1 (4.8 oz)	458
coconut mochiko filipino cake	1 piece (2.7 oz)	252
coffeecake iced	1 piece (1.6 oz)	175
cream puff custard filled chocolate frosted	1 (3.9 oz)	293
eclair	1 (3.5 oz)	262
french apple tart	1 (3.5 oz)	302
fruitcake	1 slice (1.5 oz)	139
funnel cake	1 (3.2 oz)	276
gingerbread	1 piece (2.4 oz)	213

FOOD	PORTION	CALS
jelly roll	1 slice (1.8 oz)	146
jelly roll lemon filled	1 slice (3 oz)	210
napoleon	1 mini (1 oz)	123
napoleon	1 (3 oz)	348
panettone	½₂ cake (2.9 oz)	300
petit fours	2 (0.9 oz)	120
pineapple upside down	1 piece (4.2 oz)	387
pound	1 slice (1 oz)	120
pound fat free	1 slice (2 oz)	160
sacher torte	1 slice (2.2 oz)	240
sacher torte chocolate + apricot jam	1 serv	430
strawberry shortcake	1 serv (4.1 oz)	211
strudel apple	1 piece (2.2 oz)	175
strudel cheese	1 piece (2.2 oz)	195
strudel cherry	1 piece (2.2 oz)	179
sweet potato w/ glaze	1 piece (2.7 oz)	275
tiramisu	1 piece (5.1 oz)	409
tiramisu	1 cake (4.4 lbs)	5732
torte chocolate ganache	1 slice (3.5 oz)	400
trifle w/ cream	6 oz	291
white w/ coconut icing	1 slice (3.9 oz)	399
zucchini bread	1 slice (1.4 oz)	150

CAKE ICING

chocolate	¼ cup	269
vanilla	¼ cup	322
Jiffy		
Fudge Frosting	¼ cup	150
White Frosting	¼ cup	150
Manischewitz		
Dairy Free Chocolate	2 tbsp (1.2 oz)	138
Naturally Nora		
Frosting Mix Chocolate as prep	½₂ pkg	150
Frosting Mix Vanilla as prep	½₂ pkg	170

CAKE MIX

Bisquick		
Heart Smart	⅓ cup	140
Carbolite		
Cheesecake Chocolate as prep	⅛ cake	260

FOOD	PORTION	CALS
Don's Chuck Wagon		
All Purpose Batter Mix	¼ cup	100
Jiffy		
Devil's Food as prep	⅕ cake	220
Golden Yellow as prep	⅕ cake	220
White Cake as prep	⅕ cake	210
King Arthur		
Cinnamon Buns Kit not prep	½ cup	240
Naturally Nora		
Cheerful Chocolate as prep	1/12 pkg	300
Sunny Yellow as prep	1/12 pkg	280
Surprising Stars as prep	1/12 pkg	300
CALABAZA		
fresh	½ cup	32
CALZONE (see SANDWICHES)		
CANADIAN BACON		
grilled	2 slices (1.6 oz)	87
Applegate Farms		
Natural	2 slices (2 oz)	90
Boar's Head		
Canadian Bacon	2 oz	70
Celebrity		
98% Fat Free	3 slices (1.8 oz)	60
Jones		
Slices	3	70
Organic Prairie		
Hardwood Smoked	1 oz	40
Wellshire		
Sliced	2 oz	20
CANADIAN BACON SUBSTITUTES		
Yves		
Meatless Canadian Bacon	2 slices (2 oz)	80
CANDY		
butterscotch	1 piece (6 g)	24
candied cherries	1 (4 g)	12
candied citron	1 oz	89
candied lemon peel	1 oz	90
candied orange peel	1 oz	90

FOOD	PORTION	CALS
candied pineapple slice	1 slice (2 oz)	179
candy corn	1 oz	105
caramels	1 piece (8 g)	31
caramels chocolate	1 piece (6 g)	22
carob bar	1 (3.1 oz)	453
dark chocolate	1 oz	150
fondant	1 piece (0.6 oz)	57
fondant chocolate coated	1 piece (0.4 oz)	40
fondant mint	1 oz	105
fruit pastilles	1 tube (1.4 oz)	101
fudge brown sugar w/ nuts	1 piece (0.5 oz)	56
fudge chocolate marshmallow	1 piece (0.7 oz)	84
fudge chocolate marshmallow w/ nuts	1 piece (0.8 oz)	96
fudge chocolate w/ nuts	1 piece (0.7 oz)	81
fudge peanut butter	1 piece (0.6 oz)	59
fudge vanilla w/ nuts	1 piece (0.5 oz)	62
gumdrops	10 sm (0.4 oz)	135
gumdrops	10 lg (3.8 oz)	420
hard candy	1 oz	106
jelly beans	10 sm (0.4 oz)	40
jelly beans	10 lg (1 oz)	104
lollipop	1 (6 g)	22
marzipan	1 oz	128
milk chocolate	1 bar (1.55 oz)	226
milk chocolate crisp	1 bar (1.45 oz)	203
milk chocolate w/ almonds	1 bar (1.45 oz)	215
nougat nut cream	0.5 oz	49
organic dark chocolate w/ raisins & pecans	1.4 oz	220
peanut bar	1 (1.4 oz)	209
peanut brittle	1 oz	128
peanuts chocolate covered	10 (1.4 oz)	208
peanuts chocolate covered	1 cup (5.2 oz)	773
praline	1 piece (1.4 oz)	177
pretzels chocolate covered	1 (0.4 oz)	50
pretzels chocolate covered	1 oz	130
sesame crunch	20 pieces (1.2 oz)	181
sweet chocolate	1 bar (1.45 oz)	201
sweet chocolate	1 oz	143
taffy	1 piece (0.5 oz)	56
toffee	1 piece (0.4 oz)	65

FOOD	PORTION	CALS
truffles	1 piece (0.4 oz)	59
3 Musketeers		
Bar	1 (2.1 oz)	260
Fun Size	3 (1.6 oz)	190
Miniatures	7 (1.4 oz)	170
Anastasia		
Coco Rhum Bites	2 (1 oz)	110
Andes		
Dark Chocolate Covered Cherries	2 (1 oz)	110
Thins Cherry Jubilee	8 (1.3 oz)	200
Thins Creme De Menthe	8 (1.3 oz)	200
Annabelle's		
Skinny Hunk Chewy Nougat	1 bar (1 oz)	100
Baby Ruth		
Fun Size	2 (1.3 oz)	170
Snack Bars	2 (1.3 oz)	170
Bartons		
Cashew Toppers	1 (1 oz)	140
Baskin-Robbins		
Soft Candy Mint Chocolate Chip	2 (0.3 oz)	40
Sugar Free Hard Candy Cookies 'N Cream	4 (0.6 oz)	40
Benecol		
Smart Chews Caramel	1 piece	20
Betty Crocker		
Fruit Gushers Rockin' Blue Raspberry	1 pkg (0.9 oz)	90
Blow Pop		
Regular	1 (0.6 oz)	60
Brach's		
Bridge Mix	16 pieces	190
Candy Corn	26 pieces	140
Caramel Clusters	3 pieces	210
Circus Peanuts	6 pieces	160
Fruit Rippers Berry Punch	1 pkg (0.5 oz)	60
Fruit Slices	3 pieces	150
Malts	15 pieces	190
Mellowcreme Pumpkins	6 pieces	130
Milk Maid Caramels	4 pieces	160
Mint Patties	3 pieces	140
Orange Slices	2 pieces	130
Peanut Butter Meltaways	3 pieces	200

FOOD	PORTION	CALS
Root Beer Barrels	3 pieces	70
Spearmint Leaves	5 pieces	130
Spice Drops	12 pieces	130
Sprinkles	17 pieces	200
Star Brites Butterscotch	3 pieces	60
Stars	10 pieces	200
Wild'N Fruity Gummi Bears	14 pieces	140
Breath Savers		
Sugar Free Peppermint	1 piece	5
Butterfinger		
Bar	1 (2.1 oz)	270
Crisps	1 bar (1.8 oz)	250
Crisps Minis	4 (1.5 oz)	220
Minis	4 (1.4 oz)	180
Cadbury		
Milk Chocolate Fruit & Nut	10 sq (1.4 oz)	200
Milk Chocolate Roast Almond	7 sq (1.4 oz)	210
Royal Dark	10 sq (1.4 oz)	220
Cella's		
Milk Chocolate Covered Cherries	2 (1 oz)	120
Chargers		
Chocolate Covered Espresso Beans	1 pkg (0.5 oz)	60
Charleston Chews		
Chocolate	1 bar (1.9 oz)	230
Vanilla	1 bar (1.9 oz)	230
Charms		
Fluffy Stuff Cotton Candy	1 pkg (0.6 oz)	70
Sour Balls	1 (5 g)	20
Squares	2 pieces	20
Chew-ets		
Peanut Chews Original Dark	3 pieces	170
ChocoSoy		
Soy Milk Chocolate	1 piece (0.4 oz)	50
Choward's		
Mints All Flavors	3 (5 g)	20
Chuao Chocolatier		
Choco Pod Banana	1 (0.4 oz)	50
Choco Pod Passion	1 (0.4 oz)	50
CocoaVia		
Dark Chocolate Blueberry & Almond Bar	1 (0.8 oz)	100

FOOD	PORTION	CALS
Dark Chocolate Covered Almonds	1 pkg (1 oz)	140
Dark Chocolate Crispy Bar	1 (0.7 oz)	90
Dark Chocolate Original Bar	1 (0.8 oz)	80
Milk Chocolate Almond Bar	1 (0.8 oz)	110
Milk Chocolate Bar	1 (0.8 oz)	110
Milk Chocolate Covered Raisins	1 pkg (1 oz)	150
Coffee Rio		
Coffee Candy All Flavors	4 pieces	60
Crispy Cat		
Roasted Peanut	1 bar (1 oz)	220
Dare		
RealFruit Gummies All Flavors	8 pieces (1.4 oz)	120
Dots		
All Flavors	12 (1.5 oz)	140
Dove		
Dark Chocolate Covered Almonds	13 pieces	210
Dark Chocolate Cranberry Almond	⅓ pkg (1.2 oz)	170
Dark Chocolate Miniatures	5 pieces	210
Milk Chocolate	⅓ bar	180
Milk Chocolate w/ Almonds	⅓ bar	190
Milk Chocolate Covered Almonds	13 pieces	220
Milk Chocolate Miniatures	5	220
Milk Chocolate Miniatures w/ Caramel	5 pieces	200
E. Guittard		
Bar Quevedo Bittersweet 65% Cacao	1 (2 oz)	290
Bar Sur Del Lago Bittersweet 65% Cacao	1 (2 oz)	290
Eclipse		
Mints Sugarless All Flavors	3 pieces	5
Emily's		
Espresso Beans Dark Chocolate Covered	26 (1.4 oz)	220
Endangered Species		
Dark Chocolate w/ Espresso Beans	½ bar (1.5 oz)	200
Dark Chocolate w/ Hazelnut Toffee	½ bar (1.5 oz)	220
Milk Chocolate w/ Cherries	½ bar (1.5 oz)	230
Organic Dark Chocolate	½ bar (0.7 oz)	100
Organic Dark Chocolate w/ Tangerine	½ bar (0.7 oz)	100
Organic Milk Chocolate w/ Key Lime	½ bar (0.7 oz)	110
Enjoy Life		
Boom Choco Boom Dark Chocolate Dairy Nut Soy Free	1 bar (1.4 oz)	200

FOOD	PORTION	CALS
Equal Exchange		
Organic Chocolate Espresso Bean	1 bar (1.4 oz)	216
Organic Milk Chocolate	1 bar (1.4 oz)	230
Organic Very Dark Chocolate	1 bar (1.4 oz)	220
Estee		
Fructose Sweetened Dark Chocolate	½ bar (1.4 oz)	200
Fructose Sweetened Milk Chocolate	½ bar (1.4 oz)	230
Fructose Sweetened Milk Chocolate w/ Almonds	½ bar (1.4 oz)	230
Fructose Sweetened Milk Chocolate w/ Crisp Rice	½ bar (1.2 oz)	370
Fructose Sweetened Peanut Butter Cups	5	200
Peanut Brittle	⅓ box (1.3 oz)	210
Sugar Free Assorted Fruit	3	15
Sugar Free Butterscotch	4	15
Sugar Free Gourmet Jelly Beans	26	70
Sugar Free Gum Drops Assorted Fruit	11	110
Sugar Free Gummy Bears Assorted Fruit	17	70
Sugar Free Peppermint	3	15
Sugar Free Sour Citrus Slices	9	60
Sugar Free Toffee	4	15
Sugar Free Tropical Fruit	3	15
Ethel's		
Truffles Assorted	4	200
Fauchon		
Assortment Truffles	3 (1.3 oz)	160
Chocolate Assortment	3 pieces (1.1 oz)	170
Ferrero Rocher		
Candy	3 pieces (1.3 oz)	220
Figamajigs		
Fig Candy Drops Dark Chocolate Covered	1 pkg (1.4 oz)	150
Fig Candy Drops Orange & Yellow Chocolate Covered	1 pkg (1.4 oz)	150
Frooties		
Chewy Candy Fruit Flavored	12 pieces (1.3 oz)	104
Fruitzels		
Assorted	7 pieces	120
Ghirardelli		
Squares Milk Chocolate w/ Caramel Filling	3 (1.6 oz)	220
Squares Mint Indulgence	3 (1.6 oz)	210

FOOD	PORTION	CALS
Squares 60% Cacao Dark Chocolate	4 (1.5 oz)	220
Squares 60% Cacao Dark Chocolate w/ Caramel	3 (1.6 oz)	220
Godiva		
Sugar Free Chocolate	1 bar (1.5 oz)	190
Sugar Free Chocolate w/ Almonds	1 bar (1.5 oz)	200
Sugar Free Dark Chocolate	1 bar (1.5 oz)	190
Truffles Assorted	2 (1.4 oz)	210
Goetze's		
Caramel Creams	3 pieces	130
Green & Black's		
Organic Chocolate Fairtrade Maya Gold	1 bar (3.5 oz)	526
Organic Dark Chocolate	1 bar (3.5 oz)	551
Organic Dark Chocolate Mint	1 bar (3.5 oz)	478
Organic Dark Chocolate w/ Hazelnuts & Currants	1 bar (3.5 oz)	513
Organic Milk Chocolate	1 bar (3.5 oz)	523
Organic Milk Chocolate Caramel	1 bar (3.5 oz)	495
Organic Milk Chocolate Raisins & Hazelnuts	1 bar (3.5 oz)	556
Organic Milk Chocolate Whole Almonds	1 bar (3.5 oz)	578
Organic White Chocolate	1 bar (3.5 oz)	573
Guylian		
Twists Milk Chocolate Truffle	5 pieces (1.2 oz)	230
Twists Original Praline	4 pieces (1.2 oz)	200
Hammond's		
Root Beer Drops	3 (0.6 oz)	60
Hershey's		
Bliss Dark Chocolate	3 (0.8 oz)	100
Bliss Milk Chocolate	6 (1.5 oz)	210
Cacao Reserve 65% Cacao Dark	3 sq (1.3 oz)	180
Cacoa Reserve 35% Cacao Milk Chocolate w/ Hazelnuts	3 sq (1.3 oz)	220
Chocolate Miniatures Sugar Free	5 pieces (1.4 oz)	170
Chocolate w/ Almonds Miniatures Sugar Free	5 pieces (1.4 oz)	180
Dark Chocolate Miniatures Sugar Free	5 pieces (1.4 oz)	190
Kisses	1	25
Milk Chocolate	1 bar (1.4 oz)	210
Milk Chocolate w/ Almonds	1 bar (1.4 oz)	230
Miniature Assorted	5 (1.5 oz)	210
Nuggets Cookies 'N' Creme	4	190

FOOD	PORTION	CALS
Nuggets Dark Chocolate w/ Almonds	4	220
Nuggets Milk Chocolate	4	230
Pot Of Gold	3 pieces	130
Sticks Special Dark	1 (0.4 oz)	60
Jay's		
Cotton Candy	1 pkg (2 oz)	220
Jelly Belly		
Jelly Beans Sugar Free	35	80
Jolly Rancher		
All Flavors	4 pieces	60
Lollipops All Flavors	1 (0.6 oz)	60
Sugar Free	4 pieces (0.6 oz)	35
Joyva		
Halvah Chocolate Covered	1 serv (2 oz)	380
Halvah Marble	1 serv (2 oz)	390
Junior		
Caramels	1 box (1.4 oz)	170
Mints	1 box (1.4 oz)	170
Kellogg's		
Fruit Flavored Snacks Hello Kitty	10 pieces	100
Fruit Flavored Snacks Winnie The Pooh	1 pkg	80
Fruit Streamers Watermelon Madness	1 pkg (0.8 oz)	80
Fruit Twistables Triple Cherry Explosion	1 pkg (0.8 oz)	70
Gamester Rolls All Varieties	1 pkg (0.7 oz)	80
Yogos Crazy Berries	1 pkg (0.8 oz)	90
KitKat		
Bar	1 (0.5 oz)	73
Kopali		
Organic Dark Chocolate Covered Espresso Beans	½ pkg (1 oz)	120
Lance		
Chewz Strawberry	1 pkg (1.1 oz)	120
Peanut Bar	1 (2.3 oz)	340
Legacy Chocolates		
Truffles Assorted	1 piece (0.5 oz)	90
Let's Do Organic		
Black Licorice Bars	1 (0.9 oz)	80
Black Licorice Chews	8 (1.4 oz)	130
Gummi Bears	1 pkg (0.9 oz)	80

FOOD	PORTION	CALS
Lifesavers		
Variety	4 pieces	60
Lindt		
Lindor Truffles 60% Extra Dark	3 pieces	210
Petits Desserts Assorted	4 (1.3 oz)	210
Love Candy		
Dark Chocolate	1 bar (1.5 oz)	190
Milk Chocolate	1 bar (1.5 oz)	200
Yogurt Supreme	1 bar (1.5 oz)	190
M&M's		
Almond	1 pkg (1.3 oz)	200
Dark Chocolate	1 pkg (1.7 oz)	240
Milk Chocolate	1 pkg (1.7 oz)	240
Minis	1 pkg (1.1 oz)	150
Peanut	1 pkg (1.7 oz)	250
Peanut Butter	1 pkg (1.6 oz)	240
Mamba		
Fruit Flavor	6 (0.9 oz)	170
Sour	6 (0.9 oz)	100
Mentos		
Sugar Free Mixed Berries	1 piece	5
Mike & Ike		
All Flavors	1 pkg (2 oz)	200
Milkfuls		
Candy	6 (1.4 oz)	170
Milky Way		
Bar	1 (2 oz)	260
Fun Size	2 bars (1.2 oz)	150
Midnight	1 bar (1.8 oz)	220
Midnight Minis	5 (1.4 oz)	180
Milk Chocolate Covered Caramels	5 (1.5 oz)	200
Minis	5 (1.5 oz)	190
Mr. Goodbar		
Bar	1 (1.75 oz)	270
Mrs. Fields		
Decadent Chocolates	3 pieces (1.8 oz)	240
Munch		
Nut Bar	1 (1.42 oz)	220
Necco		
Banana Splits	4 (1.4 oz)	150

FOOD	PORTION	CALS
Clark Junior Bar	1 (0.5 oz)	60
Conversation Hearts Tiny	40 (1.4 oz)	160
Double Dipped Peanuts	15 (1.4 oz)	200
Junior Assorted Wafers	1 roll (0.5 oz)	50
Mary Janes	5 (1.4 oz)	160
Mint	1 piece	12
Mint Juleps	4 (1.4 oz)	150
Nonpareils	10 (1.4 oz)	190
Squirrel Nut Caramel	5 (1.6 oz)	170
Nestle		
Crunch Stix	1 (0.6 oz)	90
Newman's Own		
Organic Chocolate Cups Dark Chocolate Peanut Butter	1 pkg (1.2 oz)	180
Organic Chocolate Cups Milk Chocolate Peanut Butter	1 pkg (1.2 oz)	180
Organic Chocolate Cups Peppermint	1 pkg (1.2 oz)	170
Organic Chocolate Sweet Dark	½ bar (¼ oz)	200
Organic Chocolate Sweet Dark Espresso	½ bar (1.4 oz)	200
Organic Chocolate Sweet Dark Orange	½ bar (1.4 oz)	200
Organic Milk Chocolate	½ bar (1.4 oz)	210
Nibs		
Licorice	9 pieces	35
Nutty Ducky's		
Cashew Brittle	4 pieces (1.6 oz)	240
Cashew Brittle Dark Chocolate	2 pieces (1.5 oz)	220
Peanut Brittle	4 pieces (1.6 oz)	230
Peanut Brittle Milk Chocolate	2 pieces (1.5 oz)	220
Odense		
Marzipan	2 tbsp (1.4 oz)	170
Pure De-Lite		
Caramel Crisp	1 bar	120
Pure Fun		
Organic Vegan Barrels Of Fun Root Beer Float	2 (0.5 oz)	60
Organic Vegan Candy Canes	1 (0.5 oz)	62
Organic Vegan Chocolate Meltdowns All Flavors	3 (0.6 oz)	70
Organic Vegan Citrus Slices All Flavors	3 (0.6 oz)	60
Organic Vegan Cotton Candy All Flavors	¼ pkg (0.5 oz)	60
Organic Vegan Jaw Boulders All Flavors	2 (0.5 oz)	58

FOOD	PORTION	CALS
Organic Vegan Pure Pops All Flavors	3 (0.6 oz)	60
Raisinets		
Candy	3 pkg (1.7 oz)	200
Reese's		
Bites	16 pieces	220
Clusters	3 (1.5 oz)	220
FastBreak	1 bar (0.7 oz)	90
Peanut Butter Cups Miniatures	5 (1.4 oz)	210
Peanut Butter Cups Miniatures Sugar Free	5 pieces (1.4 oz)	170
Peanut Butter Cups Snack Size	1 piece (0.5 oz)	80
Peanut Butter Cups Sugar Free	1 piece (1.5 oz)	180
White Peanut Butter Cups Miniatures	4 pieces (1.4 oz)	210
White Peanut Butter Cups Miniatures Sugar Free	5 pieces (1.4 oz)	180
Riesen		
Candy	4 (1.3 oz)	170
Robin Eggs		
Large	2 pieces	70
Russell Stover		
Assorted	3 pieces (1.4 oz)	170
Low Carb Pecan Delights	1 piece (1 oz)	130
Private Reserve Triple Chocolate Mousse	3 pieces (1.3 oz)	220
Private Reserve Vanilla Bean Brulee	3 pieces (1.3 oz)	180
Scharffen Berger		
Semisweet 60% Cacao	1 bar (2 oz)	320
Sencha Naturals		
Green Tea Mints All Flavors	3	5
Shaman Chocolates		
Organic Extra Dark Chocolate 82% Cacao	½ bar (1 oz)	158
Organic Milk Chocolate w/ Macadamia Nuts & Hawaiian Pink Sea Salt	½ bar (1 oz)	91
Skittles		
Original Fruit	1 pkg (2.2 oz)	250
Slim-Fast		
Protein Snack Chews Peanut Butter	1 pkg (0.9 oz)	100
Smile Chocolatiers		
Choclatea Ginger Tea Milk Chocolate 37% Cacao	½ bar (1.5 oz)	230
Choclatea Herbal Chai Tea Dark Chocolate 64% Cacao	½ bar (1.5 oz)	220

FOOD	PORTION	CALS
Choclatea Pistachio Green Tea White Chocolate	½ bar (1.5 oz)	240
Choclatea Pomegranate White Tea Very Dark Chocolate 72% Cacao	½ bar (1.5 oz)	220
Choclatea White Tea Very Dark Chocolate 72% Cacao	½ bar (1.5 oz)	220
Smucker's		
Jelly Beans	25	150
Snickers		
Almond	1 (1.8 oz)	230
Bar	1 (2.07 oz)	280
Cruncher	1 bar (1.6 oz)	220
Cruncher Fun Size	3 (1.4 oz)	230
Miniatures	4 (1.3 oz)	170
Sour Patch		
Connectors	1.5 oz	150
Kids Soft & Chewy	1 pkg (1 oz)	100
Starburst		
Baja California	1 pkg	240
Jellybeans	¼ cup	160
Original Fruit	1 pkg	240
Sour Fruit	1 pkg	240
Sugar Babies		
Candy	30 pieces (1.5 oz)	180
Chocolate	19 pieces (1.4 oz)	180
Sugar Daddy		
Pop	1 lg (1.7 oz)	200
Swedish Fish		
Aqua Life	1.5 oz	140
Original	20 pieces (1.5 oz)	140
Take 5		
Snack Size	2 pieces	220
The Chocolate Traveler		
Wedges Bittersweet	4 pieces	130
Wedges Dark Chocolate Coffee	4 pieces	130
Wedges Dark Chocolate Mint	4 pieces	130
Wedges Dark Chocolate Orange	4 pieces	120
Wedges Dark Chocolate Raspberry	4 pieces	120
Wedges Dark Chocolate Tiramisu	4 pieces	120
Wedges Milk Chocolate	4 pieces	130

FOOD	PORTION	CALS
Wedges Milk Chocolate Dulce De Leche	4 pieces	120
Wedges White Chocolate	4 pieces	140
Wedges White Chocolate Creme Brulee	4 pieces	140
Thorntons		
Chocolates Summer Collection	1	65
Toblerone		
Bittersweet Chocolate w/ Honey & Almond Nugget	⅓ bar (1.2 oz)	170
Toffifay		
Candy	5 (1.4 oz)	200
Tootsie Roll		
Midgees	6	140
Mini Chews	30 pieces (1.4 oz)	170
Pops	1 (0.6 oz)	60
Pops Caramel Apple	1 (0.6 oz)	60
Twix		
Fun Size	1 (0.6 oz)	80
Peanut Butter	1 bar	280
Twizzlers		
Chocolate	1 piece	25
Licorice	1 piece	30
Strawberry Snack Size	3 pkgs	130
Sugar Free	4 pieces (1.5 oz)	130
Vere		
75% Chocolate Gluten Free	1 sm bar	80
Brownie Box Coconut Gluten Free Vegan	3 pieces (1.4 oz)	210
Brownie Box Peanut Butter Gluten Free	3 pieces (1.3 oz)	180
Brownie Box Walnut Gluten Free	3 pieces (1.3 oz)	190
Clusters Chocolate Almond Gluten Free Vegan	2 pieces (1.3 oz)	210
Clusters Chocolate Coconut Gluten Free Vegan	3 pieces (1.7 oz)	280
Clusters Chocolate Rice Gluten Free Vegan	3 pieces (1.3 oz)	170
Clusters Chocolate Seed Gluten Free Vegan	2 pieces (1.3 oz)	210
Wafers Cacao Nibs Gluten Free Vegan	2 (1.1 oz)	170
Wafers Espresso Gluten Free Vegan	3 (1.6 oz)	250
Wafers Pink Peppercorn Gluten Free Vegan	3 (1.6 oz)	250
Wafers Spicy Pepita Gluten Free	2 (1.1 oz)	170
Wafers Tamari Almond Gluten Free Vegan	2 (1.2 oz)	170
Weight Watchers		
English Toffee Squares	3 pieces	160

FOOD	PORTION	CALS
Mint Patties	2	100
Peanut Butter Crunch	4 pieces	180
Pecan Crowns	3 pieces	150
Werther's		
Caramel Milk Chocolate	6 (1.3 oz)	230
Original	3 (0.5 oz)	60
Original Sugar Free	5 (0.5 oz)	40
Whitman's		
Sampler	3 pieces (1.4 oz)	220
Whoppers		
Malted Milk Balls	18 pieces	190
York		
Peppermint Patty	3 (1.4 oz)	150
Peppermint Patty Sugar Free	3 (1.3 oz)	110
Yummy Earth		
Organic Lollipops All Flavors	3	70
Zero		
Bar	1	70
CANTALOUPE		
dried	3.5 pieces (1.4 oz)	140
fresh cubed	1 cup	57
fresh half	½	94
Del Monte		
Fresh	¼ melon (4.7 oz)	50
CAPERS		
capers	1 tbsp	2
CARAWAY		
seed	1 tbsp	22
CARDAMOM		
ground	1 tsp	6
CARDOON		
fresh cooked w/o salt	1 serv (3.5 oz)	22
fresh shredded	1 cup (6.2 oz)	30
Frieda's		
Cardoon	1 cup	15
Ocean Mist		
Cardone Fresh Shredded	1 cup (6.2 oz)	36

FOOD	PORTION	CALS
CARIBOU		
roasted	3 oz	142
CARISSA		
fresh	1	12
CAROB		
carob mix	3 tsp	45
carob mix as prep w/ whole milk	9 oz	195
flour	1 tbsp	14
flour	1 cup	185
Bob's Red Mill		
Powder Toasted	2 tsp	25
Tree Of Life		
Chips Malt Sweetened	50 (0.5 oz)	70
CARP		
fresh cooked	3 oz	138
fresh cooked	1 fillet (6 oz)	276
fresh raw	3 oz	108
roe raw	1 oz	37
roe salted in olive oil	2 tbsp (1 oz)	40
CARROT JUICE		
canned	6 oz	73
Bolthouse Farms		
Carrot Juice	8 oz	70
Hollywood		
100% Juice	1 can (12 oz)	120
Lakewood		
Organic	6 oz	73
Luvli Juices		
Zingy Carrot	1 bottle (10 oz)	145
Naked Juice		
Just Carrot	8 oz	80
Odwalla		
100% Juice	8 oz	70
CARROTS		
CANNED		
slices	½ cup	17
slices low sodium	½ cup	17

FOOD	PORTION	CALS
Allens		
Tiny Sliced	½ cup	35
Del Monte		
Savory Sides Honey Glazed	½ cup	70
Sliced	½ cup	35
Glory		
Seasoned Honey	½ cup	50
Tillen Farms		
Crispy Carrots Pickled	5 pieces (1 oz)	30
FRESH		
baby raw	1 (0.5 oz)	6
raw	1 (2.5 oz)	31
raw shredded	½ cup	24
slices cooked	½ cup	35
Bolthouse Farms		
Matchstix	3 oz	35
Earthbound Farm		
Organic Tops On	1 (2.7 oz)	35
Organic w/ Organic Ranch Dip	1 pkg (2.2 oz)	90
Frieda's		
Gold	⅔ cup (3 oz)	35
Grimmway		
Baby	3 oz	38
Nature's Gold		
Fresh	1 med (2.7 oz)	40
River Ranch		
Shredded	¾ cup	35
FROZEN		
slices cooked	½ cup	26
Birds Eye		
Steam & Serve Carrots & Cranberries	1 cup	130
C&W		
Whole Baby	⅔ cup	35
Green Giant		
Honey Glazed	1 cup	90
Joy Of Cooking		
Bite Size	½ cup (3.3 oz)	70
CASABA		
cubed	1 cup	45
fresh	⅒	43

FOOD	PORTION	CALS
CASHEWS		
cashew butter w/o salt	1 tbsp	94
dry roasted w/ salt	18 nuts (1 oz)	160
oil roasted w/ salt	1 oz	163
oil roasted w/o salt	1 oz	163
Arrowhead Mills		
Organic Cashew Butter	2 tbsp	160
Frito Lay		
Salted	3 tbsp	160
Good Sense		
Jumbo Honey Roasted	¼ cup	170
Jumbo Roasted & Salted	¼ cup	190
Kettle		
Butter Creamy Unsalted	2 tbsp	160
Lance		
Cashews	1 pkg (1.5 oz)	270
Navitas Naturals		
Cashews	1 oz	160
O.N.E.		
Cashew Juice	1 bottle (11 oz)	140
Peeled Snacks		
Nut Picks Cashew Later	1 pkg (1 oz)	180
Planters		
Chocolate Lovers Milk Chocolate	10 pieces (1.5 oz)	230
Dry Roasted	19 pieces (1 oz)	160
Organic	23 pieces (1 oz)	170
Sunfood		
Organic	1 oz	164
Tree Of Life		
Cashew Butter Creamy	2 tbsp	180
CASSAVA		
fresh	3.5 oz	120
CATFISH		
channel breaded & fried	3 oz	194
wolffish atlantic baked	3 oz	105
Simmons		
Farm Raised	4 oz	140
CAULIFLOWER		
flowerets fresh	1 (0.5 oz)	3

FOOD	PORTION	CALS
flowerets fresh cooked w/o salt	3 (2 oz)	12
fresh	1 cup	25
fresh cooked w/o salt	1 cup	29
fresh head small	1 (9.2 oz)	66
frzn cooked w/o salt	1 cup	34
green fresh	1 cup	20
green fresh small head	1 (11.4 oz)	101
pickled	¼ cup	14
pickled chow chow	¼ cup	74
Birds Eye		
Steamfresh Garlic Cauliflower	1 cup (2.4 oz)	40
Green Giant		
Cheese Sauce	½ cup	50
Mann's		
Cauliettes Fresh	1 serv (3 oz)	20
River Ranch		
Florets Fresh	1 cup	20
TAKE-OUT		
batter dipped fried	1 piece (0.9 oz)	55
batter dipped fried	1 cup	178
w/ cheese sauce	1 cup	249

CAVIAR

black or red	2 tbsp	81

CELERY

fresh	1 lg stalk (2.2 oz)	9
pickled	½ cup	10
raw diced	½ cup	8
seeds	1 tsp	1
strips	1 cup	17
Dole		
Stalks	2 med (3 oz)	20
Earthbound Farm		
Organic Hearts	2 stalks (3.9 oz)	20
Frieda's		
Celery Root	¾ cup	35
River Ranch		
Sticks Fresh	4 (3 oz)	15
TAKE-OUT		
creamed	½ cup	87

FOOD	PORTION	CALS
stir fried	½ cup	30
stuffed w/ cheese	1 (5 inch)	38

CELERY JUICE
juice	1 cup	42

CELTUCE
raw	3.5 oz	22

CEREAL
bran flakes	¾ cup	90
corn flakes	1¼ cups	110
farina as prep w/ water	¾ cup	88
granola	½ cup	285
oatmeal instant as prep w/ water	1 cup (8.2 oz)	138
oatmeal regular & quick as prep w/ water	¾ cup (6.1 oz)	149
oatmeal regular & quick not prep	⅓ cup (0.9 oz)	104
puffed rice	1 cup	56
puffed wheat	1 cup	44
shredded mini wheats	1 cup	107
shredded wheat rectangular	1 biscuit (0.8 oz)	85
Alti Plano		
Hot Cereal Chai Almond	1 pkg	210
Hot Cereal Oaxacan Chocolate	1 pkg	170
Hot Cereal Orange Date	1 pkg	180
Hot Cereal Regular	1 pkg	190
Hot Cereal Spiced Apple Raisin	1 pkg	160
Instant Quinoa Hot Cereal Spiced Apple Raisin	1 pkg	160
Instant Quinoa Organic Hot Cereal Oaxacan Chocolate	1 pkg	170
Alvarado Street Bakery		
Plain Granola	½ cup	220
Arrowhead Mills		
Organic Amaranth Flakes	1 cup	140
Organic Kamut Flakes	1 cup	120
Organic Multigrain Flakes	1 cup	170
Organic Nature O's	1 cup	130
Organic Puffed Corn	1 cup	60
Organic Puffed Millet	1 cup	60
Organic Puffed Wheat	1 cup	60
Organic Rice Flakes Sweetened	1 cup	180
Organic Shredded Wheat	1 cup	190

FOOD	PORTION	CALS
Organic Spelt Flakes	1 cup	120
Back To Nature		
Energy Start Hi Protein Crunch	½ cup	170
Flax & Fiber Crunch	1 cup	200
Granola Apple Blueberry	½ cup	200
Granola Classic	½ cup	180
Granola French Vanilla	½ cup	220
Heart Basics Organic Apple Cinnamon Harvest	¾ cup	180
Multigrain Harvest	1 cup	210
Oat & Soy Crisp	¾ cup	180
Strawberry & Seven Grains	1 cup	210
Barbara's Bakery		
Alpen No Sugar Added	⅔ cup	200
Organic Breakfast O's Fruit Juice Sweetened	1 cup	120
Organic Brown Rice Crisps Fruit Juice Sweetened	1 cup	120
Organic Corn Flakes Fruit Juice Sweetened	1 cup	110
Organic Wild Puffs	1 cup	100
Organic Wild Puffs Fruity Punch	1 cup	110
Organic Ultima High Fiber	½ cup	90
Organic Ultima Pomegranate	½ cup	100
Puffins Cinnamon	⅔ cup	100
Puffins Originals	¾ cup (0.9 oz)	90
Shredded Oats Bite Size	1¼ cups (2 oz)	220
Shredded Wheat	2 biscuits (1.4 oz)	140
Bear Naked		
Apple Cinnamon	¼ cup	140
Banana Nut	¼ cup	140
Fruit And Nut	¼ cup	140
Peak Protein	½ cup	200
Bob's Red Mill		
Farina Creamy Brown Rice not prep	¼ cup	150
Muesli Old Country	¼ cup	110
Natural Granola No Fat	½ cup	180
Organic Right Stuff Hot Cereal 6 Grain not prep	¼ cup	140
Rolled Oats Gluten Free not prep	½ cup	160
Cascadian Farm		
Organic Clifford Crunch	1 cup	100
Organic Granola Oats & Honey	⅔ cup	230

FOOD	PORTION	CALS
Chappaqua Crunch		
Original Granola	⅓ cup	115
Simply Granola w/ Raisins	⅓ cup	120
Simply Granola w/ Raspberries	⅓ cup	110
CoCo Wheats		
Hot Cereal	⅓ cup	200
Country Choice Organic		
Multigrain Hot Cereal not prep	½ cup	130
Oats Old Fashioned not prep	½ cup	150
Oats Quick not prep	½ cup	150
Dorset Cereals		
Berries & Cherries	½ cup	150
Simply Delicious Muesli	½ cup	200
Super Cranberry Cherry & Almond	½ cup	200
Earthbound Farm		
Organic Granola Maple Almond	½ cup	260
Enjoy Life		
Allergen Gluten Free Granola Cinnamon	½ cup	160
EnviroKidz		
Organic Orangutan O's	¾ cup	120
Fantastic		
Oatmeal Big Cup Apple Cinnamon	1 pkg	270
Oatmeal Big Cup Maple Raisin 3 Grain	1 pkg	270
General Mills		
Cheerios	1 cup	110
Cheerios Crunch Oat Cluster	¾ cup	100
Cheerios Yogurt Burst Strawberry	¾ cup	120
Cheerios Yogurt Burst Vanilla	¾ cup	120
Chex Whole Grain Chocolate	¾ cup	130
Curves	¾ cup	100
Fiber One	½ cup (1 oz)	60
Fiber One Raisin Bran Clusters	1 cup (2 oz)	170
Total Honey Clusters	¾ cup	170
Total Raisin Bran	1 cup	170
Total Whole Grain	¾ cup (1 oz)	100
Trix	1 cup (1.1 oz)	120
Glucerna		
Crunchy Flakes 'N Raisins	1 pkg (1.6 oz)	140
Crunchy Flakes 'N Strawberries	1 pkg (1.5 oz)	150

FOOD	PORTION	CALS
Glutino		
Gluten Free Apple Cinnamon	½ cup	120
Gluten Free Honey Nut	½ cup	130
Gram's Gourmet		
Crunch Granolas All Flavors	½ cup	349
Grandy Oats		
Organic Granola Classic	½ cup	252
Organic Granola Low Fat Cranberry Chew	½ cup	191
Organic Granola Mainely Maple	½ cup	204
Health Valley		
Empower	1 cup	200
Granola Low Fat Tropical Fruit	⅔ cup	180
Heart Wise	1 cup	200
Organic Cherry Lemon Blast Ems	¾ cup	120
Organic Golden Flax	¾ cup	190
Organic Multigrain Apple Cinnamon Square Ems	1¼ cup	210
Organic Oat Bran O's	¾ cup	100
Rice Crunch-Ems	1 cup	110
Hodgson Mill		
Hot Cereal Bulgur Wheat w/ Soy not prep	¼ cup	115
Hot Cereal Oat Bran not prep	¼ cup	120
Honest Foods		
Granola Planks Maple Almond Crunch	½ bar (2 oz)	250
Kashi		
7 Whole Grain Flakes	1 cup	180
7 Whole Grain Honey Puffs	1 cup	120
7 Whole Grain Nuggets	½ cup	210
7 Whole Grain Pilaf as prep	½ cup	170
GoLean	1 cup	140
GoLean Crunch!	1 cup	190
GoLean Crunch! Honey Almond Flax	1 cup	200
GoLean Instant Hot Cereal Creamy Truly Vanilla	1 pkg	150
GoLean Instant Hot Cereal Hearty Honey & Cinnamon	1 pkg	150
Good Friends	1 cup	170
Granola Mountain Medley	½ cup	220
Heart To Heart Instant Oatmeal Golden Brown Maple	1 pkg	160

FOOD	PORTION	CALS
Heart To Heart Instant Oatmeal Raisin Spice	1 pkg	150
Heart To Heart Oat Flakes & Blueberry Clusters	1¼ cups	200
Heart To Heart Toasted Oat	¾ cup	110
Honey Sunshine	¾ cup (1.1 oz)	100
Mighty Bites All Flavors	1 cup	110
Organic Promise Autumn Wheat	1 cup	190
Organic Promise Cinnamon Harvest	1 cup	190
Organic Promise Strawberry Fields	1 cup	120
Vive Probiotic Digestive Wellness	1¼ cups	170
Kellogg's		
All-Bran	½ cup	80
All-Bran Extra Fiber	½ cup	50
Apple Jacks	1 cup	130
Caramel Nut Crunch	1 cup	210
Cocoa Krispies	¾ cup	120
Complete Oat Bran Flakes	¾ cup	110
Corn Flakes	1 cup	100
Corn Pops	1 cup	120
Cracklin' Oat Bran	¾ cup	200
Crispix	1 cup	110
Frosted Flakes	¾ cup	120
Frosted Flakes ⅓ Less Sugar	1 cup	120
Fruit Harvest	¾ cup	120
Fruit Loops	1 cup	120
Fruit Loops ⅓ Less Sugar	1¼ cups	120
Granola Low Fat w/ Raisins	⅔ cup	230
Honey Smacks	¾ cup	100
Mini-Wheat Frosted	5 (1.8 oz)	180
Mueslix Raisins Dates & Almonds	⅔ cup	200
Organic Mini Wheats Frosted	24 pieces	190
Organic Raisin Bran	1 cup	190
Organic Rice Krispies	1¼ cups	120
Product 19	1 cup	100
Raisin Bran	1 cup	190
Rice Krispies	1¼ cups	120
Smart Start Antioxidants	1 cup	190
Smart Start Healthy Heart	1¼ cups	230
Smorz	1 cup	120
Special K	1 cup	110

FOOD	PORTION	CALS
Special K Fruit & Yogurt	¾ cup	120
Special K Low Carb Lifestyle Protein Plus	¾ cup	100
Special K Red Berries	1 cup	110
Special K Vanilla Almond	¾ cup	110
Keto		
Hot Cereal Apple Cinnamon	2 scoops	150
Hot Cereal Strawberry & Creme	2 scoops	150
Liquid Cereal		
Apple & Cinnamon	1 can (11 oz)	160
Chocolate	1 can (11 oz)	170
Fruit	1 can (11 oz)	150
Peanut Butter	1 can (11 oz)	170
Lundberg		
Purely Organic Hot'n Creamy Rice	⅓ cup	190
Malt-O-Meal		
Balance	¾ cup	120
Cinnamon Toasters	¾ cup	130
Colossal Crunch	¾ cup	120
Creamy Hot Wheat not prep	3 tbsp	130
Crispy Rice	1¼ cups	130
Frosted Flakes	¾ cup	120
Frosted Mini Spooners	1 cup	190
Honey & Oat Blenders	¾ cup	120
Honey Buzzers	1⅓ cup	110
Instant Oatmeal Apple & Cinnamon	1 pkg	130
Instant Oatmeal Cinnamon & Spice	1 pkg	170
Instant Oatmeal Maple & Brown Sugar	1 pkg	160
Original Hot Wheat not prep	3 tbsp	130
Puffed Rice	1 cup	60
Raisin Bran	1 cup	220
Mom's Best Naturals		
Oatmeal Instant	1 pkg	160
Raisin Bran	1 cup	230
Toasted Wheat-fuls	1 cup	200
Toasty O's	1 cup	120
Natural Ovens		
Great Granola	½ cup	250
Nature's Path		
Optimum Organic ReBound	¾ cup	190
Organic Flax Plus Pumpkin Raisin Crunch	¾ cup	200

FOOD	PORTION	CALS
Organic Granola Pomegran Plus	½ cup	140
Organic Smart Bran	⅔ cup	90
Organic Zen Instant Oatmeal Cranberry Ginger	1 pkg	150
Nature's Plus		
Organic Oatmeal Hemp Plus	1 pkg	160
Newman's Own		
Sweet Enough Honey Flax Flakes	¾ cup	100
Sweet Enough Honey Nut O's	¾ cup	110
Sweet Enough Wheat Puffs	¾ cup	100
Perky's		
Nutty Flax	¾ cup	230
PerkyO's Original	¾ cup	120
Post		
100% Bran	½ cup (0.8 oz)	80
Bran Flakes	1 cup	100
Cocoa Pebbles	¾ cup (1 oz)	110
Golden Crisp	¾ cup (1 oz)	110
Grape Nuts O's	1 cup (1 oz)	120
Grape-Nuts	2 oz	200
Grape-Nuts Trail Mix Crunch	1 cup (1.7 oz)	170
Great Grains Raisins Dates & Pecans	¾ cup (2 oz)	210
Honey Bunches Of Oats	¾ cup	130
Honey Bunches Of Oats Peaches	1 cup	120
Honey Bunches Of Oats Strawberry	¾ cup	120
Honeycomb	1⅓ cups (1 oz)	120
LiveActive Mixed Berry Crunch	1 cup	190
LiveActive Nut Harvest Crunch	1 cup	220
Oreo O's	1 cup	110
Raisin Bran	1 cup (2 oz)	190
Selects Banana Nut Crunch	1 cup (2 oz)	240
Selects Blueberry Morning	2 oz	220
Shredded Wheat Frosted	2 oz	180
Shredded Wheat 'N Bran	2 oz	200
Shredded Wheat Original	2 biscuits (1.6 oz)	160
Shredded Wheat Spoon Size	1 cup	170
Toasties Corn Flakes	1 cup (1 oz)	100
Quaker		
Instant Oatmeal Cinnamon & Spice	1 pkg	170
Instant Oatmeal Cinnamon Roll	1 pkg	160
Instant Oatmeal Crunch Maple & Brown Sugar	1 pkg	190

FOOD	PORTION	CALS
Instant Oatmeal Crunch Mixed Berry	1 pkg	190
Instant Oatmeal Express Baked Apple	1 pkg	200
Instant Oatmeal For Kids Dinosaur Eggs	1 pkg	190
Instant Oatmeal Lower Sugar Maple & Brown Sugar	1 pkg	120
Instant Oatmeal Maple Brown Sugar w/ Pecans	1 pkg	160
Instant Oatmeal Nutrition For Women Golden Brown Sugar	1 pkg	170
Instant Oatmeal Organic Regular	1 pkg	100
Instant Oatmeal Regular	1 pkg	100
Instant Oatmeal Simple Harvest Apples w/ Cinnamon	1 pkg	150
Instant Oatmeal Strawberries & Cream	1 pkg	130
Instant Oatmeal Supreme Apple Raisin	1 pkg	150
Instant Oatmeal Supreme Cinnamon Pecan	1 pkg	180
Instant Oatmeal Take Heart Golden Maple	1 pkg	160
Instant Oatmeal Weight Control Banana Bread	1 pkg	160
Life	¾ cup	120
Life Cinnamon	¾ cup	120
Life Honey Graham	¾ cup	120
Life Vanilla Yogurt Crunch	1¼ cups	210
Oat Bran Hot Cereal not prep	½ cup	150
Old Fashioned Oats not prep	½ cup	150
Quick Oats Sun Country Iron Fortified	1 pkg	150
Ralston		
100% Hot Wheat	⅓ cup	150
Apple Dapples	1 cup	120
Cocoa Crumbles	1 cup	120
Confruity Crisp	¾ cup	110
Corn Biscuits	1 cup	110
Corn Flakes	1 cup (1 oz)	100
Crisp Crunch	¾ cup	120
Crisp Crunch Berry Treats	1 cup	120
Crisp Rice	1¼ cups	120
Enriched Bran Flakes	¾ cup	90
Farina	3 tbsp	120
Freaky Fruits	1 cup	120
Frosted Flakes	¾ cup	120
Fruit Rings	1 cup	120

FOOD	PORTION	CALS
Grits	¼ cup	140
Instant Oats Bananas & Cream	1 pkg	130
Magic Stars	¾ cup	120
Oats & More w/ Almonds	¾ cup	130
Oats Instant	1 pkg	100
Oats Instant Apples & Cinnamon	1 pkg	130
Oats Instant Blueberries & Cream	1 pkg	130
Oats Instant Cinnamon & Spice	1 pkg	170
Oats Instant For Kids Cinnawow	1 pkg	140
Oats Instant For Kids Maplicious & Brown Sugar	1 pkg	150
Oats Instant For Kids Roarin' Raspberry	1 pkg	150
Oats Instant For Kids Strawberries & Stars	1 pkg	140
Oats Instant Maple Brown Sugar	1 pkg	160
Oats Instant Peaches & Cream	1 pkg	130
Oats Instant Raisins & Spice	1 pkg	150
Oats Instant Strawberries & Cream	1 pkg	140
Oats Old Fashioned	½ cup	150
Oats Quick	½ cup	140
Raisin Bran	1 cup	200
Rice Biscuits	1¼ cups	120
Shredded Wheat Frosted Bite Size	1¼ cups	200
Silly Spheres	1½ cups	110
Tasteeos	1 cup	110
Tasteeos Apple Cinnamon	¾ cup	120
Tasteeos Honey Nut	1 cup	120
South Beach		
Crunch Strawberry Harvest	1 cup	170
Crunch Vanilla Almond	1 cup	180
Granola Clusters Cherry Almond	1 pkg (1 oz)	130
Granola Clusters Mixed Berry	1 pkg (1 oz)	130
Stark Sisters		
Granola Lo-Fat Raspberry Blueberry	½ cup	230
Granola Nutty Maple	½ cup	250
Granola Original Maple Almond	½ cup	240
Sunbelt		
Granola Low Fat Cinnamon & Raisins	½ cup	250
Udi's		
Granola BanaBerry	¼ cup (1.1 oz)	120
Granola Hawaiian	¼ cup (1.1 oz)	120

FOOD	PORTION	CALS
Granola Muesli	¼ cup (1.1 oz)	120
Granola Nuggets	¼ cup (1.1 oz)	150
Granola Original	¼ cup (1.1 oz)	130
Weetabix		
Organic	2 biscuits (1.2 oz)	120
Organic Crispy Flakes	¾ cup	110
Wheatena		
Toasted Wheat	⅓ cup	160
YogActive		
Probiotic High Fibre Wheat Strawberry Raspberry	⅔ cup	160
Probiotic Kiwi	⅔ cup	120
Probiotic Strawberry	⅔ cup	130
Probiotic Strawberry Dark Chocolate	⅔ cup	130
Zoe's		
Granola Cinnamon Raisin	½ cup	190
Granola Cranberries Currants	½ cup	190
Granola Honey Almond	½ cup	190
O's Cinnamon	¾ cup	120
O's Honey	¾ cup	120
O's Natural	¾ cup	120
CEREAL BARS (see also ENERGY BARS)		
Aristo		
Acai Blueberry Lime	1 (1.3 oz)	130
Pomegranate & Cranberry	1 (1.3 oz)	140
Attune		
Wellness Yogurt & Granola Lemon Creme	1 (1.4 oz)	180
Wellness Yogurt & Granola Strawberry Bliss	1 (1.4 oz)	180
Back To Nature		
Bakery Squares Banana Walnut	1 (1.1 oz)	130
Chewy Trail Mix Cherry Pecan	1 (1 oz)	120
Fruit & Grain Apple	1 (1.1 oz)	110
Barbara's Bakery		
Fruit & Yogurt Cherry Apple	1	150
Nature's Choice Blueberry	1 (1.3 oz)	150
Organic Crunchy Granola Cinnamon Crisp	2 (1.5 oz)	190
Cascadian Farm		
Organic Chewy Granola Fruit & Nut	1 (1.2 oz)	140
CocoaVia		
Dark Chocolate Almond	1 (0.8 oz)	90

FOOD	PORTION	CALS
Country Choice Organic		
Oatmeal Squares Apple Cinnamon	1 (2 oz)	210
Oatmeal Squares Maple	1 (2 oz)	210
Enjoy Life		
Allergen Gluten Free Caramel Apple	1 (1 oz)	110
Entenmann's		
Multi-Grain Real Strawberry	1 (1.3 oz)	140
EnviroKidz		
Crispy Rice Panda Peanut Butter	1 (1 oz)	110
Estee		
Rice Crunchy Chocolate	1	60
Rice Crunchy Chocolate Chip	1	70
Rice Crunchy Vanilla	1	70
General Mills		
Team Cheerios Strawberry	1	160
Trix	1	160
Glenny's		
Organic Muesli Chocolate Chip	1 (1.6 oz)	170
Organic Muesli Raisins & Dates	1 (1.6 oz)	170
Slim Carb Bars Brownie Cheesecake	1 (1.3 oz)	130
Slim-1 w/ Acai Very Berry Blast	1 (1.1 oz)	100
Slim-1 w/ Green Tea Double Fudge	1 (1.1 oz)	100
Slim-1 w/ Hoodia Peanut Butter Caramel	1 (1.1 oz)	100
Glutino		
Gluten Free Breakfast Bar Apple	1 (1.4 oz)	120
Gluten Free Breakfast Bar Chocolate	1 (1.4 oz)	110
Gluten Free Organic Chocolate & Peanut	1 (1 oz)	110
Gluten Free Organic Wildberry	1 (1 oz)	100
Health Valley		
Cafe Creations Cinnamon Danish	1 (1.4 oz)	130
Date Almond Low Fat	1 (1.5 oz)	150
Granola Chocolate Chip Low Fat	1 (1.5 oz)	160
Granola Moist & Chewy Dutch Apple	1 (1 oz)	100
Granola Trail Mix Cranberries Nuts & Yogurt Chips	1 (1.2 oz)	140
Organic Fig Cobbler	1 (1.4 oz)	130
Organic Raspberry Tarts	1 (1.4 oz)	150
Organic Strawberry Cobbler	1 (1.3 oz)	130
Peanut Butter & Grape	1 (1.3 oz)	130

FOOD	PORTION	CALS
Hershey's		
Crispy Rice Peanut Butter	1 (0.5 oz)	60
Honest Foods		
Cran Lemon Zest	1 (2.2 oz)	240
Farmer's Trail Mix	1 (2.2 oz)	240
Kashi		
TLC Chewy Granola Honey Almond Flax	1 (1.2 oz)	140
TLC Chewy Trail Mix	1 (1.2 oz)	140
TLC Soft Baked Apple Spice	1 (1.2 oz)	110
TLC Soft Baked Blackberry Graham	1 (1.2 oz)	110
TLC Soft Baked Ripe Strawberry	1 (1.2 oz)	110
Kellogg's		
All-Bran Brown Sugar Cinnamon	1	130
All-Bran Honey Oat	1	130
All-Bran Oatmeal Raisin	1	120
Crunchy Nut Sweet & Salty Chocolatey Almond	1 (1.1 oz)	160
FiberPlus Antioxidants Chocolate Chip	1 (1.2 oz)	120
FiberPlus Antioxidants Dark Chocolate Almond	1 (1.2 oz)	130
Nutri-Grain Apple Cinnamon	1	140
Nutri-Grain Banana Muffin	1	170
Nutri-Grain Chewy Granola Chocolatey Chunk	1	110
Nutri-Grain Cinnamon Raisin Muffin	1	170
Nutri-Grain Yogurt Vanilla	1	140
Smart Start Healthy Heart Cinnamon	1 (1.4 oz)	150
Snack Bites	1 pkg (0.8 oz)	90
Special K Chocolatey Drizzle	1 (0.8 oz)	90
Special K Meal Bar Chocolate Peanut Butter	1 (1.6 oz)	190
Special K Snack Bar Chocolate Peanut	1 (0.9 oz)	110
Special K Strawberry	1 (0.8 oz)	90
Special K Vanilla Crisp	1 (0.8 oz)	90
KeriBar		
Vegan Apple Peanut Butter	1 (1.4 oz)	140
Vegan Cherry Almond	1 (1.4 oz)	140
Vegan Strawberry Chocolate Chip	1 (1.4 oz)	130
Kind		
Almond & Coconut	1	193
Almonds & Apricot In Yogurt	1	208

FOOD	PORTION	CALS
Banana & Oatbran	1	160
Nut Delight	1	203
Walnut & Date	1	150
Kudos		
Granola Chocolate Chip	1 (1 oz)	120
Granola Peanut Butter	1	130
Granola w/ M&M's	1	100
Granola w/ Snickers	1	100
Lean Body		
Hi-Protein Granola Peanuts 'N Chocolate	1 (2.8 oz)	340
Natural Ovens		
Great Granola Mixed Fruit	1 (1.4 oz)	150
Nature Valley		
Chewy Granola Blueberry Yogurt	1	140
Chewy Granola Lemon Yogurt	1	140
Chewy Granola Vanilla Yogurt	1	140
Chewy Trail Mix Granola Apple Cinnamon	1	140
Chewy Trail Mix Granola Fruit & Nut	1	140
Chewy Trail Mix Granola Mixed Berry	1	140
Crunchy Granola Apple Crisp	1	140
Crunchy Granola Banana Nut	2	190
Crunchy Granola Maple Brown Sugar	2	180
Crunchy Granola Peanut Butter	2	160
Crunchy Granola Roasted Almond	2	190
Heart Healthy Chewy Granola Honey Nut	1	160
Heart Healthy Granola Oatmeal Raisin	1	150
Sweet & Salty Granola Almond	1	160
Sweet & Salty Granola Peanut	1	170
Nutri-Grain		
Nutri-Grain Blueberry	1	140
Nutri-Grain Mixed Berry	1	140
Post		
Honey Bunches Of Oats Banana Nut	1 (1.2 oz)	140
Honey Bunches Of Oats Oatmeal Raisin	1 (1.2 oz)	130
Quaker		
Breakfast Bar Apple Crisp	1 (1.3 oz)	130
Breakfast Bar Graham Strawberry	1 (1 oz)	120
Breakfast Bar Iced Raspberry	1 (1.3 oz)	130
Breakfast Bites Iced Raspberry	1 pkg (1.3 oz)	130
Breakfast Bites Strawberry	1 pkg (1.3 oz)	130

FOOD	PORTION	CALS
Chewy Chocolate Chip	1 (0.8 oz)	100
Chewy Cookies & Cream	1 (0.8 oz)	90
Chewy 90 Calorie Cinnamon Sugar	1 (1 oz)	90
Chewy 90 Calorie Honey Nut	1 (0.8 oz)	90
Chewy Dipps Peanut Butter	1 (1 oz)	150
Chewy Low Fat S'mores	1 (1 oz)	110
Crunchy Granola Oats & Berries	1 (1 oz)	130
Oatmeal To Go Oatmeal Raisin	1 (2.1 oz)	220
Oatmeal To Go Raspberry Streusel	1 (2.1 oz)	220
Q-Smart Cranberry Vanilla Almond	1 (1 oz)	120
Trail Mix Cranberry Raisin & Almond	1 (1.2 oz)	150
Revolution Foods		
Jammy Sammy Apple Cinnamon & Oatmeal	1 (1 oz)	100
Organic Jammy Sammy PB & Grape	1 (1 oz)	110
Organic Jammy Sammy PB & Strawberry	1 (1 oz)	110
Rice Krispies		
Split Stix Chocolatey	1 (1 oz)	130
Split Stix Original	1 (1 oz)	120
Treats Original	1 (0.8 oz)	90
South Beach		
100 Calorie Chocolate Delight	1 (1 oz)	100
100 Calorie Peanut Butter Chocolate Chip	1 (1 oz)	100
100 Calorie Snack Bar Mixed Berry	1 (1 oz)	100
Fiber Fit Granola Mocha	1 (1.2 oz)	120
Fiber Fit Granola S'Mores	1 (1.2 oz)	120
High Protein Chocolate	1 (1.2 oz)	140
High Protein Cranberry Almond	1 (1.2 oz)	140
High Protein Maple Nut	1 (1.2 oz)	140
High Protein Peanut Butter	1 (1.2 oz)	140
Wings Of Nature		
Organic Apple Cinnamon	1 (1.2 oz)	119
Organic Cafe Mocha Coffee	1 (1.2 oz)	153
Organic Cappuccino Coffee	1 (1.2 oz)	153
Yotta		
Apple Cinnamon	1 (1.2 oz)	120
Cherry	1 (1.2 oz)	120
Orange	1 (1.2 oz)	120

CHAMPAGNE

champagne	1 serv (3.5 oz)	84
mimosa	1 serv	117

FOOD	PORTION	CALS
punch	1 serv (4 oz)	73
sekt german champagne	1 serv (3.5 oz)	84

CHAYOTE
fresh cooked	1 cup	38
raw	1 (7 oz)	49
raw cut up	1 cup	32

CHEESE (see also CHEESE DISHES, CHEESE SUBSTITUTES, COTTAGE CHEESE, CREAM CHEESE, NEUFCHATEL)

american	1 oz	93
american cheese spread	1 oz	82
beaufort	1 oz	115
bel paese	1 oz	112
blue	1 oz	100
blue crumbled	1 cup (4.7 oz)	477
bocconcini smoked	1 oz	90
brick	1 oz	105
brie	1 oz	95
cacio di roma sheep's milk cheese	1 oz	130
caerphilly	1.4 oz	150
camembert	1 oz	85
cantal	1 oz	105
caraway	1 oz	107
chabichou	1 oz	95
chaource	1 oz	83
cheddar	1 oz	114
cheddar low fat	1 oz	49
cheddar low sodium	1 oz	113
cheddar reduced fat	1.4 oz	104
cheddar shredded	1 cup	455
cheshire	1 oz	110
cheshire reduced fat	1.4 oz	108
colby	1 oz	112
colby low fat	1 oz	49
colby low sodium	1 oz	113
comte	1 oz	114
coulommiers	1 oz	88
crottin	1 oz	105
derby	1.4 oz	161
edam	1 oz	101

FOOD	PORTION	CALS
edam reduced fat	1.4 oz	92
emmentaler	1 oz	115
feta	1 oz	75
fontina	1 oz	110
frais	1.6 oz	51
gjetost	1 oz	132
gloucester double	1.4 oz	162
goat fresh	1 oz	23
goat hard	1 oz	128
gorgonzola	1 oz	107
gouda	1 oz	101
grana padano shaved	1 tbsp	20
gruyere	1 oz	117
lancashire	1.4 oz	149
leicester	1.4 oz	160
limburger	1 oz	93
lymeswold	1.4 oz	170
maroilles	1 oz	97
monterey	1 oz	106
morbier	1 oz	99
mozzarella fresh	1 oz	80
mozzarella part skim	1 oz	72
muenster	1 oz	104
parmesan grated	1 tbsp	23
parmesan hard	1 oz	111
picodon	1 oz	99
pimento	1 oz	106
pont l'eveque	1 oz	86
port du salut	1 oz	100
provolone	1 oz	100
pyrenees	1 oz	101
quark 20% fat	1 oz	33
quark 40% fat	1 oz	48
quark made w/ skim milk	1 oz	22
queso anejo	1 oz	106
queso asadero	1 oz	101
queso chihuahua	1 oz	106
queso fresco	1 oz	41
queso manchego	1 oz	107
queso panela	1 oz	74

FOOD	PORTION	CALS
raclette	1 oz	102
reblochon	1 oz	88
ricotta part skim	½ cup (4.4 oz)	171
ricotta whole milk	½ cup (4.4 oz)	216
romadur 40% fat	1 oz	83
romano	1 oz	110
roquefort	1 oz	105
rouy	1 oz	95
saint marcellin	1 oz	94
saint nectaire	1 oz	97
saint paulin	1 oz	85
sainte maure	1 oz	99
selles sur cher	1 oz	93
stilton blue	1.4 oz	164
stilton white	1.4 oz	145
swiss	1 oz	107
swiss processed	1 oz	95
tilsit	1 oz	96
tome	1 oz	92
triple creme	1 oz	113
vacherin	1 oz	92
wensleydale	1.4 oz	151
whey cheese	1 oz	126
yogurt cheese	1 oz	80
Applegate Farms		
Organic Cheddar Milk	1 slice (0.7 oz)	85
Organic Muenster Kase	1 slice (0.8 oz)	85
Yogurt Cheese w/ Probiotics	1 slice (0.7 oz)	80
Athenos		
Traditional	¼ cup	90
Traditional Reduced Fat	¼ cup	70
Back To Nature		
Organic American Slices	1 slice (0.7 oz)	80
Organic Cheddar Cubes	8 pieces (1.1 oz)	130
Organic Cheddar Shredded	¼ cup	110
Organic Mozzarella Shredded	¼ cup	80
Organic White Cheddar Slices Reduced Fat	1 slice (0.7 oz)	60
BelGioioso		
Mozzarella Fresh	1 in cube (1 oz)	80

FOOD	PORTION	CALS
Boar's Head		
American	1 oz	100
American 25% Lower Sodium 25% Lower Fat	1 oz	90
ButterKase	1 oz	100
Cheddar Sharp	1 oz	110
Colby Jack	1 oz	110
Cream Havarti	1 oz	110
Creamy Blue	1 oz	90
Double Gloucester Yellow	1 oz	110
Edam	1 oz	90
Feta	1 oz	60
Gouda	1 oz	110
Lacey Swiss	1 oz	90
Longhorn Colby	1 oz	110
Monterey Jack	1 oz	100
Mozzarella	1 oz	90
Muenster	1 oz	100
Muenster Low Sodium	1 oz	100
Provolone 42% Lower Sodium	1 oz	100
Provolone Picante Sharp	1 oz	100
Swiss No Salt Added	1 oz	110
Cabot		
Cheddar	1 oz	110
Cheddar Horseradish	1 oz	110
Cheddar Light 50% Reduced Fat	1 oz	70
Cheddar Light 50% Reduced Fat Omega-3	1 oz	70
Cheddar Light 75% Reduced Fat	1 oz	60
Cheddar Shake	2 tsp	25
Cheddar Tomato Basil	1 oz	110
Monterey Jack	1 oz	110
Pepper Jack 50% Reduced Fat	1 oz	70
Swiss Slices	1 (1 oz)	110
Cantare		
Baked Brie En Croute	1 oz	100
Connoisseur		
Asiago Spread	1 tbsp	90
Brie Spread	2 tbsp	90
Gorgonzola Spread	1 tbsp	90
Wheel Asiago Pesto	2 tbsp	90
Wheel Swiss Bacon	2 tbsp	90

FOOD	PORTION	CALS
Cracker Barrel		
Fontina	1 slice (0.7 oz)	80
Sharp Cheddar 2% Milk	1 oz	90
Crystal Farms		
American Singles	1 slice (0.7 oz)	70
American Singles 2%	1 slice (0.7 oz)	50
American Singles Fat Free	1 slice (0.7 oz)	30
Blue Crumbled	2 tbsp	100
Cheese Curds	8 pieces (1 oz)	110
Cheezoids Sticks	1 piece (0.8 oz)	70
Danish Havarti	1 oz	110
Deli Slices Muenster	1 slice (0.8 oz)	80
Deli Slices Swiss	1 slice (0.7 oz)	80
Feta Crumbled	¼ cup	90
Gorgonzola Crumbled	2 tbsp	100
It's So Cheesy Cheddar Aerosol	2 tbsp	90
Little Chunks To Go	1 pkg (0.7 oz)	80
Marble Jack	1 oz	110
Parmesan Grated	2 tsp	25
Pepper Jack	1 oz	110
Ricotta	¼ cup	90
Shredded Mexican 4 Cheese	¼ cup	100
Shredded Mozzarella	¼ cup	80
Shredded Pizza Blend	¼ cup	100
Shredded Sharp Cheddar	¼ cup	110
Smoked Gouda	1 oz	100
String	1 piece (1 oz)	80
Dragone		
Mozzarella Whole Milk	1 oz	90
Parmesan Wedge	1 oz	100
Ricotta Part Skim	¼ cup (2.2 oz)	90
Easy Cheese		
American	2 tbsp (1.1 oz)	90
Cheddar	2 tbsp (1.1 oz)	90
Fage		
Feta	1 oz	80
Finlandia		
Muenster	1 slice (1.1 oz)	120
Swiss Thin Sliced	1 slice (0.5 oz)	55

FOOD	PORTION	CALS
Formaggio		
Fresh Mozzarella	1 oz	90
Fresh Made		
Farmers Cheese Nonfat	2 tbsp	15
Friendship		
Farmer	2 tbsp (1 oz)	50
Farmer No Salt Added	2 tbsp (1 oz)	50
Frigo		
Mozzarella Part Skim	1 oz	80
Parmesan Shredded	¼ cup (1 oz)	100
Ricotta Whole Milk	¼ cup (2.2 oz)	110
Romano Shredded	¼ cup (1 oz)	100
Heluva Good Cheese		
Cheddar Extra Sharp	1 oz	110
Horizon Organic		
American	1 slice (0.7 oz)	60
Cheddar	1 oz	110
Monterey Jack	1 oz	100
Shred Mexican	¼ cup	110
Shred Parmesan	1 tbsp	20
Slice Provolone	1 slice (0.7 oz)	70
Sticks Colby	1 (1 oz)	110
String Mozzarella	1 stick (1 oz)	80
J.L. Kraft		
Spreadable Feta & Spinach	2 tbsp	80
Jordan's		
Provolone	1 slice (1 oz)	100
Kraft		
Cheddar Extra Sharp	1 oz	120
Cheddar Sharp Shredded 2% Milk	¼ cup	80
LiveActive 1% Milk Cheddar Cubes	7 (1 oz)	90
LiveActive 2% Milk Marbled Colby & Monterey Jack	1 stick (1 oz)	90
LiveActive Cheddar Cheese Sticks	1 (1 oz)	120
LiveActive Colby & Monterey Jack Cubes	7 (1 oz)	110
LiveActive Mozzarella Sticks	1 (1 oz)	80
Shredded Mexican Style Cheddar & Monterey Jack	¼ cup	110
Singles American 2%	1 (0.7 oz)	50

FOOD	PORTION	CALS
Land O Lakes		
American	1 slice (0.7 oz)	70
Chedarella	1 oz	110
Cheddar	1 oz	110
Snack 'N Cheese To Go Cheddar Mild	1 serv (0.7 oz)	80
Snack 'N Cheese To Go Cheddar Mild Reduced Fat	1 serv (0.5 oz)	60
Snack 'N Cheese To Go Co-Jack	1 serv (0.7 oz)	80
Snack 'N Cheese To Go Co-Jack Reduced Fat	1 serv (0.7 oz)	60
Swiss	1 oz	110
Laughing Cow		
Cheese Bites Light	6 pieces (0.8 oz)	35
Creamy French Onion Light	1 wedge	35
Creamy Garlic & Herb Light	1 wedge (0.7 oz)	35
Creamy Swiss Light Original	1 wedge (0.7 oz)	35
Creamy Swiss Original	1 wedge (0.7 oz)	50
Mini Babybel Bonbel	1 piece (0.7 oz)	70
Mini Babybel Gouda	1 piece (0.7 oz)	80
Mini Babybel Light Original	1 piece (0.7 oz)	50
Mini Babybel Mild Cheddar	1 piece (0.7 oz)	70
Mini Babybel Original	1 piece (0.7 oz)	70
Lifeway		
Farmer's Kefir	2 tbsp	25
Farmer's Kefir Lite	2 tbsp	25
Sweet Kiss Peach	1 oz	45
Meza		
Baked Brie In Pastry w/ Cranberries & Spiced Almonds	1 oz	110
Miller's		
Mozzarella	1 slice (1 oz)	81
Mont Chevre		
Assorted Crottins	1 oz	70
Mt Vikos		
Feta Sheep & Goat Milk	1 oz	80
Organic Valley		
Blue Crumbles	1 oz	100
Cheddar Mild	1 oz	110
Feta	1 oz	60
Monterey Jack Shredded	¼ cup	80
Muenster	1 slice (0.7 oz)	80

FOOD	PORTION	CALS
Provolone	1 slice (0.7 oz)	70
Swiss	1 oz	110
Polly-O		
Mozzarella Part Skim	1 oz	70
Mozzarella Shredded	¼ cup	90
Ricotta Part Skim	¼ cup	90
President		
Feta	1 oz	90
Rouge Et Noir		
Breakfast	1 oz	90
Brie Garlic	1 oz	90
Brie Pesto	1 oz	90
Brie Tomato Basil	1 oz	90
Brie Triple Creme	1 oz	110
Camembert	1 oz	90
Le Petit Bleu	1 oz	110
Le Petit Chevre	1 oz	90
Marin French Blue	1 oz	110
Marin French Gold	1 oz	110
Schlosskranz	1 oz	85
Saladena		
Goat Crumbles	¼ cup	80
Sap Sago		
Fat Free Cheese Grated	1 tsp	10
Sargento		
4 Cheese Italian Shredded	¼ cup	80
4 Cheese Mexican Reduced Fat Shredded	¼ cup (1 oz)	80
American Burger	1 slice (0.7 oz)	70
Bistro Blends Shredded Mozzarella w/ Sun Dried Tomato & Basil	¼ cup	90
Blue Crumbled	¼ cup (1 oz)	100
Cheddar Chipotle Shredded	¼ cup	100
Cheddar Chipotle Sticks	1 (0.7 oz)	80
Cheddar Mild Cubes	7 (1 oz)	120
Cheddar Mild Shredded Reduced Fat	¼ cup (1 oz)	80
Cheddar White Vermont Sharp	1 slice (0.7 oz)	80
Cheddar White Vermont Sharp Shredded	¼ cup (1 oz)	110
Cheese Dips Cheddar & Buttery Pretzels	1 pkg (3.8 oz)	360
Cheese Dips Cheddar & Tortilla Chips	1 pkg (3 oz)	320
Colby-Jack Shredded	¼ cup (1 oz)	110

FOOD	PORTION	CALS
Fancy 6 Cheese Italian Shredded	¼ cup	90
Jarlsberg	1 slice (0.8 oz)	80
Monterey Jack Shredded	¼ cup (1 oz)	110
Mozzarella Reduced Fat Shredded	¼ cup (1 oz)	80
Mozzarella Shredded	¼ cup (1 oz)	80
Muenster	1 slice (0.7 oz)	80
Nacho & Taco Shredded	¼ cup (1 oz)	110
Parmesan Grated	2 tsp (5 g)	25
Parmesan Shredded	2 tsp	20
Pepper Jack	1 slice (0.7 oz)	80
Provolone	1 slice (0.7 oz)	70
Provolone Reduced Fat	1 slice (0.7 oz)	50
Ricotta Fat Free	¼ cup	50
Ricotta Light	¼ cup	60
Ricotta Whole Milk	¼ cup	90
String	1 piece (1 oz)	80
String Light	1 piece (0.7 oz)	50
Swiss Reduced Fat	1 slice (0.7 oz)	80
Swiss Shredded	¼ cup (1 oz)	110
Swiss Thick Slice	1 slice (1 oz)	110
Swiss Thin Sliced	1 slice (0.6 oz)	70
Smart Balance		
Cheddar Shredded	1 oz	80
Mozzarella Shredded	1 oz	80
Sorrento		
Mozzarella Fresh	1 oz	90
Mozzarella w/ Tomato & Basil Shredded	¼ cup	80
Stella		
3 Cheese Italian Shredded	¼ cup	100
Asiago Wedge	1 oz	110
Gorgonzola Wedge	1 oz	100
Kasseri Wedge	1 oz	110
Treasure Cave		
Blue Cheese Crumbled	¼ cup (1 oz)	100
Feta Crumbled	¼ cup (1 oz)	60
Gorgonzola Crumbled	¼ cup (1 oz)	100
Weight Watchers		
String Light	1 stick (0.8 oz)	50
Wholesome Valley		
Organic American	1 slice (0.7 oz)	50

FOOD	PORTION	CALS
CHEESE DISHES		
Alexia		
Mozzarella Stix	2 pieces	120
Farm Rich		
Cheese Sticks Breaded	2 (2.1 oz)	210
Mozzarella Bites Breaded	4 (2.2 oz)	150
Original Cheese Bites Breaded	7 (2.1 oz)	180
Fillo Factory		
Tyropita Cheese Fillo Appetizers	3 (3 oz)	230
Stouffer's		
Welsh Rarebit	¼ pkg (2.5 oz)	140
TAKE-OUT		
fondue	½ cup (3.8 oz)	247
fried mozzarella sticks	3 (4.6 oz)	503
souffle	1 serv (7 oz)	504
welsh rarebit	1 slice	228
CHEESE SUBSTITUTES		
mozzarella	1 oz	70
Playfood		
Cheesey Cheese	1 oz	60
Rice		
American Flavor	1 slice (0.7 oz)	50
Shreds Mozzarella Flavor	⅓ cup (1 oz)	70
Vegan American Flavor	1 slice (0.7 oz)	45
Sheese		
Blue Style	1 oz	100
Cheddar Style Medium	1 oz	100
Creamy Mexican	2 tbsp	80
Creamy Original	2 tbsp	80
Super Stix		
Mozzarella Flavor	1 (1 oz)	70
Vegan Gourmet		
Cheese Alternative Cheddar	1 oz	50
Cheese Alternative Monterey Jack	1 oz	70
Cheese Alternative Mozzarella	1 oz	70
Cheese Alternative Nacho	1 oz	45
Veggie		
American Flavor	1 slice (0.6 oz)	40
Grated Parmesan Flavor	2 tsp	15
Mozzarella Flavor	1 slice (0.7 oz)	40

FOOD	PORTION	CALS
Pepper Jack Flavor	1 oz	60
Shreds Cheddar Flavor	1 oz	70

CHERIMOYA
fresh	1	515

CHERRIES
CANNED
maraschino	¼ cup (1.4 oz)	66
maraschino	1 (4 g)	7
sour in heavy syrup	½ cup	116
sour in light syrup	½ cup	94
sour water packed	½ cup	44
sweet juice pack	½ cup	68
sweet pitted in heavy syrup	½ cup	105
sweet water pack	½ cup	57

Chukar Cherries
Cherry Jubilee Dessert Sauce	1 tbsp	40

Del Monte
Sweet Dark Pitted In Heavy Syrup	½ cup	100

DRIED
bing unsulfured	¼ cup	130
montmorency tart pitted	⅓ cup	160
tart	½ cup	200
yogurt covered	¼ cup	170

Bob's Red Mill
Tart	⅓ cup	140

Chukar Cherries
Bing	3 tbsp	130
Bing Chocolate Covered	3 tbsp (1.4 oz)	180
Cabernet Dark Chocolate Covered	2 tbsp (1.5 oz)	180
Columbia River Tart	⅓ cup	120
Rainier	3 tbsp	130
Totally Tart	⅓ cup	140

De-Lite
Tart	1 oz	95

Eden
Montmorency	¼ cup	140

Emily's
Dark Chocolate Covered	11 (1.4 oz)	180

FOOD	PORTION	CALS
Frieda's		
Bing	¼ cup (1.4 oz)	120
Tart	⅓ cup (1.4 oz)	150
Good Sense		
Cherries	⅓ cup	145
Peeled Snacks		
Fruit Picks Cherry-Go-Round	1 pkg (1.5 oz)	130
Sunsweet		
Tart & Sweet	¼ cup (1.4 oz)	100
FRESH		
sour	1 cup	52
sour pitted	1 cup	78
sweet	20	86
Rainier		
Sweet Premium Northwest	1 cup	90
Super Cherry		
Rainier	21	90
FROZEN		
sour unsweetened	½ cup	36
sweet sweetened	½ cup	115
CHERRY JUICE		
tart cherry concentrate	1 cup	140
Eden		
Organic Montmorency	8 oz	140
Froose		
Cheerful Cherry	1 box (4.2 oz)	80
HP		
Tart Montmorency Concentrate	1 oz	80
L&A		
Black Cherry 100% Juice	8 oz	180
Old Orchard		
100% Pure Tart Cherry	8 oz	140
Smart Juice		
Organic 100% Juice Tart Cherry	8 oz	130
Tart Is Smart		
Tart Cherry Concentrate	1 oz	80
CHERVIL		
seed	1 tsp	1

FOOD	PORTION	CALS
CHESTNUTS		
chinese steamed	3 (1 oz)	43
creme de marrons	1 oz	73
japanese roasted	1 oz	57
ready-to-eat vacuum packed	5 (1 oz)	40
roasted	3 (1 oz)	70
Gefen		
Whole Roasted & Peeled	¼ cup (1.4 oz)	52
CHEWING GUM		
bubble gum	1 block	20
stick	1 piece	7
sugarless	1 piece	5
Bazooka		
Bubble Gum	1 piece (4 g)	15
Big Red		
Gum	1 piece	10
Brach's		
Abra Cabubble	1 piece	45
Choward's		
Scented Gum	3 pieces	10
Doublemint		
Gum	1 piece	10
Dubble Bubble		
Gumball	1 piece	10
Eclipse		
Flash All Flavors	1 piece	0
Sugarless All Flavors	2 pieces	5
Extra		
Sugar Free All Flavors	1 piece	5
Sugar Free Bubble Gum	1 piece	5
Flare		
Warming Cinnamon	1 piece	5
Juicy Fruit		
Gum	2 pieces	10
Orbit		
Sugarfree Citrusmint	1 piece	<5
White Melon Breeze	2 pieces	5
Skittles		
Bubble Gum	2 pieces	10

FOOD	PORTION	CALS
SteviaDent		
Gum	2 pieces	3
Stride		
All Flavors	1 piece	<5
Trident		
Extra Care	1 piece	<5
Splash Strawberry Lime	1 piece	<5
Winterfresh		
Gum	1 stick	10
Thin Ice Mountain Rush	1 piece	0
Wrigley's		
Spearmint	1 stick	10
CHIA SEEDS		
dried	1 oz	134

CHICKEN (see also CHICKEN DISHES, CHICKEN SUBSTITUTES, DINNER, HOT DOG)

FOOD	PORTION	CALS
CANNED		
chicken spread	1 serv (2 oz)	88
meat drained	1 can (5 oz)	230
w/ broth	½ can (2.5 oz)	117
Swanson		
Chunk Breast In Water	2 oz	50
Tyson		
Premium Chunk	½ can (2 oz)	60
Premium Chunk Breast	½ can (2 oz)	60
Valley Fresh		
Chunk White	2 oz	70
White & Dark Chunk	2 oz	80
FRESH		
back w/ skin roasted bones removed	1 (3.7 oz)	318
back w/o skin roasted bones removed	1 (2.8 oz)	191
breast w/ skin battered fried bones removed	½ breast (4.9 oz)	364
breast w/ skin floured fried bones removed	1 (3.4 oz)	218
breast w/ skin roasted bones removed	½ breast (3.4 oz)	193
breast w/ skin stewed bones removed	½ breast (3.9 oz)	202
breast w/o skin fried bones removed	½ breast (3 oz)	161
breast w/o skin roasted bones removed	½ breast (3 oz)	142
breast w/o skin stewed bones removed	1 (3.3 oz)	143
breast roasted diced	1 cup (5 oz)	231

FOOD	PORTION	CALS
broiler/fryer w/ skin roasted bones removed	½ (10.5 oz)	715
capon meat & skin roasted bones removed	½ (1.4 lbs)	1459
cornish hen w/ skin roasted	1 (9 oz)	668
cornish hen w/ skin roasted	½ (4.5 oz)	335
cornish hen w/o skin roasted	½ (4 oz)	147
cornish hen w/o skin roasted	1 (7.7 oz)	295
dark meat w/o skin roasted diced	1 cup (5 oz)	287
drumstick w/ skin battered floured & fried bones removed	1 (1.7 oz)	120
drumstick w/ skin battered fried bones removed	1 (2.5 oz)	193
drumstick w/ skin roasted bones removed	1 (1.8 oz)	112
drumstick w/ skin stewed bones removed	1 (2 oz)	116
drumstick w/o skin fried bones removed	1 (1.5 oz)	82
drumstick w/o skin roasted bones removed	1 (1.5 oz)	76
drumstick w/o skin stewed bones removed	1 (1.6 oz)	78
feet cooked	1 (1.2 oz)	73
ground crumbled fried	3 oz	161
ground patty cooked	1 sm (1.7 oz)	114
ground patty cooked	1 med (2.1 oz)	142
ground patty cooked	1 lg (2.8 oz)	190
meat & skin stewed bones removed	¼ chicken (4.6 oz)	372
neck w/ skin battered fried	1 (1.8 oz)	172
neck w/ skin fried	1 (1.3 oz)	120
neck w/ skin simmered	1 (1.3 oz)	94
roaster meat & skin roasted bones removed	¼ chicken (8.4 oz)	535
skin battered fried from ½ chicken	6.7 oz	749
skin floured fried from ½ chicken	2 oz	281
skin roasted from ½ chicken	2 oz	254
skin stewed from ½ chicken	2.5 oz	261
tail cooked	1 (1 oz)	84
thigh w/ skin battered & fried bones removed	1 (3 oz)	238
thigh w/ skin floured & fried bones removed	1 (2.2 oz)	162
thigh w/ skin roasted bones removed	1 (2.2 oz)	153
thigh w/ skin stewed bones removed	1 (2.4 oz)	158
thigh w/o skin fried bones removed	1 (1.8 oz)	113
thigh w/o skin roasted bones removed	1 (1.8 oz)	109
thigh w/o skin stewed bones removed	1 (1.9 oz)	107
wing w/ skin battered & fried bones removed	1 (1.7 oz)	159
wing w/ skin floured & fried bones removed	1 (1.1 oz)	103

FOOD	PORTION	CALS
wing w/ skin roasted bones removed	1 (1.2 oz)	99
wing w/o skin fried bones removed	1 (0.7 oz)	42
wing w/o skin roasted bones removed	1 (0.7 oz)	43
wing w/o skin stewed bones removed	1 (0.8 oz)	43
Murray's		
Whole Lean	4 oz	170
Tyson		
Breasts Boneless Skinless	4 oz	110
Cornish Hen	1 serv (4 oz)	200
Drumsticks	4 oz	150
Thigh Cutlets Boneless Skinless	4 oz	130
Whole Cut Up	4 oz	220
Wings	4 oz	220
FROZEN		
breast roll roasted	2 oz	75
fajita strips	1 (0.3 oz)	13
patty cooked	1 (3.5 oz)	287
Barber		
Buffalo Fingers	1 (3.3 oz)	160
Nuggets 4 Cheese Stuffed	3 (3 oz)	230
Nuggets Cheddar & Bacon Stuffed	3 (3 oz)	240
Potato Chip Sticks	2 (4.5 oz)	350
Ian's		
Fingers	3	190
Nuggets	5	190
Nuggets Allergy Free	5	190
Patties	1 (3.4 oz)	220
Organic Prairie		
Ground	4 oz	200
Whole Young Small	4 oz	260
Tyson		
Any'tizers Barbeque Style Wings	3 (3.2 oz)	200
Any'tizers Homestyle Chicken Fries	7 (3.2 oz)	230
Any'tizers Popcorn Chicken	6 (2.8 oz)	220
Breast Pattie	1 (2.6 oz)	180
Cordon Bleu	1 piece (5.9 oz)	380
Diced Strips	1 serv (3 oz)	90
Kiev	1 piece (5.9 oz)	480
Weaver		
Breast Strips	3	230

FOOD	PORTION	CALS
Breast Tenders	5	240
Buffalo Popcorn Chicken	7	230
Crispy Breast Strips	2	220
Crispy Mini Drums	5	250
Croquettes	2 + gravy	230
Honey Batter Breast Tenders	5	220
Hot Wings Buffalo Style	3	190
Nuggets	4	210
Patties Breast	1	170
Patties Italian	1	210
Patties Original	1	180
Wings Honey BBQ	3	200
Wellshire		
Chicken Bites Dinosaur Shaped Gluten Free	5	160
READY-TO-EAT		
Applegate Farms		
Organic Roasted	2 oz	60
Boar's Head		
Breast Hickory Smoked	2 oz	60
Breast Oven Roasted	2 oz	60
Butterball		
Breast Oven Roasted Thin Sliced	4 slices (2 oz)	50
Breast Strips Oven Roasted	½ pkg (3 oz)	90
Carl Buddig		
Chicken Sliced	2 oz	85
Healthy Ones		
Oven Roasted 97% Fat Free	4 slices (2 oz)	60
Hillshire Farm		
Smoked Breast	6 slices (2 oz)	60
Oscar Mayer		
Breast Oven Roasted Thin Sliced	⅓ pkg (2 oz)	60
Breast Strips Breaded	½ pkg (3 oz)	170
Breast Strips Grilled	½ pkg (3 oz)	110
Perdue		
Short Cuts Chicken Breast Honey Roasted	½ cup (2.5 oz)	90
Short Cuts Chicken Strips Fajita Style	½ cup	90
Short Cuts Grilled Chicken Breast	½ cup (2.5 oz)	90
Short Cuts Grilled Italian	½ cup	90
Short Cuts Grilled Lemon Pepper	½ cup (2.5 oz)	80

FOOD	PORTION	CALS
Sara Lee		
Breast Oven Roasted	4 slices (2 oz)	45
Tyson		
Chicken Strips Fajita	1 serv (3 oz)	110
Honey Roasted Breast	2 slices (1.6 oz)	50
Hot Wings Buffalo Style	4	220
Roasted Whole Chicken Lemon Pepper	1 serv (3 oz)	120
Salad Kit Chunk Chicken	1 pkg (3.4 oz)	210
TAKE-OUT		
chicken tenders	4 (2.2 oz)	180

CHICKEN DISHES
FROZEN
Barber		
Broccoli & Cheese Reduced Fat	1 piece (5.5 oz)	250
Cordon Bleu	1 piece (6 oz)	370
Cordon Bleu Reduced Fat	1 piece (5.5 oz)	260
Creme Brie & Apple	1 piece (6 oz)	350
Kiev	1 piece (6 oz)	430
Mashed Potato Stuffed	1 piece (6 oz)	340
Skinless Breast Stuffed	1 piece (6 oz)	280
Maple Leaf Farms		
Chicken Breast Stuffed Broccoli & Cheese	1 serv (6 oz)	340
MIX		
Chicken Helper		
Asian Chicken Fried Rice as prep	1 cup	250
Classic Creamy Chicken & Noodles as prep	1 cup	280
Jambalaya as prep	1 cup	280
REFRIGERATED		
Lunchables		
Chicken Shake-Up	1 pkg	220
Tyson		
Chicken Breast Medallions In White Wine & Garlic Sauce	1 serv (5 oz)	140
Ventera		
Rollatini w/ Rice Stuffing & Marsala Wine Sauce	1 serv + sauce (6 oz)	230
Wellshire		
Shredded Chicken In BBQ Sauce	¼ cup	70
TAKE-OUT		
arroz con pollo	1 serv (16 oz)	579

FOOD	PORTION	CALS
barbecued pulled chicken	1 serv (9 oz)	312
boneless breast w/ apple stuffing	1 serv (5 oz)	260
breast & wing breaded & fried	2 pieces (5.7 oz)	494
buffalo wing + sauce	2 (1.7 oz)	147
cacciatore breast + sauce	1 serv (5.9 oz)	323
cacciatore drumstick + sauce	1 serv (3.2 oz)	172
cacciatore thigh + sauce	1 serv (3.8 oz)	204
cacciatore wing + sauce	1 serv (2.1 oz)	113
chicharrones de pollo	3 (2.6 oz)	289
chicken & dumplings	1 cup (8.6 oz)	368
chicken & noodles in cream sauce	1 cup (8 oz)	323
chicken a la king	1 cup (8.5 oz)	465
chicken breast parmigiana	1 serv (5.8 oz)	278
chicken cordon bleu + sauce	1 serv (8 oz)	504
chicken creole w/o rice	1 cup (8.6 oz)	187
chicken kiev breast meat	1 serv (9 oz)	653
chicken meatloaf	1 lg slice (5 oz)	243
chicken paprikash	1½ cups	296
chicken pie w/ top crust	1 slice (5.6 oz)	472
chicken satay + peanut sauce	2 skewers	239
creamed chicken	1 cup (8.5 oz)	388
croquette	1 (2.2 oz)	159
curry	1 cup (8.3 oz)	288
curry breast half + sauce	1 (7 oz)	244
curry drumstick + sauce	1 (3.7 oz)	129
curry thigh + sauce	1 (4.4 oz)	154
curry wing + sauce	1 (2.4 oz)	84
drumstick & thigh breaded & fried	2 pieces (5.2 oz)	431
fricassee	1 cup (8.6 oz)	322
groundnut stew hkatenkwan	1 serv (15.7 oz)	576
jamaican jerk wings	4 (9.9 oz)	709
jambalaya w/ sausage & rice	1 cup (8.6 oz)	393
kobete turkish chicken w/ pastry	1 serv	513
sancocho de pollo dominican chicken stew	1 serv	702
stew	1 cup (8.8 oz)	176
tandoori chicken breast	1 serv	260
tandoori chicken leg & thigh	1 serv	300
tetrazzini	1 cup (8.6 oz)	369

FOOD	PORTION	CALS
CHICKEN SUBSTITUTES		
Boca		
Chik'n Nuggets	1 serv (3 oz)	180
Chik'n Patties	1 (2.5 oz)	160
Chicken Free Chicken		
Country Smoked	2 oz	80
Gardenburger		
Chik'n Grill	1 (2.5 oz)	100
Lightlife		
Smart Cutlet Seasoned Chicken	1 (4 oz)	180
Smart Menu Chick'n Nuggets	4	220
Smart Menu Chick'n Patties	1	160
Smart Menu Chick'n Strips	1 serv (3 oz)	80
Loma Linda		
Fried Chik'n w/ Gravy	2 pieces (2.8 oz)	150
Morningstar Farms		
Chik'n Roasted Herb	1 patty (2.2 oz)	110
Meal Starters Chik'n Strips	12 (3 oz)	140
Quorn		
Cutlets	1 (3.5 oz)	200
Gruyere Cutlet	1 (4 oz)	260
Naked Cutlet	1 (2.4 oz)	80
Nuggets	3–4 (3 oz)	180
Patties	1 (2.6 oz)	160
Tenders	1 cup (3 oz)	90
Veat		
Chick'n Free Nuggets	1 serv (2.5 oz)	140
Vegetarian Breast	1 (1.8 oz)	90
Viana		
Veggie Chickin Fillets	1 (3.7 oz)	260
Veggie Chickin Nuggets	3 (2.6 oz)	200
Worthington		
FriChik Original	2 pieces (3.2 oz)	140
Meatless Chicken Style	1 slice (2 oz)	90
Yves		
Meatless Chicken Burger	1 (2.6 oz)	100
Meatless Smoked Chicken Slices	4 (2.2 oz)	100
CHICKPEAS		
CANNED		
chickpeas	1 cup	285

FOOD	PORTION	CALS
Allens		
Garbanzo Beans	½ cup	120
Eden		
Organic Garbanzo	½ cup	130
Green Giant		
Garbanzo Beans	½ cup	100
Progresso		
ChickPeas	½ cup	100
DRIED		
cooked	1 cup	269
Arrowhead Mills		
Organic Dried Chickpeas not prep	¼ cup	160
REFRIGERATED		
Sabra		
Balela Vinaigrette	2 oz	100
Spicy Armenian Salad	2 oz	50
CHICORY		
endive fresh chopped	½ cup	4
greens raw chopped	½ cup	21
root raw	1 (2.1 oz)	44
roots raw cut up	½ cup (1.6 oz)	33
witloof head raw	1 (1.9 oz)	9
witloof raw	½ cup (1.6 oz)	8
Frieda's		
Belgian Endive	2 cups	115
CHILI		
powder	1 tbsp	24
Ahh!Gourmet		
Wriggly Sambal Chili Sauce Paste	4 tbsp	170
Allergaroo		
Gluten Free Chili Mac	1 pkg (8 oz)	240
Boca		
Chili w/ Ground Burger	1 pkg (9.4 oz)	150
Bush's		
ChiliMagic Chili Starter as prep	1 cup	250
Original No Beans	1 cup	240
Comfort Care		
Vegetarian White	1 cup (8 oz)	150

FOOD	PORTION	CALS
Del Monte		
Sauce	1 tbsp	20
Fantastic		
3 Bean	1 pkg (8 oz)	180
Vegetarian Mix not prep	¼ cup	100
Health Valley		
Chunky Spicy Vegetarian No Salt Added	1 cup	150
Vegetarian Spicy	1 cup	150
Heinz		
Chili Sauce	1 tbsp (0.6 oz)	20
Hunt's		
Family Favorites Chili	¼ cup (2.2 oz)	25
Lean Cuisine		
Cafe Classics Three Bean Chili	1 pkg (10 oz)	260
Lightlife		
Smart Chili	1 pkg	200
McCormick		
Mexican Style Chili Powder	¼ tsp	0
McIlhenny		
Original Recipe	½ cup	50
Mimi's Gourmet		
Organic Vegan Gluten Free 3 Bean w/ Rice	1 pkg (11.5 oz)	270
Organic Vegan Gluten Free Black Bean & Corn	1 pkg (10.5 oz)	250
Organic Vegan Gluten Free White Bean	1 pkg (10.5 oz)	230
Pacific Foods		
Beef Steak w/ Beans	1 cup	250
Ro-Tel		
Chili Fixin's	½ cup	35
Spice Hunter		
Powder Blend Salt Free	¼ tsp	0
Stagg		
Chunkero w/ Beans	1 cup	300
Classic w/ Beans	1 cup	330
Country Blend	1 cup	330
Country Blend w/ Beans	1 cup	330
Ranch House Chicken w/ Beans	1 cup	290
Silverado Beef w/ Beans	1 cup	230
Turkey Ranchero w/ Beans	1 cup	240
Vegetable Garden Four Bean	1 cup	200

FOOD	PORTION	CALS
Worthington		
Vegetarian	1 cup	280
TAKE-OUT		
chiles rellenos cheese filled	1 (5 oz)	365
chili con carne w/ beans	1 cup	264
chili con carne w/ beans & chicken	1 cup (8.9 oz)	218
con carne w/ beans & rice	1 cup	298
vegetarian con carne	1 cup	272

CHILI PEPPER (see PEPPERS)

CHINESE FOOD (see ASIAN FOOD)

CHINESE PRESERVING MELON

cooked	½ cup	11

CHIPS (see also SNACKS)

FOOD	PORTION	CALS
apple chips	10 (0.8 oz)	101
banana	1 oz	147
carrot	28 (1 oz)	95
corn	1 oz	147
plantain	1 oz	158
potato salted	1 oz	155
potato sticks	1 pkg (1 oz)	148
potato sticks	½ cup (0.6 oz)	94
potato unsalted	1 oz	152
potato unsalted reduced fat	1 oz	138
soy	1 oz	107
sweet potato	1 oz	141
taro	10 (0.8 oz)	115
tortilla lowfat baked	1 oz	118
tortilla lowfat unsalted	1 oz	118
tortilla white corn	1 oz	139
tortilla yellow corn	1 oz	139
Athenos		
Pita Chips Original	11 (1 oz)	120
Bachman		
Potato Golden Crisps	1 pkg (1 oz)	150
Bravos!		
Tortilla Nacho Cheese	1 oz	150
Brothers-All-Natural		
Potato Crisps Fresh Onion & Garlic	1 pkg	45

FOOD	PORTION	CALS
Potato Crisps Original w/ Sea Salt	1 pkg	45
Butterfield		
Potato Sticks Shoestring	1 pkg (1.7 oz)	250
Cape Cod		
Potato 40% Reduced Fat	19	130
Potato Beachside BBQ	19	150
Potato Classic	19	150
Potato Fresh Garden Herb Reduced Fat	19	130
Potato Jalapeno & Cheddar	19	140
Potato No Salt	19	150
Potato Robust Russet	19	150
Potato Salt & Vinegar	19	150
Potato Sea Salt & Cracked Pepper	19	140
Tortilla Reduced Carb	10	140
Tortilla Veggie	12	140
Corazonas		
Tortilla Jalapeno Jack	1 oz	140
Tortilla Original	1 oz	140
Tortilla Salsa Picante	1 oz	140
Doritos		
Baked Cooler Ranch	15 (1 oz)	120
Baked Nacho Cheesier	15	120
Cooler Ranch	12	140
Four Cheese	12	140
Guacamole	12	150
Light Nacho Cheesier	11	90
Natural White Nacho Cheese	11	150
Ranchero	12	150
Rollitos Cooler Ranch	17	140
Rollitos Zesty Taco	17	150
Toasted Corn	13	140
Eatsmart		
Cafe Fries Malt Vinegar & Sea Salt	1 oz	150
Cafe Fries Tangy Tomato & Spices	1 oz	150
CheddAirs	1 oz	135
Soy Crisps Parmesan Garlic & Olive Oil	1 oz	160
Soy Crisps Tomato Romano & Olive Oil	1 oz	160
Veggie Crisps	1 oz	140
Veggie Crisps Cheddar & Jalapeno	1 oz	130
Veggie Crisps Sundried Tomato & Pesto	1 oz	140

FOOD	PORTION	CALS
Eden		
Brown Rice Chips	25	150
Sea Vegetable Chips	25	140
Vegetable	25	130
Wasabi	25	130
Flat Earth		
Baked Fruit Crisps Apple Cinnamon Grove	14 (1 oz)	130
Baked Fruit Crisps Peach Mango Paradise	14 (1 oz)	130
Baked Fruit Crisps Wild Berry Patch	14 (1 oz)	130
Baked Veggie Crisps Farmland Cheddar	14 (1 oz)	130
Baked Veggie Crisps Garlic & Herb Field	14 (1 oz)	130
Baked Veggie Crisps Tangy Tomato Ranch	14 (1 oz)	130
FoodShouldTasteGood		
Tortilla Buffalo	10 (1 oz)	130
Tortilla Chocolate Gluten Free	1 pkg (1 oz)	140
Tortilla Multigrain Gluten Free	1 pkg (1 oz)	140
Tortilla Sweet Potato Gluten Free	10 (1 oz)	130
French's		
Potato Sticks Barbecue	¾ cup	160
Potato Sticks Cheddar	¾ cup	170
Potato Sticks Original	¾ cup	190
Fritos		
Corn Chips King Size	12	160
Original	32	160
Scoops	10	160
Twists	23	150
Garden Of Eatin'		
Organic Pita Baked Brown Sugar & Cinnamon	8	120
Organic Tortilla Blue Corn	7	140
Organic Tortilla Blue Corn No Salt Added	16	140
Organic Tortilla White Corn	7	140
Glenny's		
Organic Soy Barbeque	1 oz	110
Organic Soy Creamy Ranch	1 oz	110
Soy Crisps Apple Cinnamon	½ pkg (0.6 oz)	70
Soy Crisps Caramel	½ pkg (1.3 oz)	70
Soy Crisps Low Fat Lightly Salted	½ pkg (0.6 oz)	70
Soy Crisps No Salt	½ pkg (0.6 oz)	70
Soy Crisps Salt & Pepper	½ pkg (0.6 oz)	70
Soy Crisps White Cheddar	½ pkg (0.6 oz)	70

FOOD	PORTION	CALS
Spud Delites Sea Salt	1 pkg (1.1 oz)	100
Veggie Fries	½ pkg (0.6 oz)	70
Zen Health Tortilla Crisps Original	1 oz	110
Guiltless Gourmet		
Tortilla Blue Corn	18 (1 oz)	120
Tortilla Chili Lime	18 (1 oz)	120
Tortilla Chipotle	18 (1 oz)	123
Tortilla Yellow Corn	18 (1 oz)	120
Tortilla Yellow Corn Unsalted	18 (1 oz)	120
Jay's		
Potato	1 oz	150
Kettle		
Bakes Potato Aged White Cheddar	1 oz	120
Bakes Potato Hickory Honey Barbeque	1 oz	120
Bakes Potato Lightly Salted	1 oz	120
Krinkle Cut Potato Barbeque	1 oz	150
Krinkle Cut Potato Dill & Sour Cream	1 oz	150
Krinkle Cut Potato Lightly Salted	1 oz	150
Krinkle Cut Potato Salt & Fresh Ground Pepper	1 oz	150
Organic Tortilla Blue Corn	1 oz	140
Organic Tortilla Brown Rice & Black Bean w/ Garlic & Onions	1 oz	120
Organic Tortilla Fire Roasted Chili	1 oz	140
Organic Tortilla Five Grain Yellow Corn	1 oz	140
Organic Tortilla Lightly Salted Yellow Corn	1 oz	140
Organic Tortilla Little Dippers	1 oz	140
Organic Tortilla Sesame Blue Moons	1 oz	150
Potato Cheddar Beer	1 oz	150
Potato Honey Dijon	1 oz	150
Potato Sea Salt & Vinegar	1 oz	150
Potato Spicy Thai	1 oz	150
Potato Unsalted	1 oz	150
Potato Yogurt & Green Onion	1 oz	150
Lay's		
Baked KC Masterpiece	11 (1 oz)	120
Baked Sour Cream & Onion	12 (1 oz)	120
Chile Limon	1 oz	150
Classic	1 pkg (1 oz)	150
Deli Style Original	17 (1 oz)	150
Dill Pickle	20 (1 oz)	160

FOOD	PORTION	CALS
Flamin' Hot	17 (1 oz)	160
KC Masterpiece BBQ	15 (1 oz)	150
Kettle Cooked Jalapeno	15 (1 oz)	140
Kettle Cooked Mesquite BBQ	18 (1 oz)	140
Kettle Cooked Original	22 (1 oz)	150
Kettle Cooked Sea Salt & Vinegar	18 (1 oz)	140
Light Fat Free KC Masterpiece	20 (1 oz)	75
Light Fat Free Original	20 (1 oz)	75
Limon	17 (1 oz)	150
Natural Country BBQ	14 (1 oz)	150
Natural Sea Salt & Vinegar	16 (1 oz)	150
Natural Sea Salted	16 (1 oz)	150
Original Baked	11 (1 oz)	110
Salt & Vinegar	17 (1 oz)	150
Sour Cream & Onion	17 (1 oz)	160
Stax	13 (1 oz)	160
Wavy	11 (1 oz)	150
Wavy Au Gratin	13 (1 oz)	150
Wavy Hickory Barbecue	13 (1 oz)	150
Wavy Ranch	12 (1 oz)	150
Lundberg		
Rice Chips Original Sea Salt	1 oz	140
Rice Chips Sesame Seaweed	1 oz	140
Rice Chips Wasabi	1 oz	140
Madhouse Munchies		
Potato Sea Salt	16	150
Potato Sea Salt & Vinegar	16	150
Tortilla White	9	140
Manny's		
Organic Tortilla Blues	1 oz	150
Tortilla No Salt Added	1 oz	150
Maui		
Shrimp Chips	17	140
Mexi-Snax		
Tortilla Multi-Grain Blue	15 (1 oz)	140
Tortilla Pico De Gallo	15 (1 oz)	140
Tortilla Salted	15 (1 oz)	140
Tortilla Tamari	15 (1 oz)	130
Michael Season's		
Potato Crisps Thin Baked Low Fat	14	120

FOOD	PORTION	CALS
Potato Kettle Style Reduced Fat	18	130
Potato Reduced Fat	20	140
Potato Reduced Fat Unsalted	20	140
Moore's		
Corn Chips	1 oz	160
New York Deli		
Potato Kettle Cooked	1 oz	150
Popchips		
Corn Hint Of Butter	23 (1 oz)	120
Potato Barbeque	19 (1 oz)	120
Potato Original	22 (1 oz)	120
Rice Sea Salt	19 (1 oz)	120
Rice Wasabi	20 (1 oz)	120
Pringles		
Jalapeno	15 (1 oz)	150
Loaded Baked Potato	15 (1 oz)	150
Minis Cheddar Cheese	1 pkg	120
Minis Original	1 pkg	120
Original	14 (1 oz)	160
Pizza	15 (1 oz)	150
Select Cinnamon Sweet Potato	28 (1 oz)	150
Select Parmesan Garlic	28 (1 oz)	140
Snack Stacks Original	1 pkg	140
Revolution Foods		
Organic Popalongs Whole Grains Cheesy Cheese	16 (0.7 oz)	90
Organic Popalongs Whole Grains Original	16 (0.7 oz)	100
Organic Popalongs Whole Grains Simply Cinnamon	16 (0.7 oz)	100
Robert's American Gourmet		
Soy Crisps Country Barbecue	1 oz	130
Ruffles		
Baked Original	10	120
Cheddar & Sour Cream	11	160
KC Masterpiece Mesquite BBQ	11	150
Light Cheddar & Sour Cream	15	75
Light Original	17	70
Original	12	160
Potato Crisps	16	160
Reduced Fat Sea Salted	15	140

FOOD	PORTION	CALS
Sour Cream & Onion	11	160
Salba Smart		
Organic Blue Corn Omega-3 Enriched	1 oz	104
Santitas		
White Corn	9	130
Yellow Corn	9	130
Snyder's Of Hanover		
Kosher Dill	1 oz	140
MultiGrain Sunflower	1 oz	140
MultiGrain Sunflower Southwestern Cheddar	1 oz	140
MultiGrain Tortilla Lightly Salted	1 oz	130
MultiGrain Tortilla Strips Flaxseed Gold	1 oz	140
Organic Veggie Crisps	1 oz	140
Potato Original	1 oz	150
Sweet Potato Baked	1 oz	110
Tortilla Pounder Multi-Grain	1 oz	130
Tortilla White Corn	1 oz	140
Solea		
Polenta Corn	1 oz	120
Potato Olive Oil Sea Salt	1 oz	120
Stacy's		
Pita Chips Multigrain	1 pkg	140
Pita Chips Parmesan Garlic & Herb	1 oz	140
Pita Chips Texarkana Hot	1 oz	130
Soy Thin Chips Sticky Bun	18 (1 oz)	130
Soy Thin Crisps Simply Cheese	18 (1 oz)	130
SunChips		
French Onion	10	140
Original	1 pkg (1 oz)	140
Tastee		
Potato Yukon Gold	1 oz	130
Terra		
Exotic Vegetable Original	14 (1 oz)	150
Exotic Vegetable Zesty Tomato	14 (1 oz)	150
Kettles Potato Sea Salt & Pepper	15 (1 oz)	140
Parsnip Chips	12 (1 oz)	150
Potato Au Natural	18 (1 oz)	150
Potato Blues	1 oz	130
Potato Frites Sea Salt & Vinegar	1 oz	150
Potato Golds Original	1 oz	130

FOOD	PORTION	CALS
Potato Potpourri	1 oz	140
Potato Red Bliss	1 oz	140
Stix Original Exotic Vegetable	1 oz	150
Sweet Potato	17 (1 oz)	160
Sweets & Beets	16 (1 oz)	150
Taro	1 oz	140
Thunder		
Potato Buffalo Wing w/ Blue Cheese	22 (1 oz)	150
Sour Cream & Onion	22 (1 oz)	150
Tostitos		
Blue Corn	6	140
Crispy Rounds	13	140
Gold	6	140
Light Restaurant Style	6	90
Restaurant Style	6	130
Santa Fe	7	140
Scoops	13	140
Yellow Corn	6	140
Utz		
Pita Natural w/ Sea Salt	1 oz	120
Potato	20 (1 oz)	150
Potato Baked	1 oz	110
Potato BBQ	20 (1 oz)	150
Potato Grandma Kettle	1 oz	140
Potato Homestyle Kettle	1 oz	140
Potato Kettle Classics	20 (1 oz)	150
Potato Mystic Kettle	1 oz	150
Potato Mystic Kettle Reduced Fat	1 oz	130
Potato Natural Lightly Salted Kettle	1 oz	140
Potato No Salt Added	20 (1 oz)	150
Potato Onion & Garlic	1 oz	150
Potato Ripple	20 (1 oz)	150
Sweet Potato Kettle Classics	20 (1 oz)	150
Tortilla Baked	10	120
Tortilla Organic Yellow Corn	1 oz	140
Vegetable Natural Exotic Medley	1 oz	160
Wise		
Dipsy Doodles Corn Chips	1 oz	160
Potato	1 pkg (1 oz)	150
Potato Lightly Salted	1 oz	150

FOOD	PORTION	CALS
Potato Ridgies	1 oz	150
Potato Unsalted	1 oz	150

CHITTERLINGS
pork cooked	3 oz	258

CHIVES
freeze-dried	1 tbsp	1
fresh chopped	1 tbsp	1
fresh chopped	1 tsp	0

CHOCOLATE (see also CANDY, CHOCOLATE SPREAD, CHOCOLATE SYRUP, COCOA, HOT CHOCOLATE, ICE CREAM TOPPINGS, MILK DRINKS)

baking	1 oz	145
baking grated unsweetened	¼ cup	165
baking liquid unsweetened	1 oz	134
baking squares unsweetened	1 sq (1 oz)	145
chips milk chocolate	1 cup (6 oz)	862
chips semisweet	60 pieces (1 oz)	136
chips semisweet	1 cup (6 oz)	804
drink mix powder	2–3 heaping tsp	75
drink mix powder as prep w/ whole milk	9 oz	226
mexican baking	1 sq (0.7 oz)	85
Baker's		
Chips Chocolate Chunks	13 pieces (0.5 oz)	70
E. Guittard		
Chips Cappuccino	30 (0.5 oz)	80
Chips Milk Chocolate	12 (0.5 oz)	80
Chips Semisweet	30 (0.5 oz)	70
M&M's		
Baking Bits Milk Chocolate	1 tbsp	70
Baking Bits Semi-Sweet Chocolate	1 tbsp	70
Sunfood		
Organic Cacao Beans	1 oz	171
Organic Cacao Nibs	1 oz	171
Organic Powder	2 tbsp (1 oz)	120
MIX		
Nesquik		
Chocolate Powder	2 tbsp (0.6 oz)	60
Chocolate Powder No Sugar Added	2 tbsp (0.4 oz)	35

CHOCOLATE MILK (see MILK DRINKS)

FOOD	PORTION	CALS
CHOCOLATE SPREAD		
Love'n Bake		
Chocolate Schmear	2 tbsp	140
CHOCOLATE SYRUP		
chocolate fudge	1 cup (11.9 oz)	1176
chocolate fudge	1 tbsp (0.7 oz)	73
syrup	1 cup	653
syrup	2 tbsp	82
syrup as prep w/ whole milk	9 oz	232
Colac		
Chocolate Topping	1 tbsp	37
Hershey's		
Syrup	2 tbsp	100
Nesquik		
Calcium Fortified	2 tbsp (1.3 oz)	100
Smucker's		
Sundae Syrup Chocolate	2 tbsp	110
U-Bet		
Original	2 tbsp (1.4 oz)	128
CHUTNEY		
apple	1.2 oz	68
coconut	2 oz	87
fresh mint	2 oz	18
mango	¼ cup (2 oz)	227
tomato	1 oz	90
Chukar Cherries		
Curried Cherry	1 tbsp	30
Patak's		
Major Grey	1 tbsp	60
Mango Hot	1 tbsp	60
Mango Sweet	1 tbsp	60
Robert Rothschild Farm		
Hot Peach & Apple	2 tbsp	45
School House Kitchen		
Bardshar	1 oz	80
Wild Thymes Farm		
Apricot Cranberry Walnut	1 tbsp	16
Plum Currant Ginger	1 tsp	20

FOOD	PORTION	CALS
CILANTRO		
fresh	¼ cup	1
fresh sprigs	5 (5 g)	1
Dorot		
Chopped Cube frzn	1 cube (4 g)	5
CINNAMON		
cinnamon sugar	1 tsp	16
ground	1 tsp	6
sticks	0.5 oz	39
CISCO		
raw	3 oz	84
smoked	1 oz	50
CLAMS		
CANNED		
liquid only	1 cup	6
liquid only	3 oz	2
meat only	1 cup	236
meat only	3 oz	126
Brunswick		
Baby	2 oz	50
Bumble Bee		
Baby	¼ cup	50
Chopped	¼ cup	25
Minced	¼ cup	25
Smoked	¼ cup	130
Chicken Of The Sea		
Chopped	¼ cup	30
Minced	¼ cup	30
Whole Baby	¼ cup	30
Orleans		
Clam Juice	1 tbsp	0
Polar		
Baby	¼ cup	30
FRESH		
cooked	3 oz	126
cooked	20 sm	133
raw	3 oz	63
raw	20 sm (6.3 oz)	133
raw	9 lg (6.3 oz)	133

FOOD	PORTION	CALS
FROZEN		
Mrs. Paul's		
Fried	18 (3 oz)	270
TAKE-OUT		
breaded & fried	20 sm	379
CLEMENTINE JUICE		
Izze		
Sparkling Clementine	8 oz	100
CLEMENTINES		
Cuties		
Fresh	2 (6 oz)	80
Haddon House		
In Light Syrup	½ cup	80
Sunkist		
Fresh	2	80
Tina		
Fresh	1	50
CLOVES		
ground	1 tsp	7
COCOA (see also HOT CHOCOLATE)		
cocoa butter	1 tbsp	120
powder unsweetened	1 tbsp	12
COCONUT		
dried sweetened shredded	¼ cup	116
dried toasted	1 oz	168
dried unsweetened	1 oz	187
fresh from 1 coconut	14 oz	1405
fresh shredded	¼ cup	71
Bob's Red Mill		
Shredded	3 tbsp	120
Frieda's		
White	¼ cup (1.4 oz)	140
Let's Do Organic		
Organic Reduced Fat Shredded	1 can (0.5 oz)	70
Shredded	3 tbsp (0.5 oz)	110
Prosperity		
Organic Coconut Flax Butter Garlic & Onion	1 tbsp	140

FOOD	PORTION	CALS
COCONUT JUICE		
coconut water fresh	½ cup	23
creamed sweetened canned	½ cup	264
milk canned	½ cup	276
A Taste Of Thai		
Coconut Milk	⅓ cup	140
Lite Coconut Milk	⅓ cup	45
Goya		
Coconut Water	1 can (11.8 oz)	120
Let's Do Organic		
Creamed	1 oz	220
Milk	¼ cup	100
O.N.E.		
Natural Coconut Water	1 box (11 oz)	60
Vita Coco		
Coconut Water	1 box (11 oz)	65
Coconut Water w/ Fruit Juice All Flavors	1 box (11 oz)	110
COD		
atlantic canned	3 oz	89
atlantic canned	1 can (11 oz)	327
atlantic dried	3 oz	246
atlantic fresh cooked	1 fillet (6.3 oz)	189
atlantic fresh cooked	3 oz	89
atlantic fresh raw	3 oz	70
pacific fresh baked	3 oz	95
roe canned	1 oz	34
roe tarama	3.5 oz	547
Mrs. Paul's		
Fillets Lightly Breaded	1 (4 oz)	220
TAKE-OUT		
roe baked w/ butter & lemon juice	1 oz	36
COFFEE (see also COFFEE BEVERAGES, COFFEE SUBSTITUTES)		
INSTANT		
decaffeinated as prep	8 oz	2
decaffeinated powder	1 rounded tsp	4
powder	1 rounded tsp	4
REGULAR		
brewed	8 oz	2
roasted beans	1 oz	64

FOOD	PORTION	CALS
Flavia		
English Breakfast	1 bag	0
Espresso Roast	1 bag	0
French Roast	1 bag	0
French Vanilla	1 bag	0
Soy Java		
All Flavors	1 tbsp	20
Spava		
Calm Decaffeinated	1 cup	0

COFFEE BEVERAGES

FOOD	PORTION	CALS
America's Best Brew		
Iced Coffee All Flavors	8 oz	110
Cafe Sepia		
House Blend	1 bottle (6.2 oz)	80
Mocha	1 bottle (6.2 oz)	70
Cinnabon		
Latte Caramel Nut	1 can (8 oz)	170
Latte Cinnamon Vanilla	1 can (8 oz)	170
Lattes All Flavors	1 can (9.5 oz)	190
Click		
Espresso Protein Drink as prep	2 scoops (1.1 oz)	120
Cool Java		
Cappuccino Dark Roast	1 bottle (11 oz)	190
Cappuccino French Vanilla	1 bottle (11 oz)	190
Cappuccino Mocha	1 bottle (11 oz)	190
Double Bean Elixir		
Coffee Soda All Flavors	8 oz	90
Double Hit		
Maximum Energy Coffee Drink	1 can (12 oz)	80
Frappio		
Iced Coffee Energy Drink	1 can (15 oz)	260
Froid		
Original or French Vanilla	1 bottle (11 oz)	180
General Foods		
International Coffees Cafe Francais	1 serv	60
International Coffees Cafe Vienna	1 serv	70
International Coffees Cafe Vienna Sugar Free	1 serv	30
International Coffees Creme Caramel	1 serv	60
International Coffees French Vanilla Cafe	1 serv	60

FOOD	PORTION	CALS
International Coffees French Vanilla Sugar & Fat Free Decaffeinated	1 serv	30
International Coffees French Vanilla Sugar Free	1 serv	30
International Coffees Italian Cappuccino	1 serv	50
International Coffees Orange Cappuccino	1 serv	70
International Coffees Suisse Mocha	1 serv	60
International Coffees Suisse Mocha Decaffeinated Sugar Free	1 serv	30
International Coffees Suisse Mocha Sugar Free	1 serv	30
International Coffees Swiss White Chocolate	1 serv	70
International Coffees Vanilla Creme Decaffeinated	1 serv	60
International Coffees Vanilla Creme Decaffeinated Sugar Free	1 serv	35
International Coffees Viennese Chocolate Cafe	1 serv	50
Godiva		
Latte French Vanilla	1 bottle (12 oz)	200
Mocha Dark Chocolate	1 bottle (16 oz)	200
Iced 'Spresso		
Ultra Light American Vanilla	1 bottle (9.5 oz)	90
Ultra Light Espresso Latte	1 bottle (9.5 oz)	70
Loco-Joe		
Iced Coffee	1 box (8.25 oz)	160
O.N.E.		
Coffee Berry	1 bottle (11 oz)	107
Shock		
Latte	8 oz	150
Triple Latte	1 can (8 oz)	125
Triple Mocha	1 can (8 oz)	125
Starbucks		
DoubleShot	1 (6.5 oz)	140
Stomping Grounds		
Latte Caramel not prep	⅓ cup	70
Latte Espresso not prep	⅓ cup	35
Latte Mocha not prep	⅓ cup	60
Latte Vanilla not prep	⅓ cup	60
Tully's Coffee		
Bellaccino All Flavors	1 bottle (9.5 oz)	210

FOOD	PORTION	CALS
Wolfgang Puck		
Gourmet Heated Lattes All Flavors	1 can (10 oz)	100
TAKE-OUT		
cafe amaretto w/ alcohol	1 serv	192
cafe au lait	1 cup (8 oz)	77
cafe brulot	1 cup	48
cafe brulot w/ alcohol	1 serv	130
cafe con leche	1 cup (6 oz)	104
cappuccino	1 cup (8 oz)	77
cuban coffee w/ rum & creme de cacao	1 (9 oz)	112
dutch coffee w/ gin	1 (7 oz)	181
espresso	1 cup (4 oz)	2
french coffee w/ orange liqueur & kahlua	1 (8 oz)	232
irish coffee	1 serv (8 oz)	209
italian coffee w/ strega	1 (7 oz)	163
latte w/ skim milk	1 serv (13 oz)	88
latte w/ whole milk	1 serv (14 oz)	143
mocha	1 serv (17 oz)	403
puerto rican coffee w/ rum & kahlua	1 (8 oz)	166
turkish	1 cup (4 oz)	50

COFFEE SUBSTITUTES
Pixie

Mate Latte Chai	½ cup (4 oz)	80
Mate Latte Dark Roast	½ cup (4 oz)	70
Mate Latte Mocha	½ cup (4 oz)	70
Mate Latte Original	½ cup (4 oz)	70

Teeccino

Herbal Coffee All Flavors	1 cup	15

COFFEE WHITENERS
Coffee-Mate

Half & Half Original	2 tbsp	40
Half & Half Vanilla	2 tbsp	60
Latte Classic	2 tbsp	100
Latte Mocha	2 tbsp	90
Latte Vanilla	2 tbsp	90
Liquid All Flavors	1 tbsp	40
Liquid French Vanilla Fat Free	1 tbsp	10
Liquid Original	1 tbsp	20
Liquid Original Fat Free	1 tbsp	10

FOOD	PORTION	CALS
Liquid Original Low Fat	1 tbsp	10
Original Lite Powder	1 tsp	10
Original Powder	1 tsp	10
Sugar Free All Flavors	1 tbsp	15
Farmland		
Nondairy Creamer	2 tbsp	40
Hood		
Country Creamer Non Dairy	1 tbsp	20
International Delight		
Amaretto	1 tbsp	40
Fat Free Amaretto	1 tbsp	30
Fat Free French Vanilla	1 tbsp	30
Fat Free Irish Creme	1 tbsp	30
French Vanilla	1 tbsp	45
Sugar Free French Vanilla	1 tbsp	20
WildWood		
Soymilk Creamer Plain	1 tbsp	15

COLESLAW
Dole

Classic Cole Slaw	1½ cups (3 oz)	25
Fresh Express		
3 Color Deli	1½ cups	20
Kit w/ Sweet & Creamy Dressing	3 cups	120
Old Fashioned	2 cups	25
Mann's		
Broccoli Cole Slaw w/o Dressing	1 serv (3 oz)	25
River Ranch		
Country Homestyle Kit	1 cup	140
Honey Dijon Peppercorn Kit	1 cup	120
Mix	1¼ cups	25
TAKE-OUT		
coleslaw w/ dressing	¾ cup	147
vinegar & oil coleslaw	3.5 oz	150

COLLARDS

fresh cooked	½ cup	17
frzn chopped cooked	½ cup	31
raw chopped	½ cup	6
Allens		
Seasoned	½ cup	35

FOOD	PORTION	CALS
Glory		
Green Fresh	2 cups	25
Seasoned canned	½ cup	35
Sensibly Seasoned canned	½ cup	20

COOKIES
MIX

FOOD	PORTION	CALS
chocolate chip	1 (0.56 oz)	79
oatmeal	1 (0.6 oz)	74
oatmeal raisin	1 (0.6 oz)	74
Aunt Paula's		
Low Carb Chef Peanut Butter as prep	1	66
Bob's Red Mill		
Gluten Free Chocolate Chip as prep	2	260
Keto		
Chocolate Chip as prep	1	47
Oatmeal Raisin as prep	2	59
King Arthur		
Chocolate Chip Whole Grain not prep	2 tbsp	90
Nature's Path		
Organic Chocolate Chip	⅒ pkg	150
Pillsbury		
Ready To Bake Chocolate Chip Sugar Free	1	90
READY-TO-EAT		
animal crackers	1 (2.5 g)	11
animal crackers	11 (1 oz)	126
animal crackers	1 box (2.4 oz)	299
australian anzac biscuit	1	98
butter	1 (5 g)	23
chocolate chip	1 (0.4 oz)	48
chocolate chip	1 box (1.9 oz)	233
chocolate chip low fat	1 (0.25 oz)	45
chocolate chip low sugar low sodium	1 (0.24 oz)	31
chocolate chip soft-type	1 (0.5 oz)	69
chocolate w/ creme filling	1 (0.35 oz)	47
chocolate w/ creme filling chocolate coated	1 (0.60 oz)	82
chocolate w/ creme filling sugar free low sodium	1 (0.35 oz)	46
chocolate w/ extra creme filling	1 (0.46 oz)	65
chocolate wafer	1 (0.2 oz)	26
cream cheese	1 (1.1 oz)	141

FOOD	PORTION	CALS
digestive biscuits plain	2	141
fig bars	1 (0.56 oz)	56
fortune	1 (0.28 oz)	30
fudge	1 (0.73 oz)	73
gingersnaps	1 (0.24 oz)	29
graham	1 sq (0.24 oz)	30
graham chocolate covered	1 (0.49 oz)	68
graham honey	1 (0.24 oz)	30
hermits	1 (1 oz)	117
jumbles coconut	1 (1 oz)	121
ladyfingers	1 (0.38 oz)	40
macaroons	1 (0.8 oz)	97
madeleines	1 (0.8 oz)	86
marshmallow chocolate coated	1 (0.46 oz)	55
marshmallow pie chocolate coated	1 (1.4 oz)	165
molasses	1 (0.5 oz)	65
neapolitan tri-color cookie	1 (0.6 oz)	79
oatmeal	1 (0.6 oz)	81
oatmeal soft-type	1 (0.5 oz)	61
oatmeal raisin	1 (0.6 oz)	81
oatmeal raisin low sugar no sodium	1 (0.24 oz)	31
oatmeal raisin soft-type	1 (0.5 oz)	61
peanut butter sandwich	1 (0.5 oz)	67
peanut butter sandwich sugar free low sodium	1 (0.35 oz)	54
peanut butter soft-type	1 (0.5 oz)	69
pinenut cookies	1 (1.1 oz)	134
raisin soft-type	1 (0.5 oz)	60
reginette queen's biscuit	1 (0.8 oz)	86
shortbread	1 (0.28 oz)	40
shortbread pecan	1 (0.49 oz)	79
spritz	1 (0.4 oz)	42
sugar	1 (0.52 oz)	72
sugar low sugar sodium free	1 (0.24 oz)	30
sugar wafers w/ creme filling	1 (0.12 oz)	18
sugar wafers w/ creme filling sugar free sodium free	1 (0.14 oz)	20
toll house original	1 (0.8 oz)	105
vanilla sandwich	1 (0.35 oz)	48
vanilla wafers	1 (0.21 oz)	28
zeppole	1 (0.8 oz)	78

FOOD	PORTION	CALS
ABC		
Vegan Colossal Chocolate Chip	1 (2.1 oz)	240
Vegan Double Chocolate Decadence	1 (2.1 oz)	240
Vegan Luscious Lemon Poppyseed	1 (2.1 oz)	240
Vegan Mac The Chip	1 (2.1 oz)	250
Vegan Peanut Butter Chocolate Chip	1 (2.1 oz)	240
Vegan Phenomenal Pumpkin Spice	1 (2.1 oz)	220
Alex & Dani's		
Original Hazelnut	3 (1 oz)	130
Annie's Homegrown		
Bunny Grahams All Flavors	26	130
Archway		
Frosty Lemon	1 (0.9 oz)	110
Fruit Filled Raspberry	1 (0.8 oz)	90
Arico		
Gluten Free Casein Free Almond Cranberry	1 bar (1.4 oz)	140
Gluten Free Casein Free Double Chocolate	1 (0.9 oz)	100
Gluten Free Casein Free Lemon Ginger	1 (0.9 oz)	90
Gluten Free Casein Free Peanut Butter	1 bar (1.4 oz)	160
Arrowroot		
Biscuit	1 (5 g)	20
Back To Nature		
Chocolate Chunk	2	130
Crispy Oatmeal	2	120
Sandwich Chocolate & Mint Creme	2	130
Sandwich Classic Creme	2	130
Bahlsen		
Butter Leaves	7 (1 oz)	140
Hit Minis Chocolate Filled	5 (1.2 oz)	170
Nuss Dessert	3 (1.1 oz)	170
Barbara's Bakery		
Fig Bars Traditional	1	60
Fig Bars Wheat Free	1	60
Organic 100 Calorie Mini Ginger	1 pkg (0.9 oz)	100
Snackimals Chocolate Chip	10	120
Snackimals Wheat Free Oatmeal	10	120
Barnum's		
Animal Crackers	10 (1 oz)	120
Bolands		
Custard Creams	1	62

FOOD	PORTION	CALS
Breaktime		
Ginger	4 (1 oz)	130
Oatmeal	4 (1 oz)	130
Brown & Haley		
Almond Roca	6 (1 oz)	110
Buzz Strong's		
Real Coffee	1 (1.2 oz)	150
Cameo		
Sandwich Creme	2 (1 oz)	130
Chips Ahoy!		
Chocolate Chip	1 pkg (1.4 oz)	190
Mini	1 pkg (1.2 oz)	170
Reduced Fat	1 pkg (1.1 oz)	140
Comfort Care		
Cabin Hearth Chocolate Chip	1 (2 oz)	250
Cabin Hearth Oatmeal Peach	1 (2 oz)	200
Cabin Hearth Oatmeal Raisin	1 (2 oz)	200
Country Choice Organic		
Fit Kids Snackin' Grahams Chocolate	18 (1 oz)	110
Oatmeal Chocolate Chip	1 (0.8 oz)	100
Oatmeal Raisin	1 (0.8 oz)	100
Crummy		
Organic Chocolate Chip	1 (2 oz)	240
Organic Lavender Chocolate Chip	1 (2 oz)	240
Dare		
Lemon Creme	1 (0.7 oz)	100
Maple Leaf Creme	1 (0.6 oz)	80
David's		
Hamantash Raspberry	1 (0.7 oz)	85
De Beukelaer		
Pirouline	8 (1 oz)	130
DiCamillo		
Biscotti DiPrato	5 (1 oz)	130
Divvies		
Chocolate Chip Vegan	1	130
Oatmeal Raisin Vegan	1	120
Doritos		
Barras De Coco	5	120
Dove		
Beyond Chocolate Chunk	1 (0.7 oz)	110

FOOD	PORTION	CALS
Chocolate Walnut Rendezous	1 (0.7 oz)	110
Milk Chocolate Moment	3 (1.1 oz)	160
Mint Chocolate Serenade	3 (1.1 oz)	160
Earthbound Farm		
Organic Ginger Snaps	2	120
Elite		
Tea Biscuits Chocolate	4	80
Emily's		
Fortune Dark Chocolate Covered	2 (1.4 oz)	140
Graham Cracker Milk Chocolate Covered	1 (1 oz)	150
Enjoy Life		
Allergen Gluten Free Gingerbread Spice	2 (1 oz)	100
Allergen Gluten Free No Oats Oatmeal	2 (1 oz)	120
Allergen Gluten Free Snickerdoodle	2 (1 oz)	130
Snack Bar Sunbutter Crunch	1 (1 oz)	140
Entenmann's		
Original Chocolate Chip	3	140
Soft Baked Chocolate Chunk	1 (1.3 oz)	190
Estee		
Fructose Sweetened Chocolate Chip	4	160
Fructose Sweetened Lemon	4	160
Fructose Sweetened Sandwich Chocolate	3	170
Fructose Sweetened Sandwich Original	3	170
Fructose Sweetened Sandwich Peanut Butter	3	190
Fructose Sweetened Vanilla	4	160
Fructose Sweetened Vanilla Sandwich	3	170
Sugar Free Chocolate Chip	3	110
Sugar Free Lemon	3	110
Sugar Free Wafer Chocolate Creme	4	150
Sugar Free Wafer Lemon Creme	4	150
Sugar Free Wafer Peanut Butter Creme	4	150
Sugar Free Wafer Strawberry Creme	4	150
Sugar Free Wafer Vanilla Creme	4	150
Fauchon		
Assorted Chocolate	4 (2 oz)	330
Fox's		
Golden Crunch Creams	1	75
French Meadow Bakery		
Gluten Free Chocolate Chip	1 (1.3 oz)	190

FOOD	PORTION	CALS
Frieda's		
Asian Almond	2 (1 oz)	170
Gak's Snacks		
Organic Brownie Chip	1 (1 oz)	130
Organic Chocolate Chip	1 (1 oz)	140
Organic Oatmeal	1 (1 oz)	120
Gamesa		
Animalitos	14	110
Arcoiris Marshmallow	2	120
Arcoiris Merengue	6	200
Emperador Chocolate	2	120
Emperador Fresa	2	120
Emperador Limon	6	270
Emperador Vanilla	2	120
Hawaianas	3	130
Marias	8	120
Ricanelas	8	140
Roscas	3	130
Sugar Wafers Chocolate	3	160
Sugar Wafers Strawberry	3	160
Ginger Snaps		
Cookies	4 (1 oz)	120
Girl Scout		
Cafe Cookies	5	150
Lemon Cooler Reduced Fat	5	130
Samoas	2	150
Tagalongs	2	130
Thin Mints	4	140
Trefoils	4	130
Gluten-Free Pantry		
Gluten Free Buckwheat Raisin	1 (1 oz)	140
Gluten Free Chocolate Chunk	1 (1 oz)	140
Glutino		
Gluten Free Wafers Chocolate	4	160
Gluten Free Wafers Lemon	3	150
Gottena		
Exquisit	5	170
Gourmet Pastries		
Kourabiethes Butter Almond	1 (1.1 oz)	150
Phoenicia Honey & Spice	1 (1.3 oz)	140

FOOD	PORTION	CALS
Grandma's		
Homestyle Big Chocolate Chip	1 (1.4 oz)	190
Homestyle Big Fudge Chocolate Chip	1 (1.4 oz)	170
Homestyle Big Oatmeal Raisin	1 (1.4 oz)	180
Homestyle Big Peanut Butter	1 (1.4 oz)	200
Mini Vanilla Creme	9	150
Peanut Butter Sandwich	5	210
Rich N'Chewy Chocolate Chip	1 pkg	270
Vanilla Creme Sandwich	5	210
Health Valley		
Mini Mint Chocolate Chip	4 (1 oz)	120
Oatmeal Raisin	1 (0.8 oz)	90
Raisin Oatmeal Low Fat	3	110
White Chocolate Chunk	1 (1 oz)	140
Healthy Handfuls		
Organic Crocodile Cookies	1 pkg (1 oz)	130
Organic Koala Krackers	1 pkg (1 oz)	120
Home Free		
Organic Chocolate Chip	1 (1 oz)	140
Organic Oatmeal	1 (1 oz)	120
Honey Maid		
Grahams Honey	1 (1.1 oz)	130
Grahams Honey Low Fat	1 (1.1 oz)	120
Jacob's		
Oat Crumbles Chocolate & Pecan	1	107
Joseph's		
Almond Sugar Free	4	100
Chocolate Chip Sugar Free	4	95
Lemon Sugar Free	4	95
Oatmeal Chocolate Chip w/ Pecans Sugar Free	4	100
Peanut Butter Sugar Free	4	95
Kashi		
TLC Happy Trail Mix	1 (1 oz)	130
TLC Oatmeal Raisin Flax	1 (1 oz)	130
TLC Oatmeal Dark Chocolate	1 (1 oz)	130
Kedem		
Tea Biscuits Orange	2	32

FOOD	PORTION	CALS
Keebler		
100 Calorie Pack RightBites Sandies Shortbread	1 pkg (0.7 oz)	100
Animal Crackers Frosted	8	150
Chips Deluxe Chocolate Lovers	1	90
Chips Deluxe Coconut	2	150
Chips Deluxe Fudge Stripes	1	100
Chips Deluxe Original	1 pkg (2 oz)	300
Chocolate Dip & Cookie Sticks	1 pkg (1 oz)	130
Danish Wedding	4	130
Dipping Delights Cheesecake	1	90
E.L. Fudge Original	1	90
Fudge Shoppe Fudge Stripes	3	150
Fudge Shoppe Grasshoppers	4	140
Fudge Shoppe Mint Creme Filled	2	160
Graham Honey	8 (1 oz)	110
Graham Original	8 (1 oz)	130
Oatmeal Country Style	2	130
Sandies Drops Butter Pecan	4	140
Sandies Fudge Drops	4 (1 oz)	140
Sandies Pecan Shortbread Reduced Fat	1	80
Scooby-Doo Graham Sticks	9	130
S'mores Snack	1 pkg (0.8 oz)	110
Soft Batch Chocolate Chip	1	80
Vanilla Wafers	8	140
Vienna Fingers	2	150
Vienna Fingers Reduced Fat	2	140
Khaya		
Krunchi Orange & Chocolate	5 (1.53 oz)	240
Shortbread Grapeseed	13 (1.15 oz)	193
Shortbread Orange Rooibos	13 (1.15 oz)	259
La Choy		
Fortune	4 (1 oz)	110
Lance		
Oatmeal Creme	1 (2.5 oz)	300
Van-O-Lunch	1 pkg (1.6 oz)	230
Late July		
Organic Sandwich Dark Chocolate	3 (1.2 oz)	150
Organic Sandwich Vanilla Bean w/ Green Tea	2 (0.8 oz)	110

FOOD	PORTION	CALS
Laura's Wholesome Junk Food		
Anna Banana Split	1	105
Gluten Free Charlotte's Chocolate Chip	2	120
Gluten Free Sally's Raisin	2	110
Lemon Vanilla	2	120
Oatmeal Chocolate Chip	2	110
Oatmeal Raisin	2	100
Wheat Free X-Treme Chocolate Fudge	2	110
Lean Body		
Cookie Bar Hi-Protein S'Mores	1 (3.2 oz)	360
Lee's		
Dreamy Mallows	2	150
Leibniz		
Butter Biscuits	6	130
Liz Lovely		
Vegan Cowboy	½ cookie (1.3 oz)	190
Vegan Cowgirl	½ cookie (1.5 oz)	210
Vegan Ginger Snapdragons	½ cookie (1.5 oz)	190
Lorna Doone		
Shortbread	4 (1 oz)	140
LU		
Le Chocolatier	3 (1 oz)	150
Le Fondant	4 (1.1 oz)	170
Le Petit Beurre	4 (1.2 oz)	140
Le Petit Ecolier Milk Chocolate	2 (0.9 oz)	130
Le Petit Fruit Strawberry	5 (1.2 oz)	110
Pim's Sensation Bar Chocolate	1	110
Shortbread	2 (1 oz)	140
M&M's		
Milk Chocolate	1 pkg (1.15 oz)	150
Mallomars		
Cookies	2	120
Miss Meringue		
Chocolettes Crunchy Chocolate	4	110
Chocolettes Strawberry Vanilla	4	130
Classiques Cappuccino	4	110
Classiques Chocolate Chip	4	120
Classiques Dulce De Leche Artisan	4	110
Macaroons Traditional	1 (1.3 oz)	180
Madeleines Traditional	2 (1.2 oz)	160

FOOD	PORTION	CALS
Minis Vanilla	13 (1.1 oz)	110
Minis Vanilla Sugar Free	13	35
Montana Monster Munchies		
Original	½ (1.4 oz)	177
Raisin	½ (1.4 oz)	172
Moon Pie		
Mini All Flavors	1 pkg (1.2 oz)	130
Murray's		
Sugar Free Chocolate Sandwich	3 (1 oz)	130
Sugar Free Chocolate Chip	3 (1.1 oz)	160
Sugar Free Fudge Dipped Grahams	4 (1 oz)	150
Sugar Free Ginger Snap	7 (1.1 oz)	130
Sugar Free Oatmeal	3 (1.1 oz)	140
Sugar Free Shortbread	8 (1 oz)	130
Nabisco		
100 Calorie Pack Alpha-Bits Mini	1 pkg	100
100 Calorie Pack Barnum's Animal Choco	1 pkg	100
100 Calorie Pack Lorna Doone	1 pkg	100
100 Calorie Pack Teddy Grahams Mini Cinnamon	1 pkg	100
Biscos Sugar Wafers	8 (1 oz)	140
Social Tea	6	140
Nana's		
No Gluten Berry Vanilla	1 bar (1.2 oz)	130
No Gluten Chocolate	1 (3.5 oz)	360
No Gluten Ginger	1 (3.5 oz)	360
No Gluten Nana Banana	1 bar (1.2 oz)	130
No Wheat Oatmeal Raisin	1 (3.5 oz)	280
Vegan Chocolate Chip	1 (4 oz)	320
Vegan Peanut Butter	1 (4 oz)	360
Vegan Sunflower	1 (3.5 oz)	380
Natural Ovens		
Oatmeal Raisin	1 (1.3 oz)	120
Nature's Path		
Organic Signature Lemon Poppyseed	4	130
Organic Animal Vanilla	9	120
New York Style		
Biscotti Almond	3 (1 oz)	130

FOOD	PORTION	CALS
Newman's Own		
Organic Champion Chip Chocolate Chocolate Chip	4	160
Organic Champion Chip Chocolate Chip	4	160
Organic Champion Chip Double Chocolate Mint Chip	4	160
Organic Champion Chip Espresso Chocolate Chip	4	150
Organic Champion Chip Orange Chocolate Chip	4	160
Organic Champion Chip Wheat Free Dairy Free	4	160
Organic Fig Newmans Fat Free	2	120
Organic Fig Newmans Low Fat	2	140
Organic Fig Newmans Wheat Free Dairy Free	2	120
Organic Newman-O's Chocolate Creme	2	130
Organic Newman-O's Ginger-O's	2	120
Organic Newman-O's Mint Creme	2	130
Organic Newman-O's Original	2	130
Organic Newman-O's Tops & Bottoms	6	120
Organic Newman-O's Wheat Free Dairy Free	2	130
Newtons		
Fig	2 (1.1 oz)	110
Fig 100% Whole Grain	2 (1.3 oz)	130
Fig Fat Free	2 (1 oz)	90
Raspberry	2 (1 oz)	100
Nilla Wafers		
Cookies	1 oz	140
Reduced Fat	1 oz	110
Nonni's		
Biscotti Cioccolati	1 (0.8 oz)	110
Biscotti Limone	1 (0.8 oz)	110
Biscotti Original	1 (0.7 oz)	90
NutraBalance		
High Fibre	1 (0.7 oz)	90
Nutter Butter		
Bites	1 pkg (1.2 oz)	170
Sandwich Cookie	1 (1 oz)	130
Oreo		
Cakesters	2 (2 oz)	250

FOOD	PORTION	CALS
Cakesters Mini Golden 100 Calorie Pack	1 pkg (0.8 oz)	100
Double Stuff	1 (1 oz)	140
Mini	1 pkg (1.2 oz)	160
Sandwich Cookie	2 (1.2 oz)	160
Pepperidge Farm		
Chantilly Raspberry	2	120
Chessmen	3 (0.9 oz)	120
Dark Chocolate Mint Chocolate Chunk	1	140
Gingerman	4	130
Medallion Milk Chocolate	5	160
Milano	3	180
Milano French Vanilla	2	130
Milano Mint Chocolate Covered	4	130
Milano Sugar Free	3	170
Nantucket Chocolate Dipped	1	150
Nantucket Dark Chocolate Chunk	1	140
Pirouettes Cappuccino	2	120
Pirouettes Chocolate Mint	2	120
Pirouettes Vanilla Cream	3 (1.1 oz)	133
Sausalito Milk Chocolate Macadamia Nut	1	140
Shortbread	2	140
Soft Baked Milk Chocolate	1	150
Soft Baked Oatmeal Cranberry	1	130
Soft Baked Sugar	1	140
Tahiti	2	170
Verona Apricot Raspberry	3	140
Polar		
Fortune	2	56
Quaker		
Breakfast Cookie Oatmeal Raisin	1	180
Right Direction		
Chocolate Chip	1	60
Ruger		
Wafers Vanilla	3 (1 oz)	160
SnackWell's		
Cookie Cakes Chocolate Mint	1 (0.6 oz)	50
Creme Sandwich	1 pkg (1.7 oz)	210
Devil's Food Fat Free	1 (0.5 oz)	50
Sugar Free Lemon Creme	2 (1.1 oz)	130
Sugar Free Shortbread	2 (1 oz)	130

FOOD	PORTION	CALS
Snikiddy		
Cherry Oaties	1 pkg (0.8 oz)	110
South Beach		
Fiber Fit Double Chocolate Chunk	1 pkg (0.8 oz)	100
Fiber Fit Oatmeal Chocolate Chunk	1 pkg (0.8 oz)	100
Wafer Sticks Dark Chocolate Hazelnut Creme	1 pkg	100
Wafer Sticks Dark Chocolate Peanut Butter	1 pkg	100
Stella D'Oro		
100 Calorie Pack Breakfast Treats Original	1 pkg (0.8 oz)	100
Almond Delight	1 (1 oz)	150
Angelica Goodies	1 (0.7 oz)	90
Anginetti	4 (1.1 oz)	130
Biscotti Almond	1 (0.7 oz)	90
Biscotti French Vanilla	1 (0.7 oz)	90
Breakfast Treats Chocolate	1 (0.9 oz)	110
Breakfast Treats Original	1 (0.7 oz)	90
Coffee Treats Almond Toast	2 (0.9 oz)	100
Coffee Treats Angel Wings	3 (1 oz)	160
Coffee Treats Anisette Sponge	2 (0.9 oz)	90
Coffee Treats Anisette Toast	3 (1.2 oz)	130
Coffee Treats Roman Egg Biscuits	1 (1.1 oz)	130
Egg Jumbo	3 (1.2 oz)	120
Lady Stella	3 (1 oz)	130
Margherite	2 (1 oz)	130
Swiss Fudge	3 (1.2 oz)	170
Teddy Grahams		
Chocolate	24 (1.1 oz)	130
Honey	24 (1 oz)	130
Temptations		
Chocolate Alps	1 bar (1.6 oz)	170
Chocolate Mocha	1 bar (1.6 oz)	170
No Gluten Chocolate Rush	1 bar (1.6 oz)	170
Voortman		
Chinese Almond	1 (0.9 oz)	130
Coconut Delight	1 (0.6 oz)	90
Dutch Creme	1 (0.8 oz)	110
Fudge Swirl	1 (0.6 oz)	80
Gingerboy	1 (0.7 oz)	100
Maple Leaf	1 (0.6 oz)	90
Molasses	1 (1 oz)	110

FOOD	PORTION	CALS
Oatmeal Apple	1 (0.7 oz)	90
Peanut Delight	1 (0.9 oz)	130
Shortbread	1 (0.6 oz)	90
Sugar Free Chocolate Chip	1 (0.7 oz)	80
Sugar Free Lemon Wafers	3 (1 oz)	130
Sugar Free Vanilla Creme	2 (0.7 oz)	100
Sugar Free Wafers Peanut Butter	4 (1 oz)	150
Sugar Free Wafers Vanilla	3 (1 oz)	130
Turnover Blueberry	1 (0.9 oz)	110
Turnover Cherry	1 (0.9 oz)	110
Turnover Strawberry	1 (0.9 oz)	110
Wafer Chocolate Covered	1 (0.7 oz)	100
Wafer Vanilla	3 (1 oz)	140
Wafers Mini Chocolate	5 (1 oz)	130
Walkers		
Shortbread	1	100
Whippet		
Original	2 (1.2 oz)	150
World Of Grains		
Apple Cinnamon	1 pkg	130
Cranberry	1 pkg	130
Multigrain	1 pkg	130
Zwieback		
Toast	1 (8 g)	35
REFRIGERATED		
chocolate chip	1 (0.42 oz)	59
chocolate chip unbaked	1 oz	126
oatmeal	1 (0.4 oz)	56
oatmeal raisin	1 (0.4 oz)	56
peanut butter	1 (0.4 oz)	60
peanut butter dough	1 oz	130
sugar	1 (0.42 oz)	58
sugar dough	1 oz	124
Pillsbury		
Chocolate Chip	2 (1.3 oz)	170
Gingerbread	2 (1.1 oz)	170
Oatmeal Chocolate Chip	2 (1.3 oz)	170
Peanut Butter	2 (1 oz)	130
S'Mores	2 (1.3 oz)	160
Sugar	2 (1.3 oz)	170

FOOD	PORTION	CALS
TAKE-OUT		
biscotti w/ nuts chocolate dipped	1 (1.3 oz)	117
black & white	1 lg (3 oz)	302
finikia	1 (1.2 oz)	171
koulourakia butter cookie twist	1 (0.9 oz)	113
linzer tart	1 (2.4 oz)	280
CORIANDER		
cilantro fresh	1 tsp (2 g)	tr
leaf dried	1 tsp	2
leaf fresh	¼ cup	1
seed	1 tsp	5
CORN		
CANNED		
cream style	½ cup	93
w/ red & green peppers	½ cup	86
white	½ cup	66
yellow	½ cup	66
Del Monte		
Cream Style	½ cup	60
Cream Style No Salt Added	½ cup	60
Fiesta	½ cup	50
Gold & White	½ cup	80
Savory Sides In Butter Sauce	½ cup	90
Savory Sides Santa Fe	½ cup	70
Summer Crisp	½ cup	70
White	½ cup	60
Green Giant		
Mexicorn	⅓ cup	70
Super Sweet Yellow & White	⅓ cup	60
Orchids		
Whole Young Spears	½ cup (4.6 oz)	25
FRESH		
white cooked	½ cup	89
white raw	½ cup	66
yellow cooked	1 ear (2.7 oz)	83
yellow cooked	½ cup	89
yellow raw	1 ear (3 oz)	77
yellow raw	½ cup	66

FOOD	PORTION	CALS
FROZEN		
cooked	½ cup	67
on the cob cooked	1 ear (2.2 oz)	59
Birds Eye		
Steamfresh Singles Super Sweet	1 pkg (3.2 oz)	80
Steamfresh Southwestern	⅔ cup (2.9 oz)	90
Steamfresh Sweet Mini Corn On The Cob	1 (3 oz)	90
C&W		
Cheddar Bacon	½ cup	130
Early Harvest Supersweet Petite	⅔ cup	70
Salsa Corn	1 cup	90
Europe's Best		
Baby Sweet	⅔ cup	50
Glory		
Savory Accents Fried Corn	½ cup	110
Green Giant		
Cream Style	½ cup	110
Nibblers On-The-Cob	1 (2.1 oz)	70
Niblets & Butter Sauce Low Fat	⅔ cup	110
Pictsweet		
Cut Corn	⅔ cup	100
Roast Works		
Flame Roasted Cob Corn	1 cob (3 oz)	130
Stouffer's		
Souffle	½ pkg (6 oz)	150
TAKE-OUT		
fritters	1 (1 oz)	62
on the cob w/ butter cooked	1 ear	155
scalloped	1 cup	257

CORN CHIPS (see CHIPS)

CORNISH HEN (see CHICKEN)

CORNMEAL

cornmeal mush as prep w/ water	1 cup	223
cornmeal yellow	½ cup (2.2 oz)	236
whole grain blue	½ cup (1.9 oz)	201
yellow self-rising	½ cup (3 oz)	296
Indian Head		
Stone Ground	¼ cup	100

FOOD	PORTION	CALS
Martha White		
White Self Rising	3 tbsp (1.1 oz)	100
Yellow	3 tbsp (1.1 oz)	110
McKenzie's		
Hush Puppies	1 serv (1.9 oz)	190
Quaker		
Quick Grits not prep	¼ cup	130
TAKE-OUT		
corn pone	1 piece (2.1 oz)	128
fritter puerto rican style	1 (1.4 oz)	109
harina de maiz con coco	½ cup	383
harina de maize con leche	1 cup	295
hush puppies	1 (0.8 oz)	74
johnnycake	1 piece (1.7 oz)	134
CORNSTARCH		
cornstarch	1 cup (4.5 oz)	488
Argo		
Cornstarch	1 tbsp	30
Bob's Red Mill		
Cornstarch	1 tbsp	30
Kingsford's		
Cornstarch	1 tbsp	30
COTTAGE CHEESE		
creamed	1 cup (7.4 oz)	217
creamed	4 oz	117
creamed w/ fruit	4 oz	140
dry curd	1 cup (5.1 oz)	123
dry curd	4 oz	96
lowfat 1%	4 oz	82
lowfat 1%	1 cup (7.9 oz)	164
lowfat 2%	1 cup (7.9 oz)	203
lowfat 2%	4 oz	101
Breakstone's		
Fat Free	½ cup	80
LiveActive	1 pkg (4 oz)	90
LiveActive Mixed Berries	1 pkg (4 oz)	120
Cabot		
Cottage Cheese	½ cup	100
No Fat	½ cup	70

FOOD	PORTION	CALS
Friendship		
1% Lowfat	½ cup	90
1% Lowfat No Salt Added	½ cup	90
1% Lowfat Whipped	½ cup	90
2% Digestive Health	½ cup	90
2% Pot Style	½ cup	90
4% California Style	½ cup	110
Nonfat	½ cup	80
Hood		
4% Fat w/ Pineapple	½ cup	130
Fat Free	½ cup	80
Low Fat	½ cup	90
Low Fat No Salt Added	½ cup	90
Low Fat w/ Peaches	½ cup	110
Horizon Organic		
Lowfat	½ cup	100
Regular	½ cup	120
Knudsen		
LiveActive Pineapple	1 pkg (4 oz)	110
Land O Lakes		
1% Lowfat	½ cup (4 oz)	90
2% Lowfat	½ cup (3.7 oz)	100
Cottage Cheese	½ cup (3.7 oz)	110
Fat Free	½ cup (4 oz)	80
Light N'Lively		
Lowfat	½ cup	80
Nancy's		
Organic Lowfat	½ cup	80
Organic Valley		
Low Fat	½ cup	100
COTTONSEED		
kernels roasted	1 tbsp	51
COUSCOUS		
cooked	1 cup (5.5 oz)	176
dry	1 cup (6.1 oz)	650
Hodgson Mill		
Whole Wheat not prep	⅓ cup	210
Marrakesh Express		
Mango Salsa as prep	1 cup	190

FOOD	PORTION	CALS
Mushroom as prep	1 cup	190
Plain as prep	1 cup	270
Near East		
Mediterranean Curry as prep	1 cup	220
Original Plain as prep	1 cup	190
Parmesan as prep	1 cup	220
Toasted Pine Nut as prep	1 cup	230
Wild Mushroom & Herb as prep	1 cup	230
Rice Select		
All Varieties not prep	¼ cup	150
CRAB		
CANNED		
blue	½ cup	67
blue drained	1 can (6.5 oz)	124
Ace Of Diamonds		
Fancy w/ Leg Meat	¼ cup (2 oz)	40
Brunswick		
Crabmeat 15% Leg	2 oz	40
Fancy Lump	2 oz	45
Bumble Bee		
Lump	¼ cup	40
Pink	¼ cup	35
White	¼ cup	40
Chicken Of The Sea		
Fancy	½ can (2 oz)	40
Lump	½ can (2 oz)	35
Madam		
Crab Meat	½ cup	40
Polar		
Claw Meat	¼ cup (2 oz)	37
Jumbo Lump Meat	¼ cup (2 oz)	39
Terry's		
Crabmeat	¼ cup	40
FRESH		
alaska king meat only steamed	3 oz	82
blue cooked flaked	1 cup (4 oz)	120
dungeness steamed	3 oz	94
queen steamed	3 oz	98

FOOD	PORTION	CALS
FROZEN		
Mama Belle's		
Crab Cakes Maryland Style	1 (2 oz)	100
Margaritaville		
Coral Reef Cakes + Sauce	1	200
Mrs. Paul's		
Deviled Crab Cakes	1 (3 oz)	220
Phillips Seafood		
Crab Cakes	1 (3 oz)	160
Crab Meat Stuffing	1 serv (3.5 oz)	170
Mini Cakes	4	160
Slammers	2	150
TAKE-OUT		
alaska king leg steamed	1 leg (4.7 oz)	130
baked	1 (3.8 oz)	160
cakes	2 (4.2 oz)	186
crab imperial	1 crab (6.8 oz)	289
crab salad	1 serv (5.5 oz)	285
crab thermidor	1 serv (6.4 oz)	456
deviled	1 serv (4.5 oz)	254
dungeness steamed	1 crab (4.5 oz)	140
empanada de jueyes	1 (4.4 oz)	341
fried crab puffs	4 (3.2 oz)	323
kenagi korean crab cooked	1 serv (3 oz)	71
salmorejo de jueyes (in tomato sauce)	1 serv (4.5 oz)	215
soft-shell breaded & fried	1 med (2.3 oz)	216
taco de jueyes	1 (4.2 oz)	266

CRACKER CRUMBS

FOOD	PORTION	CALS
cracker meal	1 cup	440
graham cracker crumbs	1 cup	355
Honey Maid		
Graham Cracker Crumbs	2½ tbsp (0.6 oz)	70
Keebler		
Graham	¼ cup	93
Kellogg's		
Corn Flake Crumbs	6 tbsp (1.2 oz)	120

CRACKERS

FOOD	PORTION	CALS
melba toast round	1	12
oyster cracker	¼ cup	48

FOOD	PORTION	CALS
saltines	1	13
water biscuits	3	92
zwieback	1 oz	107
34 Degrees		
Crispbread Sesame	19 (1.1 oz)	140
Annie's Homegrown		
Cheddar Bunnies BBQ	50	130
Cheddar Bunnies Original	50	150
Cheddar Bunnies Ranch	50	130
Cheddar Bunnies Whole Wheat	50	130
Athenos		
Pita Chips Whole Wheat	11 (1 oz)	120
Back To Nature		
Classic Rounds	5	70
Crispy Wheats	17	130
Rice Thin Sesame Ginger	16	120
Rice Thin White Cheddar	16	120
Barbara's Bakery		
Rite Rounds Lite Original	5 (0.5 oz)	60
Wheatines Original	4	60
Better Cheddars		
Original	1.1 oz	160
Blue Diamond		
Nut-Thins Almond	16	130
Nut-Thins Hazelnut	16	130
Nut-Thins Pecan	16	130
Bremner Wafers		
Cracked Wheat	7 (0.5 oz)	70
Original	7 (0.5 oz)	70
Soup & Chili Crackers	50 (0.5 oz)	60
Breton		
Garden Vegetable	4 (0.7 oz)	100
Minis Cheddar Cheese	20 (0.7 oz)	100
Brown Rice Snaps		
Cheddar	6	60
Original Tamari Seaweed	9	60
Unsalted Plain	8	60
Cheese Nips		
Cheddar	1 pkg (1.2 oz)	170

FOOD	PORTION	CALS
Cheetos		
Cheddar	1 pkg	240
Chicken Biskit		
Original	1.1 oz	160
Dare		
Crackers	3 (0.5 oz)	70
Original	4 (0.7 oz)	90
Reduced Fat & Salt	5 (0.7 oz)	80
Doritos		
Jalapeno Cheese	1 pkg	230
Nacho Cheesier	1 pkg	240
Dr. Kracker		
Flatbread Klassic Seed	1 (1 oz)	120
Flatbread Pumpkin Seed Cheddar	1 (1 oz)	120
Flatbread Seeded Spelt	1 (1 oz)	120
Flatbread Seedlander	1 (1 oz)	120
Flatbread Spelt Sunflower Cheddar	1 (1 oz)	120
Krispy Grahams	5 (1 oz)	110
Eden		
Brown Rice	8 (1.1 oz)	120
Nori Nori Rice	15 (1 oz)	110
Foods Alive		
Golden Flax Maple & Cinnamon	5	150
Golden Flax Mexican Harvest	5	150
Golden Flax Onion Garlic	5	140
Golden Flax Organic Hemp	5	130
Golden Flax Regular	5	150
Gamesa		
Sabrisas	11	150
Glutino		
Gluten Free	4 (0.5 oz)	70
Gluten Free Rusks	2 (0.7 oz)	80
GrainsFirst		
Autumn Harvest	7 (1.1 oz)	140
Grissol		
Crispy Baguettes Garden Herb	8 (1 oz)	110
Health Valley		
Organic Bruschetta Vegetable	4	70
Organic Cracked Pepper	4	70
Organic Cracker Stix Garlic Herb	8	70

FOOD	PORTION	CALS
Organic Whole Wheat	4	70
Healthy Handfuls		
Lucky Duckies Cheddar Cheese	1 pkg (1 oz)	100
Jacob's		
Table Cracker Bran	1	33
Kashi		
TLC Country Cheddar	18 (1 oz)	130
TLC Honey Sesame	15 (1 oz)	130
TLC Natural Ranch	15 (1 oz)	130
TLC Original 7 Grain	15 (1 oz)	130
TLC Party Mediterranean Bruschetta	4	120
TLC Snack Fire Roasted Vegetable	5	130
Keebler		
Club Multi-Grain	4	70
Club Original	4	70
Club Reduced Fat	5	70
Club Snack Sticks	12	130
Puffed Original	24	140
Sandwich Cheese & Peanut Butter	1 pkg (1.4 oz)	200
Sandwich Toast & Peanut Butter	1 pkg (1.4 oz)	200
Sandwich Wheat & Cheddar	1 pkg (1.3 oz)	190
Toasteds Harvest Wheat	16	130
Toasteds Sesame	5	80
Toasteds Wheat	5	80
Town House Bistro	2	80
Town House FlipSides Original	5	70
Town House Original	5	80
Town House Reduced Fat	6	60
Town House Reduced Sodium	5	80
Town House Toppers	3	70
Wheatables 33% Less Fat	19	140
Wheatables Original	17	140
Zesta Saltine Fat Free	5	60
Zesta Saltine Original	5	60
Kitchen Table Bakers		
Aged Parmesan	3	80
Everything	3	80
Garlic	3	80
Jalapeno	3	80

FOOD	PORTION	CALS
Lance		
Captain Wafers	4	70
Nekot	1 pkg (1.7 oz)	240
Nipchee	1 pkg (1.4 oz)	190
Peanut Butter On Wheat	1 pkg (1.4 oz)	200
Toastchee	1 pkg (1.5 oz)	220
Toastchee Reduced Fat	1 pkg (1.4 oz)	180
Late July		
Organic Classic Rich	4 (0.5 oz)	70
Organic Classic Saltine	4 (0.5 oz)	60
Mary's Gone Crackers		
Wheat Free Gluten Free Black Pepper	13 (1 oz)	140
Wheat Free Gluten Free Onion	13 (1 oz)	140
Wheat Free Gluten Free Original Seed	13 (1 oz)	140
Milton's		
Multi-Grain	2	70
Nabisco		
Garden Harvest Apple Cinnamon	16 (1 oz)	120
Garden Harvest Banana	16 (1 oz)	120
Garden Harvest Tomato Basil	16 (1 oz)	120
Garden Harvest Vegetable Medley	16 (1 oz)	120
Vegetable Thins	21 (1 oz)	150
Water Original	4	60
Wheat	4	90
Nature's Path		
Signature Tamari Flax	15	110
New York Style		
Crispini Seeds & Spice	6	120
Panetini Original	2	80
Panetini Three Cheese	2	80
Pita Chips Garlic	7	130
Pita Chips Natural Whole Wheat	7	120
Nonni's		
Panetini Roasted Garlic	5 (1 oz)	120
Panetini Sun Dried Tomato Basil	5 (1 oz)	120
Orkney		
Oatcakes Thin	4 (1.8 oz)	227
Pepperidge Farm		
100 Calorie Pack Goldfish Cheddar	1 pkg	100
100 Calorie Pack Goldfish Pretzel	1 pkg	100

FOOD	PORTION	CALS
Goldfish Cinnamon Graham	1 pkg	210
Goldfish Pizza	55	140
Goldfish Reduced Sodium Cheddar	60	140
Goldfish w/ Whole Grain	55	140
Snack Sticks Pumpernickel	15	120
Water Crackers	4	60
Wheat Crisps Spicy Salsa	16	140
Peter Pan		
Peanut Butter Cheese	1 pkg	210
Peanut Butter Toast	1 pkg	210
Premium		
Saltines Fat Free	5 (0.5 oz)	60
Saltines Low Sodium	0.5 oz	80
Saltines Multigrain	5 (0.5 oz)	60
Saltines Original	0.5 oz	60
Saltines Unsalted Tops	5	60
Ritz		
Crackers	0.5 oz	80
Low Sodium	0.5 oz	80
Reduced Fat	5 (0.5 oz)	70
Whole Wheat	0.5 oz	70
San-J		
Brown Rice Black Sesame	5	140
Brown Rice Sesame	5	130
Brown Rice Tamari	6	170
Sara Lee		
Cracked Pepper Trio	7	130
English Water	7	130
Harvest Vegetable	6	140
Sociables		
Original	0.5 oz	70
South Beach		
Whole Wheat	1 pkg	100
Triscuit		
Deli-Style Rye	1 oz	120
Original	1 oz	120
Reduced Fat	1 oz	120
True North		
Peanut Crunches	¼ cup (1 oz)	150
Pistachio Crisps	12 (1 oz)	140

FOOD	PORTION	CALS
Utz		
Cheese Peanut Butter	6	200
Vegetable Thins		
Original	1 oz	150
Vinta		
Original	3 (0.7 oz)	100
Wasa		
Crisp'N Light 7 Grain	3	60
Fiber Rye	1	30
Hearty Rye	1	45
Light Rye	2 (0.6 oz)	60
Oats	1	60
Sourdough Rye	1	35
Water Crackers		
Original	6 (0.5 oz)	60
Westminster		
Oyster	1 pkg (0.5 oz)	66
Wheat Thins		
100% Whole Grain	1 oz	140
Low Sodium	1.1 oz	150
Original	1.1 oz	150
Reduced Fat	1 oz	130
Wheatsworth		
Crackers	5 (0.5 oz)	80
Wisecrackers		
Low Fat Roasted Garlic	10	110
CRANBERRIES		
cranberry orange relish	¼ cup	118
cranberry sauce	¼ cup	109
dried	½ cup	85
dried organic	⅓ cup	120
fresh chopped	1 cup	13
fresh whole	1 cup	11
sauce	1 slice (2 oz)	86
Chukar Cherries		
North Cove Dried	¼ cup	100
De-Lite		
Dried Sweetened	1 oz	92
Earthbound Farm		
Organic Dried	⅓ cup	130

FOOD	PORTION	CALS
Eden		
Organic Dried	⅓ cup	140
Emily's		
Milk Chocolate Covered	¼ cup (1.4 oz)	180
Fool		
Cranberry Spread	1 tbsp	30
Frieda's		
Dried	⅓ cup (1.4 oz)	110
Fruitaceuticals		
OmegaCrans Dried	¼ cup	91
Good Sense		
Cranberries 'N More	¼ cup	170
Dried Sweetened	½ cup	130
Lollipop Tree		
Cranberry Curd	1 tbsp	50
Mariani		
Dried Sweetened	⅓ cup	130
Newman's Own		
Organic Dried	¼ cup	130
Ocean Spray		
Craisins	⅓ cup	130
Sunsweet		
Dried	⅓ cup (1.5 oz)	140
Tree Of Life		
Organic Jellied	¼ cup (2.5 oz)	100
Wild Thymes Farm		
Cranberry Fig Sauce	1 tsp	19
Original Cranberry Sauce	1 tbsp	21

CRANBERRY BEANS

canned	½ cup	108
dried cooked w/o salt	½ cup	120
Goya		
Roman Beans Dried not prep	¼ cup (1.4 oz)	80

CRANBERRY JUICE

cranberry juice cocktail low calorie w/ vitamin C	8 oz	46
cranberry juice cocktail w/ vitamin C	8 oz	137
unsweetened	8 oz	116

FOOD	PORTION	CALS
Apple & Eve		
100% Juice	8 oz	130
Lakewood		
Organic	6 oz	50
Organic Light	6 oz	45
Langers		
Cranberry 100	8 oz	140
Nantucket Nectars		
Cranberry Cocktail	8 oz	130
Northland		
100% Juice No Sugar Added	8 oz	130
Ocean Spray		
White Cran Peach	8 oz	120
Old Orchard		
Cocktail	8 oz	140
Ssips		
Cocktail	1 box (7 oz)	110
CRAYFISH		
cooked	3 oz	97
raw	8 crayfish	24
raw	3 oz	76
CREAM (see also WHIPPED TOPPINGS)		
clotted cream	2 tbsp (1 oz)	164
creme fraiche	2 tbsp (1 oz)	100
half & half	1 cup (8.5 oz)	315
half & half	1 tbsp (0.5 oz)	20
heavy whipping	1 tbsp (0.5 oz)	52
heavy whipping whipped	1 cup (4.1 oz)	411
light coffee	1 cup (8.4 oz)	496
light coffee	1 tbsp (0.5 oz)	29
light whipping	1 tbsp (0.5 oz)	44
light whipping cream whipped	1 cup (4.2 oz)	345
Cabot		
Whipped	2 tbsp	15
Coffee-Mate		
Half & Half Fat Free	2 tbsp	20
Hood		
Half & Half	2 tbsp	40
Light	1 tbsp	30

FOOD	PORTION	CALS
Simply Smart Fat Free Half & Half	2 tbsp	15
Whipping Cream	1 tbsp	45
Horizon Organic		
Half & Half	2 tbsp	35
Heavy Whipping	1 tbsp	50
Land O Lakes		
Aerosol Whipped Light Cream	2 tbsp (0.2 oz)	20
Half & Half	2 tbsp (1.1 oz)	35
Half & Half Fat Free	2 tbsp (1.1 oz)	20
Heavy Whipping	1 tbsp (0.5 oz)	50
Organic Valley		
Half & Half	2 tbsp (1 oz)	40
Straus		
Organic Whipping Cream	1 tbsp (0.5 oz)	52
CREAM CHEESE		
cream cheese	1 oz	99
cream cheese	1 pkg (3 oz)	297
Back To Nature		
Organic Cream Cheese	⅛ pkg (1 oz)	100
Boar's Head		
Cream Cheese	2 tbsp (1 oz)	100
Connoisseur		
Wheel Mango Peach	2 tbsp	110
Wheel Wild Blueberry	2 tbsp	100
Crystal Farms		
Regular	1 oz	90
Tub	2 tbsp	100
Whipped	2 tbsp	70
Earth Balance		
Brick	2 tbsp	80
Tub	2 tbsp	80
Horizon Organic		
Reduced Fat	2 tbsp	70
Spreadable	2 tbsp	110
Lifeway		
Lox & Onion	2 tbsp	80
Vegetable	2 tbsp	80
Whipped	2 tbsp	80
Nancy's		
Organic	2 tbsp	95

FOOD	PORTION	CALS
Organic Valley		
Cream Cheese	1 oz	100
Soft	2 tbsp	90
Philadelphia		
⅓ Less Fat	1 oz	70
Fat Free	1 oz	30
Original	1 oz	100
Whipped	2 tbsp	60

CREAM CHEESE SUBSTITUTES
Vegan Gourmet

Alternative Cream Cheese	2 tbsp (1 oz)	90
WholeSoy & Co.		
Soy Cream Cheese Organic Original or Flavored	2 tbsp	70

CREAM OF TARTAR
cream of tartar	1 tsp	8

CREPES
basic crepe unfilled	1 (7 in)	112
Ekizian		
Chickpea Crepe	1 (7 in) 1.5 oz	212
Frieda's		
Ready-To-Use	1 (0.5 oz)	30

CROAKER
atlantic breaded & fried	3 oz	188
atlantic raw	3 oz	89

CROCODILE
cooked	3 oz	78

CROISSANT
apple	1 (2 oz)	145
cheese	1 (2 oz)	236
plain	1 (2 oz)	232
plain mini	1 (1 oz)	115
Sara Lee		
Croissant	1 (1.5 oz)	170
Petite	2 (2 oz)	230
TAKE-OUT		
w/ egg & cheese	1 (4.5 oz)	368

FOOD	PORTION	CALS
w/ egg cheese & bacon	1 (4.5 oz)	413
w/ egg cheese & ham	1 (5.3 oz)	474
w/ egg cheese & sausage	1 (5.6 oz)	523

CROUTONS
plain	1 cup (1 oz)	122
seasoned	1 cup (1.4 oz)	186
Cardini's		
Italian	2 tbsp	30
Edward & Sons		
Organic Lightly Salted	2 tbsp	30
Fresh Gourmet		
Butter & Garlic	7 (7 g)	35
Cheese & Garlic	12 (0.5 oz)	70
Classic Caesar	6 (7 g)	35
Cornbread Sweet Butter	½ cup (1 oz)	110
Country Ranch	6 (7 g)	35
Fat Free Garlic Caesar	12 (7 g)	30
Italian Seasoned	6 (7 g)	35
Organic Seasoned	5 (7 g)	30
Pepperidge Farm		
Whole Grain Seasoned	6	30
Zesty Italian	6	30
Rothbury Farms		
Seasoned	2 tbsp	30

CUCUMBER
fresh peeled	1 med (7 oz)	24
fresh sliced	1 cup	14
fresh w/ peel sliced	½ cup	34
Frieda's		
Japanese	⅔ cup	10
Seedless Hothouse	⅔ cup	110
TAKE-OUT		
cucumber & onion salad w/ vinegar	1 cup	52
cucumber raita	1 serv (3.3 oz)	40
cucumber salad w/ oil & vinegar	1 cup	183
cucumber salad w/ sour cream dressing	1 cup	68
kimchee	½ cup (1.8 oz)	36
tzatziki	½ cup (3.4 oz)	72

FOOD	PORTION	CALS
CUMIN		
seed	1 tsp (2 g)	8
seed	1 tbsp (6 g)	22
CURRANT JUICE		
black currant nectar	7 oz	110
red currant nectar	7 oz	108
CurrantC		
Black Currant Juice	8 oz	130
CURRANTS		
black fresh	½ cup	36
zante dried	½ cup	204
Sun-Maid		
Zante	¼ cup	130
CURRY		
curry powder	1 tsp	7
paste	1 tube (6 oz)	465
A Taste Of Thai		
Curry Paste Green	1 tsp	15
Curry Paste Panang	1 tsp	25
Curry Paste Red	1 tsp	20
Curry Paste Yellow	1 tsp	30
Helen's Kitchen		
Indian Curry w/ Tofu Steaks & Rice	1 pkg (9 oz)	300
Patak's		
Curry Paste Biryani	2 tbsp	180
Garam Masala Paste	2 tsp	130
Tandoori Paste	2 tbsp	30
Vegetable Curry w/ Rice Rich Creamy Coconut	1 pkg	400
Vegetable Curry w/ Rice Rich Tomato & Onion	1 pkg (10.5 oz)	290
Vegetable Curry w/ Rice Tangy Lemon & Cilantro	1 pkg	300
Vindaloo Paste	2 tbsp	160
Spice Hunter		
Curry Seasoning Salt Free	¼ tsp	0
TastyBite		
Green Curry Vegetables & Jasmine Rice	1 pkg (12 oz)	320
Yellow Curry Vegetables & Jasmine Rice	1 pkg (12 oz)	380
TAKE-OUT		
beef curry	1 cup	432

FOOD	PORTION	CALS
beef kurma	1 serv (10 oz)	611
chicken curry ½ breast	1 serv	160
chicken curry boneless	1 serv (6.2 oz)	219
chicken curry leg & thigh	1 serv	180
chickpea curry	1 serv (8.3 oz)	305
eggplant curry	1 serv (8 oz)	241
lamb curry	1 cup	257
mixed vegetable curry	1 serv (7.7 oz)	398
pea & potato curry	1 serv (7 oz)	284
pork vindaloo curry	1 serv	620
potato curry	1 serv (5.5 oz)	791
sambhar dhal curry	1 serv (10 oz)	177

CUSK

fillet baked	3 oz	106

CUSTARD
MIX

as prep w/ 2% milk	½ cup (4.7 oz)	148
as prep w/ whole milk	½ cup (4.7 oz)	163
flan as prep w/ 2% milk	½ cup (4.7 oz)	135
flan as prep w/ whole milk	½ cup (4.7 oz)	150

READY-TO-EAT
Kozy Shack

Flan	1 pkg (4 oz)	145

TAKE-OUT

baked	½ cup (5 oz)	148
flan	½ cup (5.4 oz)	220
flan de calabaza	1 piece (3.5 oz)	225
flan de coco	1 piece (4.2 oz)	340
tocino del cielo heaven's delight	1 cup	856
zabaione	½ cup (57.2 g)	135

CUTTLEFISH

steamed	3 oz	134

DANDELION GREENS

fresh cooked	½ cup	17
raw chopped	½ cup	13

Frieda's

Dandelion Greens	2 cups	40

FOOD	PORTION	CALS
DANISH PASTRY		
READY-TO-EAT		
Entenmann's		
Danish Ring Walnut	⅙ ring (2 oz)	260
TAKE-OUT		
cheese	1 (2.5 oz)	266
cinnamon	1 (5 oz)	572
fruit	1 (5 oz)	527
lemon	1 (2.5 oz)	263
raisin nut	1 (2.3 oz)	280
DATES		
deglet noor chopped	¼ cup (1.3 oz)	104
deglet noor dried	1 (7 g)	20
jujube dried	1 oz	75
jujube fresh	1 oz	30
jujube preserved in sugar	1 oz	91
medjool	1 (0.8 oz)	66
Bob's Red Mill		
Dried Crumbles	⅓ cup	130
Earthbound Farm		
Organic Dried	6 (1.4 oz)	120
Frieda's		
Medjool	2 to 3 (1.4 oz)	120
SunDate		
Fancy Medjool	3 (1.4 oz)	120
Sunsweet		
California Pitted	5 to 6 (1.4 oz)	120
Tree Of Life		
Deglate Noor Pitted	5 (1.5 oz)	120
Organic Medjool	5 (1.5 oz)	120
DEER (see VENISON)		
DELI MEATS/COLD CUTS (see also BEEF, CHICKEN, HAM, MEAT SUBSTITUTES, TURKEY)		
barbecue loaf pork & beef	1 slice (0.8 oz)	40
beerwurst beef	2 oz	155
berliner pork & beef	1 slice (0.8 oz)	53
blood sausage	1 slice (0.9 oz)	95
bologna beef	1 slice (1 oz)	88
bologna beef lowfat	1 slice (1 oz)	57

FOOD	PORTION	CALS
bologna beef reduced sodium	1 slice (1 oz)	88
bologna beef & pork	1 slice (1 oz)	87
bologna beef & pork lowfat	1 slice (1 oz)	64
braunschweiger pork	1 slice (1 oz)	92
corned beef brisket	2 oz	90
dutch brand loaf pork & beef	1 slice (1.3 oz)	104
headcheese pork	1 slice (1.6 oz)	71
honey loaf pork & beef	1 slice (1 oz)	35
lebanon bologna beef	2 slices (1 oz)	105
mortadella beef & pork	1 slice (0.5 oz)	47
olive loaf pork	2 slices (2 oz)	134
pastrami beef	1 slice (1 oz)	41
peppered loaf pork & beef	1 slice (1 oz)	41
pepperoni pork & beef	15 slices (1 oz)	135
picnic loaf pork & beef	1 slice (1 oz)	65
salami cooked beef & pork	1 slice (0.8 oz)	58
salami hard pork	3 slices (0.9 oz)	14
salami hard pork & beef less sodium	1 slice (1 oz)	113
sandwich spread pork & beef	¼ cup	141
summer sausage thuringer cervelat	2 oz	203
Applegate Farms		
Organic Genoa Sliced	1 oz	100
Boar's Head		
Abruzzese Hot & Sweet	1 oz	100
Bologna 25% Lower Sodium	2 oz	150
Bologna Beef	2 oz	150
Bologna Garlic	2 oz	150
Bologna Lebanon	2 oz	100
Bologna Pork & Beef	2 oz	150
Braunschweiger Lite	2 oz	120
Capocollo Hot & Sweet	1 oz	80
Dutch Loaf	2 oz	150
Liverwurst Smoked	2 oz	170
Mortadella	2 oz	160
Olive Loaf	2 oz	130
Pastrami	2 oz	70
Pickle & Pepper Loaf	2 oz	150
Prosciutto	1 oz	60
Salami Beef	2 oz	120
Salami Cooked	2 oz	130

FOOD	PORTION	CALS
Salami Hard	1 oz	110
Sopressata Hot & Sweet	1 oz	100
Spiced Ham	2 oz	120
Butterball		
Turkey Bologna	1 slice (1 oz)	60
Turkey Ham	1 slice (1 oz)	35
Carl Buddig		
Beef	2 oz	90
Corned Beef	2 oz	90
Healthy Ones		
Pastrami 97% Fat Free	4 slices (2 oz)	60
Hebrew National		
Bologna Beef	1 slice (1 oz)	80
Bologna Lean Beef	4 slices (2 oz)	90
Salami Beef	3 slices (2 oz)	150
Salami Lean Beef	4 slices (2 oz)	90
Oscar Mayer		
Salami Beef	3 slices (1.8 oz)	150
Sara Lee		
Corned Beef	1 slice (2 oz)	50
Pastrami	2 slices (1.6 oz)	60
Salami Genoa	4 slices (1 oz)	110
Salami Hard	4 slices (1 oz)	120
Wellshire		
Salami Genoa	1 oz	100
Salami Hard	1 oz	100
Sopressata Sliced	1 oz	100
DILL		
seed	1 tsp	6
sprigs fresh	5 (0.3 oz)	0
weed dry	1 tbsp	8

DINNER (*see also* ASIAN FOOD, CURRY, PASTA DINNERS, POT PIE, SPANISH FOOD)

Banquet		
Turkey Meal	1 meal (9.25 oz)	290
Betty Crocker		
Complete Meals Chicken & Buttermilk Biscuits	⅕ pkg (5.4 oz)	280
Complete Meals Stroganoff	⅕ pkg (5 oz)	200

FOOD	PORTION	CALS
Birds Eye		
Steamfresh Meals For Two Asian Chicken Vegetable Medley	½ pkg (11.9 oz)	290
Steamfresh Meals For Two Grilled Chicken Marinara	½ pkg (11.9 oz)	360
Steamfresh Meals For Two Sweet & Spicy Chicken	½ pkg (11.9 oz)	370
Voila! Pasta Primavera w/ Chicken	1⅔ cups	250
Voila! Shrimp Scampi	1¾ cups	190
Voila! Southwestern Chicken	2 cups	250
Boston Market		
Glazed Rotisserie Chicken w/ Mashed Potatoes Gravy Vegetables	1 pkg (16 oz)	390
Meatloaf w/ Mashed Potatoes & Gravy	1 pkg (16 oz)	880
C&W		
Stir Fry Feast Pot Sticker + Sauce	2 cups	200
Stir Fry Feast Ultimate + Sauce	1½ cups	190
Campbell's		
Supper Bakes Cheesy Chicken w/ Pasta	⅙ pkg	170
Supper Bakes Garlic Chicken w/ Pasta	⅙ pkg	220
Supper Bakes Savory Pork Chops w/ Herb Stuffing	⅙ box	160
Supper Bakes Traditional Roast Chicken w/ Stuffing	⅙ pkg	160
Contessa		
Beef Goulash not prep	1¾ cups	210
Chicken Alfredo not prep	1¾ cups	330
Chicken Cacciatore not prep	1¾ cups	230
Fantastic		
Ginger Shiitake w/ Rice Noodles	1 pkg (7.4 oz)	340
Fillo Factory		
Organic Fillo Pie Eggplant & Red Pepper	1 serv (5 oz)	230
Glory		
Savory Singles Chicken & Dumplings	1 pkg	290
Savory Singles Chicken Smoked Sausage & Rice Casserole	1 pkg	440
Savory Singles Ham & Sausage Jambalaya	1 pkg	400
Savory Singles Turkey & Gravy w/ Cornbread Stuffing	1 pkg	440

FOOD	PORTION	CALS
Glutino		
Gluten Free Chicken Pomodoro w/ Brown Rice & Vegetables	1 pkg (9.1 oz)	190
Gluten Free Chicken Ranchero w/ Brown Rice	1 pkg (9.1 oz)	180
Golden Cuisine		
Beef Stew	1 pkg	350
Boneless Pork Patty	1 pkg	504
Breaded Baked Fish w/ Rice Pilaf	1 pkg	300
Chicken Cacciatore	1 pkg	417
Chicken & Noodles	1 pkg	331
Chicken Parmesan	1 pkg	430
Chicken w/ Marinara Sauce	1 pkg	329
Meatloaf Patty & Gravy	1 pkg	340
Mesquite Chicken	1 pkg	320
Pot Roast w/ Gravy	1 pkg	343
Salisbury Steak & Mushroom Sauce	1 pkg	350
Swedish Meatballs	1 pkg	440
Turkey Tetrazzini	1 pkg	304
Green Giant		
Create A Meal Stir Fry Sweet & Sour as prep	1 cup	280
Skillet Meal Chicken Teriyaki as prep	1½ cups	240
Healthy Choice		
Beef Merlot	1 pkg	240
Beef Pot Roast w/ Gravy	1 pkg (11 oz)	310
Beef Stroganoff	1 pkg	320
Beef Teriyaki	1 pkg	310
Beef Tips Portabello	1 pkg	300
Blackened Chicken	1 pkg	300
Boneless Beef Ribs w/ Classic BBQ Sauce	1 pkg	360
Cafe Steamers Beef Merlot	1 pkg (10 oz)	220
Cafe Steamers Cajun Style Chicken & Shrimp	1 pkg (10.4 oz)	250
Cafe Steamers Chicken Margherita	1 pkg (10 oz)	340
Cafe Steamers Creamy Dill Salmon	1 pkg (9.8 oz)	240
Cafe Steamers Grilled Basil Chicken	1 pkg (10.6 oz)	290
Cafe Steamers Grilled Whiskey Steak	1 pkg (9.4 oz)	250
Charbroiled Beef Patty	1 pkg	310
Cheesy Rice & Chicken	1 pkg	250
Chicken Breast & Vegetables	1 pkg	260
Chicken Broccoli Alfredo	1 pkg	300
Chicken Carbonara	1 pkg	290

FOOD	PORTION	CALS
Chicken Margherita	1 pkg	340
Chicken Parmigiana	1 pkg (11.6 oz)	350
Chicken Piccata	1 pkg	260
Chicken Teriyaki	1 pkg	270
Chicken Tuscany	1 pkg	340
Country Breaded Chicken	1 pkg	370
Country Glazed Chicken	1 pkg	230
Country Herb Chicken	1 pkg (11.35 oz)	240
Creamy Herb Roasted Chicken	1 pkg	240
Fresh Mixers Southwestern Chicken	1 pkg (7.9 oz)	310
Grilled Basil Chicken	1 pkg	330
Grilled Chicken Breast & Pasta	1 pkg	250
Grilled Chicken Breast w/ Mashed Potatoes	1 pkg	190
Grilled Chicken Caesar	1 pkg	300
Grilled Chicken Marinara	1 pkg	270
Grilled Steak w/ Roasted Garlic Sauce	1 pkg	220
Grilled Turkey Breast	1 pkg	250
Grilled Whiskey Steak	1 pkg	280
Herb Baked Fish	1 pkg	360
Homestyle Chicken & Pasta	1 pkg	250
Honey Glazed Chicken	1 pkg	320
Lemon Pepper Fish	1 pkg (10.7 oz)	310
Mandarin Chicken	1 pkg (9.1 oz)	240
Mesquite Chicken BBQ	1 pkg	300
Mixed Grills Chicken Honey BBQ w/ Dipping Sauce	1 pkg	380
Mixed Grills Chicken Honey Mustard w/ Dipping Sauce	1 pkg	360
Mixed Grills Chicken Teriyaki w/ Dipping Sauce	1 pkg	340
Mixed Grills Chicken Tomato Garlic w/ Dipping Sauce	1 pkg	370
Mixed Grills Steak BBQ Sauce	1 pkg	420
Mixed Grills Steak Teriyaki w/ Dipping Sauce	1 pkg	350
Mixed Grills Steak w/ Zesty Steak Sauce	1 pkg	350
Oriental Style Beef	1 pkg	310
Oriental Style Chicken	1 pkg	240
Oven Roasted Beef	1 pkg	280
Princess Chicken	1 pkg	310
Roast Turkey Breast	1 pkg	220

FOOD	PORTION	CALS
Roasted Chicken Breast	1 pkg	280
Roasted Chicken Chardonnay	1 pkg	290
Salisbury Steak	1 pkg (12.5 oz)	360
Salisbury Steak w/ Red Skin Mashed Potatoes	1 pkg	200
Sesame Chicken	1 pkg	260
Slow Roasted Turkey Breast w/ Mashed Potatoes	1 pkg	210
Sweet & Sour Chicken	1 pkg (12 oz)	430
Traditional Meatloaf	1 pkg	300
Traditional Turkey Breast	1 pkg	300
Tuna Casserole	1 pkg	270
Ian's		
Chicken Finger Meal Allergen Free	1 pkg (7 oz)	368
Chicken Nugget Meal	1 pkg (8 oz)	440
Fish Stick Meal	1 pkg (8.4 oz)	480
Hamburger Meal	1 pkg (7 oz)	296
Pizza Meal	1 pkg (6.7 oz)	340
Popcorn Turkey Dog Meal Allergen Free	1 pkg (7 oz)	442
Joy Of Cooking		
Braised Beef Tips & Egg Noodles	1 cup (7.7 oz)	220
Roasted Herb Chicken	1 cup (7.7 oz)	170
Kashi		
Black Bean Mango	1 pkg (10 oz)	340
Lemon Rosemary Chicken	1 pkg (10 oz)	330
Lime Cilantro Shrimp	1 pkg (10 oz)	250
Southwest Style Chicken	1 pkg (10 oz)	240
Sweet & Sour Chicken	1 pkg (10 oz)	320
Kid Cuisine		
All Star Chicken Breast Nuggets	1 meal	460
Bug Safari Chicken Breast Nuggets	1 meal	450
Carnival Corn Dog	1 meal	430
Deep Sea Adventure Fish Sticks	1 meal	400
Fiesta Beef Taco Dippers	1 meal	370
Pop Star Popcorn Chicken	1 meal	410
Lean Cuisine		
Cafe Classics Baked Chicken Florentine	1 pkg (8 oz)	200
Cafe Classics Baked Lemon Pepper Fish	1 pkg (9 oz)	220
Cafe Classics Beef Peppercorn	1 pkg (8.75 oz)	220
Cafe Classics Beef Portabello	1 pkg (9 oz)	200
Cafe Classics Beef Pot Roast	1 pkg (9 oz)	190

FOOD	PORTION	CALS
Cafe Classics Bowl Creamy Basil Chicken	1 pkg (10.5 oz)	310
Cafe Classics Bowl Grilled Chicken Caesar	1 pkg (9 oz)	270
Cafe Classics Chicken Carbonara	1 pkg (9 oz)	280
Cafe Classics Chicken & Vegetables	1 pkg (10.5 oz)	240
Cafe Classics Chicken L'Orange	1 pkg (9 oz)	230
Cafe Classics Chicken Marsala	1 pkg (8.1 oz)	140
Cafe Classics Chicken Parmesan	1 pkg (10.9 oz)	280
Cafe Classics Chicken Tuscan	1 pkg (12 oz)	300
Cafe Classics Chicken w/ Almonds	1 pkg (8.5 oz)	260
Cafe Classics Chicken w/ Basil Cream Sauce	1 pkg (8.5 oz)	270
Cafe Classics Fiesta Grilled Chicken	1 pkg (9.5 oz)	250
Cafe Classics Garlic Beef & Broccoli	1 pkg (9 oz)	170
Cafe Classics Glazed Chicken	1 pkg (8.5 oz)	220
Cafe Classics Glazed Turkey Tenderloins	1 pkg (9 oz)	260
Cafe Classics Grilled Chicken	1 pkg (9.4 oz)	160
Cafe Classics Grilled Chicken w/ Teriyaki Glaze	1 pkg (10 oz)	270
Cafe Classics Herb Roasted Chicken	1 pkg (8 oz)	190
Cafe Classics Honey Dijon Grilled Chicken	1 pkg (8 oz)	220
Cafe Classics Honey Mustard Chicken	1 pkg (8 oz)	250
Cafe Classics Honey Roasted Pork	1 serv (9.5 oz)	230
Cafe Classics Mandarin Chicken	1 pkg (9 oz)	270
Cafe Classics Meatloaf w/ Gravy & Whipped Potatoes	1 pkg (9.4 oz)	280
Cafe Classics Orange Peel Chicken	1 pkg (12 oz)	390
Cafe Classics Oven Roasted Beef	1 pkg (9.25 oz)	210
Cafe Classics Roasted Garlic Chicken	1 pkg (8.8 oz)	200
Cafe Classics Roasted Turkey & Vegetables	1 pkg (8 oz)	150
Cafe Classics Roasted Turkey Breast	1 pkg (12 oz)	280
Cafe Classics Roasted Turkey Breast w/ Dressing	1 pkg (9.75 oz)	270
Cafe Classics Salisbury Steak	1 pkg (12.5 oz)	310
Cafe Classics Salisbury Steak w/ Mac & Cheese	1 pkg (9.5 oz)	280
Cafe Classics Sesame Chicken	1 pkg (9 oz)	330
Cafe Classics Southern Beef Tips	1 pkg (8.75 oz)	250
Cafe Classics Steak Tips Dijon	1 pkg (12 oz)	320
Cafe Classics Steak Tips Portabello	1 pkg (7.5 oz)	180
Cafe Classics Stuffed Cabbage	1 pkg (9.5 oz)	200
Cafe Classics Swedish Meatballs	1 pkg (9.1 oz)	290
Cafe Classics Sweet & Sour Chicken	1 pkg (10 oz)	300
Cafe Classics Three Cheese Chicken	1 pkg (8 oz)	230

FOOD	PORTION	CALS
Comfort Classics Baked Chicken	1 pkg (8.6 oz)	230
Dinnertime Selects Balsamic Glazed Chicken	1 pkg (12 oz)	400
Dinnertime Selects Chicken Florentine	1 pkg (13.25 oz)	420
Dinnertime Selects Chicken Portabello	1 pkg (12 oz)	370
Dinnertime Selects Lemon Garlic Shrimp	1 pkg (12 oz)	350
Skillet Beef Teriyaki & Rice	1 serv	190
Spa Cuisine Chicken Mediterranean	1 pkg (10.5 oz)	240
Spa Cuisine Chicken In Peanut Sauce	1 pkg (9 oz)	280
Spa Cuisine Chicken Pecan	1 pkg (9 oz)	260
Spa Cuisine Lemon Chicken	1 pkg (9 oz)	290
Spa Cuisine Lemongrass Chicken	1 pkg (9.4 oz)	240
Spa Cuisine Pork w/ Cherry Sauce	1 pkg (8.25 oz)	260
Spa Cuisine Rosemary Chicken	1 pkg (8.25 oz)	230
Spa Cuisine Salmon w/ Beef	1 pkg (9.5 oz)	360
Mon Cuisine		
Vegan Moroccan Couscous	1 pkg (10 oz)	280
Vegan Veal Schnitzel In Sauce	1 pkg (10 oz)	300
Vegetarian Stuffed Cabbage In Tomato Sauce	1 pkg (10 oz)	220
Moosewood		
Organic Vegetarian Moroccan Stew	1 pkg (10 oz)	150
Organic Bistro		
Chicken Citron	1 pkg (13.5 oz)	490
Ginger Chicken	1 pkg (13.25 oz)	490
Jamaican Shrimp Cakes	1 pkg (12 oz)	380
Savory Turkey	1 pkg (12 oz)	430
Sockeye Salmon Cakes	1 pkg (12.2 oz)	600
Spiced Chicken Morocco	1 pkg (12.2 oz)	390
Wild Salmon	1 pkg (13.1 oz)	500
Organic Classics		
Chicken Marsala w/ Mashed Potatoes	1 pkg (9.5 oz)	330
Jamaican Style Jerk Chicken w/ Wehani Rice	1 pkg (9.5 oz)	270
Lemon Chicken w/ Wehani Rice	1 pkg (9.5 oz)	320
Pacific Foods		
Beef Steak Stew	1 cup	250
Chicken Stew	1 cup	200
Quorn		
Meat Free Simply Saute Indian	½ pkg	240
Meat Free Simply Saute Mexican	½ pkg	340
Meat Free Simply Saute Thai	½ pkg	240

FOOD	PORTION	CALS
Savvy Faire		
Baja Jack Scramble	1 pkg (8.2 oz)	370
Braised Beef	1 pkg (9.4 oz)	320
Herb Crusted Chicken	1 pkg (9.7 oz)	430
Seeds Of Change		
Chicken Teriyaki	1 pkg (10 oz)	300
Mushroom Wild Pilaf	1 pkg (11 oz)	350
Seven Grain Pilaf	1 pkg (11 oz)	390
Shady Brook		
Roasted Carved Turkey	1 pkg (18.6 oz)	550
South Beach		
Beef & Broccoli & Asian Style Noodles	1 pkg	320
Caprese Style Chicken w/ Cauliflower & Broccoli	1 pkg	250
Cashew Chicken w/ Sugar Snap Peas	1 pkg	360
Chicken Alfredo A La Roma	1 pkg	270
Chicken Basilico w/ Rotini	1 pkg	280
Chicken Santa Fe Style Rice & Beans	1 pkg (8.9 oz)	340
Garlic Herb Chicken w/ Green Beans Almondine	1 pkg	250
Garlic Parmesan Chicken w/ Penne	1 pkg	290
Garlic Sesame Beef w/ Cauliflower Sugar Snap Peas & Peppers	1 pkg	250
Kung Pao Chicken Breast Strips w/ Peppers & Broccoli	1 pkg	300
Meatloaf w/ Gravy	1 pkg (8.9 oz)	210
Orange Beef Slices & Brown Rice In Sauce w/ Broccoli & Carrots	1 pkg	260
Roasted Turkey	1 pkg (9.4 oz)	240
Savory Beef w/ Cheesy Broccoli	1 pkg	240
Savory Pork w/ Pecans & Green Beans	1 pkg	260
Szechwan Pork & Asian Noodles In Sauce	1 pkg	270
Stouffer's		
Beef Stew	1 pkg (11 oz)	280
Beef Stroganoff	1 pkg (9.75 oz)	380
Chicken A La King	1 pkg (11.5 oz)	360
Corner Bistro Burbon Steak Tips	1 pkg (12 oz)	520
Corner Bistro Sesame Chicken	1 pkg (12.63 oz)	510
Country Fried Beef Steak	1 pkg (16 oz)	610
Creamed Chipped Beef	½ pkg (5.5 oz)	140
Fish Filet	1 pkg (9 oz)	400

FOOD	PORTION	CALS
Fried Chicken Breast	1 pkg (8.88 oz)	360
Green Pepper Steak	1 pkg (10.5 oz)	240
Grilled Chicken Teriyaki	1 pkg (9.38 oz)	300
Grilled Lemon Pepper Chicken	1 pkg (9 oz)	240
Meatloaf	1 pkg (6 oz)	560
Pork Cutlet	1 pkg (10 oz)	370
Roast Pork	1 pkg (9.5 oz)	320
Roast Turkey Breast	1 pkg (16 oz)	390
Salisbury Steak	1 pkg (16 oz)	470
Stuffed Pepper	1 pkg (10 oz)	220
Swedish Meatballs	1 pkg (11.5 oz)	560
Swanson		
Chicken & Dumplings	1 cup	230
Chicken A La King	1 can	270
Tamarind Tree		
Alu Chole	1 pkg (9.25 oz)	320
Channa Dal Masala	1 pkg (9.25 oz)	290
Dal Makhani	1 pkg (9.25 oz)	350
Navratan Korma	1 pkg (9.25 oz)	370
Palak Paneer	1 pkg (9.25 oz)	350
Saag Chole	1 pkg (9.25 oz)	330
Vegetable Jalfrazi	1 pkg (9.25 oz)	280
Taste Above		
Meatless Zesty BBQ w/ Veggie Beef & Rice	1 pkg (10 oz)	280
TastyBite		
Beans Marsala & Basmati Rice	1 pkg (12 oz)	426
Spinach Dal & Basmati Rice	1 pkg (12 oz)	372
Stir Fry Vegetables & Jasmine Rice	1 pkg (12 oz)	450
Vegetable Supreme & Basmati Rice	1 pkg (12 oz)	317
Yves		
Meatless Santa Fe Beef	1 pkg (10.5 oz)	360
DIP		
spinach sour cream	¼ cup	155
Blue Bunny		
Incrediples	2 tbsp	30
Incrediples Taco Fiesta	2 tbsp	30
Spicy Buffalo	2 tbsp	30
Bravos!		
Salsa	2 tbsp	15
Salsa Con Queso	1 tbsp	25

FOOD	PORTION	CALS
Cabot		
French Onion	2 tbsp	50
Ranch	2 tbsp	50
Cedarlane		
Organic Five Layer Mexican	2 tbsp	60
Eatsmart		
Flame Roasted Salsa Con Queso	2 tbsp	35
Garden Style Sweet Salsa	2 tbsp	20
Jalapeno & Lime Tres Bean	2 tbsp	25
Fritos		
Bean	2 tbsp	40
Chili Cheese	2 tbsp	45
Hot Bean	2 tbsp	40
Jalapeno Cheddar	2 tbsp	50
Mild Cheddar	2 tbsp	60
Guiltless Gourmet		
Black Bean Mild	2 tbsp (1.1 oz)	40
Kraft		
Green Onion	2 tbsp	60
LiteHouse		
Avocado	2 tbsp	140
Caramel Low Fat	1 tbsp	110
Caramel Original	2 tbsp	110
Dilly	2 tbsp	150
Fruit Dip Chocolate Yogurt	2 tbsp	110
Fruit Dip Vanilla Yogurt	2 tbsp	60
Lite Ranch Veggie	2 tbsp	70
Organic Ranch	2 tbsp	130
Marie's		
French Onion Roasted	2 tbsp	100
Guacamole	2 tbsp	40
Honey Vanilla Cream Fruit Dip	2 tbsp	60
Spinach Parmesan	2 tbsp	90
Marzetti		
Veggie Dip Light Veggie	1 pkg (3.25 oz)	170
Veggie Fat Free Ranch	2 tbsp	35
Naturally Fresh		
Caramel	2 tbsp	100
Chocolate	2 tbsp	70
Cream Cheese Strawberry	2 tbsp	90

FOOD	PORTION	CALS
Ranch Lite	2 tbsp	80
Ranch Vegetable	2 tbsp	120
Phillips Seafood		
Crab & Spinach	2 tbsp	50
Maryland Crab	2 tbsp	70
Road's End Organics		
Nacho Cheese Gluten Free	2 tbsp	20
Robert Rothschild Farm		
Artichoke	2 tbsp	60
Ruffles		
French Onion	¼ cup	200
Ranch	2 tbsp	60
Snyder's Of Hanover		
Three Bean	2 tbsp	25
Utz		
Jalapeno Cheddar	2 tbsp	260
Sour Cream & Onion	2 tbsp	60
Wild Thymes Farm		
Indian Vindaloo Curry	1 tbsp	12
Indonesian Peanut Sauce	1 tbsp	32
Wise		
French Onion	2 tbsp	60
Nacho Cheese	2 tbsp	50
DOCK		
fresh cooked	3½ oz	20
raw chopped	½ cup	15
DOUGHNUTS		
chocolate glazed	1 med (1.5 oz)	175
chocolate w/ chocolate icing	1 med (2 oz)	218
creme filled	1 (3 oz)	307
custard filled	1 (2.3 oz)	235
french cruller glazed	1 med (1.4 oz)	169
jelly filled	1 (3 oz)	289
old fashioned plain	1 med (2 oz)	226
oriental okinawan	1 (0.6 oz)	75
plain chocolate frosted	1 med (1.5 oz)	194
plain glazed	1 med (1.6 oz)	192
whole wheat sugared	1 med (1.6 oz)	162

FOOD	PORTION	CALS
Entenmann's		
Crumb	1	260
Frosted Devil's Food	1	310
Glazed	1	260
Glazed Popems	4	220
Mini Frosted	1 (1 oz)	150
Plain Old Fashion	1	230
PoP'ettes Chocolate Frosted	3 (2.2 oz)	330
Super Bakery		
Daily Donut	1 (2.2 oz)	250
Proballs Slam Powdered Baseballs	1 (1.3 oz)	130
DRINK MIXERS		
whiskey sour mix	2 oz	55
whiskey sour mix not prep	1 pkg (0.6 oz)	64
McIlhenny		
Bloody Mary Mix as prep	1 cup	70
DRUM		
freshwater baked	3 oz	130
freshwater fillet baked	5.4 oz	236
DUCK		
boneless roasted	½ duck (7.8 oz)	444
boneless w/o skin roasted	3.5 oz	201
boneless w/o skin roasted diced	1 cup (4.9 oz)	281
chinese pressed	3 oz	162
chinese pressed	1 cup (4.9 oz)	267
pekin breast boneless w/ skin roasted	1 (4.2 oz)	242
pekin breast w/o skin broiled	3 oz	133
pekin leg w/ skin w/o bone roasted	1 (3.2 oz)	200
pekin leg w/o skin & bone roasted	1 (2.6 oz)	134
w/ skin & bone roasted	½ duck (13 oz)	1287
w/ skin & bone roasted	1 serv (6 oz)	583
Grimaud Farms		
Muscovy Duck Confit	1 serv (3 oz)	170
Muscovy Duck Whole	1 serv (3.7 oz)	200
TAKE-OUT		
breast battered & fried bone removed	½ (3.2 oz)	199
leg battered & fried bone removed	1 (2.5 oz)	155
wing roasted bone removed	1 (1.1 oz)	101

FOOD	PORTION	CALS
DUMPLING		
Kahiki		
Potstickers Chicken	5 (3.3 oz)	230
Samosas Coconut Curry Chicken	4 (2.8 oz)	170
Pepperidge Farm		
Apple	1	250
Peach	1	320
Traveling Chef		
Potstickers Chicken + Dipping Sauce	5 pieces + 1 tbsp sauce	285
TAKE-OUT		
apple	1 (6.7 oz)	661
bread dumpling	1 lg	330
cherry	1 (2.7 oz)	238
cornmeal	1 (2.8 oz)	134
fried pork	1 (3.5 oz)	338
fried puerto rican style	1 med (1.1 oz)	117
gyoza potstickers vegetable	8 (4.9 oz)	210
peach	1 (2.7 oz)	253
piroshki meat filled	1 (3.4 oz)	348
steamed meat	1 (1.3 oz)	41
DURIAN		
fresh	3.5 oz	141
EDAMAME (see SOYBEANS)		
EEL		
fresh cooked	1 fillet (5.6 oz)	375
fresh cooked	3 oz	200
raw	3 oz	156
smoked	3.5 oz	330
EGG (see also EGG DISHES, EGG SUBSTITUTES)		
CHICKEN		
hard or soft cooked	1	77
pickled	1	72
poached	1	73
scrambled plain	2	199
sunny side up	2	155
white cooked	1	17
yolk cooked	1	55

FOOD	PORTION	CALS
Crystal Farms		
In Shell Pasteurized	1	70
Peeled Hard Cooked	1	70
Davidson's		
Pasteurized Shell Eggs	1 lg	75
Egg-Land's Best		
Extra Large	1 (2 oz)	80
Large	1	70
Organic Brown	1	70
Eggology		
100% Organic Egg Whites	¼ cup	30
Gold Circle Farms		
Cage Free	1 lg	70
Good Earth Organics		
Organic Instant Whites	1 pkg (0.5 oz)	50
Horizon Organic		
Jumbo	1 (2.2 oz)	90
Land O Lakes		
Farm Fresh Brown Extra Large	1 (1.8 oz)	70
Organic Valley		
Egg Whites Pasteurized	¼ cup	25
Large Omega-3	1	70
Pete & Gerry's		
Organic Large	1 (1.8 oz)	70
Sunny Fresh		
Eggs ASAP!	2	140
Tree Of Life		
White Large Natural Omega-3	1 (1.8 oz)	70
OTHER POULTRY		
duck 100 year old	1 (1 oz)	49
duck cooked	1 (2.5 oz)	129
duck preserved hard core	1 (1.8 oz)	80
duck preserved soft core	1 (1.8 oz)	80
duck salted	1 (1 oz)	54
goose cooked	1 (5 oz)	265
quail canned	1 (0.3 oz)	14
quail cooked	1 (0.5 oz)	24
turkey raw	1 (2.8 oz)	135

FOOD	PORTION	CALS

EGG DISHES
Aunt Jemima
Eggs & Sausage	1 pkg (6.2 oz)	370
Omelet Ham & Cheese	1 pkg (5.2 oz)	250

Cedarlane
Zone Omelette Cheese	1 pkg (10.4 oz)	350

Jimmy Dean
Breakfast Bowls D-Lights Sausage	1 pkg	230
Breakfast Bowls Eggs Potato & Ham	1 pkg	390
Breakfast Bowls Eggs Potatoes Sausage & Cheddar Cheese	1 pkg	490
Breakfast Skillets Bacon as prep	1 serv (4.5 oz)	370
Breakfast Skillets Ham as prep	1 serv (4.5 oz)	270
Breakfast Skillets Smoked Sausage as prep	1 serv (4.5 oz)	380
Omelets Ham & Cheese	1 (4.2 oz)	280
Omelets Sausage & Cheese	1 (4.3 oz)	270

TAKE-OUT
deviled	1 half	62
eggs benedict	2	825
omelet cheese	3 eggs	387
omelet mushroom	3 eggs	251
omelet mushroom & onion	3 eggs	294
omelet plain	3 eggs	338
omelet spanish	3 eggs	496
omelet spinach	3 eggs	279
omelet western	3 eggs	355
salad	½ cup	353
scotch egg	1 (4.2 oz)	301
tortilla de amarillo omelet w/ plantain	3 eggs	536

EGG ROLLS
egg roll wrapper fresh	1	83

Blue Horizon Organic
Spring Rolls Chinese Shrimp	3 (2.1 oz)	130
Spring Rolls Indian	3 (2.1 oz)	110
Spring Rolls Thai	3 (2.1 oz)	110
Spring Rolls Thai Shrimp	3 (2.1 oz)	130

Frieda's
Egg Roll Wrappers	2 (1.6 oz)	130

Kahiki
Chicken	1 (3 oz)	160

FOOD	PORTION	CALS
Chipotle Lime Chicken	1 (3 oz)	170
Lemongrass Chicken Stix	3 (2.6 oz)	100
Pork & Shrimp	1 (3 oz)	140
Vegetable	1 (3 oz)	90
Lean Cuisine		
Cafe Classics Vegetable	1 pkg (9 oz)	310
Nasoya		
Egg Roll Wrapper	3	170
Pagoda		
Sweet & Sour Chicken	1 (2.7 oz)	170
Phillips		
Spring Rolls Crab & Shrimp w/ Sauce	3 (3.75 oz)	220
TAKE-OUT		
chicken	1 (3 oz)	140
lobster	1 (4.8 oz)	270
meat & shrimp	1 (4.8 oz)	320
pork & shrimp	1 (5 oz)	300
shrimp	1 (3 oz)	170
spicy pork	1 (3 oz)	200
vegetable	1 (3 oz)	170
EGG SUBSTITUTES		
Better'n Eggs		
All Whites	¼ cup	30
Ham & Cheese	¼ cup	45
Original	¼ cup (2 oz)	30
Plus	¼ cup	35
Three Cheese	¼ cup	45
Bob's Red Mill		
Egg White Dried	2 tsp	15
Vegetarian Egg Replacer	1 tbsp	30
Egg Beaters		
Original	¼ cup	30
EggPro		
Powder	1 tbsp	15
Fantastic		
Tofu Scrambler not prep	1 tbsp	35
Horizon Organic		
Liquid Egg	¼ cup	35
Quick Eggs		
Fat Free Cholesterol Free	¼ cup	30

FOOD	PORTION	CALS
EGGNOG		
eggnog	1 qt	1368
eggnog	1 cup	342
eggnog flavor mix as prep w/ milk	9 oz	260
Farmland		
Egg Nog	½ cup	180
Hood		
Fat Free Sugar Free	1 cup	110
Golden	½ cup	180
Light	½ cup	140
Horizon Organic		
Lowfat	½ cup	140
Organic Valley		
Ultra Pasteurized	½ cup	180
Straus		
Organic Cream Top	4 oz	160
TAKE-OUT		
eggnog	1 cup	306
EGGPLANT		
cubed cooked w/ oil	1 cup	133
pickled	½ cup	33
slices grilled	1 (2 oz)	36
Cedarlane		
Eggplant Mediterranean	1 pkg (10 oz)	230
Celentano		
Eggplant Parmigiana	1 serv (7 oz)	330
Frieda's		
Chinese	⅔ cup (3 oz)	20
Japanese Nasu	⅔ cup (3 oz)	20
Peloponnese		
Baba Ganoush	2 tbsp	40
Sabra		
Baba Ghanoush	2 oz	50
Stonewall Kitchen		
Eggplant Spread	1 tbsp	25
TastyBite		
Punjab Eggplant	½ pkg (5 oz)	144
TAKE-OUT		
baba ghannouj	¼ cup	55
caponata	2 tbsp (1 oz)	30

FOOD	PORTION	CALS
iman bayildi eggplant w/ onion & tomato	1 serv (15.6 oz)	345
indian eggplant runi	1 serv	180
moussaka	1 serv (9 oz)	372
papoutsaki little shoes	1 serv (15.5 oz)	245
tempura	1 serv (1.5 oz)	118

ELDERBERRIES
fresh	1 cup	105

ELDERBERRY JUICE
elderberry	7 oz	76

ELK
eye of round roasted	3.5 oz	151
ground cooked	3.5 oz	143
Natural Frontier Foods		
Filet	1 (4 oz)	140

ENERGY BARS (*see also* CEREAL BARS, NUTRITION SUPPLEMENTS)
Activex		
Organic All Flavors	1 (1.6 oz)	200
All In One		
All Flavors	1 (1.8 oz)	180
Amino Vital		
Fit Apple Pie	1 (1.76 oz)	150
Fit Chocolate Peanut	1 (1.76 oz)	190
Fit Toasted Nut Cranberry	1 (1.76 oz)	180
Atkins		
Morning Start Apple Crisp	1	170
Morning Start Blueberry Muffin	1	160
Morning Start Chocolate Chip Crisp	1	160
Attune		
Wellness Chocolate Crisp	1 (0.7 oz)	100
Wellness Cool Mint Chocolate	1 (0.7 oz)	100
Balance		
100 Calories Peanut Butter Crisp	1 (1 oz)	100
100 Calories Vanilla Crisp	1 (1 oz)	100
Carbwell Chocolate Fudge	1 (1.8 oz)	190
Gold Chocolate Peanut Butter	1 (1.8 oz)	210
Gold S'mores Crunch	1 (1.8 oz)	210
Organic Apricot Mango Crisp	1 (1.6 oz)	180
Organic Cranberry Pomegranate Crisp	1 (1.6 oz)	180

FOOD	PORTION	CALS
Original Almond Brownie	1 (1.8 oz)	200
Original Mocha Crisp	1 (1.8 oz)	200
Pure Banana Cashew	1 (1.6 oz)	180
Pure Cherry Pecan	1 (1.6 oz)	190
Belly-bar		
Baby Needs Chocolate	1	170
Berry Nutty Cravings	1	170
Mellow Oat	1	180
Boomi Bar		
Almond Protein Plus	1	270
Cashew Almond Delicacy	1	260
Cranberry Apple	1	210
Merry Macadamia	1	220
Pistachio Pineapple	1	200
Bora Bora		
Organic Cranberry Crunch	1 (1.4 oz)	170
Organic Peanut Peanut	1 (1.4 oz)	230
Organic Sesame Raisin	1 (1.4 oz)	170
Choice		
Berry Almond Crispy	1	50
Fudge Brownie	1	140
Peanut Butter Crispy	1	60
Peanutty Chocolate	1	140
Clif		
Banana Nut Bread	1 (2.4 oz)	250
Builders Chocolate Mint	1 (2.4 oz)	270
Builders Peanut Butter	1 (2.4 oz)	270
Carrot Cake	1 (2.4 oz)	240
Chocolate Brownie	1 (2.4 oz)	240
Chocolate Chip	1 (2.4 oz)	250
Cool Mint Chocolate	1 (2.4 oz)	250
Crunchy Peanut Butter	1 (2.4 oz)	250
Mojo Mixed Nuts	1 (1.6 oz)	220
Mojo Mountain Mix	1 (1.6 oz)	200
Nectar Cinnamon Pecan	1 (1.6 oz)	170
Nectar Lemon Vanilla Cashew	1 (1.6 oz)	180
Oatmeal Raisin Walnut	1 (2.4 oz)	240
ZBar Peanut Butter	1 (1.3 oz)	140
Glucerna		
All Flavors	1 (0.7 oz)	80

FOOD	PORTION	CALS
Gnu		
Flavor & Fiber Banana Walnut	1 (1.4 oz)	130
Flavor & Fiber Chocolate Brownie Bar	1 (1.4 oz)	140
Hooah!		
Chocolate Crisp	1 (2.29 oz)	280
JojoBar		
Chocolate Cashew	1 (1.8 oz)	220
Peanut Butter & Jelly	1 (1.8 oz)	220
Kashi		
GoLean Chocolate Almond Toffee	1 (2.7 oz)	290
GoLean Cookies 'N Cream	1 (2.7 oz)	290
GoLean Crunchy Chocolate Peanut	1 (1.8 oz)	180
GoLean Malted Chocolate Chip	1 (2.7 oz)	290
GoLean Oatmeal Raisin Cookie	1 (2.7 oz)	280
GoLean Peanut Butter & Chocolate	1 (2.7 oz)	290
GoLean Roll Caramel Peanut	1 (1.9 oz)	200
GoLean Roll Fudge Sundae	1 (1.9 oz)	190
TLC Chewy Granola Cherry Dark Chocolate	1 (1.2 oz)	120
TLC Crunchy Granola Honey Toasted 7 Grain	1 (1.4 oz)	180
TLC Crunchy Granola Pumpkin Spice	1 (1.4 oz)	180
TLC Crunchy Granola Roasted Almond	1 (1.4 oz)	180
LaraBar		
Apple Pie	1	190
Banana Cookie	1	210
Cashew Cookie	1	230
Cherry Pie	1	190
Chocolate Coconut Chew	1	220
Ginger Snap	1	220
Jocolat	1 (1 oz)	110
Lean Body		
Gold Caramel Cookie Twist	1 (2.9 oz)	330
Living Harvest		
Organic Hemp Protein Forbidden Fruit	1 (1.6 oz)	170
Luna		
Caramel Nut Brownie	1 (1.7 oz)	190
Chai Tea	1 (1.7 oz)	180
Dulce De Leche	1 (1.7 oz)	180
Iced Oatmeal Raisin	1 (1.7 oz)	180
Key Lime Pie	1 (1.7 oz)	180
LemonZest	1 (1.7 oz)	180

FOOD	PORTION	CALS
Nutz Over Chocolate	1 (1.7 oz)	180
Mommy Munchies		
Chocolate Mint	1 (1.8 oz)	180
Cinnamon Bun	1 (1.8 oz)	180
Mrs. May's		
Trio Blueberry	1 (1.2 oz)	170
Trio Tropical	1 (1.2 oz)	170
Nature's Path		
Optimum Blueberry Flax & Soy	1 (2 oz)	200
Optimum Cranberry Ginger & Soy	1 (2 oz)	200
Optimum Peanut Butter	1 (2 oz)	230
Optimum Pomegran Cherry	1 (2 oz)	230
Optimum ReBound	1 (2 oz)	190
Nutiva		
Organic Flax & Raisin	1 (1.4 oz)	200
Organic Flaxseed Flax Chocolate	1 (1.4 oz)	200
Original Organic Hempseed	1 (1.4 oz)	210
Odwalla		
Berries GoMega	1	220
Carrot	1	220
Choco-walla	1	240
Cranberry C Monster	1	220
Super Protein	1	230
Superfood	1	230
Oh Mama!		
Chocolate Peanut Butter	1 (1.8 oz)	190
Frosted White Lemon	1 (1.8 oz)	180
Frosted White Raspberry	1 (1.8 oz)	180
Perfect 10		
Bliss Apricot	1 (1.8 oz)	215
Bliss Cranberry	1 (1.8 oz)	215
Natural Apricot	1 (1.8 oz)	205
Natural Cranberry	1 (1.8 oz)	164
Natural Lemon	1 (1.8 oz)	210
PowerBar		
Harvest Apple Cinnamon Crisp	1 (2.3 oz)	240
Harvest Chunky Cherry Crunch	1 (2.3 oz)	240
Harvest Dipped Double Chocolate Crisp	1 (2.3 oz)	250
Harvest Dipped Oatmeal Raisin Cookie	1 (2.3 oz)	250
Harvest Dipped Toffee Chocolate Chip	1 (2.3 oz)	250

FOOD	PORTION	CALS
Harvest Peanut Butter Chocolate Chip	1 (2.3 oz)	240
Harvest Strawberry Crunch	1 (2.3 oz)	230
Performance Apple Cinnamon	1 (2.3 oz)	230
Performance Banana	1 (2.3 oz)	230
Performance Cappuccino	1 (2.3 oz)	230
Performance Chocolate	1 (2.3 oz)	230
Performance Chocolate Peanut Butter	1 (2.3 oz)	240
Performance Cookies & Cream	1 (2.3 oz)	240
Performance Malt Nut	1 (2.3 oz)	230
Performance Oatmeal Raisin	1 (2.3 oz)	230
Performance Peanut Butter	1 (2.3 oz)	230
Performance Strawberry Cream	1 (2.3 oz)	230
Performance Vanilla Crisp	1 (2.3 oz)	230
Performance Wild Berry	1 (2.3 oz)	230
Protein Plus Carb Select Chocolate	1 (2.5 oz)	260
Protein Plus Carb Select Chocolate Caramel Crunch	1 (2.6 oz)	270
Protein Plus Carb Select Chocolate Peanut Butter	1 (2.5 oz)	270
Protein Plus Carb Select Peanut Caramel	1 (2.6 oz)	270
Protein Plus Chocolate Fudge Brownie	1 (2.7 oz)	270
Protein Plus Chocolate Peanut Butter	1 (2.7 oz)	290
Protein Plus Cookies & Cream	1 (2.7 oz)	290
Protein Plus Vanilla Yogurt	1 (2.7 oz)	290
Triple Treat Caramel Peanut Crisp	1 (1.9 oz)	220
Triple Treat Caramel Peanut Fusion	1 (1.9 oz)	230
Triple Treat Chocolate Caramel Fusion	1 (1.9 oz)	230
Triple Treat Chocolate Peanut Butter Crisp	1 (1.9 oz)	220
Prana Bar		
Apricot Goji	1 (1.7 oz)	220
Coconut Acai	1 (1.7 oz)	220
Pear Ginseng	1 (1.7 oz)	220
Pria		
Carb Select Caramel Nut Brownie	1 (1.7 oz)	170
Carb Select Chocolate Mocha Crisp	1 (1.7 oz)	130
Carb Select Chocolate Peanut Butter Crisp	1 (1.7 oz)	130
Carb Select Cookies N' Caramel	1 (1.7 oz)	170
Carb Select Peanut Butter Caramel Nut	1 (1.7 oz)	170
Chocolate Peanut Crunch	1 (1 oz)	110
Complete Nutrition Chocolate Mint Crisp	1 (1.6 oz)	170

FOOD	PORTION	CALS
Complete Nutrition Chocolate Peanut Butter Crisp	1 (1.6 oz)	170
Complete Nutrition French Vanilla Crisp	1 (1.6 oz)	170
Creme Caramel Crisp	1 (1 oz)	110
Double Chocolate Cookie	1 (1 oz)	110
French Vanilla Crisp	1 (1 oz)	110
Mint Chocolate Cookie	1 (1 oz)	110
Strawberry Shortcake	1 (1 oz)	110
PureFit		
Almond Crunch	1 (2 oz)	230
Peanut Butter Crunch	1 (2 oz)	240
Resource		
Mini Nutrition Bar	1	90
Sencha Naturals		
Green Tea Bar Lively Lemongrass	1 (2 oz)	220
Green Tea Bar Original	1 (2 oz)	220
Simply Nutrilite		
Sweet & Salty	1 (1.6 oz)	170
Slim-Fast		
Classic Meal Bar Chocolate Cookie Dough	1	220
Classic Meal Bar Milk Chocolate Peanut	1	220
High Protein Granola Bar Chocolate Chip	1	190
High Protein Granola Bar Peanut	1	200
Low Carb Breakfast Bar Apple Cobbler	1	180
Low Carb Breakfast Bar Peanut Butter	1	190
Low Carb Snack Bar Caramel Nut	1	120
Low Carb Snack Bar Coconut Almond	1	120
Low Carb Snack Bar Peanut Butter Crunch	1	120
Optima Meal Bar Apple Crisp	1	180
Optima Meal Bar Caramel Crispy Peanut	1	220
Optima Meal Bar Chewy Granola Trail Mix	1	210
Optima Snack Bar Banana Nut Muffin	1	150
Optima Snack Bar Blueberry Muffin	1	140
Optima Snack Bar Chocolate Peanut Nougat	1	120
Optima Snack Bar Oatmeal Raisin Cookie	1	120
Snickers Marathon		
Chewy Chocolate Peanut	1 (1.9 oz)	210
Solo GI		
Berry Bliss	1 (1.6 oz)	190
Chocolate Charger	1 (1.6 oz)	190

FOOD	PORTION	CALS
Mint Mania	1 (1.6 oz)	190
Peanut Power	1 (1.6 oz)	200
South Beach		
Energy Mix	1 pkg (1 oz)	160
SoyJoy		
Fruit & Soy Bar Berry	1 (1.1 oz)	130
Fruit & Soy Bar Mango Coconut	1 (1.1 oz)	140
Fruit & Soy Bar Raisin Almond	1 (1.1 oz)	130
T.H.E. Bar		
Granola Raisin	1 (1.8 oz)	200
Think5		
Red Berry	1 (2.5 oz)	240
Red Berry Chocolate Covered	1 (2.8 oz)	290
ThinkPink		
Blueberry Dark Chocolate	1 (2.1 oz)	240
Lemon Burst	1 (2.1 oz)	230
Peanut Butter Caramel	1 (2.1 oz)	230
White Chocolate Raspberry	1 (2.1 oz)	240
Zoe's		
Chocolate Delight	1 (1.7 oz)	190
Chocolate Peanut Butter Bliss	1 (1.7 oz)	200
Heavenly Apple	1	180
Peanut Butter Paradise	1 (1.7 oz)	190

ENERGY DRINKS

FOOD	PORTION	CALS
180		
Blue w/ Acai	1 can (8.2 oz)	120
Blue w/ Acai Low Calorie	1 can (8.2 oz)	15
Orange Citrus Blast	1 can (8.2 oz)	120
Orange Citrus Blast Sugar Free	1 can (8.2 oz)	5
Red w/ Gogi	1 can (8.2 oz)	130
1In3Trinity		
Energy Drink	1 can (8.4 oz)	10
Accelerade		
All Flavors	8 oz	80
Amino Vital		
Amino Acid Supplement All Flavors	8 oz	35
Pro Fruit Punch	8 oz	35
Pro Tropic Fruit	8 oz	40
Puredge All Flavors	8 oz	50

FOOD	PORTION	CALS
Arizona		
Diet Green Tea Energy Drink	8 oz	10
Green Tea Energy Drink	8 oz	100
Pomegranate Lite	8 oz	70
B52		
Zero Sugar Citrus Berry	8 oz	10
Bally Blast		
Energy Drink	1 can (8.3 oz)	120
Sugar Free	1 can (8.3 oz)	10
Banzai		
Energy Drink	8 oz	120
Bawls		
Guarana	8 oz	90
Guaranexx Sugar Free	1 bottle (10 oz)	0
Beaver Buzz		
Citrus	1 can	140
Black Hole		
Blueberry	8 oz	100
Citrus	8 oz	110
Bliss		
Energy Drink	1 can (8.4 oz)	110
Low Carb	1 can (8.4 oz)	26
Bloom		
All Flavors	1 can (10.5 oz)	100
Blox		
Black Cherry	8 oz	86
Orange Rush	8 oz	103
Original	8 oz	105
Blu Fuel		
Energy Drink	1 can (10 oz)	133
BooKoo		
Energy Drink	8 oz	110
Shot All Flavors	1 can (5.57 oz)	80
Zero Carb	8 oz	0
Boost		
Beauty	1 bottle (12 oz)	220
High Protein Vanilla	8 oz	240
Youth	1 bottle (12 oz)	200
Boozer		
Hangover Remedy	1 can (8.4 oz)	110

FOOD	PORTION	CALS
Brain Toniq		
Functional Drink	1 can (8.4 oz)	80
Brain Twist		
Flu & Cold Defense All Flavors	8 oz	70
C1.5		
Extreme	1 can (8.4 oz)	120
Caballo Negro		
Double Kick	8 oz	120
Energy Drink	1 can (8.4 oz)	120
Cascabel		
Energy Drink	1 can (8.4 oz)	110
Sugar Free	1 can (8.4 oz)	10
Celsius		
Ginger Ale	1 bottle (12 oz)	10
Orange	1 bottle (12 oz)	10
Cheetah		
Energy Drink	1 can (12 oz)	80
Choice		
Chocolate	1 can (8 oz)	220
Vanilla	1 can (8 oz)	220
Cintron		
Citrus Mango	8 oz	110
Citrus Mango Sugar Free	8 oz	0
Coca-Cola		
Zero	8 oz	1
Coolah		
Original	8 oz	120
Cytomax		
Sport Drinks All Flavors	1 bottle (20 oz)	130
Defcon3		
Healthy Energy Soda	1 can (12 oz)	45
Defense		
Effervescent Supplement	1 can	150
Diablo		
Energy Drink	1 can (8.7 oz)	151
DNA Energy		
Low Carb Citrus	8 oz	0
Double Hit		
Maximum Energy Coffee Drink Sugar Free	1 can (12 oz)	0

FOOD	PORTION	CALS
Dr. Tim's		
ISO-5	1 bottle (11.2 oz)	60
Jungle Juice	1 bottle (4 oz)	20
Emu		
Energy Drink	1 bottle (8.4 oz)	170
EQ Thirst Equalizer		
All Flavors	8 oz	60
Everlast		
High Energy Citrus Blast	1 can (8.3 oz)	140
Freedom		
Energy Drink	1 can (12 oz)	160
Full Throttle		
Energy Drink	8 oz	100
Fury	8 oz	110
Function		
Alternative Energy	8 oz	60
Brainiac Carambola Punch	8 oz	60
Urban Detox Citrus Prickly Pear	8 oz	60
Youth Trip Acai Grape	8 oz	60
Fuze		
Refresh Banana Coconut	8 oz	90
Refresh Peach Mango	8 oz	90
Refresh Strawberry Banana	8 oz	100
Slenderize Cranberry Raspberry	8 oz	5
Slenderize Low Carb Tropical Punch	8 oz	5
Slenderize Tangerine Grapefruit	8 oz	10
Vitalize Blackberry Grape	8 oz	100
Vitalize Orange Mango	8 oz	100
Gatorade		
All Flavors	8 oz	50
Ginger Orange	8 oz	110
Lemonade All Flavors	8 oz	50
Rain All Flavors	8 oz	50
X-Factor All Flavors	8 oz	50
Gleukos		
Preformance All Flavors	8 oz	70
Go Fast		
Energy Drink	1 can (8.4 oz)	90
Light	1 can (8.4 oz)	20
Sportsman's	1 can (8.4 oz)	90

FOOD	PORTION	CALS
Guaraviton		
Energy Drink	8 oz	98
Guayaki		
Organic Empower Mint	8 oz	38
Organic Raspberry Revolution	8 oz	50
Organic Unsweetened	8 oz	15
Guru		
Energy Drink	1 can (8.3 oz)	100
Lite	1 can (8.3 oz)	5
Happy Bunny		
Spaz Juice	1 can (8.4 oz)	110
Her Energy		
Pink Lemonade	1 can (8.4 oz)	130
Pink Lemonade Sugar Free	1 can (8.4 oz)	0
Hiball		
All Flavors	1 bottle (10 oz)	10
Hiro		
Thermo	1 can (8.33 oz)	10
Vitality	1 can (8.33 oz)	10
Hooah!		
Soldier Fuel All Flavors	1 can (12 oz)	160
Hydrive		
All Flavors	1 bottle (11.2 oz)	25
Iron Energy		
All Flavors	8 oz	90
Jet Set		
Club Soda	1 can (12 oz)	0
Ginger Ale	1 can (12 oz)	150
Original	1 can (12 oz)	105
Tonic Water	1 can (12 oz)	150
King 888		
Original	8 oz	110
Sugar Free	8 oz	0
Krank'd		
All Flavors	1 bottle (16 oz)	80
Liv Naturals		
All Flavors	8 oz	70
Lost		
Big Gun	6 oz	100
Five-O	8 oz	70

FOOD	PORTION	CALS
Perfect 10	8 oz	10
Marquis Platinum		
Vitality Drink	1 can	30
Mix1		
All Flavors	1 bottle (11 oz)	200
Monster		
Energy Assault	8 oz	100
Energy Drink	8 oz	100
Khaos Energy Juice	8 oz	90
Lo Carb	8 oz	10
Mr. Re		
Restorative	1 can (11 oz)	80
Nexcite		
Herbal Fizz	1 bottle	72
NOS		
High Performance	1 bottle (11 oz)	150
Ocean Spray		
Cranergy Cranberry Life	1 bottle (12 oz)	50
Cranergy Raspberry Cranberry Lift	1 bottle (12 oz)	50
Odwalla		
Berries GoMega	8 oz	160
Mo' Beta	8 oz	150
Super Protein Original	8 oz	190
Superfood	8 oz	130
Wellness	8 oz	150
OOBA		
All Flavors	8 oz	90
Pickle Juice		
Dill	8 oz	0
Sport	8 oz	7
Pimpjuice		
Energy Drink	1 can (8 oz)	140
PJ Tight	1 can (8 oz)	20
Power Trip		
Xtreme	1 can (10.5 oz)	140
Powerade		
Arctic Shatter	8 oz	64
Fruit Punch	8 oz	65
Green Squall	8 oz	64
Jagged Ice	8 oz	65

FOOD	PORTION	CALS
NASCAR Grape	8 oz	64
Olympic Citrus	8 oz	63
Option All Flavors	8 oz	10
PowerBar		
Endurance Sport Drink	1 pkg (0.6 oz)	70
Performance Recovery Drink	1 pkg (0.8 oz)	90
Purity Organic		
Acerola Cherry	1 bottle	60
Pomegranate Blueberry	1 bottle	60
Pomegranate Raspberry	1 bottle	60
Quench Aid		
Berry	1 pkg	10
Dragonfruit	1 pkg	10
Rawlings EX2		
Sustained Energy	1 can (8.4 oz)	132
Red Eye		
Classic	1 bottle (12 oz)	208
Extreme	1 bottle (12 oz)	140
Gold	1 bottle (12 oz)	208
Passion	1 bottle (12 oz)	149
Platinum	1 bottle (12 oz)	149
Rehab		
Recovery Supplement	1 can (12 oz)	150
Resurrect		
Daily Detox & Anti-Hangover Elixir	1 can (12 oz)	5
Rip It		
Citrus X	8 oz	130
Citrus X Sugar Free	8 oz	0
Energy Fuel	8 oz	130
Energy Lite	8 oz	0
Rockstar		
Energy Cola	8 oz	120
Energy Drink	8 oz	140
Juiced	8 oz	90
Ronin		
Diet	1 can (16 oz)	15
Original	1 can (16 oz)	180
Rox		
Energy Drink	1 can	110
Zero	1 can	10

FOOD	PORTION	CALS
Rumba		
Energy Juice	8 oz	120
Simply Nutrilite		
Berry Antioxidant	1 can (8.4 oz)	120
Slim-Fast		
Classic Ready-To-Drink Creamy Milk Chocolate	1 can	220
Classic Ready-To-Drink French Vanilla	1 can	220
High Protein Ready-To-Drink All Flavors	1 can	190
Low Carb Diet Ready-To-Drink All Flavors	1 can	190
Snapple A Day		
Meal Replacement All Flavors	1 bottle (11.5 oz)	210
SoBe		
Drive	8 oz	120
Karma	8 oz	120
Lean Diet Citrus	8 oz	5
Sol Mate		
All Flavors	1 bottle	90
Source Burn		
2	8 oz	130
Energy Drink	8 oz	140
Sugar Free	8 oz	10
Speed Zone		
Energy Drink	1 can (8.4 oz)	110
Steaz		
Organic Fuel	8 oz	90
Stewie's		
Domination Serum	1 can (8.45 oz)	110
Mind Erase Elixir	1 can (8.45 oz)	100
Stinger		
All Flavors	1 can (8.4 oz)	130
Sugar Free All Flavors	1 can (8.4 oz)	0
Sum Poosie		
Energy Drink	1 bottle (12 oz)	170
Swing Juice		
Energy Drink	8 oz	60
Tantra		
Erotic	1 can (8.4 oz)	130
T-Fusion		
Energy Tea	8 oz	0

FOOD	PORTION	CALS
The Beast		
Energy Drink	1 can (8.3 oz)	120
Therafizz		
Energy	1 pkg	8
Vitamin C	1 pkg	5
Tornado		
Energy Drink	8 oz	110
Vault		
Energy Drink	8 oz	120
Venga		
Brainstorm	8 oz	130
Calorie Burn	8 oz	10
Energize	8 oz	100
Health&Zen	8 oz	80
ViB		
Chill-N	1 can (8 oz)	40
Who's Your Daddy		
Original	8 oz	110
Sugar Free	8 oz	0
Wide Open Performance		
Energy Drink	1 can (8.3 oz)	120
Xcyto		
Sugar Free	1 can (12.5 oz)	10
XL		
Diet	1 can (8.8 oz)	10
Energy Drink	1 can (8.8 oz)	113
Xtazy		
All Flavors	1 can	160
Youth Juice		
Drink	2 oz	10
Zenergize		
Chill	1 tablet	2
Energy+	1 tablet	2
Hydrate	1 tablet	2
ENGLISH MUFFIN		
READY-TO-EAT		
apple cinnamon	1	138
crumpet	1 (1.5 oz)	80
granola	1	155
mixed grain	1	155

FOOD	PORTION	CALS
plain	1	134
plain toasted	1	133
raisin cinnamon	1	138
sourdough	1	134
wheat	1	127
whole wheat	1	134
Crystal Farms		
English Muffin	1	130
Food For Life		
7 Sprouted Grains	1	160
Ezekiel 4:9 Cinnamon Raisin	1	160
Ezekiel 4:9 Sprouted Grain	1	160
Genesis 1:29 Original	1	180
Pepperidge Farm		
100% Whole Wheat	1	140
Original	1	130
Rudi's Organic Bakery		
MultiGrain w/ Flax	1 (2 oz)	130
Whole Grain Wheat	1 (2 oz)	120
Sara Lee		
Heart Healthy Wheat w/ Honey	1	140
Original w/ Whole Grain	1	140
Thomas'		
100 Calories	1	100
Corn	1	150
Griller Multi Grain	1 (3.2 oz)	210
Griller Onion	1 (3.2 oz)	200
Hearty Grains 100% Whole Wheat	1	120
Hearty Grains Honey Wheat	1	130
Light Multi Grain	1	100
Oatmeal & Honey	1	130
Original	1	120
Original Whole Grain	1	130
Raisin Cinnamon	1	140
Sandwich Size Original	1	190
TAKE-OUT		
w/ butter	1 (2.2 oz)	189
w/ cheese & sausage	1 (4 oz)	393
w/ egg cheese & canadian bacon	1 (4.8 oz)	289
w/ egg cheese & sausage	1 (5.8 oz)	487

FOOD	PORTION	CALS
EPAZOTE		
fresh	1 tbsp (1 g)	tr
fresh sprig	1 (2 g)	1
EPPAW		
raw	½ cup	75
FALAFEL		
Near East		
Falafel Patties Vegetarian as prep	2.5	220
Sabra		
Burger	1 (1.8 oz)	90
VeggieLand		
FalafelBurger	1 (4 oz)	190
TAKE-OUT		
falafel	1 (1.2 oz)	57
FAT (see also BUTTER, BUTTER SUBSTITUTES, MARGARINE, OIL)		
bacon grease	1 tbsp	116
beef shortening	1 tbsp	115
beef suet	1 oz	242
chicken	1 tbsp (0.4 oz)	115
duck	1 tbsp (0.4 oz)	113
goose	1 tbsp	115
goose	1 oz	257
lamb new zealand	1 oz	182
lard	1 cup (205 g)	1849
lard	1 tbsp (13 g)	115
meat pan drippings	½ tbsp	124
pork raw	1 oz	230
salt pork	1 cube (1 oz)	215
shortening	1 tbsp	113
shortening	1 cup	1812
turkey	1 tbsp	116
ucuhuba butter	1 tbsp	120
whale blubber	1 oz	244
Crisco		
Butter Flavor	1 tbsp	110
Shortening	1 tbsp	110
Earth Balance		
Natural Shortening	1 tbsp	130

FOOD	PORTION	CALS
Nebraska Land		
Pork Fatback	0.5 oz	110
Smart Balance		
Shortening	1 tbsp	110
Spectrum		
Organic Shortening	1 tbsp	110
FAVA BEANS		
canned	½ cup	91
fava fresh cooked	½ cup	94
Progresso		
Fava Beans	½ cup (4.6 oz)	100
FEIJOA		
fresh	1 (1.75 oz)	25
puree	1 cup	119
FENNEL		
fresh bulb	1 (8.2 oz)	73
fresh sliced	1 cup	27
leaves	1 oz	7
seed	1 tsp	7
stir fried	1 cup	85
Ocean Mist		
Fennel Sweet Anise Sliced Fresh	1 cup	27
FENUGREEK		
seed	1 tsp	12
FIBER		
apple fiber	0.5 oz	40
Benefiber		
Supplement	1 pkg (4 g)	20
Metamucil		
Natural Fiber Regular Flavor	1 rounded tsp (7 g)	25
UniFiber		
Natural Fiber	1 pkg (4 g)	4
Wellements		
Fiber-Psyll	1 scoop (0.5 oz)	55
FIDDLEHEAD FERNS		
fresh	3.5 oz	34

FOOD	PORTION	CALS
FIG JUICE		
Smart Juice		
Organic 100% Juice	8 oz	131
FIGS		
canned in heavy syrup	½ cup	114
canned in light syrup	½ cup	87
canned water pack	½ cup	66
dried california	½ cup (3.5 oz)	200
dried cooked	½ cup	139
dried small	1 (1.4 oz)	30
dried whole	1 (8 g)	21
fresh large	1 (2.2 oz)	47
Blue Ribbon		
California Figs	1 pkg (1.5 oz)	120
Figamajigs		
Chocolate Covered Bar	1 bar (1.4 oz)	130
Chocolate Covered Bar w/ Almonds	1 bar (1.4 oz)	150
Hermes		
Organic Adriatic Fig Spread	1 tbsp	60
Nuta Figs		
Mission	¼ cup (1.4 oz)	110
Orchard Choice		
Mission	4–5 (1.4 oz)	110
Trucco		
Kalamata	2	100
FIREWEED		
leaves chopped	1 cup (0.8 oz)	24
FISH (see also individual names, FISH SUBSTITUTES, SUSHI)		
CANNED		
Beach Cliff		
Fish Steaks In Louisiana Hot Sauce	1 can (3.7 oz)	160
Fish Steaks In Mustard Sauce	1 can (3.7 oz)	160
Fish Steaks In Soybean Oil	1 can (3.7 oz)	200
Fish Steaks w/ Hot Green Chilies	1 can (3.7 oz)	160
Fish Steaks w/ Jalapeno Peppers	1 can (3.7 oz)	130
Brunswick		
Fish Steaks In Louisiana Hot Sauce	1 can (3.7 oz)	160
Fish Steaks In Mustard Sauce	1 can (3.7 oz)	160
Fish Steaks In Soybean Oil	1 can (3.7 oz)	200

FOOD	PORTION	CALS
Fish Steaks In Spring Water	1 can (3.7 oz)	150
Fish Steaks w/ Hot Tabasco Peppers	1 can (3.7 oz)	220
Seafood Snacks Golden Smoked	1 can (3.2 oz)	170
Seafood Snacks In Lemon & Cracked Pepper	1 can (3.2 oz)	160
Seafood Snacks In Louisiana Hot Sauce	1 can (3.2 oz)	140
Seafood Snacks In Teriyaki Sauce	1 can (3.2 oz)	160
Seafood Snacks In Tomato & Basil Sauce	1 can (3.2 oz)	140
Seafood Snacks Kippered	1 can (3.2 oz)	160
Chicken Of The Sea		
Fish Steaks	½ can (2 oz)	70
FROZEN		
breaded fillet	1 (2 oz)	155
sticks	1 stick (1 oz)	76
Dr. Praeger's		
Breaded Fillets	1 (2.1 oz)	100
Fishies	3 (1.5 oz)	90
Gorton's		
Classic Crispy Battered Fillets	2	230
Classic Crunchy Golden Fillets	2	140
Fillets Beer Battered	2 (3.6 oz)	250
Fillets Breaded Lemon Herb	2 (3.6 oz)	240
Fillets Potato Crunch	2 (3.6 oz)	240
Fish Sticks Classic Breaded	6	290
Grilled Fillets Cajun Blackened	1 (3.8 oz)	100
Grilled Fillets Lemon Pepper	1 (3.7 oz)	100
Tenders Original Batter	3 pieces (3.6 oz)	230
Ian's		
Fillets	1 (3.4 oz)	260
Fish Sticks	5 pieces	190
Fish Sticks Allergy Free	5 pieces	190
Van de Kamp's		
Battered Tenders	4 (4 oz)	210
Crisp & Healthy Breaded Fish Sticks	6 (3.6 oz)	140
Crunchy Fillets	2 (3.5 oz)	230
Sticks	6 (4 oz)	260
TAKE-OUT		
fish cake	1 (4.7 oz)	166
jamaican brown fish stew	1 serv	426
kedgeree	5.6 oz	242
mousse	1 serv (3.5 oz)	185

FOOD	PORTION	CALS
stew	1 cup (7.9 oz)	157
taramasalata	2 tbsp	124
FISH OIL		
cod liver	1 tbsp	123
herring	1 tbsp	123
menhaden	1 tbsp	123
salmon	1 tbsp	123
sardine	1 tbsp	123
shark	1 oz	270
whale beluga	1 oz	252
whale bowhead	1 oz	252
Cormega		
Omega-E Orange	1 pkg	20
Spectrum		
Cod Liver Oil w/ Lemon	1 tsp	40
FISH PASTE		
fish paste	2 tsp	15
FLAXSEED		
Arrowhead Mills		
Organic	3 tbsp (1 oz)	140
Bob's Red Mill		
Flaxseed Meal	2 tbsp	60
Carringon Farms		
Organic Flax Paks	1 pkg (0.4 oz)	50
Flax USA		
Flax Sprinkles	2 tbsp (0.5 oz)	70
Hodgson Mill		
Milled	2 tbsp	60
Natural Ovens		
Flax Complete Supplement	1 tbsp (0.4 oz)	60
Tree Of Life		
Flax Seed	3 tbsp (1 oz)	140
FLOUNDER		
FRESH		
cooked	3 oz	99
cooked	1 fillet (4.5 oz)	148

FOOD	PORTION	CALS
FROZEN		
Mrs. Paul's		
Fillets Lightly Breaded	1 (2.7 oz)	150
TAKE-OUT		
breaded & fried	3.2 oz	211
stuffed w/ crab	1 piece (7.6 oz)	332
FLOUR		
all-purpose self-rising	½ cup (2.2 oz)	221
all-purpose unbleached	½ cup (2.2 oz)	228
arrowroot	½ cup (2.2 oz)	228
bread flour	½ cup (2.4 oz)	247
buckwheat whole groat	½ cup (2.1 oz)	201
cake	½ cup (2.4 oz)	248
carob	1 tbsp (0.2 oz)	13
carob	½ cup (1.8 oz)	114
chickpea besan	½ cup (1.6 oz)	178
peanut low fat	½ cup (1.1 oz)	128
potato	½ cup (2.8 oz)	286
rice brown	½ cup (2.8 oz)	287
rice white	½ cup (2.8 oz)	289
rye dark	½ cup (2.2 oz)	207
rye light	½ cup (1.8 oz)	187
soy lowfat	½ cup (1.5 oz)	165
triticale whole grain	½ cup (2.3 oz)	220
white all-purpose enriched bleached	½ cup (2.2 oz)	228
whole wheat	½ cup (2.1 oz)	203
Arrowhead Mills		
Organic Barley	⅓ cup	95
Organic Brown Rice	⅓ cup	130
Organic Kamut	⅓ cup	130
Organic Oat	⅓ cup	120
Organic Rye	¼ cup	110
Organic Spelt	⅓ cup	130
Organic Unbleached White	¼ cup	120
Organic White Rice	⅓ cup	120
Bob's Red Mill		
Brown Rice	¼ cup	140
Corn	¼ cup	160
Graham	¼ cup	120
Kamut Organic	¼ cup	94

FOOD	PORTION	CALS
Sorghum Sweet White Gluten Free	¼ cup	120
Spelt	¼ cup	120
Whole Wheat	¼ cup	110
Whole Wheat Hard White Organic	¼ cup	120
Domata Living Flour		
Gluten Free Casein Free	¼ cup	110
Gold Medal		
All Purpose	¼ cup (1 oz)	100
Self Rising	¼ cup (1 oz)	100
Whole Wheat	¼ cup (1 oz)	100
Wondra	¼ cup (1 oz)	100
Heckers		
All Purpose Unbleached	¼ cup	100
Hodgson Mill		
Best For Bread	¼ cup	100
Buckwheat	¼ cup	100
Oat Bran Flour	¼ cup	110
Kentucky Kernel		
Seasoned Flour	4 tsp	36
King Arthur		
All Purpose	¼ cup	110
All Purpose Unbleached	¼ cup	110
Organic Artisan	¼ cup	110
Organic White Whole Wheat	¼ cup	100
Organic Whole Wheat	½ cup	110
Self-Rising	¼ cup	120
White Whole Wheat	¼ cup	100
Whole Wheat	¼ cup	110
Lundberg		
Brown Rice	¼ cup	110
Manitoba Harvest		
Hemp Seed Flour	¼ cup	120
FOOD COLORS		
blue	1 tsp	0
orange	1 tsp	0
red	1 tsp	tr
yellow	1 tsp	tr
FRENCH BEANS		
dried cooked	1 cup	228

FOOD	PORTION	CALS
FRENCH FRIES (see POTATOES)		
FRENCH TOAST		
french toast frzn	1 slice (2 oz)	126
Aunt Jemima		
Cinnamon	2 slices (4 oz)	240
Whole Grain	2 slices (4 oz)	240
Eggo		
Toaster Sticks Original	2	220
Farm Rich		
Original Sticks	5 (4.2 oz)	330
Ian's		
Sticks	5 (3.2 oz)	250
TAKE-OUT		
plain	1 slice	151
sticks	5 (4.9 oz)	513
w/ butter	2 slices	356
FROG LEGS		
frog legs	3 oz	175
TAKE-OUT		
as prep w/ seasoned flour & fried	1 (0.8)	70
FRUCTOSE		
Bob's Red Mill		
Fructose	1 tsp	15
Estee		
Fructose	1 tsp	15
Packet	1 pkg	10
Tree Of Life		
Fructose	1 tsp (4 g)	15
FRUIT DRINKS (see also individual names, SMOOTHIES, YOGURT DRINKS)		
MIX		
Bio Fruit		
Mix	1 scoop (8 g)	42
Crystal Light		
LiveActive On The Go	1 pkg	10
Sugar Free All Flavors as prep	1 serv	5
Luna		
Dragonfruit Kiwi	1 pkg	50
Pomegranate Berry	1 pkg	50

FOOD	PORTION	CALS
South Beach		
Tide Me Over Strawberry Banana	1 pkg	30
Tide Me Over Tropical Breeze	1 pkg	30
Tang		
Orange Pineapple as prep	1 serv (8 oz)	100
Orange Strawberry as prep	1 serv (8 oz)	110
READY-TO-DRINK		
fruit punch	6 oz	87
After The Fall		
Banana Casablanca	8 oz	150
Mango Montage	8 oz	150
Apple & Eve		
100% Cranberry Apple Juice	8 oz	100
Mango Mangosteen	8 oz	120
Brazsoy		
Fruit Juice w/ Soy	8 oz	94
Capri Sun		
Fruit Punch	1 pkg (7 oz)	90
Crayons		
Kiwi Strawberry	1 bottle (12 oz)	130
Outrageous Orange Mango	1 bottle (12 oz)	140
Redder Than Ever Fruitpunch	1 bottle (12 oz)	130
Crystal Light		
Strawberry Kiwi Sugar Free	8 oz	5
Drenchers		
Super Fruit Endurance Grape Apple	8 oz	120
Super Juice Fit N' Lean Heart Healthy Tropical Passion	8 oz	10
Super Juice Fit N' Lean Power Protein Orange Cream	8 oz	20
Super Juice Immunity Fruit & Veggie Berry	8 oz	110
Essn		
Sparkling Blood Orange & Cranberry	1 can (8.4 oz)	160
Feel Good Drinks		
Spritz Cranberry & Lime No Sugar Added	1 bottle	159
Spritz Orange & Passionfruit No Sugar Added	1 bottle	151
Spritz Pink Citrus No Sugar Added	1 bottle	159
Firefly		
Chill Out De-stress Drink	1 bottle (11.2 oz)	100
De-tox Morning After Drink	1 bottle (11.2 oz)	104

FOOD	PORTION	CALS
Five Alive		
Citrus	8 oz	120
Fizz Ed.		
Pomegranate Cherry	1 can (8.4 oz)	90
Frutzzo		
Organic 100% Juice Pomegranate Acai	1 bottle (12 oz)	140
Organic 100% Juice Pomegranate Passionfruit	1 bottle (12 oz)	140
GoodBelly		
Black Currant Probiotic Drink	8 oz	120
Blueberry Acai Probiotic Drink	1 bottle (2.7 oz)	50
Cranberry Watermelon Probiotic Drink	8 oz	100
Peach Mango Probiotic Drink	1 bottle (2.7 oz)	50
Strawberry Rosehips Probiotic Drink	1 bottle (2.7 oz)	50
Hawaiian Punch		
Bodacious Berry	8 oz	110
Fruit Juicy Red	8 oz	80
Green Berry Rush	8 oz	120
Mazin Melon Mix	8 oz	110
Tropical Vibe	8 oz	110
Wild Purple Smash	8 oz	110
Hog Wash		
All Flavors	1 bottle (10 oz)	37
Hood		
Fruit Punch	1 cup	120
Juici		
Sparkling All Flavors	1 bottle (12 oz)	105
Juicy Juice		
Harvest Surprise Orange Mango	8 oz	130
Kagome		
Burgundy Berry Blossom	8 oz	100
Golden Peach Garden	8 oz	100
Orange Carrot Blossom	8 oz	100
Purple Roots & Fruits	8 oz	130
L&A		
Pineapple Coconut	8 oz	140
Lakewood		
Lean Green	6 oz	90
Organic Acai Amazon Berry	6 oz	95
Land O Lakes		
Juice Cranberry Apple	1 cup (8 oz)	120

FOOD	PORTION	CALS
Minute Maid		
Berry Kiwi	1 can (12 oz)	160
Cranberry Grape	8 oz	150
Light Mango Tropical	8 oz	5
Light Orange Tangerine	8 oz	15
Orange Tangerine	8 oz	110
Pomegranate Blueberry 100% Juice	8 oz	120
Tropical Punch Chilled	8 oz	110
Naked Juice		
Berry Blast	8 oz	120
Blue Machine	8 oz	170
Green Machine	8 oz	130
Mango Acai	8 oz	190
Power C	8 oz	120
Protein Zone	8 oz	210
Red Machine	8 oz	160
Strawberry Banana C	8 oz	120
Very Berry	8 oz	130
Very Pro Berry	8 oz	190
Well Being	8 oz	140
Nantucket Nectars		
100% Juice Peach Orange	8 oz	130
100% Juice Pomegranate Cherry	8 oz	120
Kiwi Berry	8 oz	120
Organic Banana Mango Carrot	8 oz	140
Pineapple Orange Guava	8 oz	120
Newman's Own		
Orange Mango Tango	8 oz	150
Noble		
Organic 100% Juice Orange Tangerine	8 oz	120
Northland		
Cranberry Blueberry	1 cup (8 oz)	140
NutraShake		
Fruit Punch Plus Fiber	1 pkg (8 oz)	120
Ocean Spray		
Ruby Tangerine	8 oz	120
Odwalla		
Quenchers AntioxiDance	8 oz	90
Quenchers B Berrier	8 oz	120

FOOD	PORTION	CALS
OKF		
Sparkling Fresh Guava	1 bottle (8.3 oz)	20
Sparkling Fresh Peach	1 bottle (8.3 oz)	50
Old Orchard		
100% Juice Pomegranate Black Currant	8 oz	130
100% Juice Pomegranate Cherry	8 oz	140
Cocktail Apple Passion Mango	8 oz	120
Healthy Balance Apple Kiwi Strawberry	8 oz	30
Phat Phruit		
Peach Mango	8 oz	40
Pineapple Orange	8 oz	40
Sabor Latino		
Guava Mango Drink	1 box (7 oz)	110
Nectar Strawberry Banana + Calcium	8 oz	150
Pina Colada	8 oz	130
Snapple		
Cranberry Raspberry	8 oz	120
Diet Carrot Apple	8 oz	10
Diet Plum-A-Granate	8 oz	0
Go Bananas	8 oz	120
Kiwi Strawberry	8 oz	110
Snapricot Orange	8 oz	120
Ssips		
Cherry Berry	1 box (7 oz)	110
Sun Shower		
100% Juice Nectarine Mango	8 oz	93
Sundia		
Tropical Medley	½ cup	70
Tree Ripe		
Organic Fruit Punch	8 oz	150
TreeTop		
Apple Grape No Sugar Added	8 oz	130
Tropicana		
Fruit Punch	1 cup	130
Light Fruit Punch	8 oz	10
Orange Tangerine Juice	8 oz	110
Orchard Berry	8 oz	110
Organic Orchard Medley	8 oz	120
Twister Berry Blast	8 oz	120
Twister Citrus Spark	8 oz	120

FOOD	PORTION	CALS
Twister Fruit Fury	8 oz	120
Twister Light Strawberry Spiral	8 oz	40
V8		
Light Peach Mango	8 oz	50
Splash Berry Blend	8 oz	70
Splash Diet Berry Blend	8 oz	10
Splash Mango Peach	8 oz	80
V-Fusion Pomegranate Blueberry	8 oz	100
Vruit		
Apple Carrot	1 box (8.45 oz)	120
Berry Veggie	1 box (8.45 oz)	110
Orange Veggie	1 box (8.45 oz)	110
Tropical Blend	1 box (8.45 oz)	110
Wadda Juice		
All Flavors	1 bottle (4 oz)	25
Walnut Acres		
Organic Orange Carrot	8 oz	110
Welch's		
White Grape Peach 100% Juice	8 oz	160

FRUIT MIXED (see also individual names)
CANNED

FOOD	PORTION	CALS
fruit cocktail in heavy syrup	½ cup	93
fruit cocktail juice pack	½ cup	56
fruit cocktail water pack	½ cup	40
fruit salad in heavy syrup	½ cup	94
fruit salad in light syrup	½ cup	73
fruit salad juice pack	½ cup	62
fruit salad water pack	½ cup	37
mixed fruit in heavy syrup	½ cup	92
tropical fruit salad in heavy syrup	½ cup	110
Del Monte		
Carb Clever Fruit Cocktail	½ cup	40
Fruit Cocktail In 100% Juice	½ cup	60
Fruit Cocktail In Extra Light Syrup	½ cup	60
Fruit Cocktail In Heavy Syrup	½ cup	100
Fruit Naturals Tropical Medley	½ cup	70
Orchard Select Premium Mixed	½ cup	80
SunFresh Citrus Salad	½ cup	80

FOOD	PORTION	CALS
Dole		
Mixed Fruit Light Syrup	½ cup (4.3 oz)	80
Tropical Fruit Salad	½ cup	80
Liberty Gold		
Fruit Cocktail In Heavy Syrup	½ cup	90
Polar		
Mixed Fruit Light Syrup	½ cup (4.9 oz)	50
DRIED		
mixed	11 oz pkg	712
Brothers-All-Natural		
Crisps Strawberry Banana	1 pkg (0.42 oz)	45
Fruitaceuticals		
PomaCrans	¼ cup	100
Fun-Yums		
Fresh Crispy Mixed Fruit	1 serv (0.9 oz)	25
Goodniks		
Fruit Medley	¼ cup	110
Mariani		
Berries 'N Cherries	¼ cup	140
Revolution Foods		
Organic Mashups Tropical	1 pkg (3.2 oz)	60
Sun-Maid		
Mixed	¼ cup	100
Sunsweet		
Berry Blend	¼ cup (1.4 oz)	120
Orchard Mix	¼ cup (1.4 oz)	100
Tropical Mix	⅓ cup	150
FROZEN		
mixed fruit sweetened	1 cup	245
FRUIT SNACKS		
fruit leather	1 bar (0.8 oz)	81
fruit leather pieces	1 pkg (0.9 oz)	92
fruit leather pieces	1 oz	97
fruit leather rolls	1 sm (0.5 oz)	49
fruit leather rolls	1 lg (0.7 oz)	73
Bare Fruit		
Bananas & Cherries	1 pkg (0.6 oz)	55
Betty Crocker		
Fruit By The Foot All Flavors	1 roll	80

FOOD	PORTION	CALS
Funky Monkey		
Bananamon	1 pkg (1 oz)	110
Carnaval Mix	1 pkg (1 oz)	110
Jivealime	1 pkg (1 oz)	110
Purple Funk	1 pkg (1 oz)	120
Jelly Belly		
Fruit Snacks	1 pkg (2.5 oz)	220
Peeled Snacks		
Fruit & Nuts FigSated	⅓ cup	150
Fruit & Nuts Plu-what?	⅓ cup	150
Revolution Foods		
Organic Mashups Berry	1 pkg (3.2 oz)	40
Sharkies		
Organic Energy Fruit Chews All Flavors	1 pkg (1.8 oz)	170
Stretch Island		
Fruit Leather Bountiful Blueberry	1 pkg (0.5 oz)	45
Fruit Leather Harvest Grape	1 pkg (0.5 oz)	45
Fruit Leather Mango Sunrise	1 pkg (0.5 oz)	45
Fruit Leather Truly Tropical	1 pkg (0.5 oz)	45
Organic Smooshed Fruit Apple	1 piece (0.4 oz)	40
Organic Smooshed Fruit Strawberry	1 piece (0.4 oz)	40
Tahitian Noni		
Soft Chews Raspberry	1 pkg (2 oz)	240
Tropicana		
Fruit Wise Bars All Flavors	1 bar (1.4 oz)	140
Fruit Wise Strips All Flavors	1 strip (0.7 oz)	70
Welch's		
Fruit'N Yogurt Strawberry	1 pkg (0.9 oz)	90
Mixed Fruit	1 pkg (0.9 oz)	80
GARLIC		
clove	1	4
fresh chopped	1 tbsp	18
powder	1 tsp	9
Dorot		
Crushed Cubes frzn	1 cube (4 g)	7
Frieda's		
Elephant	1 tbsp	5
Vinegar Marinated	1 oz	30
McCormick		
Garlic Salt	¼ tsp	0

FOOD	PORTION	CALS
Spice World		
Ajo Garlic Clove	1 (3 g)	5
GEFILTE FISH		
sweet	1 piece (1.5 oz)	35
Mrs. Adler's		
Pike'n Whitefish	1 piece (1.8 oz)	50
Ungar's		
Gefilte Fish	2 slices (1.8 oz)	83
Lite	2 slices (2.4 oz)	80
No Sugar	2 slices (1.8 oz)	70
GELATIN		
READY-TO-EAT		
Del Monte		
Mandarin Orange In Lite Orange Gel	1 pkg (4.5 oz)	60
Mixed Fruit In Cherry Gel	1 pkg (4.5 oz)	90
Peaches In Lite Strawberry Banana Gel	1 pkg (4.5 oz)	60
Peaches In Peach Gel	1 pkg (4.5 oz)	90
Peaches In Raspberry Gel	1 pkg (4.5 oz)	90
Hunt's		
Snack Pack Juicy Gels Raspberry Mixed Berry	1 serv (3.5 oz)	100
Snack Pack Juicy Gels Strawberry	1 serv (3.5 oz)	100
Snack Pack Juicy Gels Strawberry Orange	1 serv (3.5 oz)	100
Snack Pack Tropical Punch	1 serv (3.5 oz)	100
Jell-O		
Sugar Free Lemon Lime	1 serv (3.2 oz)	10
Kozy Shack		
Gel Treats Cherry	1 pkg (4 oz)	85
Gel Treats Lemon Lime	1 pkg (4 oz)	85
Gel Treats Orange	1 pkg (4 oz)	85
Gel Treats Strawberry	1 pkg (4 oz)	85
Gel Treats Sugar Free Orange	1 pkg (4 oz)	11
Gel Treats Sugar Free Strawberry	1 pkg (4 oz)	11
GIBLETS		
capon simmered	1 cup (5 oz)	238
chicken fried	1 cup (5 oz)	402
chicken simmered	1 cup (5 oz)	289
turkey simmered	1 cup (5 oz)	243

FOOD	PORTION	CALS
GINGER		
ground	1 tsp	6
pickled	0.5 oz	5
preserved	1.5 oz	34
root fresh	5 slices	9
root fresh sliced	¼ cup	19
Eden		
Pickled w/ Shiso Leaves	1 tbsp	20
Frieda's		
Crystallized	9 pieces (1.1 oz)	100
Galanga Thai Ginger	⅔ cup	60
McCormick		
Crystallized	¼ tsp	15
Tree Of Life		
Crystallized Pieces	7 (1.4 oz)	150
GINKGO NUTS		
canned	1 oz	32
dried	1 oz	99
raw	1 oz	52
GINSENG		
dried	1 oz	90
fresh	1 oz	28
GIZZARDS		
chicken simmered	1 cup (5 oz)	212
turkey simmered	1 (3 oz)	103
GNOCCHI		
Racconto		
Potato Whole Wheat as prep w/o salt	1 cup (5.8 oz)	248
Vantia		
Gnocchi Whole Wheat	¾ cup	210
GOAT		
roasted	3 oz	122
GOJI BERRIES		
dried	1 oz	106
Kopali		
Organic Dark Chocolate Covered	½ pkg (1 oz)	120

FOOD	PORTION	CALS
Navitas Naturals		
Dried	1 oz	90
Sunfood		
Organic	1 oz	90
Superfood Snacks		
Organic Chocolate Goji Treats	3 pieces (1.4 oz)	150
Tree Of Life		
Organic	1 oz	110
GOJI JUICE		
Arthur's		
Goji Plus	1 bottle (11 oz)	210
Gojilania		
Organic	8 oz	110
GOOSE		
boneless roasted	2.7 oz	231
meat only raw	6.5 oz	298
w/ skin & bone roasted	1 serv (6.6 oz)	573
wild boneless roasted diced	1 cup (4.9 oz)	426
GOOSEBERRIES		
canned in light syrup	1 cup	184
fresh	1 cup	66
Kopali		
Organic Goldenberry	1 pkg (1.8 oz)	150
Navitas Naturals		
Cape Gooseberry Dried	1 oz	80
GRAINS		
Kashi		
7 Whole Grain Pilaf Fiery Fiesta	1 cup (4.9 oz)	210
7 Whole Grain Pilaf Moroccan Curry	1 cup (4.9 oz)	220
7 Whole Grain Pilaf Original	1 cup (4.9 oz)	220
GRAPE JUICE		
bottled unsweetened	1 cup	154
Apple & Eve		
Vintage Concord	8 oz	150
Cascadian Farm		
Organic frzn as prep	8 oz	150
First Blush		
All Flavors	8 oz	154

FOOD	PORTION	CALS
Juicy Juice		
Harvest Surprise	8 oz	120
Kedem		
100% Juice	8 oz	150
Lakewood		
Organic Concord	6 oz	105
Langers		
Plus 100% Juice	8 oz	160
White Grape Plus 100% Juice	8 oz	160
Nantucket Nectars		
Grapeade	8 oz	140
Organic Concord Grape	8 oz	130
Newman's Own		
Gorilla Grape	8 oz	140
Old Orchard		
100% Juice White	8 oz	160
Tang		
Drink Mix as prep	1 serv (8 oz)	110
Tree Ripe		
Organic 100% Juice	6 oz	120
Tropicana		
Grape	1 bottle (14 oz)	270
Walnut Acres		
Organic	8 oz	120
Welch's		
100% Juice	8 oz	170
100% White	8 oz	160
Light White Grape	8 oz	70
GRAPE LEAVES		
canned	1 (4 g)	3
fresh raw	1 (3 g)	3
Sabra		
Stuffed Meatless	1	45
TAKE-OUT		
dolmas w/ beef & rice	1 (0.7 oz)	50
dolmas w/ lamb & rice	1 (0.7 oz)	56
dolmas w/ rice	1 (2 oz)	92

FOOD	PORTION	CALS
GRAPEFRUIT		
CANNED		
juice pack	½ cup	46
unsweetened	1 cup	93
water pack	½ cup	44
Del Monte		
Fruit Naturals Red	½ cup	60
SunFresh Red	½ cup	80
SunFresh White In Real Fruit Juice	½ cup	45
FRESH		
pink	½	37
pink sections	1 cup	69
red	½	37
red sections	1 cup	69
white	½	39
white sections	1 cup	76
Ocean Spray		
Sweet Ruby	½ med (5.4 oz)	60
Sunkist		
Fresh	½ med	60
Oroblanco	½	100
GRAPEFRUIT JUICE		
fresh	1 cup	96
frzn as prep	1 cup	102
frzn not prep	6 oz	302
sweetened	1 cup	116
Apple & Eve		
Ruby Red	8 oz	130
Crystal Light		
Sunrise Ruby Red as prep	1 serv (8 oz)	5
Izze		
Sparkling Grapefruit	8 oz	160
Minute Maid		
Frozen + Calcium	8 oz	100
Ruby Red	8 oz	130
Odwalla		
100% Juice	8 oz	90
Sundia		
Ruby	½ cup	70

FOOD	PORTION	CALS
Tao Tea		
Grapefruit Lemon Fusion	8 oz	72
Tropicana		
Sweet	8 oz	130
GRAPES		
muscadine	10–12 (3.5 oz)	76
scuppernongs	10–12 (3.5 oz)	68
seedless red or green	1 cup	110
seedless red or green	20	69
thompson seedless in heavy syrup	½ cup	93
thompson seedless water pack	½ cup	49
w/ seeds green or red	1 cup	106
w/ seeds green or red	20	80
Earthbound Farm		
Organic Black	1½ cups	190
Frieda's		
Champagne	½ cup (3 oz)	50
Revolution Foods		
Organic Mashups Grape	1 pkg (3.2 oz)	60
GRAVY		
CANNED		
beef	1 can (10 oz)	155
beef	1 cup	124
chicken	1 cup	189
mushroom	1 cup	120
turkey	1 cup	122
Boston Market		
Roasted Chicken	¼ cup	25
Campbell's		
Au Jus	¼ cup	5
Chicken	¼ cup	40
Fat Free Beef	¼ cup	15
Fat Free Turkey	¼ cup	20
Mushroom	¼ cup	20
Franco-American		
Fat Free Slow Roast Chicken	¼ cup	20
Slow Roast Chicken	¼ cup	20
Heinz		
Classic Chicken Fat Free	¼ cup	15

FOOD	PORTION	CALS
HomeStyle Classic Chicken	¼ cup	25
HomeStyle Roasted Turkey	¼ cup	25
Pacific Foods		
Natural Beef	1 cup	20
Natural Chicken	¼ cup	25
Natural Mushroom	¼ cup	20
Natural Turkey	¼ cup	25
FROZEN		
Tofurky		
Giblet & Mushroom	2 tbsp	30
MIX		
au jus as prep w/ water	1 cup	32
brown as prep w/ water	1 cup	75
chicken as prep	1 cup	83
mushroom as prep	1 cup	70
onion as prep w/ water	1 cup	77
pork as prep	1 cup	76
turkey as prep	1 cup	87
Bournvita		
Extract	2 heaping tsp	34
Bovril		
Extract	1 heaping tsp	9
Butterball		
Turkey	¼ cup (2 oz)	30
Knorr		
Au Jus Instant as prep	2 oz	10
Beef Instant as prep	2 oz	20
Brown Instant as prep	2 oz	25
Brown Low Sodium Instant as prep	2 oz	25
Chicken Instant as prep	2 oz	25
Chicken Low Sodium Instant as prep	2 oz	25
Leahey Gardens		
No Beef Brown Gluten Free	¼ cup	9
No Chicken Golden	¼ cup	18
Marmite		
Extract	1 heaping tsp	9
Road's End Organics		
Savory Herb Cholesterol Free Gluten Free	¼ cup	25
TAKE-OUT		
au jus	1 cup	62

FOOD	PORTION	CALS
giblet gravy	¼ cup	45
GREAT NORTHERN BEANS		
canned	1 cup	299
dried cooked	1 cup	209
Eden		
Organic	½ cup	110
HamBeens		
Great Northerns as prep	½ cup	120
GREEN BEANS		
CANNED		
drained	1 cup	27
Allens		
No Salt	½ cup	15
Del Monte		
Cut	½ cup	20
Cut w/ Potatoes & Ham Flavor	½ cup	30
French Style	½ cup	20
Fresh Cut Italian	½ cup	30
Whole	½ cup	20
Gertie's Finest		
Pickled	1 oz	15
Green Giant		
50% Less Sodium Cut	½ cup	20
Tillen Farms		
Crispy Dilly Beans Pickled	¼ cup	15
FRESH		
cooked w/o salt	1 cup	44
raw	1 cup	34
raw whole beans	10	17
Frieda's		
Purple Wax	⅔ cup	25
GreenLine		
Fresh Trimmed	3 oz	25
FROZEN		
cooked	1 cup	38
Birds Eye		
Steamfresh Whole	1 cup (2.9 oz)	35
C&W		
French Cut	1 cup	30

FOOD	PORTION	CALS
Cascadian Farm		
Organic Petite Whole	1 cup	25
Green Giant		
Green Bean Casserole	⅔ cup	110
Pictsweet		
Cut	⅔ cup	30
TAKE-OUT		
casserole w/ mushroom sauce	1 cup	108
pickled	½ cup	19

GREENS
Allens		
Seasoned Mixed	½ cup	45
Ready Pac		
Microwave Leafy Greens as prep	½ cup	15

GROUNDCHERRIES
fresh	½ cup	37

GROUPER
cooked	3 oz	100
cooked	1 fillet (7.1 oz)	238
raw	3 oz	78

GUAR GUM
Bob's Red Mill		
Guar Gum	1 tbsp	20

GUAVA
fresh	1	45
guava sauce	½ cup	43
Frieda's		
Fresh	1 (3 oz)	45

GUAVA JUICE
Apple & Eve		
Nectar	5 oz	130
Sabor Latino		
Nectar + Calcium	8 oz	160

GUINEA HEN
boneless w/o skin raw	½ hen (9.3 oz)	290
w/ skin raw	½ hen (12 oz)	545

FOOD	PORTION	CALS
Grimaud Farms		
Guinea Fowl	1 serv (3.7 oz)	130
HADDOCK		
fresh broiled	4 oz	127
roe raw	1 oz	37
smoked	1 oz	33
Van de Kamp's		
Battered Fillets	2 (3.6 oz)	210
TAKE-OUT		
breaded & fried	4 oz	229
HAGGIS		
scottish haggis	1 serv (6.4 oz)	473
Caledonian Kitchen		
Highland Beef	3 oz	173
Vegetarian	3 oz	190
House of Kenton		
Vegetarian	1 serv (3.5 oz)	249
MacSween		
Traditional	1 (8 oz)	260
Vegetarian	1 (8 oz)	238
HALIBUT		
atlantic & pacific cooked	½ fillet (5.6 oz)	223
atlantic & pacific cooked	3 oz	119
atlantic & pacific raw	3 oz	93
greenland baked	3 oz	203
greenland baked	5.6 oz	380
FROZEN		
Van de Kamp's		
Battered Fillets	3 (4 oz)	230
HALVA (see SESAME)		
HAM		
boneless extra lean roasted	3 oz	123
boneless roasted	3 oz	151
canned extra lean roasted	3 oz	116
canned lean roasted	3 oz	142
center slice lean & fat roasted	3 oz	173
deviled	¼ cup	188
ham salad spread	2 tbsp	65

FOOD	PORTION	CALS
patty grilled	1 patty (2 oz)	205
prosciutto	4 slices (1.3 oz)	72
sliced	3 slices (2.9 oz)	137
sliced extra lean	3 slices (2.2 oz)	69
westphalian smoked	1 oz	105
whole roasted	3 oz	207
Applegate Farms		
Organic Uncured	2 oz	70
Boar's Head		
Black Forest Smoked	2 oz	60
Deluxe	2 oz	60
Deluxe 42% Lower Sodium	2 oz	60
Fresh Seasoned	2 oz	90
Maple Glazed Honey	2 oz	60
Pepper	2 oz	60
Rosemary & Sundried Tomato	2 oz	70
Virginia Smoked	2 oz	60
Carl Buddig		
Ham Sliced	2 oz	85
Honey Ham Sliced	2 oz	90
Healthy Ones		
Honey 97% Fat Free	7 slices (2 oz)	90
Organic Prairie		
Hardwood Smoked Bone In Spiral Sliced	3 oz	110
Oscar Mayer		
Brown Sugar Thin Sliced	⅓ pkg (2 oz)	70
Lunchables Ham Bagels	1 pkg	410
Virginia Shaved	2 oz	50
Sara Lee		
Bavarian Oven Roasted Honey	2 oz	70
Brown Sugar	2 oz	70
Homestyle Baked	2 oz	60
Virginia Baked	4 slices (1.8 oz)	60
Tyson		
Glazed Maple & Brown Sugar	1 serv (5 oz)	180
Honey	2 slices (1.6 oz)	50
TAKE-OUT		
croquette	1 (2.2 oz)	149
salad	½ cup	287
spam musubi	1 serv (6 oz)	253

FOOD	PORTION	CALS
thick slice fried	1 (2.2 oz)	140

HAMBURGER
Applegate Farms
Organic Beef Cooked	1 (3 oz)	195
Organic Turkey Burger	1 (4 oz)	190

Hot Pockets
Cheeseburger	1 (4.5 oz)	310

Ian's
Mini	2 (4.6 oz)	360
Mini Cheeseburger	2 (5 oz)	420

Kid Cuisine
Cheeseburger Builder	1 meal	390

Lean Pockets
Cheeseburger	1 (4.5 oz)	280

Oscar Meyer
Lunchables All-Star Burgers	1 pkg	420

Quaker Maid
Pure Beef Patties	1 (4 oz)	240

Wellshire
Beef	1 (4 oz)	260
Turkey Burgers	1 (4 oz)	200

TAKE-OUT
cheeseburger + condiments	1 reg (4.5 oz)	347
double hamburger + condiments	1 reg (5.8 oz)	384
single patty + condiments	1 reg (4 oz)	299

HAMBURGER SUBSTITUTES (see also MEAT SUBSTITUTES)
Boca
American Flame Grilled	1 (2.5 oz)	90
Cheeseburger	1 (2.5 oz)	100
Grilled Vegetable	1 (2.5 oz)	70
Ground Burger	1 serv (2 oz)	60
Original	1 (2.5 oz)	70
Original Vegan	1 (2.5 oz)	70

Dr. Praeger's
Veggie Burger Bombay	1 (2.78 oz)	110
Veggie Burger California	1 (2.75 oz)	110
Veggie Burger California Gluten Free	1 (2.75 oz)	120

Fantastic
Natures Burger Mix not prep	¼ cup	170

FOOD	PORTION	CALS
Tofu Burger Mix not prep	3 tbsp	80
Gardenburger		
Black Bean Chipotle	1 (2.5 oz)	80
Flamed Grilled	1 (2.5 oz)	90
GardenVegan	1 (2.5 oz)	100
Original	1 (2.5 oz)	100
Portabella	1 (2.5 oz)	90
Lightlife		
Light Burgers	1 (3 oz)	120
Smart Menu Burger	1	80
Morningstar Farms		
Classic Burger	1 (2.2 oz)	150
Garden Veggie Patties	1 (2.4 oz)	100
Harvest Burger	1	140
Okara Pattie	1 (2.2 oz)	120
Vegan Burger	1 (2.5 oz)	100
Sunshine Burgers		
Garden	1 (2.6 oz)	190
Original	1 (2.6 oz)	190
Tofurky		
SuperBurgers Original	1 (3.5 oz)	120
VeggieLand		
Veggie Burger Original	1 (3.5 oz)	132
Veggie Burger Peppadew	1 (5 oz)	210
WildWood		
Organic Original Burgers Tofu-Veggie	1 (3.2 oz)	180

HAZELNUTS

FOOD	PORTION	CALS
dried blanched	1 oz	191
dried unblanched	1 oz	179
dry roasted unblanched	1 oz	188
oil roasted unblanched	1 oz	187
Chukar Cherries		
Chocolate Covered Spiced	3 tbsp (1.4 oz)	228
Kettle		
Butter Creamy Unsalted	2 tbsp	180
Love'n Bake		
Hazelnut Praline	2 tbsp	170

FOOD	PORTION	CALS
HEART		
beef simmered	3 oz	140
chicken cooked	1 (3 g)	5
chicken diced simmered	½ cup	134
lamb braised	3 oz	157
pork braised	1 (4.5 oz)	191
turkey simmered	½ cup	94
veal braised	3 oz	158
Rumba		
Beef	4 oz	130
HEARTS OF PALM		
canned	1 (1.2 oz)	9
canned	½ cup	20
Del Monte		
Hearts Of Palm	2–3 pieces	20
Native Forest		
Organic	1 oz	15
HEMP		
Living Harvest		
Organic Hemp Nuts	2 tbsp (1 oz)	170
Organic Protein Powder	2 scoops (1 oz)	110
Manitoba Harvest		
Hemp Seed Butter	2 tbsp	160
Protein Powder	2 scoops (1 oz)	134
Shelled Seed	2 tbsp	160
Nutiva		
Organic Protein Powder	2 scoops (1 oz)	120
Shelled Hempseed	2 tbsp	110
HERBAL TEA (see TEA/HERBAL TEA)		
HERBS/SPICES (see also individual names)		
cajun seasoning	1 tbsp	19
chinese five spice	1 tsp	7
garam masala	1 tsp	8
poultry seasoning	1 tsp	5
pumpkin pie spice	1 tsp	6
A Taste Of Thai		
Chicken & Rice Seasoning	¼ pkg (6 g)	15

FOOD	PORTION	CALS
Bragg		
Herb & Spice Seasoning	¼ tsp	0
Chef Paul Prudhomme's		
Magic Blackened Redfish	¼ tsp	0
Magic Fajita	¼ tsp	0
Magic Pork & Veal	¼ tsp	0
Magic Poultry	¼ tsp	0
Cut N Clean		
Greens Seasoning	1½ tsp	20
Eden		
Shake Furikake	½ tsp	5
Emeril's		
Asian Essence	½ tsp	0
Bayou Blast!	½ tsp	0
Chicken Rub	½ tsp	0
Original Essence	½ tsp	0
Steak Rub	½ tsp	0
McCormick		
Blends Bon Appetit	¼ tsp	0
Cajun Seasoning	⅛ tsp	0
Greek Seasoning	¼ tsp	0
Jamaican Jerk Seasoning	¼ tsp	0
Seafood Seasoning	¼ tsp	0
Mrs. Dash		
Grilling Blend Chicken	¼ tsp	0
Grilling Blend Steak	¼ tsp	0
Original Blend	¼ tsp	0
Tomato Basil Garlic	¼ tsp	0
Nueva Cocina		
Picadillo	2 tsp	15
Taco Fresco	2 tsp	15
Ortega		
Burrito Seasoning	1½ tsp	20
Fajita Seasoning	1½ tsp	20
Taco Seasoning	1 tbsp	20
Spice Hunter		
All Purpose Blend	¼ tsp	0
Greek Seasoning Salt Free	¼ tsp	0
HERRING		
atlantic baked	4 oz	230

FOOD	PORTION	CALS
dried salted	1 fillet (1.4 oz)	161
pickled	1 oz	74
pickled in cream sauce	1 oz	72
roe	1 tbsp	39
smoked kippered	1 oz	620
Beach Cliff		
Kippered Snacks	1 can (4 oz)	220
TAKE-OUT		
breaded fried	1 serv (4 oz)	225

HIBISCUS
flowers dried sweetened	⅓ cup	100

HICKORY NUTS
dried	1 oz	187

HOMINY
white canned	1 cup	119
yellow canned	½ cup	115
Allens		
White	½ cup	100
Bush's		
Golden	½ cup	60

HONEY
honey	1 tbsp (0.7 oz)	64
honey	¼ cup (3 oz)	258
orange blossom	1 tbsp	60
wild honey	1 tbsp	60
Comfort Care		
Raw Clover	1 tbsp (0.7 oz)	60
Dutch Gold		
Clover	1 tbsp	60
Frieda's		
Honeycomb	½ cup (3 oz)	260
Tree Of Life		
Alfalfa Honey Raw Unfiltered	1 tbsp	60
Avocado Honey Raw Unfiltered	1 tbsp (0.7 oz)	60
Buckwheat Honey Raw Unfiltered	1 tbsp	60
Tupelo Honey Raw Unfiltered	1 tbsp	60
Wholesome Sweeteners		
Organic Fair Trade Amber	1 tbsp	60

FOOD	PORTION	CALS
Organic Fair Trade Raw	1 tbsp	60

HONEYDEW
balls frzn	1 cup (8 oz)	83
fresh cut up	1 cup	61
fresh wedge	1/8 melon (4.5 oz)	45
whole fresh	1 (35 oz)	360

HORSE
roasted	3 oz	149

HORSERADISH
sauce	1 tbsp	7
wasabi root raw	1 (5.9 oz)	184
wasabi root raw sliced	1/2 cup (2.3 oz)	71
Boar's Head		
Horseradish	1 tsp (5 g)	0
Horseradish & Beets	1 tsp	0
Horseradish Sauce Pub Style	1 tsp	15
Robert Rothschild Farm		
Sauce	1 tsp	20
Sara Lee		
Horseradish Sauce	1 tbsp	20
Zatarain's		
Prepared	1 tbsp	15

HOT CHOCOLATE
mix not prep	1 pkg (1 oz)	111
mix w/ no calorie sweetener as prep w/ water	8 oz	72
mix w/ sugar as prep w/ nonfat milk	8 oz	209
mix w/ sugar as prep w/ water	8 oz	138
Nestle		
Hot Cocoa Carb Select Fat Free	1 pkg	25
Hot Cocoa Milk Chocolate	1 pkg (1 oz)	80
Starbucks		
Hot Cocoa Mix	1 pkg	130
Swiss Miss		
Cocoa Caramel as prep	1 pkg	120
Cocoa No Sugar Added as prep	1 pkg	60
Cocoa Rich Creamy as prep	1 pkg	110
Cocoa w/ Marshmallows as prep	1 pkg	120
Cocoa w/ Marshmallows Fat Free as prep	1 pkg	140

FOOD	PORTION	CALS
French Vanilla as prep	1 pkg	110
Milk Chocolate as prep	1 pkg	120
TAKE-OUT		
hot chocolate	8 oz	190
mexican hot chocolate	1 cup	173

HOT DOG (see also HOT DOG SUBSTITUTES)

FOOD	PORTION	CALS
beef	1 (1.5 oz)	149
beef & pork	1 (1.5 oz)	137
beef lowfat	1 (2 oz)	133
chicken	1 (1.5 oz)	116
fat free	1 (2 oz)	62
lowfat	1 (2 oz)	88
low sodium	1 (2 oz)	180
pork and beef cheese smokie	1 (1.5 oz)	141
turkey	1 (1.5 oz)	102
Applegate Farms		
Natural Beef	1 (1.5 oz)	80
Organic Chicken	1 (1.5 oz)	70
Ball Park		
Franks	1 (2 oz)	180
Franks Beef	1 (2 oz)	180
Franks Bun Size	1 (2 oz)	180
Franks Fat Free	1 (1.8 oz)	40
Franks Lite	1 (1.8 oz)	100
Franks Singles Cheese	1 (1.6 oz)	150
Franks Smoked White Turkey	1 (1.8 oz)	45
Grillmaster Hearty Beef	1	250
Grillmaster Smokehouse	1	210
Boar's Head		
Beef	1 (2 oz)	160
Beef Cocktail	5 (2 oz)	170
Beef Lite	1 (1.6 oz)	90
Pork & Beef	1 (2 oz)	150
Dietz & Watson		
New York Style Beef	1 (2.3 oz)	130
Healthy Choice		
Beef Low Fat	1 (1.8 oz)	70
Healthy Ones		
Beef	1 (1.8 oz)	70
Franks	1 (1.8 oz)	70

FOOD	PORTION	CALS
Hebrew National		
97% Fat Free Beef	1 (1.7 oz)	45
Beef	1 (1.7 oz)	150
Cocktail Franks	5 (2 oz)	180
Dinner Frank	1 (4 oz)	350
Franks In A Blanket	5 (2.8 oz)	290
Reduced Fat Beef	1 (1.7 oz)	120
Ian's		
Popcorn Turkey Corn Dog	5 pieces (3 oz)	237
Johnsonville		
Stadium Beef	1 (2.7 oz)	240
Organic Prairie		
Beef Uncured	1 (1.5 oz)	120
Chicken Uncured	1 (1.5 oz)	100
Pork Uncured	1 (1.5 oz)	130
Turkey Uncured	1 (1.5 oz)	80
Oscar Mayer		
Beef	1 (1.6 oz)	140
Beef Light	1 (1.6 oz)	90
Cheese Dogs	1 (1.6 oz)	140
Corn Dogs	1	210
Smokies	1 (1.8 oz)	150
State Fair		
Corn Dogs	1 (2.67 oz)	180
Wellshire		
Beef Premium	1 (2 oz)	110
Cheese Franks	1 (2 oz)	110
Chicken Franks	1 (1.6 oz)	70
Turkey Franks	1 (1.6 oz)	110
TAKE-OUT		
corndog	1	460
w/ bun chili	1	297
w/ bun plain	1	242

HOT DOG SUBSTITUTES

FOOD	PORTION	CALS
Lightlife		
Smart Dogs	1	45
Smart Franks	1 (2 oz)	110
Tofu Pups	1 (1.5 oz)	60
Loma Linda		
Big Franks	1 (1.8 oz)	110

FOOD	PORTION	CALS
Big Franks Low Fat Vegan	1 (1.8 oz)	80
Morningstar Farms		
Corn Dog Veggie	1 (2.5 oz)	170
Quorn		
Meat-Free Dogs	1 (1.5 oz)	70
Yves		
Meatless Hot Dog	1	50
Tofu Dogs	1	45
HUMMUS		
Athenos		
Original	2 tbsp	80
Roasted Garlic	2 tbsp	80
Roasted Red Pepper	2 tbsp	80
Guiltless Gourmet		
Original	2 tbsp (1.1 oz)	50
Sabra		
Hummus	2 oz	110
Hummus Spicy	½ cup	171
Tribe		
40 Spices	2 tbsp	50
French Onion	2 tbsp	50
Organic Classic	2 tbsp	50
Organic Roasted Red Peppers	2 tbsp	40
Roasted Eggplant	2 tbsp	35
Scallion	2 tbsp	50
Zesty Lemon	2 tbsp	50
Wholesome Valley		
Organic Classic	2 tbsp (1 oz)	60
Wild Garden		
Hummus Dip	2 tbsp	35
WildWood		
Organic Low Fat	2 tbsp	50
Organic Mid-Eastern	2 tbsp	65
TAKE-OUT		
hummus	¼ cup (2.2 oz)	109
HYACINTH BEANS		
dried cooked	1 cup	228

FOOD	PORTION	CALS

ICE CREAM AND FROZEN DESSERTS (*see also* ICES AND ICE POPS, SHERBET, YOGURT FROZEN)

FOOD	PORTION	CALS
chocolate	½ cup (4 oz)	143
dixie cup chocolate	1 (3.5 oz)	125
dixie cup strawberry	1 (3.5 oz)	112
dixie cup vanilla	1 (3.5 oz)	116
freeze dried ice cream chocolate strawberry & vanilla	1 pkg (0.75 oz)	158
strawberry	½ cup (4 oz)	127
vanilla	½ cup (4 oz)	132
vanilla soft serve	½ cup	111
Blue Bunny		
Bar Candy Center Crunch	1 (3.2 oz)	370
Bar English Toffee	1 (1.4 oz)	130
Bar Homemade Vanilla	1 (2.3 oz)	190
Bar Orange Dream	1 (2.1 oz)	80
Bar Strawberry Sundae Crunch	1 (2.2 oz)	170
Blendz Peanut Butter Cup	1 (4.4 oz)	270
Caramel Sundae Bite Size	4 bars (3.1 oz)	340
Chocolate	½ cup	130
Cone Bunny Tracks	1 (4.8 oz)	420
Cone The Champ Chocolate Lovers	1 (3.5 oz)	300
Cone Vanilla Nutty Sundae	1 (3 oz)	250
Cups Vanilla & Chocolate	1 (1.7 oz)	100
Mint Chip	½ cup	140
Neapolitan	½ cup	130
Orange Dream	½ cup	130
Premium All Natural Vanilla	½ cup	160
Premium Bunny Tracks	½ cup	190
Premium Butter Pecan	½ cup	150
Premium Cookies & Cream	½ cup	150
Premium Double Strawberry	½ cup	140
Premium Exquisite Mint	½ cup	170
Premium Rocky Road	½ cup	150
Premium Toasted Almond Fudge	½ cup	160
Sandwich Big Vanilla	1 (3.7 oz)	260
Sandwich Chips Galore	1 (3.4 oz)	310
Strawberry	½ cup	120
Breyers		
Butter Pecan	½ cup	150

FOOD	PORTION	CALS
Carb Smart Chocolate	½ cup	90
Carb Smart Fudge Bar	1 (3.5 oz)	100
Carb Smart Vanilla	½ cup	90
Carb Smart Vanilla Bar Chocolate Coated	1 (3 oz)	170
Cherry Vanilla	½ cup	130
Chocolate Crackle	½ cup	160
Chocolate Extra Creamy	½ cup	140
Coffee	½ cup	130
Cookies & Cream	½ cup	150
Double Churn ½ Fat Chocolate Mocha Silk	½ cup	130
Double Churn ½ Fat Creamy Vanilla	½ cup	100
Double Churn ½ Fat Mint Chocolate Chip	½ cup	130
Double Churn ½ Fat Rocky Road	½ cup	130
Double Churn Fat Free Chocolate Fudge Brownie	½ cup	110
Double Churn Fat Free Creamy Vanilla	½ cup	90
Double Churn Fat Free French Chocolate	½ cup	90
Double Churn No Sugar Added Vanilla	½ cup	80
Dulce De Leche	½ cup	150
French Vanilla	½ cup	140
Heath English Toffee	½ cup	160
Overload Very Chocolate Cherry	½ cup	120
Overload Waffle Cone	½ cup	130
Peach	½ cup	120
Sandwich Mrs. Fields Brownie	1 (6 oz)	450
Sandwich Mrs. Fields Cookie	1 (3 oz)	190
Sandwich Oreo	1 (3 oz)	170
Snickers	½ cup	170
Strawberry	½ cup	120
Strawberry Cheesecake Sara Lee	½ cup	160
Vanilla Fudge Brownie	½ cup	150
Vanilla Lactose Free	½ cup	130
Bubbies		
Mochi Mango	1 piece (1.3 oz)	110
Butterfinger		
Bar	1 (1.9 oz)	210
Celestial Seasonings		
Tea Dreams Bars Chocolate Caramel Chai	1 (2.7 oz)	240
Tea Dreams Cinnamon Apple Spice	½ cup	140
Tea Dreams Vanilla Ginger Spice Chai	½ cup	140

FOOD	PORTION	CALS
Ciao Bella		
Gelato Chocolate	1 pkg (3.5 oz)	210
Gelato Hazelnut	1 pkg (3.5 oz)	210
Gelato Vanilla	1 pkg (3.5 oz)	184
Dippin' Dots		
Banana Split	½ cup	170
Chocolate	½ cup	165
Fudge Fat Free No Sugar Added	½ cup	92
Horchata	½ cup	170
Java Delight	½ cup	170
Root Beer Float	½ cup	111
Vanilla	½ cup	170
Dove		
Beyond Vanilla	½ cup	240
Give In To Mint	½ cup	300
Irresistibly Raspberry	½ cup	240
Milk Chocolate w/ Almonds	1 bar (3.3 oz)	340
Milk Chocolate w/ Vanilla Ice Cream	1 bar (3.3 oz)	330
Miniatures Milk Chocolate w/ Vanilla Ice Cream	5 pieces (3.1 oz)	300
Triple Chocolate	1 bar (2.8 oz)	200
Unconditional Chocolate	½ cup	290
Vanilla w/ A Chocolate Soul	½ cup	290
Edy's		
Carb Benefit Butter Pecan	½ cup	170
Carb Benefit Chocolate	½ cup	150
Carb Benefit Chocolate Chip	½ cup	160
Carb Benefit Mint Chocolate Chip	½ cup	160
Carb Benefit Vanilla Bean	½ cup	140
Dips Chocolate	26 pieces	420
Dips Mint	26 pieces	420
Dips Vanilla	26 pieces	420
Grand Andes Cool Mint	½ cup	170
Grand Butter Pecan	½ cup	170
Grand Chocolate	½ cup	150
Grand Chocolate Caramel Swirl	½ cup	170
Grand Chocolate Chip	½ cup	160
Grand Chocolate Fudge Mousse	½ cup	160
Grand Chocolate Fudge Sundae	½ cup	170
Grand Coffee	½ cup	140

FOOD	PORTION	CALS
Grand Cookie Dough	½ cup	180
Grand Cookies 'N Cream	½ cup	160
Grand Double Fudge Brownie	½ cup	170
Grand Dulce De Leche	½ cup	150
Grand Espresso Chip	½ cup	150
Grand French Vanilla	½ cup	160
Grand Fudge Tracks	½ cup	180
Grand Ice Cream Sandwich	½ cup	150
Grand Mint Chocolate Chips	½ cup	170
Grand Peanut Butter Cup	½ cup	180
Grand Real Strawberry	½ cup	130
Grand Rocky Road	½ cup	170
Grand Spumoni	½ cup	150
Grand Toffee Bar Crunch	½ cup	170
Grand Toll House Cookie Swirl	½ cup	170
Grand Turtle Sundae	½ cup	160
Grand Utimate Caramel Cup	½ cup	170
Grand Vanilla	½ cup	140
Neapolitan	½ cup	140
Slow Churned Light Butter Pecan	½ cup	120
Slow Churned Light Caramel Delight	½ cup	120
Slow Churned Light Chocolate	½ cup	110
Slow Churned Light Chocolate Chip	½ cup	120
Slow Churned Light Chocolate Fudge Chunk	½ cup	120
Slow Churned Light Coffee	½ cup	105
Slow Churned Light Cookie Dough	½ cup	130
Slow Churned Light Cookies 'N Cream	½ cup	120
Slow Churned Light French Silk	½ cup	130
Slow Churned Light French Vanilla	½ cup	100
Slow Churned Light Fudge Tracks	½ cup	120
Slow Churned Light Mint Chocolate Chips	½ cup	120
Slow Churned Light Mocha Almond Fudge	½ cup	120
Slow Churned Light Neapolitan	½ cup	100
Slow Churned Light Rocky Road	½ cup	120
Slow Churned Light Strawberry	½ cup	110
Slow Churned Light Vanilla	½ cup	100
Slow Churned No Sugar Added Butter Pecan	½ cup	120
Slow Churned No Sugar Added Chocolate	½ cup	95
Slow Churned No Sugar Added Cookie Dough	½ cup	110

FOOD	PORTION	CALS
Slow Churned No Sugar Added Fat Free Chocolate Fudge	½ cup	100
Slow Churned No Sugar Added Fat Free Raspberry Vanilla Swirl	½ cup	90
Slow Churned No Sugar Added Fat Free Vanilla	½ cup	90
Slow Churned No Sugar Added Fat Free Vanilla Chocolate Swirl	½ cup	100
Slow Churned No Sugar Added Fudge Tracks	½ cup	110
Slow Churned No Sugar Added Mint Chocolate Chips	½ cup	110
Slow Churned No Sugar Added Neapolitan	½ cup	95
Slow Churned No Sugar Added Triple Chocolate	½ cup	110
Slow Churned No Sugar Added Vanilla	½ cup	90
Eskimo Pie		
Milk Chocolate	1 bar (1.8 oz)	160
Fat Boy		
Casco Nut Sundae On A Stick	1 (3 oz)	310
Casco Nut Sundae On A Stick Cherry Cordial	1 (3 oz)	300
Sandwich Chocolate	1 (3 oz)	210
Sandwich Egg Nog	1 (3 oz)	220
Sandwich Jr. Vanilla	1 (1.6 oz)	120
Sandwich Vanilla	1 (3 oz)	220
Glace De Vino		
Chocolate Amaretto Cream Sherry	½ cup	180
Raspberry Merlot Cheesecake	½ cup	180
Good Humor		
Bar Chocolate Eclair	1 (3 oz)	160
Bar Cookies & Cream	1 (3 oz)	190
Bar Vanilla Chocolate Coated	1 (4 oz)	260
Cone King Giant	1 (8 oz)	390
Cone King Vanilla	1 (4.6 oz)	250
Cone Sundae	1 (4.3 oz)	260
King Bar Heath	1 (4 oz)	310
Sandwich Oreo	1 (4.5 oz)	240
Sandwich Giant Vanilla	1 (6 oz)	220
Sandwich Vanilla	1 (3 oz)	130
Swirlwind	1 (6 oz)	160

FOOD	PORTION	CALS
GoodBody		
Chocolate Banana	1 bar (3.5 oz)	120
Chocolate Double Dutch	1 bar (3.5 oz)	130
Chocolate Peanut Butter	1 bar (3.5 oz)	180
Vanilla & Raspberry Sorbet	1 bar (3.5 oz)	120
Vanilla & Strawberry Sorbet	1 bar (3.5 oz)	120
Vanilla & Tropical Sorbet	1 bar (3.5 oz)	120
Green & Black's		
Organic Chocolate Covered Chocolate	1 bar (3.5 oz)	214
Organic Chocolate Covered Vanilla	1 bar (3.5 oz)	233
Hawaiian Punch		
Cream Surfers	1 bar	90
Healthy Choice		
Bar Sorbet & Cream	1	100
Brownie Bliss	½ cup	130
Butter Pecan Crunch	½ cup	100
Cappuccino Chocolate Chunk	½ cup	120
Caramel Fudge Brownie	½ cup	120
Cherry Chocolate Mambo	½ cup	130
Chocolate Chocolate Chunk	½ cup	120
Cookies 'N Cream	½ cup	120
Crazy Caramel	½ cup	120
Double Karma	½ cup	140
French Silk	½ cup	120
Happy Together	½ cup	150
Jumpin' Java	½ cup	130
Low Fat Bar Fudge	1	90
Low Fat Bar Mocha Fudge	1	90
Low Fat Bar Strawberry & Cream	1	90
Mint Chocolate Chip	½ cup	120
No Sugar Added Chocolate Fudge Brownie	½ cup	120
No Sugar Added Coffee Almond Fudge	½ cup	110
No Sugar Added Mint Chocolate Chip	½ cup	110
No Sugar Added Vanilla	½ cup	100
Peanut Butter Cup	½ cup	120
Praline & Caramel	½ cup	120
Rocky Road	½ cup	130
Sandwich Caramel	1	140
Sandwich Fudge Swirl	1	140
Sandwich Vanilla	1	130

FOOD	PORTION	CALS
Turtle Fudge Cake	½ cup	130
Vanilla	½ cup	110
Vanilla Bean	½ cup	120
Vanilla Caramel Fudge	½ cup	140
Hershey's		
French Vanilla	½ cup	170
Neapolitan	½ cup	160
Hood		
Butterscotch Blast	½ cup	160
Chocolate	½ cup	140
Chocolate Eclair	1 bar (2.2 oz)	150
Cookie Dough Delight	½ cup	160
Creamy Coffee	½ cup	140
Fat Free Chocolate Passion	½ cup	100
Fat Free Very Vanilla	½ cup	100
Fudge Twister	½ cup	150
Grasshopper Pie	½ cup	160
Hoodsie Cups	1 (1.7 oz)	100
Light Butter Pecan	½ cup	140
Light Creamy Vanilla	½ cup	110
Low Fat No Sugar Added Vanilla Dream	½ cup	90
Maple Walnut	½ cup	160
No Sugar Added Chocolate Chip	½ cup	100
Nutty Royale	1 cone (2.5 oz)	220
Orange Cream	1 bar (2.2 oz)	90
Sandwich Vanilla	1	180
Sandwich Vanilla Light	1 (2.2 oz)	160
Sandwich Vanilla Lowfat	1 (2.8 oz)	80
Spumoni	½ cup	140
Klondike		
Bar Caramel Pretzel	1 (4 oz)	260
Bar Original Vanilla	1 (4.5 oz)	250
Bar Reese's	1 (4 oz)	260
Bar Whitehouse Cherry	1 (4.5 oz)	250
Cone Crunchy Vanilla	1 (4.3 oz)	280
Slim A Bear 100 Calorie Sandwich Vanilla	1 (3 oz)	100
Slim A Bear Bar Vanilla	1 (4 oz)	170
Land O Lakes		
Vanilla	½ cup (2.4 oz)	150
Vanilla Light	½ cup (2.3 oz)	100

FOOD	PORTION	CALS
M&M's		
Cone	1 (2.8 oz)	250
Sandwich	1 (3 oz)	260
Vanilla Fudge	½ cup	180
Molli Coolz		
Cup Banana Cream Pie	1	120
Cup Chocolate Fusion	1	140
Cup Chocolate Peanut Butter	1	160
Ionz Cotton Candy	1 cup	100
Ionz S'mores	1 cup	110
Rocks Cherry Blue Raz & Lemon	1 cup	80
Rocks Lemon Lime	1 cup	80
Shakers Chocolate	1 (10.2 oz)	250
Natural Choice		
Organic Double Chocolate	½ cup	230
Organic Strawberry	½ cup	210
Organic Vanilla	½ cup	220
No Pudge!		
Giant Chocolate Eclair Low Fat	1 bar	110
Giant Cone Chocolate No Sugar Added	1	110
Giant Cone Cookies & Cream Low Fat	1	140
Giant Cone Fudgy Brownie Low Fat	1	140
Giant Cone Vanilla No Sugar Added	1	110
Giant Cookies & Cream Low Fat No Sugar Added	1 bar	100
Giant Fudgy Fat Free No Sugar Added	1 bar	60
Giant Sandwich Brownie Batter Low Fat	1	140
Giant Sandwich Brownie Chunk Low Fat	1	140
Giant Sandwich Vanilla & Chocolate No Sugar Added	1	130
Giant Strawberry Shortcake 98% Fat Free	1 bar	90
Popsicle		
Creamsicle	1 (2.5 oz)	100
Purely Decadent		
Dairy Free Bar Chocolate Coated Vanilla	1 (2.7 oz)	200
Dairy Free Bar Chocolate Coated Vanilla Almond	1 (2.7 oz)	210
Organic Coconut Milk Chocolate	½ cup	150
Organic Coconut Milk Vanilla Bean	½ cup	150
Organic Dairy Free Belgian Chocolate	½ cup	180

FOOD	PORTION	CALS
Organic Dairy Free Chocolate Obsession	½ cup	210
Organic Dairy Free Gluten Free Cookie Dough	½ cup	230
Organic Dairy Free Mocha Almond Fudge	½ cup	200
Organic Dairy Free Snickerdoodle	½ cup	190
Organic Dairy Free Vanilla	½ cup	170
Rice Dream		
Bar Vanilla Nutty	1 (3.3 oz)	320
Bar Vanilla w/ Chocolate Coating	1 (3 oz)	230
Carob Almond	½ cup	180
Frozen Pie Chocolate	1 (3.4 oz)	330
Mint Carob Chip	½ cup	170
Strawberry	½ cup	160
Sheer Bliss		
Bar Pomegranate	1 (3.1 oz)	260
Blissbites	2 (1.1 oz)	100
Blisswich	1 (3.3 oz)	270
Freedom	½ cup (4 oz)	290
Mediterranean Coffee	½ cup (4 oz)	260
Pomegranate	½ cup (4 oz)	290
Vanilla	½ cup (4 oz)	300
Skinny Cow		
Bar Vanilla Strawberry Sorbet Swirl	1	110
Cone Chocolate w/ Fudge	1	150
Cone Vanilla & Caramel	1	150
Fudge Bar	1	100
Sandwich Chocolate Peanut Butter	1	150
Sandwich Strawberry Shortcake	1	140
Sandwich Vanilla	1	140
Sandwich Vanilla No Sugar Added	1	140
SoDelicious		
Dairy Free Sandwich Minis Pomegranate	1 (1.4 oz)	90
Dairy Free Sandwich Mint	1 (2.2 oz)	150
Dairy Free Sandwich Vanilla	1 (2 oz)	150
Dairy Free Sugar Free Chocolate Coated Vanilla Bar	1 (2.2 oz)	150
Dairy Free Sugar Free Fudge Bar	1 (2 oz)	80
Organic Dairy Free Sandwich Neapolitan	1 (2.2 oz)	150
Soy Dream		
Butter Pecan	½ cup	140
Sandwich Lil' Dreamers Chocolate	1 (1.4 oz)	100

FOOD	PORTION	CALS
Vanilla	½ cup	140
Straus		
Organic Coffee	4 oz	240
Organic Vanilla Bean	4 oz	240
Tofutti		
Cuties Vanilla	1 (1.4 oz)	120
Turkey Hill		
Banana Split	½ cup	150
Choco Mint Chip	½ cup	160
Chocolate All Natural	½ cup	150
Chocolate Marshmallow	½ cup	160
Coconut Cream Pie	½ cup	170
Cookies 'N Cream	½ cup	150
Duetto Cherry	½ cup	120
Duetto Lemon	½ cup	120
Duetto Root Beer	½ cup	120
French Vanilla	½ cup	140
Light Banana Split	½ cup	110
Light Dulce De Chocolate	½ cup	120
Light Moose Tracks	½ cup	140
Light Vanilla Bean	½ cup	100
No Sugar Added Cherry Fudge Ripple	½ cup	80
No Sugar Added Vanilla Bean	½ cup	70
Original Vanilla	½ cup	140
Peanut Butter Ripple	½ cup	170
Rocky Road	½ cup	170
Sandwich Chocolate Chunk	1 (3.2 oz)	320
Sandwich Light Vanilla Bean	1 (2.5 oz)	160
Sandwich Vanilla Bean	1 (2.5 oz)	190
Sundae Cone Vanilla Fudge	1 (3.3 oz)	320
Tin Roof Sundae	½ cup	150
Twix		
Ice Cream	½ cup	160
Ice Cream Bar	1 (1.6 oz)	170
Weight Watchers		
English Toffee Crunch	1 bar	110
Smart Ones Giant Sundae	1 serv (8 oz)	150
TAKE-OUT		
cone vanilla light soft serve	1 (4.6 oz)	164
gelato chocolate hazelnut	½ cup (5.3 oz)	370

FOOD	PORTION	CALS
gelato vanilla	½ cup (3 oz)	211
ice cream pie no crust	1 slice (3.4 oz)	218
mud pie	⅛ pie (8 oz)	698
sundae caramel	1 (5.4 oz)	303
sundae hot fudge	1 (5.4 oz)	284
sundae strawberry	1 (5.4 oz)	269

ICE CREAM CONES AND CUPS

FOOD	PORTION	CALS
brown sugar cone	1 (10 g)	40
wafer cone	1	17
waffle cone	1 lg	121
Keebler		
Cone Sugar	1	50
Ice Creme Cone	1	15
Waffle Bowl	1	50
Waffle Cone	1	50

ICE CREAM TOPPINGS

FOOD	PORTION	CALS
butterscotch	2 tbsp (1.4 oz)	103
caramel	2 tbsp (1.4 oz)	103
marshmallow cream	1 jar (7 oz)	615
marshmallow cream	1 oz	88
nuts in syrup	2 tbsp	184
pineapple	2 tbsp (1.5 oz)	106
pineapple	1 cup (11.5 oz)	861
strawberry	1 cup (11.5 oz)	863
strawberry	2 tbsp (1.5 oz)	107
Lollipop Tree		
Hot Fudge Sauce	1 tbsp	80
Maple Walnut Cream	2 tbsp	190
Sanders		
Butterscotch Caramel	2 tbsp	90
Smucker's		
Butterscotch Caramel	2 tbsp	130
Dove Dark Chocolate	2 tbsp	140
Dove Milk Chocolate	2 tbsp	130
Dulce De Leche Milk Caramel Spread	2 tbsp	110
Hot Fudge	2 tbsp	140
Hot Fudge Sugar Free Fat Free	2 tbsp	90
Magic Shell Caramel	2 tbsp	220
Magic Shell Chocolate	2 tbsp	210

FOOD	PORTION	CALS
Magic Shell Chocolate Fudge	2 tbsp	120
Magic Shell Turtle Delight	2 tbsp	210
Magic Shell Twix	2 tbsp	210
Steel's		
Sugar Free Chocolate Fudge	2 tbsp	45
Sugar Free Peanut Butter Fudge	2 tbsp	75

ICED TEA
MIX
A La Source

Organic as prep	8 oz	90
Organic Green Tea as prep	8 oz	90
Organic Herbal Tea Red Rooibos	8 oz	80
Celestial Seasonings		
Blueberry Ice	1 cup	0
Crystal Light		
On The Go All Flavors as prep	1 serv	5
Sugar Free All Flavors as prep	1 serv	5
Lipton		
Chailatta Chocolate as prep	8 oz	120
Chailatta Hazelnut as prep	8 oz	120
Chailatta Original as prep	8 oz	120
Chailatta Vanilla as prep	8 oz	120
Decaffeinated Lemon as prep	1 serv	70
Decaffeinated Lemon Unsweetened as prep	1 serv	0
Diet Lemon as prep	1 serv	5
Diet Peach as prep	1 serv	5
Diet Raspberry as prep	1 serv	5
Green Tea as prep	1 serv	70
Lemon Sweetened as prep	1 serv	70
Sweetened All Fruit Flavors as prep	1 serv	80
To Go w/ Honey & Lemon	1 pkg	0
To Go w/ Lemon	1 pkg	0
To Go w/ Mandarin & Mango	1 pkg	0
Unsweetened as prep	1 serv	0
Nestea		
Lemon Liquid Concentrate as prep	8 oz	80
Peach Liquid Concentrate as prep	8 oz	90
Sugar Free w/ Lemon	2 tsp	5
Sweetened w/ Lemon	1⅓ tbsp	60
Unsweetened w/ Lemon	2 tsp	5

FOOD	PORTION	CALS
READY-TO-DRINK		
Anteadote		
All Flavors	8 oz	0
Arizona		
Green Tea w/ Ginseng & Honey	8 oz	70
Lemon	8 oz	90
Bina		
Lemon	8 oz	70
Peach	8 oz	114
Bolthouse Farms		
Perfectly Protein Vanilla Chai Tea w/ Soy	8 oz	160
Bombilla & Gourd		
Organic Eco Teas All Flavors	8 oz	40
Brazil Gourmet		
Nectar Tea All Flavors	8 oz	90
Nectar Tea Light Mango Passion	8 oz	60
C+Swiss		
Hemp Ice Tea	1 can (8.4 oz)	90
Cafe Sepia		
Matcha Latte	1 can (8.6 oz)	130
Crystal Light		
Sugar Free Lemon	8 oz	5
Delta Blues		
Spearmint Tea Punch	8 oz	90
Enviga		
All Flavors	1 can (12 oz)	5
Fuze		
Antioxidant Tea	8 oz	60
Green Tea	8 oz	60
White Tea	8 oz	60
Gold Peak Tea		
Green Tea Sweetened	1 bottle (16.9 oz)	170
Hawaiian		
Iced Tea	1 can (11.5 oz)	120
Honest Tea		
Assam	8 oz	17
Black Forest Berry	8 oz	25
Gold Rush	8 oz	9
Green Dragon	8 oz	30
Kashmiri Chai	8 oz	17

FOOD	PORTION	CALS
Lori's Lemon	8 oz	30
Moroccan Mint	8 oz	17
Peach Oo-La-Long	8 oz	30
Hood		
Iced Tea	1 cup	100
Inko's		
White Tea All Flavors	1 bottle (16 oz)	56
White Tea Honeysuckle	1 bottle	0
Ito En		
Apricot	8 oz	60
Green Tea Apple	8 oz	70
Mango	8 oz	50
Shencho Shot	1 can (6.4 oz)	0
White Tea Grape	8 oz	60
Joe Tea		
All Flavors	8 oz	100
Kalahari		
Rooibos Red Tea All Flavors	8 oz	50
Kombucha		
Wonder Drink Asian Pear Ginger	1 bottle (8.5 oz)	65
Wonder Drink Rooibus Red Peach	1 bottle (8.5 oz)	60
Lipton		
Diet Green Tea w/ Citrus	8 oz	0
Diet Lemon	8 oz	0
Diet Sweet	8 oz	0
Extra Sweet	8 oz	100
Green Tea w/ Citrus	8 oz	80
Green Tea w/ Honey	8 oz	70
Lemon	8 oz	90
Original Sweetened	8 oz	70
Original Unsweetened	8 oz	0
Peach	8 oz	110
Raspberry	8 oz	110
Nantucket Nectars		
Half & Half	8 oz	90
Original Lemon	8 oz	80
Nestea		
Green Tea Diet Peach	8 oz	0
Green Tea Peach	1 bottle (20 oz)	220
Lemon	1 bottle (20 oz)	210

FOOD	PORTION	CALS
Lemon Diet	8 oz	0
Sweetened	8 oz	60
Sweetened Diet Green Tea	8 oz	0
Sweetened Green Tea	8 oz	80
Old Orchard		
Green Tea w/ Lemon & Honey	8 oz	45
Green Tea w/ Pomegranate	8 oz	45
Osteo		
Fruit Tea All Flavors	1 can (12 oz)	120
Pacific Foods		
Organic Lemon	8 oz	70
Organic Peach	8 oz	70
Organic Raspberry	8 oz	70
Organic Sweetened Black Tea	8 oz	60
Organic Unsweetened Green Tea	8 oz	0
Pixie		
Black Tea Mate Lemon Ginger	8 oz	35
Yerba Mate Authentic	8 oz	30
POM		
Light Tea Pomegranate Hibiscus Green	8 oz	35
Light Tea Pomegranate Orange Blossom	8 oz	35
Light Tea Pomegranate Wildberry White	8 oz	35
Snapple		
Diet Lemonade Iced Tea	8 oz	10
Just Plain Tea	8 oz	0
Lemonade Iced Tea	8 oz	110
Lime Green Tea	8 oz	100
Mint	8 oz	110
Peach	8 oz	100
SoBe		
Lean Diet Green Tea	8 oz	0
Lean Diet Peach Tea	8 oz	5
Solebury Home		
Organic All Flavors	8 oz	33
Sri Lankan		
Apple	8 oz	70
Lemon	8 oz	60
Ssips		
Diet Green Tea w/ Honey & Ginseng	1 box (7 oz)	0
Green Tea w/ Honey & Ginseng	1 box (7 oz)	60

FOOD	PORTION	CALS
Lemon	8 oz	100
Sweet Leaf		
Diet Mint & Honey Green Tea	8 oz	0
Lemon & Lime Unsweet	8 oz	0
Original Sweet	8 oz	70
Pomegranate Green Tea	8 oz	60
T42		
A Classic Earl Grey	8 oz	60
Jamaican Ginger Green Tea	8 oz	70
Wake-Up Blend English Breakfast	8 oz	45
With Lemon	8 oz	60
Tao Tea		
Grapefruit Green Tea	8 oz	71
Lemon Green Tea	8 oz	67
True Brew		
Cranberry Orange	8 oz	72
Green Tea	8 oz	64
Sweet Tea	8 oz	76
Turkey Hill		
Decaffeinated	8 oz	80
Diet Decaffeinated	8 oz	0
Nature's Accents Blueberry Oolong	8 oz	100
Nature's Accents Chai Spiced Zero Calorie	8 oz	0
Nature's Accents Green Tea	8 oz	70
Southern Brew Extra Sweet	8 oz	90
VidaTea		
All Flavors	1 can	90
VitaZest		
Green Tea Vitamin Enriched	8 oz	0
Weil For Tea		
Gyokuro	1 can (8.6 oz)	0
Turmeric	1 can (8.6 oz)	0

ICES AND ICE POPS
Blue Bunny

FOOD	PORTION	CALS
Bar Big Fudge	1 (2.7 oz)	110
Chill Cups Double Lemon	1 (4 oz)	100
FrozFruit Creamy Coconut	1 bar (3 oz)	150
FrozFruit Strawberries & Cream	1 bar (4 oz)	190
Pop Banana	1 (1.9 oz)	35
Pop Jolly Rancher	1 (4 oz)	120

FOOD	PORTION	CALS
Pop Root Beer	1 (1.9 oz)	40
The Original Bomb	1 (1.8 oz)	50
Breeze Freeze		
100% Fruit Juice	1 (8 oz)	54
Fruit Granita	1 (8 oz)	120
Breyers		
Pure Fruit Pop Lemon Lime	1 (1.75 oz)	40
Pure Fruit Pop Pomegranate Blends	1 (1.75 oz)	40
Dippin' Dots		
Cherry Berry	½ cup	90
Watermelon	½ cup	90
Edy's		
Sherbet Berry Rainbow	½ cup	130
Sherbet Key Lime	½ cup	130
Sherbet Orange Cream	½ cup	120
Sherbet Raspberry	½ cup	130
Sherbet Swiss Orange	½ cup	150
Sherbet Tropical Rainbow	½ cup	130
Whole Fruit Creamy Coconut	1 bar	120
Whole Fruit Lemonade	1 bar	80
Whole Fruit Lime	1 bar	80
Whole Fruit Orange & Cream	1 bar	80
Whole Fruit Peach	½ cup	90
Whole Fruit Strawberry	1 bar	80
Whole Fruit Tangerine	1 bar	80
Whole Fruit Tropical	1 bar	100
Whole Fruit Wild Berry	1 bar	80
Hawaiian Punch		
Arctic Surfers	1 pop	50
Hendrie's		
Citrus N' Berry Stix	1 (1.9 oz)	15
Fudge Stix Fat Free	1 bar (1.8 oz)	70
Hood		
Hoodsie Pop	1 (3.3 oz)	60
Luigi's		
Italian Ice Cherry	1 (6 oz)	130
Italian Ice Lemon Strawberry	1 (6 oz)	120
Italian Ice No Sugar Added Lemon	1 (6 oz)	60
Italian Ice Pina Colada	1 (6 oz)	130
Swirl Blue Ribbon Lemonade	1 (6 oz)	150

FOOD	PORTION	CALS
Minute Maid		
Fruit And Cream Swirl	1 tube (3 oz)	90
Fruit Bars	1 bar	60
Mr. J		
All Flavors	1 bar (2.25 oz)	50
Natural Choice		
Organic Vegan Fruit Bars Coconut	1 (2.75 oz)	90
Organic Vegan Fruit Bars Pink Lemonade	1 (2.75 oz)	50
Organic Vegan Grape	1 (2.75 oz)	50
Organic Vegan Sorbet Blueberry	½ cup	110
Organic Vegan Sorbet Lemon	½ cup	110
Organic Vegan Sorbet Mango	½ cup	110
PickleSickle		
Pop	1 (2 oz)	3
Popsicle		
Creamsicle Pop No Sugar Added	2 (1.65 oz)	45
Creamsicle Pop Sugar Free	2 (1.65 oz)	40
Diet Soda Pops	1 (1.6 oz)	15
Firecracker	1 (1.6 oz)	35
Fudgsicle Bar	1 (2.5 oz)	100
Fudgsicle Pops No Sugar Added	1 (1.65 oz)	40
Lifesavers Pop	1 (3.5 oz)	90
Pop Ups Orange Burst	1 (2.75 oz)	90
Rainbow Pops	1 (1.65 oz)	40
Snow Cone	1 (7 oz)	30
SoDelicious		
Dairy Free Creamy Orange Bar	1 (2.2 oz)	80
Sweet Nothings		
Bar Mango Raspberry	1 (2.6 oz)	100
The Power Of Fruit		
Original Fruit Bar	1 (1.75 oz)	28
Tropicana		
Fruit Juice Bar Orange	1	45
Fruit Juice Bar Raspberry	1	45
Strawberry	1	45
Turkey Hill		
Venice Mango	½ cup	100
Venice Pomegranate Blueberry w/ Acai	½ cup	100
Wawona		
Peach	1 pop	78

FOOD	PORTION	CALS
Strawberry	1 pop	77
JACKFRUIT		
fresh	3.5 oz	70
JALAPEÑO (see PEPPERS)		
JAM/JELLY/PRESERVES		
all flavors jam	1 tbsp (0.7 oz)	48
all flavors jam	1 pkg (0.5 oz)	34
all flavors jelly	1 tbsp (0.7 oz)	52
all flavors jelly	1 pkg (0.5 oz)	38
all flavors preserve	1 tbsp (0.7 oz)	48
all flavors preserve	1 pkg (0.5 oz)	34
apple butter	1 tbsp (0.6 oz)	33
orange marmalade	1 tbsp (0.7 oz)	49
orange marmalade	1 pkg (0.5 oz)	34
strawberry jam	1 tbsp (0.7 oz)	48
Cascadian Farm		
Organic Fruit Spread Blackberry	1 tbsp	45
Organic Fruit Spread Raspberry	1 tbsp	45
Organic Sweet Orange Marmalade	1 tbsp	45
Chukar Cherries		
Preserve No Sugar Added Cherry Amaretto	1 tbsp	24
Preserve Red Sour Cherry	1 tbsp	40
Preserve Vanilla Peach	1 tbsp	28
Columbia Empire Farms		
Marionberry Seedless Preserves	1 tbsp	60
Comfort Care		
Country Apple Butter	1 tbsp (1 oz)	40
Eden		
Organic Apple Butter	1 tbsp	20
Organic Apple Cherry Butter	1 tbsp	25
Organic Cherry Butter	1 tbsp	35
El Angel		
Strawberry Marmalade	1 tbsp	25
Gedney		
State Fair Preserves Strawberry Rhubarb	1 tbsp	50
Lollipop Tree		
Butter Cranberry Pear	1 tbsp	25
Butter Pumpkin Maple Pecan	1 tbsp	30
Jam Raspberry Peach	1 tbsp	50

FOOD	PORTION	CALS
Jam Triple Cherry	1 tbsp	50
Jelly Hot Pepper	1 tbsp	60
Jelly Wasabi Lime Pepper	1 tbsp	60
Matouk's		
Guava Jam	1 tbsp	50
Mango Jam	1 tbsp	50
Polaner		
All Fruit Apricot	1 tbsp	40
All Fruit Grape	1 tbsp	40
All Fruit Pineapple	1 tbsp	40
All Fruit Raspberry Seedless	1 tbsp	40
Revolution Foods		
Organic Jelly Grape	1 tbsp (0.7 oz)	60
Organic Preserves Strawberry	1 tbsp (0.7 oz)	60
Robert Rothschild Farm		
Preserves Cherry Acai	1 tbsp	35
Smucker's		
Cider Apple Butter	1 tbsp	45
Jam Concord Grape	1 tbsp	50
Jam Red Plum	1 tbsp	50
Jam Seedless Red Raspberry	1 tbsp	50
Jam Seedless Strawberry	1 tbsp	50
Jelly Apple	2 tbsp	50
Jelly Concord Grape	1 tbsp	50
Jelly Currant	1 tbsp	50
Jelly Elderberry	1 tbsp	50
Jelly Guava	1 tbsp	50
Jelly Mixed Fruit	2 tbsp	50
Low Sugar All Flavors	1 tbsp	25
Preserves All Flavors	1 tbsp	50
Simply Fruit All Flavors	1 tbsp	40
Sugar Free All Flavors	1 tbsp	10
Tree Of Life		
Organic Fruit Spread Grape	1 tbsp (0.6 oz)	30
Organic Fruit Spread Peach	1 tbsp (0.6 oz)	30
Welch's		
Grape Jelly	1 tbsp	50

JAPANESE FOOD (*see* ASIAN FOOD, SUSHI)

JELLY (*see* JAM/JELLY/PRESERVES)

FOOD	PORTION	CALS
JERKY		
beef	1 piece (0.7 oz)	82
pork	1 strip (0.5 oz)	62
venison	1 strip (0.5 oz)	55
Applegate Farms		
Natural Joy Stick	1 (1 oz)	100
Dakota Gourmet		
Fruit Jerky Strawberry Kiwi	1	70
Frank's RedHot		
Chile 'N Lime Steak Strips	1 oz	80
Original Beef	1 oz	80
Gary West		
Beef Strips Hickory Smoked	1 oz	70
Buffalo Strips	½ pkg (1 oz)	60
Elk Strips	½ pkg (1 oz)	70
Jack Link's		
Beef Teriyaki	1 oz	80
Organic Prairie		
Beef	1 oz	75
Outpost		
Beef	1 oz	70
Beef Steak	1 pkg (0.9 oz)	60
Beef Stick	1 (0.4 oz)	60
Pemmican		
Homestyle Tender All Flavors	1 oz	80
Kippered Beef Original	1 pkg (1 oz)	60
Kippered Beef Peppered	1 pkg (1 oz)	60
Kippered Beef Sweet & Hot	1 pkg (1 oz)	70
Kippered Beef Teriyaki	1 pkg (1 oz)	60
Long Lasting Hot & Spicy	1 oz	60
Long Lasting Original	1 oz	60
Long Lasting Peppered	1 oz	60
Long Lasting Teriyaki	1 oz	70
Premium Cut Beef Jerky	1 oz	80
Premium Cut Turkey Peppered	1 oz	70
Premium Cut Turkey Sweet Smoked	1 oz	70
Shredded Beef All Flavors	¼ cup	80
Steak Tips All Flavors	1 oz	70
Slim Jim		
Beef	7 pieces	130

FOOD	PORTION	CALS
Beef Jerky Hickory Smoked	1 oz	80
Classic Handipack	1 box	210
Giant Caddy Pepperoni	1 pkg	150
Twin Pack Cheese & Pepperoni	1 pkg	150
Tanka		
Natural Buffalo Cranberry Bar	1 (1 oz)	70
Natural Buffalo Cranberry Bite	1 (0.5 oz)	35
Tofurky		
Jurky Original	4 pieces (1 oz)	100
Tony's Smokehouse		
Salmon	1 pkg (0.5 oz)	40
Wellshire		
Matt's Select Pepperoni	1 stick (0.9 oz)	90
Tom Tom Snack Hot n' Spicy Turkey	1 stick (0.8 oz)	50
JICAMA		
fresh	1 sm (12.8 oz)	139
raw sliced	1 cup	46
Frieda's		
Jicama	¾ cup	35
JUJUBE		
dried	1 oz	82
JUTE		
cooked	1 cup	32
KALE		
chopped cooked w/o salt	1 cup	36
fresh cooked w/ fat	1 cup	69
scotch chopped cooked w/o salt	1 cup	36
Allens		
Seasoned	½ cup	35
Glory		
Fresh Greens	1 serv (2.8 oz)	40
Seasoned canned	½ cup	35
KANGAROO		
kangaroo	3 oz	120
KEFIR		
kefir	8 oz	98

FOOD	PORTION	CALS
Lifeway		
Greek Style	8 oz	202
Nonfat All Fruit Flavors	8 oz	188
Nonfat Plain	8 oz	116
Organic Helios All Fruit Flavors	8 oz	160
Organic Helios Plain	8 oz	120
Organic Lowfat All Fruit Flavors	8 oz	160
Organic Lowfat Plain	8 oz	110
Original	8 oz	162
Probugs All Flavors	1 bottle	130
Slim6 All Flavors	8 oz	110
Nancy's		
Organic Lowfat Blackberry	1 cup	180
Organic Lowfat Plain	1 cup	110
Organic Lowfat Raspberry	1 cup	180
KETCHUP		
banana	1 tsp	10
ketchup	1 tbsp	15
ketchup	1 pkg (0.2 oz)	6
low sodium	1 tbsp	15
Del Monte		
Ketchup	1 tbsp	15
Estee		
No Sugar Added	1 tbsp	15
Heinz		
Ketchup	1 tbsp	15
No Salt	1 tbsp	20
Organic	1 tbsp	20
Hunt's		
Ketchup	1 tbsp	15
No Salt Added	1 tbsp	20
Squeeze	1 tbsp	15
Muir Glen		
Organic	1 tbsp	20
Steel's		
Sugar Free	1 tbsp	10
Texas Sassy		
Tequila Ketchup	1 tbsp (0.5 oz)	20
Tree Of Life		
Organic	1 tbsp (0.6 oz)	20

FOOD	PORTION	CALS
Wholemato		
Organic Agave	1 tbsp	15
KIDNEY		
beef simmered	3 oz	134
lamb braised	3 oz	116
pork braised	3 oz	128
veal braised	3 oz	139
Rumba		
Beef	4 oz	120
KIDNEY BEANS		
canned	½ cup	108
dried cooked w/o salt	½ cup	112
B&M		
Red Kidney Baked Beans	½ cup (4.6 oz)	200
Bush's		
Light Red	½ cup	110
Eden		
Chili Beans	½ cup	130
Organic	½ cup	100
Organic Cannellini	½ cup	100
Organic Refried	½ cup	80
Goya		
Dark	½ cup	90
Progresso		
Cannellini	½ cup (4.6 oz)	110
Rienzi		
Cannellini	½ cup	80
Red	½ cup	90
Van Camp's		
New Orleans	½ cup	90
KIWI		
fresh	1 med (2.6 oz)	46
fresh	1 lg (3.2 oz)	56
Zespri		
Gold	2 med	80
Green	2 med	100

FOOD	PORTION	CALS

KIWI JUICE
Auna
Kiwifruit Juice | 1 bottle (12 oz) | 120

KNISH
TAKE-OUT
cheese | 1 (2.1 oz) | 205
meat | 1 (1.8 oz) | 174
potato | 1 (2.1 oz) | 212
potato | 1 lg (7 oz) | 332

KOHLRABI
raw sliced | 1 cup | 36
sliced cooked w/o salt | 1 cup | 48
Frieda's
Kohlrabi | ⅔ cup | 25
TAKE-OUT
creamed | 1 cup | 150

KRILL
fresh | 1 oz | 22

KUMQUATS
canned in syrup | 1 | 13
fresh | 1 | 13

KUZU
Eden
Root Starch | 1 tbsp | 30

LAMB
cubed lean & fat braised | 4 oz | 253
cubed lean broiled | 4 oz | 211
ground broiled | 4 oz | 321
leg roasted | 4 oz | 213
loin chop lean & fat broiled | 1 chop (4 oz) | 222
rib chop lean & fat broiled | 1 chop (1.6 oz) | 165
rib roast baked | 4 oz | 386
shank lean & fat braised | 4 oz | 360
shoulder chop lean & fat cooked | 1 chop (5.5 oz) | 274
shoulder w/ bone braised | 4 oz | 231

FOOD	PORTION	CALS
LAMB DISHES		
TAKE-OUT		
keema w/ coconut milk	1 serv (8 oz)	380
moroccan pilaf w/ bulgur	1 serv	327
moussaka	4 in sq (16 oz)	659
shepherd's pie	1 (21.3 oz)	742
stew w/ potatoes & vegetables	1 cup	260
LAMBSQUARTERS		
chopped cooked w/ salt	1 cup	58
LECITHIN		
lecithin	1 tbsp	104
Bob's Red Mill		
Lecithin Granules	1 tbsp	60
Tree Of Life		
Granules	1 tbsp (0.3 oz)	55
LEEKS		
chopped cooked w/o salt	¼ cup	8
cooked	1 (4.4 oz)	38
freeze dried	1 tbsp	1
Frieda's		
Fresh	1 cup	50
LEMON		
fresh	1 med (4 oz)	22
peel	1 tsp	1
peel	1 tbsp	3
wedge	1 (7 g)	2
Sunkist		
Fresh	1 (2 oz)	15
True Lemon		
Crystallized Lemon	1 pkg (1 g)	0
LEMON CURD		
lemon curd made w/ egg	2 tsp	29
Lollipop Tree		
Lemon Curd	1 tbsp	50
Robert Rothschild Farm		
Lemon Curd & Tart Filling	1 tbsp	50

FOOD	PORTION	CALS
LEMON EXTRACT		
lemon extract	½ tsp	12
LEMON GRASS		
fresh	1 tbsp	5
LEMON JUICE		
bottled	1 tbsp	3
bottled	1 oz	6
fresh	1 oz	8
from 1 lemon	1.6 oz	12
from wedge	6 g	1
Essn		
Sparkling Meyer Lemon Juice	1 can (8.4 oz)	170
Izze		
Sparkling Lemon	8 oz	150
LEMONADE		
MIX		
A La Source		
Organic as prep	8 oz	110
Country Time		
Lemonade as prep	8 oz	60
Pink as prep	8 oz	60
Raspberry as prep	8 oz	80
Strawberry as prep	8 oz	80
Crystal Light		
Lemonade as prep	1 serv	5
On The Go as prep	1 pkg	5
Pink as prep	1 serv	5
READY-TO-DRINK		
Adina		
Hibiscus Lemon Bissap	8 oz	80
Apple & Eve		
Organic	8 oz	130
Crystal Light		
Sugar Free	8 oz	5
Honest Ade		
Cranberry	8 oz	50
Hood		
Lemonade	1 cup	110

FOOD	PORTION	CALS
Mike's		
Hard Lemonade	1 bottle (12 oz)	220
Minute Maid		
Chilled	8 oz	100
Lemonade	1 can (12 oz)	150
Light	8 oz	15
Naked Juice		
Just Made	8 oz	110
Nantucket Nectars		
Lemondade	8 oz	110
Nesbitt's		
Honey	1 bottle (12 oz)	180
Newman's Own		
Pink Virgin	8 oz	110
Roadside Virgin	8 oz	110
Virgin Lemon Aided	8 oz	110
Odwalla		
PomaGrand	8 oz	110
Pure Squeezed	8 oz	120
Santa Cruz		
Organic	1 can	160
Organic Raspberry	1 can	120
Simply		
Lemonade	8 oz	120
Snapple		
Lemonade	8 oz	110
Super Sour	8 oz	130
Ssips		
Lemonade	8 oz	110
Sweet Leaf		
Half & Half Lemonade Tea	8 oz	85
Original	8 oz	90
Tropicana		
Light	1 cup	10
Orchard Style	8 oz	120
Twister Light	8 oz	50
Twister Strawberry	8 oz	140
Turkey Hill		
Lemonade	8 oz	120

FOOD	PORTION	CALS
Uncle Matt's		
Organic	8 oz	120
LENTILS		
dried cooked	1 cup	230
Eden		
Organic Green w/ Onion & Bay Leaf	½ cup	90
Near East		
Lentil Pilaf as prep	1 cup	200
Sabra		
Dardara	2 oz	40
TastyBite		
Jodhpur Lentils	½ pkg (5 oz)	106
Madras Lentils	½ pkg (5 oz)	127
TAKE-OUT		
lentil loaf	1 slice (1.6 oz)	83
middle eastern lentil salad	1 serv (4.5 oz)	158
yemiser selatta ethiopian lentil salad	1 serv (3 oz)	115
LETTUCE (see also SALAD)		
arugula	6 leaves (0.4 oz)	3
arugula shredded	1 cup	5
boston	1 head (5.7 oz)	21
boston chopped	6 leaves	7
cornsalad field salad	1 cup (1.9 oz)	7
iceberg	1 lg head (26.5 oz)	106
iceberg	6 med leaves	7
iceberg shredded	1 cup	10
looseleaf outer leaves	6 (5 oz)	22
looseleaf shredded	1 cup	5
red leaf	6 leaves (3.6 oz)	16
red leaf shredded	1 cup	4
romaine	3 leaves (3 oz)	14
romaine heart	6 leaves (1.3 oz)	6
romaine shredded	1 cup	8
Andy Boy		
Romaine Hearts	6 leaves (3 oz)	20
Dole		
Classic Romaine	1½ cups (3 oz)	15
Shredded	1½ cups (3 oz)	15

FOOD	PORTION	CALS
Earthbound Farm		
Organic Baby Romaine Salad	2 cups	15
Fresh Express		
5 Lettuce Mix	3 cups	15
Lettuce Trio	2½ cups	15
Organic Baby Arugula	3 cups	20
Organic Hearts Of Romaine	1½ cups	15
Premium Romaine	2 cups	15
Shreds Iceberg	1½ cups	15
Sweet Butter	2½ cups	10
Frieda's		
Limestone	⅔ cup	10
Green Giant		
Hearts Of Romaine	6 leaves (3 oz)	14
Mann's		
Romaine Hearts	6 leaves (3 oz)	15
Ocean Mist		
Butter Leaf Shredded	1 cup (2 oz)	7
Green or Green Leaf Shredded	1 cup (1.3 oz)	5
Iceberg	⅙ head (3 oz)	15
Romaine Hearts	6 leaves	20
River Ranch		
Romaine Chopped	1½ cups	10
Romaine Hearts	1½ cups	10
LILY ROOT		
dried	1 oz	89
fresh	1 oz	32
LIMA BEANS		
CANNED		
lima beans	½ cup	95
Allens		
Baby Butter Beans	½ cup	120
Medium Green	½ cup	140
Del Monte		
Green	½ cup	80
East Texas Fair		
Green	½ cup	120
Hanover		
Butter Beans In Sauce	½ cup	100

FOOD	PORTION	CALS
DRIED		
cooked	½ cup	150
FROZEN		
C&W		
Baby	½ cup	110
Green Giant		
Baby & Butter Sauce as prep	⅔ cup	100
LIME		
fresh	1 (2.4 oz)	20
wedge	1 (8 g)	2
Sunkist		
Fresh	1 (2 oz)	20
True Lime		
Crystallized Lime	1 pkg	0
LIME JUICE		
bottled	1 oz	6
fresh	1 oz	8
from 1 lime	1.1 oz	11
Adina		
Lime Mint Mojita	8 oz	70
Honest Ade		
Limeade	8 oz	50
Minute Maid		
Light Limeade	8 oz	15
Newman's Own		
Virgin Limeade	8 oz	140
Sabor Latino		
Limeade	8 oz	160
Simply		
Limeade	8 oz	120
Sweet Leaf		
Limeade Cherry	8 oz	90
Turkey Hill		
Limonade	8 oz	120
LING		
blue raw	3.5 oz	83
fresh baked	3 oz	95
fresh fillet baked	5.3 oz	168

FOOD	PORTION	CALS

LINGCOD
baked	3 oz	93
fillet baked	5.3 oz	164

LIQUOR/LIQUEUR (see also BEER AND ALE, CHAMPAGNE, MALT, WINE)
7&7	1 serv	178
alabama slammer	1 serv	103
amaretto sour	1 serv	295
angel's kiss	1 serv	85
anisette	1 oz	111
antifreeze	1 serv	177
apricot brandy	1 oz	96
apricot sour	1 serv	164
aquavit	1 oz	65
b52	1 serv	247
b&b	1 serv	75
bahama breeze	1 serv	70
bahama mama	1 serv	153
bailey's & amaretto	1 serv	184
banana colada	1 serv	376
bay breeze	1 serv	173
bend me over	1 serv	242
benedictine	1 oz	104
betsy ross	1 serv	206
black devil	1 serv	220
black russian	1 serv	184
bloody mary	1 serv	150
blue whale	1 serv	222
bourbon & soda	1 serv (4 oz)	105
bourbon sour	1 serv	166
brandy	2 oz	255
brandy alexander	1 serv	266
brandy sour	1 serv	164
bushwacker	1 serv	286
campari	2 oz	245
cherry heering	2 oz	245
coffee liqueur	1 serv (1.5 oz)	175
cognac	1 oz	67
cosmopolitan martini	1 serv	126
creme de almonde	1 oz	102

FOOD	PORTION	CALS
creme de banana	1 oz	99
creme de cassis	1 oz	82
creme de menthe	1 serv (1.5 oz)	186
curacao liqueur	1 oz	81
daiquiri	1 serv (2 oz)	112
daiquiri banana	1 serv	277
dark & stormy	1 serv	64
doctor pepper	1 serv	95
drambuie	2 oz	225
frozen daiquiri	1 serv	393
frozen daiquiri pineapple	1 serv	186
frozen tequila screwdriver	1 serv	159
fuzzy navel	1 serv	247
gibson	1 serv (4 oz)	254
gin	1 serv (1.5 oz)	110
gin & tonic	1 serv (7.5 oz)	171
gin ricky	1 serv	114
grasshopper	1 serv	275
happy hawaiian	1 serv	434
harvey wallbanger	1 serv	198
head banger	1 serv	165
hot buttered rum	1 serv (8.8 oz)	316
hot toddy	1 serv	188
hurricane	1 serv	205
kamikaze	1 serv	136
long island iced tea	1 serv	292
lynchburg lemonade	1 serv	465
mai tai	1 serv	165
manhattan	1 serv	171
margarita	1 serv	173
margarita strawberry	1 serv	106
martini	1 serv (3 oz)	206
martini apple	1 serv	147
martini rum	1 serv	131
mellow yellow	1 serv	95
mexican grasshopper	1 serv	638
mint julep	1 serv	136
mississippi mud	1 serv	496
mudslide	1 serv	566
narragansett	1 serv	168

FOOD	PORTION	CALS
nutcracker	1 serv	730
old fashioned	1 serv	223
orange crush	1 serv	461
pain killer	1 serv	277
peppermint pattie	1 serv	344
pina colada	1 serv (4.5 oz)	245
planter's cocktail	1 serv	105
planter's punch	1 serv	233
presbyterian	1 serv	170
purple passion	1 serv	215
rob roy	1 serv	171
rum	1 serv (1.5 oz)	97
rum boogie	1 serv	134
rum cola	1 serv	209
rum highball	1 serv	170
rum punch	1 serv	448
rum screwdriver	1 serv	166
rum sour	1 serv	156
rum swizzle	1 serv	187
rusty nail	1 serv	159
sake	1 serv (1 oz)	39
salty dog	1 serv	210
scotch & soda	1 serv	104
sea breeze	1 serv	207
sex on the beach	1 serv	190
singapore sling	1 serv (4 oz)	115
slippery nipple	1 serv	142
sloe gin fizz	1 serv (2.5 oz)	132
snake bite	1 serv	362
southern comfort	1 serv (1.5 oz)	184
tequila	1 serv (1.5 oz)	117
tequila gimlet	1 serv	150
tequila sour	1 serv	156
tequila stinger	1 serv	221
tequila sunrise	1 serv (6.8 oz)	232
tom collins	1 serv (7.5 oz)	121
vermouth cassis	1 serv	97
vodka	1 serv (1.5 oz)	97
vodka gimlet	1 serv	150
vodka sour	1 serv	138

FOOD	PORTION	CALS
vodka stinger	1 serv	378
whiskey	1 serv (1.5 oz)	105
whiskey sour	1 serv (3.5 oz)	162
white russian	1 serv	290
zombie	1 serv	235
Absolut		
Vodka	1 shot (1.5 oz)	98
Bacardi		
Gold Rum	1 shot (1.5 oz)	98
Capt. Morgan's		
Original Spiced Rum	1 shot (1.5 oz)	86
Crown Royal		
Canadian Whiskey	1 shot (1.5 oz)	96
Jack Daniel's		
Old No.7 Tennessee Whiskey	1 shot (1.5 oz)	98
Jose Cuervo		
Gold Tequila	1 shot (1.5 oz)	96
Seagram's		
Gin	1 shot (1.5 oz)	120
Smirnoff		
Vodka	1 shot (1.5 oz)	96
LIVER (*see also* PATE)		
beef braised	1 slice (2.4 oz)	130
beef pan fried	1 slice (2.8 oz)	142
chicken fried	3 oz	146
chicken simmered	3 oz	142
duck raw	1 (1.5 oz)	60
goose raw	1 (3.3 oz)	125
lamb braised	3 oz	187
lamb fried	3 oz	202
moose braised	3 oz	132
pork braised	3 oz	140
turkey simmered	1 liver (2.9 oz)	227
veal braised	1 slice (2.8 oz)	154
veal pan fried	1 slice (2.4 oz)	129
Organic Prairie		
Beef	2 oz	80
Rumba		
Beef	4 oz	160

FOOD	PORTION	CALS
TAKE-OUT		
calves liver w/ onions	1 serv (5 oz)	177
LLAMA		
llama	3 oz	120
LOBSTER		
northern cooked	3 oz	83
northern cooked	1 cup	142
northern raw	3 oz	77
northern raw	1 lobster (5.3 oz)	136
spiny steamed	1 (5.7 oz)	233
spiny steamed	3 oz	122
Phillips Seafood		
Lobster Cake	1 (3 oz)	230
TAKE-OUT		
newburg	1 cup	485
LOGANBERRIES		
frzn	1 cup	80
LONGANS		
fresh	1	2
LOQUATS		
fresh	1	5
LOTUS		
root raw sliced	10 slices	45
root sliced cooked	10 slices	59
seeds dried	1 oz	94
Eden		
Dried Sliced	5 slices (0.3 oz)	35
Frieda's		
Lotus Root Fresh	1 cup	50
LOX (see SALMON)		
LUPINES		
dried cooked	1 cup	197
LYCHEES		
fresh	1	6
Frieda's		
Fresh	6 to 8 (3.5 oz)	60

FOOD	PORTION	CALS
Polar		
Lychee	1	110
MACA ROOT		
Navitas Naturals		
Powder Gelatanized	1 tsp (5 g)	20
Raw Powder	1 tsp (5 g)	20
MACADAMIA NUTS		
dry roasted w/ salt	11 nuts (1 oz)	200
oil roasted	1 oz	204
Chukar Cherries		
Extra Dark Chocolate Covered	3 tbsp (1.4 oz)	216
Emily's		
Milk Chocolate Covered	4 (1.5 oz)	260
Hawaiian Host		
White Choco	3 pieces (1.4 oz)	230
Mauna Loa		
Maui Onion & Garlic	1 pkg (1.2 oz)	230
Milk Chocolate Coated	3 pieces	230
Milk Chocolate Toffee	7 pieces	210
MACE		
ground	1 tsp	8
MACKEREL		
CANNED		
jack	1 cup	296
jack	1 can (12.7 oz)	563
Brunswick		
Jack In Water	2 oz	100
Chicken Of The Sea		
Jack In Tomato Sauce	¼ cup	70
Jack In Water	⅓ cup	90
Orleans		
Jack	¼ cup	90
Polar		
Jack	⅓ cup	90
DRIED		
Eden		
Bonito Flakes	2 tbsp	5

FOOD	PORTION	CALS
FRESH		
atlantic cooked	3 oz	223
atlantic raw	3 oz	174
jack baked	3 oz	171
jack fillet baked	6.2 oz	354
king baked	3 oz	114
king fillet baked	5.4 oz	207
pacific baked	3 oz	171
pacific fillet baked	6.2 oz	354
spanish cooked	1 fillet (5.1 oz)	230
spanish cooked	3 oz	134
spanish raw	3 oz	118
SMOKED		
atlantic	3.5 oz	296
MAHI MAHI		
fresh baked	4 oz	192
Phillips Seafood		
Coconut Mahi Mahi w/ Sauce	3 pieces	290
MALANGA		
dasheen mashed	1 cup	226
dasheen pieces boiled	1 cup	212
pieces fried	1 cup	304
root raw	1 (10.7 oz)	299
Frieda's		
Malanga	⅔ cup	90
MALT		
malt liquor	1 bottle (12 oz)	148
nonalcoholic	1 bottle (12 oz)	133
MALTED MILK		
chocolate as prep w/ milk	1 cup	179
chocolate flavor powder	3 heaping tsp (0.7 oz)	79
natural flavor as prep w/ milk	1 cup	186
natural flavor powder	3 heaping tsp (0.7 oz)	87
MAMMY-APPLE		
fresh	1	431

FOOD	PORTION	CALS
MANGO		
fresh	1	135
C&W		
Chunks	¾ cup	90
Kopali		
Organic Dried	1 pkg (1.8 oz)	140
Peeled Snacks		
Fruit Picks Go-Mango-Man-Go	1 pkg (1.4 oz)	120
Polar		
Sliced	3 pieces (5 oz)	100
Sunsweet		
Philippine dried	6 pieces (1.5 oz)	130
Thailand dried	⅓ cup (1.4 oz)	140
MANGO JUICE		
GoodBelly		
Mango Probiotic Drink	8 oz	100
Naked Juice		
Mighty Mango	8 oz	120
Old Orchard		
Nectar Cocktail	8 oz	120
MANGOSTEEN		
canned in syrup	1 cup	143
MARGARINE		
margarine butter blend	1 tbsp (0.5 oz)	101
squeeze	1 pkg (0.2 oz)	36
squeeze liquid	1 tbsp (0.5 oz)	102
stick	1 stick (4 oz)	810
stick	1 tbsp (0.5 oz)	100
tub diet	1 tbsp (0.5 oz)	26
tub fat free	1 tbsp (0.5 oz)	27
tub light	1 tbsp (0.5 oz)	59
tub salted	1 tbsp (0.5 oz)	101
whipped salted	1 tbsp (0.3 oz)	67
Benecol		
Spread Light	1 tbsp	50
Spread Regular	1 tbsp	70
Blue Bonnet		
Light Stick	1 tbsp	50
Soft Spread	1 tbsp	60

FOOD	PORTION	CALS
Soft Spread Light	1 tbsp	40
Stick	1 tbsp	80
Brummel & Brown		
Creamy Fruit Spread Strawberry	1 tbsp	50
Spread w/ Yogurt	1 tbsp	45
Crystal Farms		
60/40 Margarine Butter	1 tbsp	100
Margarine	1 tbsp	100
Earth Balance		
Butter Blend Salted	1 tbsp	100
Buttery Spread Original	1 tbsp	100
Buttery Spread Soy Garden	1 tbsp	100
Buttery Sticks Vegan	1 tbsp	100
Fleischmann's		
Soft Spread Light	1 tbsp	40
Soft Spread Original	1 tbsp	70
Soft Spread Unsalted	1 tbsp	70
Soft Spread w/ Olive Oil	1 tbsp	70
I Can't Believe It's Not Butter		
Regular Stick	1 tbsp	90
Soft Fat Free	1 tbsp	5
Soft Light	1 tbsp	50
Soft Regular	1 tbsp	80
Soft w/ Calcium	1 tbsp	50
Spray	5 sprays	0
Squeeze	1 tbsp	60
Stick Light	1 tbsp	50
Land O Lakes		
Soft	1 tbsp (0.5 oz)	100
Stick	1 tbsp (0.5 oz)	100
Move Over Butter		
Spread	1 tbsp	50
Parkay		
Light Spread	1 tbsp	50
Original Spread	1 tbsp	60
Original Stick	1 tbsp	90
Spray	5 sprays	0
Spread + Calcium	1 tbsp	45
Squeeze	1 tbsp	70
Stick Light	1 tbsp	50

FOOD	PORTION	CALS
Promise		
Buttery Spread	1 tbsp	80
Buttery Spread Activ	1 tbsp	70
Fat Free	1 tbsp	5
Light	1 tbsp	45
Light Activ	1 tbsp	45
Smart Balance		
37% Light	1 tbsp	45
67% Light	1 tbsp	80
Omega Plus w/ Flax Oil	1 tbsp	80
Spectrum		
Essential Omega	1 tbsp	80
Spread	1 tbsp	88

MARINADE (*see* SAUCE)

MARJORAM

dried	1 tsp	2

MARLIN

raw	3 oz	110

MARSHMALLOW

marshmallow	1 reg (0.3 oz)	23
marshmallow	1 cup (1.6 oz)	146

MATZO

brie	1 piece (0.5 oz)	54
egg	1 (1 oz)	109
matzo ball	1 med (1.2 oz)	48
plain	1 (1 oz)	111
whole wheat	1 (1 oz)	98
Horowitz Margareten		
Egg	1 (1.2 oz)	130
Manischewitz		
Dark Chocolate Coated Egg	½ (1.5 oz)	90
Egg	1 (1.2 oz)	120
Egg & Onion	1 (1 oz)	100
Matzo Ball Mix	2 tbsp	50
Thin Unsalted	1 (0.8 oz)	90
Streit's		
Egg	1 (1.1 oz)	120
Egg & Onion	1 (1 oz)	100

FOOD	PORTION	CALS
MAYONNAISE		
diet	1 tbsp	36
imitation	1 tbsp	35
mayonnaise	1 tbsp	99
Cains		
All Natural	1 tbsp	100
Light	1 tbsp	50
Carb Options		
Whipped Dressing	1 tbsp	50
Hellman's		
Light	1 tbsp	45
Real	1 tbsp	90
Real Canola No Cholesterol	1 tbsp	90
Reduced Fat	1 tbsp	20
W/ Extra Virgin Olive Oil	1 tbsp	50
Hollywood		
Canola	1 tbsp	100
Safflower	1 tbsp	100
Kraft		
Mayo	1 tbsp	90
Mayo w/ Olive Oil	1 tbsp	45
Miracle Whip		
Free	1 tbsp	15
Light	1 tbsp	25
Original	1 tbsp	40
Nasoya		
Fat Free Nayonaise	1 tbsp	10
Nayonaise	1 tbsp	35
Smart Balance		
Omega	1 tbsp	120
Omega Plus	1 tbsp	50
Spectrum		
Canola Squeeze	1 tbsp	100
Canola Squeeze Light Eggless Vegan	1 tbsp	35
Organic Dijon	1 tbsp	90
Organic Olive Oil	1 tbsp	100
Organic Roasted Garlic	1 tbsp	100
Organic Squeeze	1 tbsp	100
Organic Wasabi	1 tbsp	100

FOOD	PORTION	CALS
Vegenaise		
Grapeseed Oil	1 tbsp (0.5 oz)	90
Organic	1 tbsp (0.5 oz)	90
Original	1 tbsp (0.5 oz)	90

MEAT SUBSTITUTES (*see also* BACON SUBSTITUTES, CANADIAN BACON SUBSTITUTES, CHICKEN SUBSTITUTES, HAMBURGER SUBSTITUTES, JERKY MEATBALL SUBSTITUTES, SAUSAGE SUBSTITUTES, TURKEY SUBSTITUTES)

FOOD	PORTION	CALS
Fantastic		
Sloppy Joe Mix not prep	¼ cup	70
Taco Filling not prep	¼ cup	80
Gardenburger		
BBQ Riblets w/ Sauce	1 serv (5 oz)	240
Helen's Kitchen		
GardenSteak Tofu Steak	1 (3 oz)	150
Lightlife		
Balogna	4 slices (2 oz)	60
Gimme Lean Ground Beef	1 serv (2 oz)	50
Smart BBQ	¼ cup	70
Smart Cutlet Salisbury Steak	1 (4.5 oz)	130
Smart Deli Country Ham	4 slices (2 oz)	90
Smart Deli Pastrami Style	4 slices (2 oz)	60
Smart Deli Pepperoni Style	13 slices (1 oz)	45
Smart Ground Original	⅓ cup (1.9 oz)	80
Smart Ground Taco Burrito	⅓ cup (2 oz)	70
Smart Menu Crumbles	⅓ cup	80
Smart Menu Steak Strips	1 serv (3 oz)	80
Smart Tex Mex	¼ cup	50
Loma Linda		
Dinner Cuts	2 slices (3.2 oz)	90
Swiss Stake	1 piece (3.2 oz)	130
Morningstar Farms		
Meal Starters Steak Strips	12 pieces (3 oz)	140
Quorn		
Grounds	⅔ cup (3 oz)	80
Veat		
Gourmet Bites	1 serv (2.5 oz)	90
Vegetarian Fillet	1 (1.8 oz)	170
VeggieLand		
Crumbles Beef	½ cup	70
Veg-T-Balls	3 (3 oz)	113

FOOD	PORTION	CALS
Viana		
Cowgirl Veggie Steaks	1 (3.7 oz)	260
Veggie Cevapcici	4 pieces (2.8 oz)	240
Veggie Gyros	24 strips (3 oz)	220
Veggie Kebab	½ cup	210
Worthington		
Bolono	3 slices (2 oz)	80
Choplets	2 slices (3.2 oz)	90
Corned Beef Vegetarian	3 slices (2 oz)	140
Dinner Roast	1 slice (3 oz)	180
Multigrain Cutlets	2 slices (3.2 oz)	100
Prime Stakes	1 piece (3.2 oz)	120
Vegetable Skallops	½ cup (3 oz)	90
Wham	2 slices (2 oz)	110
Yves		
Meatless Beef Skewers	1 (2.8 oz)	100
Meatless Bologna	4 slices	60
Meatless Ground Round Original	⅓ cup	60
Meatless Pepperoni	6 slices	90
MEATBALL SUBSTITUTES		
meatless	2 (1.3 oz)	71
Gardenburger		
Mama Mia Meatballs	6 (3 oz)	110
Lightlife		
Smart Menu Meatless Meatballs	5	160
Loma Linda		
Tender Rounds	6 (2.8 oz)	120
Quorn		
Meatballs	4 (2.4 oz)	110
MEATBALLS		
beef	1 med (1 oz)	74
beef	1 lg (1.5 oz)	111
beef cocktail	1 (0.2 oz)	18
chicken	1 med (1 oz)	47
chicken	1 lg (1.5 oz)	71
chicken cocktail	1 (0.2 oz)	12
turkey	1 med (1 oz)	47
Butterball		
Seasoned Italian frzn	6 (3 oz)	170

FOOD	PORTION	CALS
Honeysuckle White		
Turkey Italian Style frzn	3 (3 oz)	190
Ian's		
Italian	3 (2.2 oz)	145
Mama Lucia		
Homestyle	4	207
Italian Style	4	280
Sausage Beef	8	220
Organic Classics		
Italian Beef	3 (3 oz)	180
Shady Brook		
Italian Beef	3 oz	260
Turkey Meatballs Appetizer Size + Sweet & Sour Sauce	6 + 2 tbsp sauce	235
Turkey Meatballs Italian Style	3 (3 oz)	190
Tyson		
Italian Style Chicken	6 (3 oz)	180
TAKE-OUT		
albondigas w/ sauce	3 + sauce (5.3 oz)	372
porcupine + tomato sauce	3 + sauce	160
swedish w/ cream sauce	3 + sauce (4.7 oz)	215
sweet & sour	3 + sauce (4.5 oz)	188
MELON		
sprite	1 (10.6 oz)	110
Frieda's		
Camouflage	1 cup (5 oz)	50
SpriteMelon	1 (10.5 oz)	115
Temptation	1/10 melon (4.7 oz)	55

MEXICAN FOOD (see SALSA, SPANISH FOOD, TORTILLA)

FOOD	PORTION	CALS
MILK		
CANNED		
condensed sweetened	1 oz	123
condensed sweetened	1 cup	982
evaporated	1/2 cup	169
evaporated skim	1/2 cup	99
Borden		
Sweetened Condensed Low Fat	2 tbsp	120
Carnation		
Evaporated	2 tbsp	40

FOOD	PORTION	CALS
Evaporated Lowfat 2%	2 tbsp (1 oz)	25
Meyenberg		
Evaporated Goat Milk	8 oz	145
DRIED		
buttermilk	1 tbsp	25
nonfat instant	1 pkg (3.2 oz)	244
Alba		
Instant Non-Fat as prep	1 cup	80
Bob's Red Mill		
Buttermilk Sweet Cream as prep	8 oz	60
Non Fat as prep	8 oz	80
Carnation		
Instant Nonfat as prep	1 cup	80
Meyenberg		
Instant Goat Milk as prep	1 cup	142
Organic Valley		
Buttermilk	3 tbsp	110
Nonfat	3 tbsp	90
Sanalac		
Powder	¼ cup (0.8 oz)	80
REFRIGERATED		
1%	1 cup	102
1%	1 qt	409
2%	1 cup	121
2%	1 qt	485
buffalo	7 oz	224
buttermilk	1 cup	99
buttermilk	1 qt	396
camel	7 oz	160
donkey	7 oz	86
goat	1 qt	672
goat	1 cup	168
human	1 cup	171
indian buffalo	1 cup	236
low sodium	1 cup	149
mare	7 oz	98
nonfat	1 cup	86
sheep	1 cup	264
whole	1 cup	150

FOOD	PORTION	CALS
Active Lifestyle		
Fat Free w/ Plant Sterols	8 oz	90
Borden		
Fat Free Skim	1 cup	80
Dairy Ease		
Fat Free Lactose Free	1 cup (8 oz)	90
Reduced Fat 2% Lactose Free	1 cup (8 oz)	130
Whole Lactose Free	1 cup (8 oz)	160
Farmland		
Buttermilk	8 oz	160
Fat Free	8 oz	80
Special Request 1% Plus Omega-3	8 oz	130
Special Request Skim Plus	8 oz	110
Special Request Skim Plus 100% Lactose Free	8 oz	110
Whole	8 oz	160
Friendship		
Buttermilk Lowfat	1 cup	120
Hood		
1%	1 cup	110
2%	1 cup	130
Buttermilk Fat Free	1 cup	90
Calorie Countdown 2%	8 oz	90
Calorie Countdown Fat Free	8 oz	45
Fat Free	1 cup	80
Simply Smart 0% Fat	1 cup	90
Simply Smart 1% Fat	1 cup	120
Whole	1 cup	150
Horizon Organic		
Fat Free	8 oz	90
Lactaid		
1% Lowfat	1 cup	110
2% Reduced Fat	1 cup	130
Calcium Fortified	1 cup	80
Fat Free	1 cup	90
Whole	1 cup	150
Land O Lakes		
1%	1 cup (8 oz)	100
2%	1 cup (8 oz)	120
Skim	1 cup (8 oz)	90
Whole	1 cup (8 oz)	150

FOOD	PORTION	CALS
Meyenberg		
Goat Milk	8 oz	142
Goat Milk Low Fat	8 oz	89
Organic Valley		
Fat Free	1 cup	90
Lactose Free Fat Free	1 cup	90
Whole Nonhomogenized	1 cup	150
Straus		
Organic Reduced Fat 2% Cream Top	8 oz	130
SunMilk		
Heart Healthy 1% Sunflower Oil	8 oz	120
Heart Healthy 2% Sunflower Oil	8 oz	120
Turkey Hill		
Cool Moos Whole Milk	8 oz	160
Tuscan		
Whole	8 oz	150
Welsh Farms		
Fat Free	8 oz	80
SHELF-STABLE		
Parmalat		
2% Reduced Fat	8 oz	130
Fat Free	8 oz	80
Lactose Free 2% Reduced Fat	8 oz	130
MILK DRINKS		
chocolate milk	1 cup	208
chocolate milk	1 qt	833
chocolate milk 1%	1 cup	158
chocolate milk 2%	1 cup	179
Bravo!		
Blenders Creamy Double Chocolate	1 bottle (11 oz)	180
Blenders Creamy French Vanilla	1 bottle (11 oz)	160
Cal-C		
Orange Tangerine	8 oz	70
Peach Mango	8 oz	70
Strawberry Citrus	8 oz	70
Cocio		
Chocolate	8 oz	140
CocoaVia		
Indulgence Rice Chocolate	1 bottle (5.65 oz)	150

FOOD	PORTION	CALS
Dove		
Bravo! Dark Chocolate	1 bottle	310
Bravo! Milk Chocolate	1 bottle	310
Farmland		
Really Really Good! Chocolate	8 oz	160
Hershey's		
Chocolate Fat Free	1 bottle	160
Chocolate Reduced Fat	1 bottle	200
Hood		
Calorie Countdown Chocolate 2%	8 oz	90
Chocolate	1 cup	230
Chocolate Lowfat	1 cup	170
Coffee Lowfat	1 cup	170
Horizon Organic		
Lowfat Chocolate	8 oz	170
Strawberry	8 oz	200
Land O Lakes		
2% Swiss Chocolate	1 cup (8.4 oz)	190
Chocolate Skim	1 cup (8 oz)	160
Strawberry	1 cup (8 oz)	190
Lifeway		
La Fruta All Flavors	8 oz	180
Nesquik		
Chocolate Powder as prep w/ lowfat milk	1 cup (8 oz)	180
Chocolate Powder No Sugar Added as prep w/ lowfat milk	1 cup (8 oz)	160
Ready-To-Drink Banana	1 cup (8 oz)	200
Ready-To-Drink Chocolate	1 cup (8 oz)	200
Ready-To-Drink Strawberry	1 cup (8 oz)	200
Ready-To-Drink Vanilla	1 cup (8 oz)	200
Strawberry Powder as prep w/ lowfat milk	1 cup (8 oz)	190
Organic Valley		
Buttermilk Lowfat 1%	1 cup	100
Parmalat		
Chocolate 2% Reduced Fat	1 cup	190
Quaker		
Chocolate	8 oz	140
Strawberry	8 oz	130
Vanilla	8 oz	130

FOOD	PORTION	CALS
Sipahh		
Straw Banana	1 straw	15
Straw Cookies and Cream	1 straw	15
Turkey Hill		
Cool Moos 2% Reduced Fat	8 oz	120
Cool Moos Chocolate	8 oz	180
Cool Moos Whole	8 oz	150
MILK SUBSTITUTES		
imitation milk	1 qt	600
imitation milk	1 cup	150
soy milk	1 cup	79
8th Continent		
Soymilk Chocolate	8 oz	140
Soymilk Original	8 oz	80
Soymilk Vanilla	8 oz	100
Soymilk Fat Free Original	8 oz	60
Soymilk Fat Free Vanilla	8 oz	70
Soymilk Light Chocolate	8 oz	90
Soymilk Light Original	8 oz	50
Soymilk Light Vanilla	8 oz	60
Almond Breeze		
Chocolate	8 oz	115
Original	8 oz	57
Original Unsweetened	8 oz	40
Vanilla	8 oz	91
Brazsoy		
Condensed Soy Milk	1 serv (0.7 oz)	54
Soy Cream	1 tbsp (0.5 oz)	27
DariFree		
Fat Free as prep	8 oz	70
Fat Free Chocolate as prep	8 oz	110
EdenBlend		
Organic	8 oz	120
Edensoy		
Organic Carob	8 oz	170
Organic Chocolate	8 oz	180
Organic Original	8 oz	140
Organic Original Light	8 oz	100
Organic Original Unsweetened	8 oz	120
Organic Vanilla	8 oz	150

FOOD	PORTION	CALS
Organic Vanilla Light	8 oz	110
Lifeway		
SoyTreat All Flavors	8 oz	160
Living Harvest		
Hempmilk Original	1 cup	130
Hempmilk Vanilla	1 cup	130
Lundberg		
Organic Drink Rice Original	8 oz	120
Manitoba Harvest		
Hemp Bliss Chocolate	8 oz	160
Hemp Bliss Original	1 cup	110
Hemp Bliss Vanilla	8 oz	150
Odwalla		
Soy Smart Chai	8 oz	150
Soy Smart Vanilla	8 oz	120
Soymilk Plain	8 oz	110
Soymilk Vanilla Being	8 oz	100
Organic Valley		
Soy Original	1 cup	100
Soy Unsweetened	1 cup	80
Pacific Foods		
Almond Low Fat Original	1 cup	70
Almond Low Fat Vanilla	1 cup	100
Multi Grain Low Fat Original	1 cup	160
Oat Organic Low Fat Original	1 cup	130
Oat Organic Low Fat Vanilla	1 cup	130
Rice Low Fat Plain	1 cup	130
Rice Low Fat Vanilla	1 cup	130
Soy Organic Unsweetened Original	1 cup	90
Soy Select Low Fat Plain	1 cup	70
Soy Select Low Fat Vanilla	1 cup	80
Soy Ultra	1 cup	130
Soy Ultra Plain	1 cup	120
Rice Dream		
Carob	8 oz	150
Heartwise Vanilla	8 oz	140
Horchata	8 oz	130
Original	8 oz	120
Original Enriched	8 oz	120
Vanilla Enriched	8 oz	130

FOOD	PORTION	CALS
Sno*e		
Tofu as prep	8 oz	80
Tofu Low Fat as prep	8 oz	70
Soy Dream		
Classic Vanilla	8 oz	140
Original Enriched	8 oz	100
·Vitasoy		
Classic Original	8 oz	120
Complete Original	8 oz	70
Complete Vanilla	8 oz	50
Creamy Original	8 oz	110
Green Tea Soymilk	8 oz	120
Light Chocolate	8 oz	100
Light Original	8 oz	60
Lite Vanilla	8 oz	70
Original Unsweetened	8 oz	80
Rich Chocolate	8 oz	160
Smooth Vanilla	8 oz	120
Vanilla Delight	8 oz	120
WildWood		
Organic Probiotic Soymilk Blueberry	8 oz	190
Organic Probiotic Soymilk Pomegranate	8 oz	180
Organic Soymilk Plain	8 oz	100
Organic Soymilk Unsweetened	8 oz	72
MILKFISH (AWA)		
baked	3 oz	162
MILKSHAKE		
chocolate	1 serv (10 oz)	393
malted	1 serv (10 oz)	402
vanilla	1 serv (10 oz)	379
Ben & Jerry's		
Cherry Garcia	1 bottle (8 oz)	320
Chocolate Fudge Brownie	1 bottle (8 oz)	340
Chunky Monkey	1 bottle (8 oz)	330
Buffy's Cool Cow		
Chocolate	1 pkg (8 oz)	150
Vanilla	1 pkg (8 oz)	150
Hershey's		
Chocolate	1 bottle	270

FOOD	PORTION	CALS
Cookies 'N' Cream	1 bottle	280
Strawberry	1 bottle	280
Lean Body		
Hi-Protein Chocolate Ice Cream	1 (17 oz)	260
Molli Coolz		
Shakers Vanilla as prep w/ skim milk	1 (10.2 oz)	240
Nesquik		
Ready-To-Drink Chocolate	1 cup (8 oz)	170

MILLET

cooked	1 cup (6.1 oz)	207
Arrowhead Mills		
Organic Hulled not prep	¼ cup	150

MINERAL WATER (*see* WATER)

MISO

dried	1 oz	86
miso	½ cup	284
Eden		
Hacho	1 tbsp	40
Organic Genmai	1 tbsp	25
Organic Mugi	1 tbsp	25
Organic Shiro	1 tbsp	30
Tekka	1 tsp	5

MOLASSES

blackstrap	1 tbsp (0.7 oz)	47
blackstrap	1 cup (11.5 oz)	771
molasses	1 tbsp (0.7 oz)	53
molasses	1 cup (11.5 oz)	873
Grandma's		
Robust	1 tbsp	60
Tree Of Life		
Blackstrap Unsulphured	1 tbsp	45

MONKFISH

baked	3 oz	82

MOOSE

roasted	4 oz	142

MOTH BEANS

dried cooked	1 cup	207

FOOD	PORTION	CALS
MOUSSE		
TAKE-OUT		
chocolate	½ cup	454
fish timbale	1 cup	329
MUFFIN		
MIX		
blueberry as prep	1 (1.75 oz)	149
corn as prep	1 (1.75 oz)	160
wheat bran as prep	1 (1.75 oz)	138
Glory		
Golden Sweet Corn as prep	1	170
Jiffy		
Apple Cinnamon as prep	1	190
Banana Nut as prep	1	180
Blueberry as prep	1	190
Bran w/ Dates as prep	1	170
Corn as prep	1	180
Raspberry as prep	1	180
King Arthur		
Cranberry Orange Whole Grain not prep	¼ cup	180
Martha White		
Whole Grain Apple Cinnamon not prep	¼ cup (1.2 oz)	140
Whole Grain Blueberry not prep	¼ cup (1.2 oz)	140
Yellow Corn not prep	¼ cup (1.2 oz)	140
Miracle Maize		
Country Style as prep	1	155
Sweet as prep	1	180
Miracle Muffins		
Banana w/ Splenda as prep	1	86
READY-TO-EAT		
blueberry	1 (2 oz)	158
oat bran wheat free	1 (2 oz)	154
toaster type blueberry	1	103
toaster type corn	1	114
toaster type wheat bran w/ raisins	1 (1.3 oz)	106
Fred's Incredible Muffins		
All Flavors	1 (2.5 oz)	100
Hostess		
100 Calorie Pack Mini Banana Streusel	1 pkg (1.2 oz)	100
100 Calorie Pack Mini Blueberry Streusel	1 pkg (1.2 oz)	100

FOOD	PORTION	CALS
Otis Spunkmeyer		
Apple Cinnamon	1 (4 oz)	420
VitaMuffin		
AppleBerryBran	1 (2 oz)	100
BlueBran	1 (2 oz)	100
CranBran	1 (2 oz)	100
Sugar Free Low Carb Banana Nut	1 (2 oz)	90
VitaTops Dark Chocolate Pomegranate	1 (2 oz)	100
VitaTops Deep Chocolate	1 (2 oz)	100
VitaTops Golden Corn	1 (2 oz)	100
VitaTops MultiBran	1 (2 oz)	100
TAKE-OUT		
corn	1 lg (2.5 oz)	214
raisin bran lowfat	1 (4 oz)	270
MULBERRIES		
fresh	1 cup	61
Kopali		
Organic Dark Chocolate Covered	½ pkg (1 oz)	140
Organic Dried	1 pkg (1.7 oz)	240
Navitas Naturals		
Dried	1 oz	91
MULLET		
striped cooked	3 oz	127
striped raw	3 oz	99
MUNG BEANS		
dried cooked	1 cup	213
MUNGO BEANS		
dried cooked	1 cup	190
MUSHROOMS		
CANNED		
caps	8 (1.6 oz)	12
caps pickled	6 (0.8 oz)	5
chanterelle	3.5 oz	12
pickled	1 cup	33
pieces	½ cup	20
straw	1 cup	58
Green Giant		
Pieces & Stems	½ cup	25

FOOD	PORTION	CALS
Polar		
Straw	½ cup	20
Whole Button	½ cup	30
Whole Shiitake	½ cup	30
Sunny Dell		
Portabella Sliced	½ cup	20
DRIED		
chanterelle	1 oz	25
shiitake	1 (3.6 g)	11
tree ear	½ cup (0.4 oz)	36
wood ear mok yee	½ cup (0.4 oz)	25
Eden		
Maitake Sliced	10 pieces (0.3 oz)	35
Shiitake	3 (0.4 oz)	35
Shiitake Sliced	3 pieces (0.3 oz)	35
Frieda's		
Chanterelle	2 pieces (4 g)	15
Wood Ear	3 pieces (4 g)	15
Ocean Spring		
Fresh Crispy Mixed Mushrooms	1 serv (0.9 oz)	113
FRESH		
brown italian or crimini sliced	1 cup	19
brown italian or crimini whole	1 (0.7 oz)	5
chanterelle	3.5 oz	11
enoki raw	1 lg (5 g)	2
enoki sliced	1 cup	29
enoki whole	1 cup	28
maitake diced	1 cup	26
maitake whole	1 (6.6 g)	2
morel	3.5 oz	9
oyster	1 sm (0.5 oz)	5
oyster sliced	1 cup	30
portabella raw	1 cap (3 oz)	22
portabella sliced grilled	1 cup (4.2 oz)	42
raw sliced	½ cup	8
shiitake cooked	4 (2.5 oz)	40
shiitake pieces cooked	1 cup	81
white	1 (0.6 oz)	4
white sliced cooked	1 cup	28

FOOD	PORTION	CALS
Frieda's		
Enoki	¼ pkg (1 oz)	10
Giorgio		
Mushrooms	3 oz	20
Golden Gourmet		
Beech Brown	4 oz	20
Beech White	4 oz	13
King Trumpet	4 oz	20
Maitake	4 oz	20
FROZEN		
Alexia		
Mushroom Bites	1 serv (2 oz)	110
Farm Rich		
Breaded	5 (3 oz)	120
TAKE-OUT		
battered fried	1 lg (0.6 oz)	39
creamed	1 cup	171
stuffed	1 (0.8 oz)	67
MUSKRAT		
roasted	3 oz	199
MUSSELS		
blue raw	1 cup	129
blue raw	3 oz	73
fresh blue cooked	3 oz	147
Polar		
Mussels	2 oz	60
MUSTARD		
dry	1 tsp	15
hot chinese	1 tsp	3
organic yellow	1 tsp	5
seed	1 tsp	15
yellow prepared	1 tbsp	3
Annie's Naturals		
Organic Horseradish	1 tsp	5
Boar's Head		
Delicatessen Style	1 tsp (5 g)	0
Honey	1 tsp (5 g)	10
Bone Suckin'		
Fat Free Gluten Free	1 tbsp	25

FOOD	PORTION	CALS
Country Cupboard		
Smokey Garlic or Horseradish	1 tsp	10
D'Oni		
Bold As Love Honey Habanero	1 tsp	5
Eden		
Organic Brown	1 tsp	0
Yellow	1 tsp	0
Emeril's		
Horseradish	1 tbsp	5
Smooth Honey	1 tbsp	10
French's		
Classic Yellow	1 tsp	0
Honey	1 tsp	10
Honey Dijon	1 tsp	10
Horseradish	1 tsp	5
Spicy Brown	1 tsp	5
Gulden's		
Spicy Brown	1 tsp	5
Hebrew National		
Deli	1 tsp	4
Hellman's		
Deli	1 tsp	5
Dijonnaise	1 tsp	5
Honey	1 tsp	10
Kosciusko		
Spicy Brown	1 tsp	0
Robert Rothschild Farm		
Champagne Garlic	1 tsp	6
Sara Lee		
Country Honey	1 tbsp	10
Cranberry Honey	1 tbsp	10
School House Kitchen		
Sweet Smooth Hot	1 tsp	15
Texas Sassy		
Mustard Sauce	2 tbsp (1 oz)	15
Vivi's		
Classic	1 tbsp (0.5 oz)	15
Sizzlin' Chipotle	1 tbsp (0.5 oz)	15
MUSTARD GREENS		
canned	1 cup	23

FOOD	PORTION	CALS
fresh as prep w/ fat	1 cup	50
fresh chopped boiled w/o salt	1 cup	21
fresh raw chopped	1 cup	15
frozen chopped boiled w/o salt	1 cup	28
Allen's		
Seasoned	½ cup	45
Glory		
Seasoned canned	½ cup	35
Sylvia's		
Specially Seasoned	½ cup	30

NATTO

natto	½ cup	187
House		
Natto	2 oz	120

NAVY BEANS

CANNED

beans	1 cup	296
Eden		
Organic	½ cup	110

DRIED

cooked	1 cup	259

NECTARINE

fresh	1	67
Sunsweet		
Dried	3 pieces (1.4 oz)	100

NECTARINE JUICE

Sun Shower

100% Juice	8 oz	93

NEUFCHATEL

neufchatel	1 oz	74
neufchatel	1 pkg (3 oz)	221
Back To Nature		
Organic	⅛ pkg (1 oz)	70
Organic Valley		
Soft	2 tbsp	70

FOOD	PORTION	CALS
NONI JUICE		
Lakewood		
Noni Pure Juice	2 oz	8
Tree Of Life		
100% Juice Concentrate	2 tbsp	15
NOODLES		
cellophane	1 cup	492
chow mein	1 cup (1.6 oz)	237
egg	1 cup (38 g)	145
egg cooked	1 cup (5.6 oz)	213
japanese soba cooked	1 cup (4 oz)	113
japanese somen cooked	1 cup (6.2 oz)	231
korean acorn noodles not prep	2 oz	195
rice cooked	1 cup (6.2 oz)	192
spinach/egg cooked	1 cup (5.6 oz)	211
A Taste Of Thai		
Rice Wide	2 oz	200
Annie Chun's		
Chow Mein	2 oz	200
Noodle Bowl Teriyaki	1 pkg	310
Noodle Express Chinese Chow Mein	½ pkg	160
Noodle Express Singapore Curry	½ pkg	160
Noodle Express Spicy Szechuan	½ pkg	170
Noodle Express Teriyaki	½ pkg	160
Noodle Express Thai Peanut	½ pkg	200
Rice	2 oz	210
Rice Pad Thai	2 oz	210
Azumaya		
Asian Style Thin Cut	1 cup	210
Catelli		
Egg	3 oz	317
Hodgson Mill		
Egg Whole Wheat not prep	2 oz	190
House		
Shirataki Tofu Noodles	2 oz	20
Shirataki Yam Noodles	2 oz	5
La Choy		
Chow Mein Noodles	½ cup (1 oz)	130
Rice	½ cup	130

FOOD	PORTION	CALS
Light 'N Fluffy		
Egg Extra Wide cooked	1½ cups	210
Manischewitz		
Egg Medium	1¼ cups	220
Nasoya		
Chinese	1 cup	210
Japanese	1 cup	210
Spinach	1 cup	210
No Yolks		
Extra Broad	2 oz	210

NUTMEG

FOOD	PORTION	CALS
ground	1 tsp	12
nutmeg butter	1 tbsp	120

NUTRITION SUPPLEMENTS (*see also* CEREAL BARS, ENERGY BARS, ENERGY DRINKS)

FOOD	PORTION	CALS
Amino Vital		
Jel All Flavors	1 pkg (4.9 oz)	70
Boost		
Breeze	8 oz	160
Diabetic	8 oz	250
Clif		
Shot Energy Gel All Flavors	1 pkg (1.1 oz)	100
DiabetiTrim		
Shake French Vanilla	1 pkg	90
Ensure		
Shake Creamy Milk Chocolate	1 bottle (8 oz)	250
Shake Strawberries & Cream	1 bottle (8 oz)	250
Glucerna		
Shake Creamy Chocolate Delight	1 bottle (8 oz)	200
Shake Homemade Vanilla	1 bottle (8 oz)	200
Jelly Belly		
Sport Beans Lemon Lime	1 pkg (1 oz)	100
Joint Juice		
Fitness All Flavors	1 bottle (18 oz)	10
Orange Tangerine	1 can (8 oz)	30
Tropical Fruit	1 can (8 oz)	30
PowerBar		
Powergel All Flavors	1 pkg (1.4 oz)	120

FOOD	PORTION	CALS
Pria		
Complete Shake Creamy Milk Chocolate	1 pkg (11.6 oz)	170
Complete Shake French Vanilla	1 pkg (11.6 oz)	170
Resource		
Beneprotein Protein Powder	1 scoop	25
Optisource High Protein Drink	1 box (4 oz)	100
Slim-Fast		
Optima Ready-To-Drink Creamy Milk Chocolate	1 can (11 oz)	190
Optima Shake Mix Chocolate Royale as prep w/ fat free milk	1 serv	190
Optima Shake Mix French Vanilla as prep w/ fat free milk	1 serv	200
Vitasoy		
Weight Management Meal All Flavors	1 bottle (10 oz)	200
NUTS MIXED (see also individual names)		
dry roasted w/ peanuts salted	¼ cup	203
dry roasted w/ peanuts w/o salt	¼ cup	203
oil roasted w/o peanuts salted	¼ cup	221
oil roasted w/o peanuts w/o salt	¼ cup	221
Emily's		
Roasted Mixed Nuts	¼ cup (1.3 oz)	230
Estee		
Chocolate Covered Fruit & Nut Mix Fructose Sweetened	¼ cup	210
Good Sense		
Deluxe Mix	¼ cup	180
Here's Howe		
Royal Mixed Nuts	1 oz	180
Organic Trails		
Tamari Roasted Nuts & Seeds	¼ cup	190
Peanut Better		
Mixed Nut Butter Creamy & Crunchy	2 tbsp	190
Planters		
Mixed	30 nuts (1 oz)	170
NUT-rition Energy Mix	¼ cup	180
NUT-rition Heart Healthy Mix	¼ cup	170
True North		
Clusters Pecan Almond Peanut	8 (1 oz)	170

FOOD	PORTION	CALS
OCA		
Frieda's		
Oca	½ cup	70
OCTOPUS		
dried boiled	3 oz	144
fresh steamed	3 oz	139
smoked	1 oz	40
TAKE-OUT		
ensalada de pulpo	1 cup	299
OHELOBERRIES		
fresh	1 cup	39
OIL		
almond	1 tbsp	120
almond	1 cup	1927
apricot kernel	1 tbsp	120
apricot kernel	1 cup	1927
avocado	1 tbsp	124
avocado	1 cup	1927
babassu palm	1 tbsp	120
butter oil	1 tbsp	112
butter oil	1 cup	1795
canola	1 tbsp	124
canola	1 cup	1927
coconut	1 tbsp	117
corn	1 tbsp	120
corn	1 cup	1927
cottonseed	1 tbsp	120
cottonseed	1 cup	1927
cupu assu	1 tbsp	120
garlic oil	1 tbsp	150
grapeseed	1 tbsp	120
hazelnut	1 tbsp	120
hazelnut	1 cup	1927
mustard	1 tbsp	124
mustard	1 cup	1927
oat	1 tbsp	120
olive	1 tbsp	119
olive	1 cup	1909
palm	1 tbsp	120

FOOD	PORTION	CALS
palm	1 cup	1927
palm kernel	1 tbsp	117
palm kernel	1 cup	1879
peanut	1 tbsp	119
peanut	1 cup	1909
peppermint	1 tsp	42
poppyseed	1 tbsp	120
pumpkin seed	1 oz	217
rice bran	1 tbsp	120
safflower	1 tbsp	120
safflower	1 cup	1927
sesame	1 tbsp	120
sheanut	1 tbsp	120
soybean	1 tbsp	120
soybean	1 cup	1927
sunflower	1 tbsp	120
sunflower	1 cup	1927
teaseed	1 tbsp	120
tomatoseed	1 tbsp	120
vegetable	1 tbsp	120
vegetable	1 cup	1927
walnut	1 tbsp	120
walnut	1 cup	1927
wheat germ	1 tbsp	120
Alpha		
Hazelnut	1 oz	257
Asoyia		
Soybean Ultra Low Lin	1 tbsp	129
Bell Plantation		
Extra Virgin Roasted Peanut	1 tbsp	120
Botticelli		
Olive	1 tbsp	120
Bragg		
Olive Extra Virgin	1 tbsp	120
Carapelli		
Grapeseed	1 tbsp	120
Olive Extra Virgin	1 tbsp	120
Consorzio		
Dipping Oil	1 tbsp	120
Olive Basil	1 tbsp	120

FOOD	PORTION	CALS
Olive Roasted Pepper	1 tbsp	120
Organic Extra Virgin Olive Meyer Lemon	1 tbsp	120
Crisco		
Cooking Spray Original	⅓ sec spray	0
Frying Oil Blend	1 tbsp	130
Light Olive	1 tbsp	120
Peanut	1 tbsp	120
Pure Vegetable	1 tbsp	120
Eden		
Olive Extra Virgin	1 tbsp	120
Organic Safflower	1 tbsp	120
Organic Soybean	1 tbsp	120
Toasted Sesame	1 tbsp	120
Enova		
Oil	1 tbsp	120
Hollywood		
Canola Enriched	1 tbsp	120
Peanut Enriched Gold	1 tbsp	120
Safflower Expeller Pressed	1 tbsp	120
House Of Tsang		
Mongolian Fire	1 tsp	45
Wok Oil	1 tbsp	130
Iowa Natural		
Soybean 1% Linolenic	1 tbsp	129
Kinloch Plantation		
100% Virgin Pecan	1 tbsp	130
Living Harvest		
Organic Hemp Oil	2 tbsp	250
Lucini		
Extra Virgin Premium Select	1 tbsp (0.5 oz)	120
Manitoba Harvest		
Hemp Seed Oil	1 tbsp	126
Mazola		
Corn	1 tbsp	120
No Stick Spray	⅓ sec spray	0
Pure Cooking Spray Canola All Flavors	¼ sec spray	0
Right Blend	1 tbsp	120
Vegetable	1 tbsp	120
Monini		
Grapeseed	1 tbsp (0.5 oz)	120

FOOD	PORTION	CALS
Nutiva		
Organic Coconut Extra Virgin	1 tbsp	120
Organic Hemp Cold Pressed	1 tbsp	120
Nutrium		
Soybean Low Linolenic	1 tbsp	129
Olivo		
Spray Olive Oil 100% Extra Virgin	⅓ sec spray	0
Orville Redenbacher's		
Popping & Topping	1 tbsp	120
Pacifica Culinaria		
Avocado	1 tbsp	120
Avocado Blood Orange	1 tbsp	120
Pam		
Cooking Spray All Types	⅓ sec spray	0
Organic Canola	⅓ second spray	0
Pompeian		
Olive	1 tbsp	130
Robert Rothschild Farm		
Basil Infused	1 tbsp	120
Smart Balance		
Omega Oil	1 tbsp	120
Spectrum		
Almond	1 tbsp	120
Apricot Kernel	1 tbsp	120
Avocado	1 tbsp	120
Canola Organic	1 tbsp	120
Coconut Organic	1 tbsp	120
Corn	1 tbsp	120
Grapeseed	1 tbsp	120
Grapeseed Oil Spray	⅓ sec spray	0
Hazelnut Toasted Organic	1 tbsp	120
Mediterranean Olive Organic	1 tbsp	120
Organic Extra Virgin Oil Spray	⅓ sec spray	0
Peanut	1 tbsp	120
Pumpkin Seed Organic	1 tbsp	120
Sesame Organic	1 tbsp	120
Sesame Toasted Organic	1 tbsp	120
Soy Organic	1 tbsp	120
Sunflower Organic	1 tbsp	120
Walnut	1 tbsp	120

FOOD	PORTION	CALS
Walnut Organic	1 tbsp	120
Tree Of Life		
Almond Expeller Pressed	1 tbsp (0.5 oz)	120
Avocado Expeller Pressed	1 tbsp (0.5 oz)	120
Macadamia Nut Expeller Pressed	1 tbsp (0.5 oz)	120
Organic Coconut Expeller Pressed	1 tbsp	120
Walnut Expeller Pressed	1 tbsp (0.5 oz)	120
Vistive		
Soybean Low Linolenic	1 tbsp	129
Wesson		
Canola	1 tbsp	120

OKRA
CANNED

FOOD	PORTION	CALS
pickled	6 pods (2.3 oz)	18
Allens		
Cut	½ cup	30
Glory		
Cut	½ cup	25
McIlhenny		
Spicy Pickled	1 oz	10
Trappey's		
Creole Gumbo	½ cup	35
FRESH		
cooked w/ salt	8 pods	19
luffa chinese okra cooked	1 cup	39
sliced cooked w/ salt	½ cup	18
FROZEN		
McKenzie's		
Breaded Okra	1 serv (2.8 oz)	90
Cut	1 serv (3 oz)	25
TAKE-OUT		
batter dipped fried	10 pieces (2.6 oz)	142

OLIVES

FOOD	PORTION	CALS
green	4 med	15
green	3 extra lg	15
green olive tapenade	1 tbsp	25
ripe	1 sm	4
ripe	1 lg	5
ripe	1 jumbo	7

FOOD	PORTION	CALS
ripe	1 colossal	12
spanish stuffed	5 (0.5 oz)	15
Peloponnese		
Amfissa	3	45
Ionian Green	3	25
Kalamata Pitted	5	45
Kalamata Spread	1 tsp	15
Stonewall Kitchen		
Mixed Olive Spread	1 tbsp	35

ONION
CANNED

FOOD	PORTION	CALS
cocktail	½ cup	41
Boar's Head		
Sweet Vidalia In Sauce	1 tbsp	10
French's		
Original French Fried	2 tbsp	45
DRIED		
flakes	1 tbsp	17
powder	1 tsp	7
shallots	1 tbsp	3
Bob's Red Mill		
Minced	1 tbsp	40
FRESH		
cooked w/o salt	1 sm (2 oz)	26
cooked w/o salt	1 med (3.3 oz)	41
cooked w/o salt	1 lg (4.5 oz)	56
cooked w/o salt chopped	1 tbsp	7
raw chopped	1 tbsp	4
raw chopped	½ cup	32
raw slice	1 (0.5 oz)	6
raw sliced	½ cup	23
scallions raw	1 med (0.5 oz)	5
scallions raw chopped	¼ cup	8
shallots raw chopped	¼ cup	29
sweet whole raw	1 (11.6 oz)	106
whole raw	1 sm (2.5 oz)	28
whole raw	1 med (4 oz)	44
whole raw	1 lg (5.3 oz)	60
Antioch Farms		
Vidalia	1 med	60

FOOD	PORTION	CALS
Arrowfarms		
Cipoline	2 (1.1 oz)	20
Bland Farms		
Vidalia Sweet	1 (5 oz)	60
Blue Ribbon		
Yellow	1 med (5.2 oz)	60
Christopher Ranch		
Shallots	1 (1 oz)	20
Earthbound Farm		
Organic Green Onions	¼ cup	10
Organic Red	1 med (5.2 oz)	60
Frieda's		
Cipolline	3 (3 oz)	30
Maui	⅓ cup (1.1 oz)	10
Pearl	⅔ cup (3 oz)	30
Shallots	1 tbsp (1 oz)	20
Nature's Harvest		
Onion	1 med (5.2 oz)	60
Ocean Mist		
Green Onions Chopped	¼ cup	10
OsoSweet		
Onion	1 med (5 oz)	60
FROZEN		
Alexia		
Onion Rings	6 (3 oz)	230
C&W		
Petite Whole	⅔ cup (3 oz)	30
Farm Rich		
Petals Breaded + Sauce	10 (3 oz)	200
Ian's		
Rings & Strings	5–9 pieces (2.5 oz)	152
TAKE-OUT		
creamed	1 cup	187
fried	½ cup	57
rings breaded & fried	8–9 (3 oz)	276

OPOSSUM

roasted	3 oz	188

FOOD	PORTION	CALS
ORANGE		
CANNED		
Del Monte		
SunFresh Mandarin	½ cup	80
FRESH		
california navel	1	65
california valencia	1	59
florida	1	69
peel	1 tbsp	6
sections	1 cup	85
Frieda's		
Cara Cara	1 med (5 oz)	70
Mandarin Delite	1 cup (5 oz)	60
Mandarin Page	1 cup (5 oz)	60
Mandarin Pixie	1 cup (5 oz)	60
Mandarin Satsuma	1 (5 oz)	60
Melogold	½ (6 oz)	50
Seville	1 (3 oz)	40
Sunkist		
Cara Cara Navel	1 med	80
Minneola Tangelo	1 (3.8 oz)	70
Moro	1 (5.4 oz)	70
Orange	1 med	80
Satsuma Mandarin	1 (3.8 oz)	50
ORANGE JUICE		
canned	1 cup	104
chilled	1 cup	110
fresh	1 cup	111
frzn as prep	1 cup	112
frzn not prep	6 oz	339
mandarin orange	7 oz	94
orange drink	6 oz	94
After The Fall		
24 Karrot Orange	8 oz	120
Bright & Early		
Orange Drink	8 oz	110
Crystal Light		
Sunrise Sunrise Sugar Free Mix as prep	1 serv	5
Dole		
100% Juice	8 oz	110

FOOD	PORTION	CALS
Florida's Natural		
Calcium & Vitamin D	8 oz	110
Hood		
100% Juice	1 cup	120
Italian Volcano		
Blood Orange Organic	1 serv (6.75 oz)	84
Land O Lakes		
Juice	1 cup (8 oz)	110
Juice w/ Calcium	1 cup (8 oz)	120
Minute Maid		
Country Style	8 oz	110
Heart Wise	8 oz	110
Kids+	8 oz	110
Light	8 oz	50
Original	8 oz	110
Plus Calcium	8 oz	110
W/ Extra Vitamin C & E Plus Zinc	8 oz	110
Mr. J		
100% Juice Calcium Fortified	1 pkg (4 oz)	60
Naked Juice		
Just OJ	8 oz	110
NutraBalance		
Fortified	1 pkg (4 oz)	60
Odwalla		
100% Juice	8 oz	110
Organic Valley		
W/ Calcium	1 cup	110
Simply		
Orange Calcium Fortified	8 oz	110
Orange Original	8 oz	110
Snapple		
Orangeade	8 oz	120
Ssips		
Orangeade	8 oz	120
Tang		
Orange Drink as prep	1 serv	90
Sugar Free Orange as prep	1 serv (8 oz)	5
Tree Ripe		
100% Juice + Calcium & Vitamins	8 oz	120
Organic 100% Juice	6 oz	90

FOOD	PORTION	CALS
Tropicana		
Antioxidant Advantage	8 oz	110
Calcium + Vitamin D	8 oz	110
Fiber	8 oz	120
Healthy Heart	8 oz	120
Healthy Kids	8 oz	110
Light'n Healthy w/ Calcium	8 oz	50
Light'n Healthy w/ Pulp	8 oz	50
No Pulp	8 oz	110
Orangeade	8 oz	111
Organic	8 oz	120
Uncle Matt's		
Organic 100% Juice Pulp Free	8 oz	110
Organic 100% Juice w/ Pulp	8 oz	110
Welsh Farms		
Juice	8 oz	110
TAKE-OUT		
orange julius	1 serv (24 oz)	443

OREGANO

crumbled	1 tsp	3
ground	1 tsp	6

ORGAN MEATS (*see* BRAINS, GIBLETS, GIZZARDS, HEART, KIDNEY, LIVER, SWEETBREAD)

OSTRICH

cooked	4 oz	195
cooked diced	1 cup (4.7 oz)	215
Natural Frontier Foods		
Filets	1 (4 oz)	130
Ground Lean	4 oz	130

OYSTERS

canned eastern	1 cup	112
eastern baked	6 med	47
eastern raw	6 med	50
eastern sauteed	6 med	76
smoked	6	33
Brunswick		
Smoked	1 can (3 oz)	140

FOOD	PORTION	CALS
Bumble Bee		
Smoked	¼ cup	120
Whole	¼ cup	70
Chicken Of The Sea		
Smoked In Oil	1 can (3.75 oz)	140
Smoked In Water	1 can (3.75 oz)	120
Smoked Teriyaki	1 can (3.75 oz)	120
Whole	½ can (2 oz)	80
Polar		
Whole	¼ cup	70
Whole Smoked	⅓ cup	95
TAKE-OUT		
breaded & fried	6	368
fritter	1 (1.4 oz)	121
oysters rockefeller	1 cup	302
stew	1 cup	208
PANCAKE/WAFFLE SYRUP		
lite	¼ cup	98
pancake syrup	1 pkg (2 oz)	156
pancake syrup	¼ cup	209
Aunt Jemima		
Butter Lite	¼ cup (2.1 oz)	100
Country Cupboard		
Boysenberry	¼ cup	0
Strawberry	¼ cup	0
Eggo		
Lite	¼ cup	110
Original	¼ cup	240
Estee		
Maple	¼ cup	30
Hungry Jack		
Lite	¼ cup	100
Original	¼ cup	210
Karo		
Pancake Syrup	¼ cup	240
Log Cabin		
Lite	¼ cup	100
Mrs. Butter-worth's		
Lite	¼ cup	100

FOOD	PORTION	CALS
Naturally Fresh		
Maple Mountain Sugar Free	2 tbsp	0
Smucker's		
Breakfast Syrup Sugar Free	¼ cup	30
Stonewall Kitchen		
Maine Maple	¼ cup	210
Wholesome Sweeteners		
Organic	¼ cup	240
PANCAKES		
FROZEN		
Aunt Jemima		
Buttermilk	3 (3 oz)	210
Buttermilk Low Fat	3 (3 oz)	210
Whole Grain	3 (3 oz)	230
Dr. Praeger's		
Broccoli	1 (2 oz)	80
Potato	1 (2.2 oz)	100
Eggo		
Buttermilk	3	280
Minis	11	260
Golden		
Potato Latkes	1 (1.3 oz)	70
Ian's		
Blueberry	1 (1.3 oz)	100
Pancake	1 (1.3 oz)	100
Inland Valley		
Potato	1 (2 oz)	120
Jimmy Dean		
Breakfast Bowls Pancake & Sausage Links	1 pkg	710
Griddle Cake Sandwich Sausage Egg & Cheese	1 (4 oz)	370
Original Pancakes & Sausage On A Stick	1 (2.5 oz)	110
McCain		
Homestyle BabyCakes	4 pieces (2.6 oz)	150
Pillsbury		
Blueberry	3 (4 oz)	230
Buttermilk	3 (4 oz)	240
Original	3 (4 oz)	250
Ratner's		
Potato Latkes	1 (1.5 oz)	80

FOOD	PORTION	CALS
MIX		
Arrowhead Mills		
Gluten Free Pancake & Waffle as prep	2 (5 in)	240
Batter Blaster		
Organic Original Pancake & Waffle Batter	¼ cup (2 oz)	112
Carbsense		
Buttermilk not prep	½ cup	140
Don's Chuck Wagon		
Buckwheat Mix	⅓ cup	160
Hodgson Mill		
Buckwheat not prep	⅓ cup	140
Whole Wheat Buttermilk not prep	⅓ cup	120
Hungry Jack		
Buttermilk Pancake & Waffle not prep	⅓ cup	150
Easy Pack Blueberry not prep	½ cup	200
Pancake & Waffle Extra Light & Fluffy not prep	⅓ cup	150
Potato not prep	2 tbsp	70
King Arthur		
Multi-Grain Buttermilk not prep	6 tbsp	160
TAKE-OUT		
buckwheat	1 (7 in)	142
norwegian lefse	1 (9 in) 2.7 oz	163
plain	1 (7 in)	183
potato	1 (1.3 oz)	70
w/ butter & syrup	2 (8.1 oz)	520
whole wheat	1 (7 in)	183

PANCREAS (*see* SWEETBREAD)

PANINI (*see* SANDWICHES)

PAPAYA		
fresh	1	117
fresh cubed	1 cup	54
Del Monte		
In Extra Light Syrup w/ Passion Fruit Puree	½ cup	70
Frieda's		
Mexican	1 cup (5 oz)	50
PAPAYA JUICE		
nectar	1 cup	142

FOOD	PORTION	CALS
Lakewood		
Red	8 oz	80
Yellow	8 oz	105
Langers		
Papaya Delight 100% Juice	8 oz	130
Old Orchard		
Nectar Cocktail	8 oz	120
PAPRIKA		
dried	1 tsp	1
Bob's Red Mill		
Hungarian	½ tsp	11
PARSLEY		
dried	1 tbsp	4
freeze dried	1 tbsp	1
fresh chopped	1 tbsp	1
fresh chopped	¼ cup	5
fresh sprigs	5 (1.8 oz)	18
Dorot		
Chopped Cubes frzn	1 cube (4 g)	5
Frieda's		
Parsley Root	⅔ cup	10
PARSNIPS		
fresh cooked	1 (5.6 oz)	130
fresh sliced cooked	½ cup	63
raw sliced	½ cup	50
Frieda's		
Sliced	1 cup	100
PASSION FRUIT		
purple fresh	1	18
PASSION FRUIT JUICE		
purple	1 cup	126
yellow	1 cup	149
PASTA (*see also* NOODLES, PASTA DINNERS, PASTA SALAD)		
DRY		
corn cooked	1 cup (4.9 oz)	176
elbows	1 cup	389
elbows cooked	1 cup (4.9 oz)	197

FOOD	PORTION	CALS
shells small cooked	1 cup (4 oz)	162
spaghetti cooked	1 cup (4.9 oz)	197
spinach spaghetti cooked	1 cup (4.9 oz)	182
spirals cooked	1 cup (4.7 oz)	189
vegetable cooked	1 cup (4.7 oz)	172
whole wheat all shapes cooked	1 cup	174
Amish Natural		
Fettuccine	2 oz	201
Fettuccine Fiber Rich	2 oz	200
Fettuccine Whole Wheat	2 oz	210
Annie Chun's		
Soba Noodles	2 oz	200
Barilla		
Pastina	2 oz	210
Penne	1 cup (2 oz)	200
Plus Penne	2 oz	200
Plus Rotini not prep	2 oz	210
Catelli		
All Shapes	3 oz	301
Bistro Cracked Black Pepper Fettuccine	¼ pkg	320
Bistro Italian Herb Fettuccine	¼ pkg	310
Bistro Lemon Pepper Linguine	¼ pkg	320
Bistro Rainbows	3 oz	320
Bistro Spinach Lasagne	3 oz	320
Bistro Sun Dried Tomato & Basil Spaghettini	¼ pkg	320
Bistro Vegetable Fusilli	3 oz	320
Healthy Harvest Flax Omega-3	3 oz	290
Healthy Harvest Multigrain	3 oz	310
Healthy Harvest Organic Whole Wheat	3 oz	320
Healthy Harvest Whole Wheat All Shapes	3 oz	310
Darielle		
All Shapes not prep	2 oz	160
DeBoles		
Angel Hair Rice Pasta	¼ pkg (2 oz)	210
Elbow Corn Pasta Wheat Free	⅙ pkg (2 oz)	200
Fettuccine	¼ pkg (2 oz)	210
Organic Angel Hair Whole Wheat	¼ pkg (2 oz)	210
Organic Eggless Ribbon	1 cup (2 oz)	210
Organic Fettuccine Spinach	¼ pkg (2 oz)	210
Organic Lasagna	¼ pkg (2.5 oz)	260

FOOD	PORTION	CALS
Organic Rigatoni Whole Wheat	1 cup (2 oz)	210
Rigatoni	¼ pkg (2 oz)	210
DeCecco		
Spaghetti w/ Spinach	⅛ pkg (2 oz)	200
Dreamfields		
Lasagna not prep	2 pieces (2 oz)	190
Rotini not prep	⅔ cup (2 oz)	190
Eden		
Bifun Pasta not prep	2 oz	200
Harusame Pasta not prep	2 oz	190
Kudzu	2 oz	200
Organic Gemelli Spelt & Buckwheat not prep	½ cup (2 oz)	210
Organic Ribbons Artichoke not prep	½ cup (2 oz)	210
Organic Rigatoni Kamut & Buckwheat not prep	½ cup (2 oz)	200
Organic Spaghetti 100% Whole Wheat not prep	2 oz	210
Organic Spirals Flax Rice not prep	½ cup (2 oz)	200
Organic Spirals Kamut Vegetable not prep	½ cup (2 oz)	210
Organic Spirals Rye not prep	½ cup (2 oz)	200
Organic Spirals Spinach not prep	½ cup (2 oz)	210
Organic Udon not prep	¼ pkg	200
Organic Udon Spelt not prep	¼ pkg	200
Organic Vegetable Alphabets not prep	½ cup (2 oz)	210
Organic Vegetable Shells not prep	½ cup (2 oz)	210
Organic Ziti Rigati Spelt not prep	½ cup (2 oz)	210
Soba Japanese 100% Buckwheat not prep	2 oz	200
Soba Japanese Lotus Root not prep	2 oz	190
Soba Japanese Mugwort not prep	2 oz	190
Soba Japanese Wild Yam not prep	2 oz	190
Udon Japanese not prep	2 oz	190
Udon Japanese Brown Rice not prep	2 oz	190
Food For Life		
Ezekiel 4:9 Sprouted Grain	2 oz	210
Gillian's		
Penne Brown Rice Pasta Wheat Gluten Egg Free	2 oz	200
Hodgson Mill		
Lasagna Whole Wheat not prep	2 oz	190

FOOD	PORTION	CALS
Organic Fettuccine Whole Wheat w/ Milled Flax Seed not prep	2 oz	200
Pasta Ribbons Whole Wheat not prep	2 oz	190
Spaghetti Whole Wheat not prep	2 oz	190
Veggie Bows not prep	2 oz	200
Wagon Wheels Veggie not prep	2 oz	200
Keto		
Elbows not prep	1.6 oz	108
Spaghetti not prep	1.3 oz	130
LifeStream		
Organic All Shapes	2 oz	208
Lundberg		
Organic Spaghetti Brown Rice	2 oz	210
Maddy's		
Gluten Free not prep	4 oz	310
Mueller's		
Elbow Macaroni not prep	½ cup	210
Multi Grain Rotini not prep	1 cup (2 oz)	190
Notta Pasta		
Rice Pasta All Shapes	2 oz	200
Pastalia		
Heart Health Low Carb not prep	2 oz	176
Rice Select		
Orzo Original not prep	⅓ cup	210
Ronzoni		
Elbows not prep	½ cup (2 oz)	210
Healthy Harvest Multigrain Spaghetti	⅐ pkg (2 oz)	190
Healthy Harvest Whole Wheat Blend Spaghetti	⅐ pkg (2 oz)	180
Lasagna	2½ pieces (2 oz)	210
Smart Pasta not prep	2 oz	180
San Giorgio		
Elbows not prep	½ cup	210
Wacky Mac		
Veggie All Shapes	2 oz	200
Whey Cool		
High Protein Xtreme Rotini	1 serv (2 oz)	210
FRESH		
cooked	2 oz	75
spinach cooked	2 oz	74

FOOD	PORTION	CALS
REFRIGERATED		
Buitoni		
Angel Hair	1¼ cups	230
Fettuccine	1¼ cups	240
Fettuccine Spinach	1¼ cups	260
Linguine	1¼ cups	240
Ravioletti Three Cheese	1 cup	270
Ravioli Chicken & Roasted Garlic	1¼ cups	340
Ravioli Chicken Parmesan	1¼ cups	310
Ravioli Classic Beef	1¼ cups	340
Ravioli Doublestuffed Mozzarella & Herb	1½ cups	340
Ravioli Four Cheese 100% Whole Wheat	1¼ cups	320
Ravioli Garden Vegetable	1 cup	250
Ravioli Light Four Cheese	1¼ cups	230
Tortellini Herb Chicken	1 cup	340
Tortellini Mixed Cheese	1 cup	320
Tortellini Spinach Cheese	1 cup	320
Tortellini Three Cheese	1 cup	320
Tortelloni Cheese & Roasted Garlic	1 cup	270
Tortelloni Chicken & Prosciutto	1 cup	320
Tortelloni Mozzarella & Herb	1 cup	330
Tortelloni Mozzarella & Pepperoni	1 cup	330
Tortelloni Portabello Mushroom & Cheese	1 cup	290
Tortelloni Sun Dried Tomato	1 cup	310
Tortelloni Sweet Italian Sausage	1 cup	330
Pasta Prima		
Ravioli Spinach & Mozzarella	1 cup	200
Ravioli Sun Dried Tomato & Mozzarella	1 cup	200
PASTA DINNERS (*see also* PASTA SALAD)		
CANNED		
Annie's Homegrown		
Organic All Stars	1 cup	150
Organic BernieOs	1 cup	150
Organic Cheesy Ravioli	1 cup	180
Organic P'sghetti Loops	1 cup	190
Chef Boyardee		
99% Fat Free Beef Ravioli	1 cup	170
Beef Ravioli	1 cup	240
Beefaroni	1 cup	260
Mini Ravioli	1 cup	250

FOOD	PORTION	CALS
Mini-Bites Spaghetti & Meatballs	1 cup	250
Spaghetti & Meat Balls	1 cup (9 oz)	270
SpaghettiOs		
A to Z's w/ Meatballs	1 cup	260
A to Z's w/ Sliced Franks	1 cup	230
Mini Beef Ravioli In Meat Sauce	1 cup	260
Pasta	1 cup	180
Plus Calcium	1 cup	170
FROZEN		
4Real		
Mac+Cheese	1 pkg (8 oz)	230
Meat Sauce w/ Beef Ravioli	1 pkg (8 oz)	190
Spaghetti Rings	1 pkg (8 oz)	180
Bertolli		
Meatballs Pomodoro & Penne	1 serv (12 oz)	600
Birds Eye		
Steamfresh Meals For Two Shrimp Alfredo	½ pkg (11.9 oz)	420
Steamfresh Meals For Two Shrimp Pasta Primavera	½ pkg (11.9 oz)	450
Blue Horizon Organic		
Penne Alfredo w/ Shrimp	½ pkg (9.9 oz)	430
Penne Alla Vodka w/ Shrimp	½ pkg (9.9 oz)	270
Pesto Farfalle w/ Shrimp	½ pkg (9.9 oz)	280
Scampi Rotini w/ Shrimp	½ pkg (9.9 oz)	410
Boca		
Lasagna Meatless	1 pkg (9.4 oz)	290
Cedarlane		
Zone Chicken & Vegetables Pasta & Ginger	1 pkg (10 oz)	340
Zone Lasagna Vegetable	1 pkg (10.9 oz)	310
Celentano		
Cheese Ravioli	4 (4.3 oz)	230
Contessa		
Ravioli Portobello	6 (6.7 oz)	360
Glory		
Macaroni & Cheese	1 pkg	480
Glutino		
Gluten Free Duo Mushroom Penne	1 pkg (10.5 oz)	380
Gluten Free Macaroni & Cheese	1 pkg (8.8 oz)	430
Gluten Free Penne Alfredo	1 pkg (9.1 oz)	340

FOOD	PORTION	CALS
Golden Cuisine		
Cheese Manicotti	1 pkg	360
Spaghetti & Meatballs	1 pkg	490
Tuna Casserole	1 pkg	386
Green Giant		
Skillet Meal Chicken & Cheesy Pasta as prep	1¼ cups	270
Healthy Choice		
Breaded Chicken Breast w/ Mac & Cheese	1 pkg	290
Creamy Garlic Shrimp w/ Bow Tie Pasta	1 pkg (11.5 oz)	280
Fettuccini Alfredo	1 pkg	280
Fettuccini Alfredo Chicken	1 pkg	290
Lasagna Bake	1 pkg	270
Macaroni & Cheese	1 pkg	290
Manicotti	1 pkg	280
Rigatoni w/ Broccoli & Chicken	1 pkg	270
Spaghetti w/ Meat Sauce	1 pkg	310
Stuffed Pasta Shells	1 pkg	290
Helen's Kitchen		
Farfalle & Basil Pasta w/ Tofu Steaks	1 pkg (9 oz)	320
Joy Of Cooking		
Al Dente Cavatappi Bolognese	1 cup (7.7 oz)	280
Best Loved Macaroni & Cheese	1 cup (5.4 oz)	280
Cheese Ravioli Pomodoro	1 cup (7.7 oz)	250
Creamy Fettuccine Carbonara	1 cup (7.5 oz)	330
Kashi		
Chicken Pasta Pomodoro	1 pkg (10 oz)	280
Kid Cuisine		
Cheese Blaster Mac & Cheese	1 meal	380
Twist & Twirl Spaghetti w/ Mini Meatballs	1 meal	460
Lean Cuisine		
Cafe Classics Bow Tie Pasta & Chicken	1 pkg (9.5 oz)	240
Cafe Classics Bowl Three Cheese Stuffed Rigatoni	1 pkg (10 oz)	260
Cafe Classics Cheese Lasagna w/ Chicken Breast Scallopini	1 pkg (10 oz)	290
Cafe Classics Four Cheese Cannelloni	1 pkg (9.1 oz)	260
Cafe Classics Grilled Chicken & Penne Pasta	1 pkg (12 oz)	320
Cafe Classics Jumbo Rigatoni w/ Meatballs	1 pkg (15.4 oz)	400
Cafe Classics Lasagna w/ Meat Sauce	1 pkg (10.5 oz)	310
Cafe Classics Macaroni & Beef	1 pkg (9.5 oz)	270

FOOD	PORTION	CALS
Cafe Classics Macaroni & Cheese	1 pkg (10 oz)	300
Cafe Classics Penne Pasta w/ Tomato Basil Sauce	1 pkg (10 oz)	270
Cafe Classics Roasted Chicken w/ Lemon Pepper Fettuccini	1 pkg (8.1 oz)	250
Cafe Classics Shrimp & Angel Hair Pasta	1 pkg (10 oz)	240
Cafe Classics Spaghetti w/ Meat Sauce	1 pkg (11.5 oz)	280
Cafe Classics Spaghetti w/ Meatballs	1 pkg (9.5 oz)	270
Dinnertime Selects Chicken Fettuccini	1 pkg (12 oz)	360
One Dish Favorites Alfredo Pasta w/ Chicken & Broccoli	1 pkg (10 oz)	270
One Dish Favorites Angel Hair Pasta Marinara	1 pkg (10 oz)	260
One Dish Favorites Cheese Ravioli	1 pkg (8.5 oz)	250
One Dish Favorites Chicken Fettuccini	1 pkg (9.25 oz)	280
One Dish Favorites Lasagna Cheese Florentine Bake	1 pkg (10 oz)	270
One Dish Favorites Lasagna Chicken Florentine	1 pkg (10 oz)	270
One Dish Favorites Lasagna Classic Five Cheese	1 pkg (11.5 oz)	330
Skillet Chicken Alfredo	1 serv	180
Marie Callender's		
Meat Lasagna	1 cup	240
Michelina's		
Lasagna w/ Meat Sauce	1 pkg (9 oz)	340
Milton's		
Lasagna Vegetable w/ Multi-Grain Pasta	1 cup (8 oz)	340
Mon Cuisine		
Vegetarian Spaghetti & Meatballs	1 pkg (10 oz)	360
Moosewood		
Organic Vegetarian Broccoli & Pasta Parmesan	1 pkg (10 oz)	380
Organic Vegetarian Farfalle & Spinach Pesto Sauce	1 pkg (10 oz)	370
Organic Vegetarian Spicy Penne Puttanesca	1 pkg (10 oz)	300
New York Ravioli		
Jolie Kid Shapes Ravioli Cheese	1 cup	330
Jolie Kid Shapes Ravioli Cheese & Broccoli	1 cup	340
Ravioli Four Cheese	1 cup	360
Ravioli Tomato Basil & Mozzarella	1 cup	340

FOOD	PORTION	CALS
Organic Bistro		
Pasta Puttanesca	1 pkg (12.15 oz)	330
Organic Classics		
Cajun Chicken Tetrazzine w/ Penne Pasta	1 pkg (10 oz)	370
Chicken Cacciatore w/ Penne Pasta	1 pkg (10 oz)	270
Macaroni & Meat Sauce	1 pkg (10 oz)	340
Plum Organics		
Bowtie Pasta	1 pkg (6.9 oz)	230
Cheese Filled Spinach Tortellini	1 pkg (6.9 oz)	190
Putney Pasta		
Ravioli Butternut Squash & Vermont Maple Syrup	1 cup	200
Ravioli Portobello & Grilled Onion	7 (5.2 oz)	240
Ravioli Whole Wheat Spinach & Cheese	9 (5 oz)	300
Skillet Meal Chicken Piccata	1 serv (9 oz)	300
Skillet Meal Shrimp Pesto	1 serv (9 oz)	540
Tortellini Spinach Mozzarella & Walnuts	1 cup	360
Tortellini Tri-Color Three Cheese	1 cup	340
Savvy Faire		
Lasagna Florentine	1 pkg (9.2 oz)	300
Seeds Of Change		
Chicken Fettuccine Alfredo	1 pkg (10 oz)	340
Lasagna Creamy Spinach	1 pkg (11 oz)	370
Lasagna Vegetable	1 pkg (11 oz)	310
Penne Marinara	1 pkg (11 oz)	290
South Beach		
Penne & Chicken In Roasted Red Pepper Sauce w/ Broccoli	1 pkg	290
Stouffer's		
Cheesy Spaghetti Bake	1 pkg (12 oz)	460
Chicken Parmigiana	1 pkg (13.13 oz)	460
Escalloped Chicken & Noodles	1 pkg (8 oz)	330
Homestyle Chicken & Noodles	1 pkg (12 oz)	340
Italian Sausage Stuffed Rigatoni	1 pkg (9.13 oz)	380
Lasagna Bake w/ Meat Sauce	1 pkg (11.5 oz)	380
Lasagna Vegetable	1 pkg (10.5 oz)	390
Macaroni & Beef	1 pkg (11.5 oz)	330
Macaroni & Cheese	1 cup (6 oz)	350
Manicotti Cheese	1 pkg (9 oz)	360
Shrimp Scampi	1 pkg (14 oz)	410

FOOD	PORTION	CALS
Tuna Noodle Casserole	1 pkg (10 oz)	350
Turkey Tettrazini	1 pkg (10 oz)	380
Taste Above		
Meatless Thai Peanut Coconut Sauce w/ Veggie Chicken & Vermicelli	1 pkg (10 oz)	320
Meatless Tuscan Marinara Sauce w/ Veggie Chicken & Penne Pasta	1 pkg (10 oz)	320
Weight Watchers		
Smart Ones Lasagna w/ Meat Sauce	1 pkg (10.5 oz)	300
Yves		
Meatless Lasagna	1 pkg (10.5 oz)	300
MIX		
A Taste Of Thai		
Coconut Ginger	1 cup	280
Pad Thai For Two	½ pkg	345
Peanut Noodles as prep	1 cup	330
Red Curry Noodles as prep	1 cup	280
Annie's Homegrown		
Gluten Free Rice Pasta & Cheddar as prep	1 cup	330
Organic Shells & Real Aged Wisconsin Cheddar as prep	1 cup	370
Organic Whole Wheat Shells & Cheddar as prep	1 cup	360
Organic Skillet Meals Beef Stroganoff as prep	1 cup	320
Organic Skillet Meals Cheddar & Herb Chicken as prep	1 cup	310
Organic Skillet Meals Cheese Lasagna as prep	1 cup	280
Organic Skillet Meals Cheeseburger Macaroni as prep	1 cup	350
Organic Skillet Meals Chicken Fettuccine as prep	1 cup	330
Organic Skillet Meals Creamy Tuna Spirals as prep	1 cup	260
Shells & Real Aged Wisconsin Cheddar as prep	1 cup	290
Shells & White Cheddar as prep	1 cup	290
Aramana		
Cheddar Cheeseburger as prep	1 cup	260
Creamy Chicken Alfredo as prep	1 cup	260
Mild Mexican as prep	1 cup	260

FOOD	PORTION	CALS
Back To Nature		
Alfredo & Gemelli as prep	1 cup	340
Macaroni & Cheese as prep	1 cup	320
White Cheddar & Spirals as prep	1 cup	330
Carapelli		
Penne Alfredo as prep	1 cup	240
Spirals Creamy Tomato as prep	1 cup	240
DeBoles		
Organic Macaroni & Cheese Whole Wheat as prep	1 cup	410
Pasta & Cheese as prep	1 cup	420
Rice Shells & Cheddar as prep	½ cup	260
Hamburger Helper		
Cheesy Jambalaya as prep	1 cup	330
Keto		
Macaroni & Cheese not prep	1 serv	112
Knorr		
Pasta & Sauce Jalapeno Jack as prep	1 cup	230
Pasta Sides w/ Whole Grains Alfredo as prep	⅔ cup	300
Kraft		
Bistro Deluxe Sundried Tomato Parmesan as prep	1 cup	300
La Bella Vita		
Chicken & Lemon Borsellini as prep	1 cup	270
Near East		
Basil & Herb as prep	1 cup	240
Spicy Tomato as prep	1 cup	230
Pasta Roni		
Angel Hair w/ Herbs as prep	1 cup	310
Chicken as prep	1 cup	300
Chicken Quesadilla as prep	1 cup	310
Fettuccine Alfredo as prep	1 cup	450
Nature's Way Mushrooms In Cream Sauce as prep	1 cup	280
Sour Cream & Chives as prep	1 cup	310
Stroganoff as prep	1 cup	350
Road's End Organics		
Mac & Cheese Dairy Free Gluten Free as prep	1 cup	310
Shells & Cheese as prep	1 cup	330

FOOD	PORTION	CALS
Whey Cool		
High Protein Macaroni & Cheese as prep	1 serv	260
REFRIGERATED		
Country Crock		
Elbow Macaroni & Cheese	1 cup	380
SHELF-STABLE		
Allergaroo		
Gluten Free Spaghetti	1 pkg (8 oz)	220
Gluten Free Spyglass Noodles	1 pkg (8 oz)	230
Betty Crocker		
Bowl Appetit! Cheddar Broccoli Pasta	1 bowl (2.8 oz)	330
Bowl Appetit! Garlic Parmesan Pasta	1 bowl (2.8 oz)	320
Healthy Choice		
Fresh Mixers Ziti & Meat Sauce	1 pkg (6.9 oz)	340
TastyBite		
Peanut Sauce w/ Noodles	1 pkg (10 oz)	530
TAKE-OUT		
bami goreng indonesian noodle dish	1 cup	170
lasagna meatless	1 piece (9 oz)	356
lasagna w/ meat	1 piece (8 oz)	362
lasagna w/ vegetables	1 serv (9 oz)	315
macaroni & cheese w/ ham	1 cup	542
manicotti cheese filled & marinara sauce	1 (5 oz)	229
manicotti cheese filled & meat sauce	1 (5 oz)	239
pasta w/ pesto sauce	1 cup	370
ravioli cheese & spinach filled & cream sauce	1 cup	362
ravioli cheese w/ tomato sauce	1 cup	335
ravioli meat filled & marinara sauce	1 cup	372
rigatoni w/ sausage sauce	¾ cup	260
spaghetti w/ red clam sauce	1 cup	285
spaghetti w/ sauce & meatballs	2 cups	670
spaghetti w/ white clam sauce	1 cup	456
tortellini cheese w/ tomato sauce	1 cup	332
tortellini meat filled & marinara sauce	1 cup	281
tortillini spinach filled & marinara sauce	1 cup	238

PASTA SALAD
MIX
Dole

FOOD	PORTION	CALS
Veggie Pasta Salads Broccoli Ranch	1½ cups	230
Veggie Pasta Salads Cheddar Bacon Ranch	1½ cups	370

FOOD	PORTION	CALS
Veggie Pasta Salads Garden Vegetable	1½ cups	240
Veggie Pasta Salads Italian Herb	1½ cups	270
TAKE-OUT		
pasta salad w/ crab vegetables mayonnaise	1 cup	317
tortellini salad cheese filled & vinaigrette dressing	1 cup	333

PATE
chicken liver canned	1 tbsp	26
duck pate	1 oz	96
fish pate	1 oz	76
liver w/ truffle	1 serv (2 oz)	183
mushroom anchovy pate	1 can (2.25 oz)	130
pate de foie gras smoked canned	1 tbsp	60
pork pate	1 oz	107
pork pate en croute	1 oz	91
rabbit pate	1 oz	66
shrimp	1 can (2.25 oz)	140
Patchwork		
All Flavors	2 oz	270

PEACH
CANNED
halves in heavy syrup	1 half	60
halves in light syrup	1 half	44
halves juice pack	1 half	34
halves water pack	1 half	18
peach sauce	½ cup	120
spiced in heavy syrup	1 fruit	66
spiced in heavy syrup	1 cup	180
Del Monte		
Carb Clever Sliced	½ cup	30
Freestone Lite Slices	½ cup	60
Freestone Sliced	½ cup	100
Fruit Naturals Chunks	½ cup	70
Halves In Heavy Syrup	½ cup	100
Orchard Select Sliced Cling	½ cup	80
Sliced In 100% Juice	½ cup	60
Sliced Light Syrup Raspberry Flavor	½ cup	80
Liberty Gold		
Sliced Cling In Heavy Syrup	½ cup	100

FOOD	PORTION	CALS
Polar		
White	½ cup	70
S&W		
Slices Lightly Sweetened Juice	½ cup	80
Yellow Cling In Heavy Syrup	½ cup	100
DRIED		
halves	10	311
halves	1 cup	383
halves cooked w/ sugar	½ cup	139
halves cooked w/o sugar	½ cup	99
Crispy Green		
Crispy Peaches	1 pkg (0.36 oz)	38
Mrs. May's		
Fruit Chips	1 pkg	35
FRESH		
peach	1	37
sliced	1 cup	73
FROZEN		
slices sweetened	1 cup	235
C&W		
Ultimate Sliced	¾ cup	50
PEACH JUICE		
nectar	1 cup	134
After The Fall		
Georgia Peach	8 oz	130
Froose		
Playful Peach	1 box (4.2 oz)	80
PEANUT BUTTER		
chunky	2 tbsp	188
chunky	1 cup	1520
chunky w/o salt	2 tbsp	188
chunky w/o salt	1 cup	1520
smooth	2 tbsp	188
smooth	1 cup	1517
smooth w/o salt	2 tbsp	188
smooth w/o salt	1 cup	1517
Arrowhead Mills		
Organic Creamy	2 tbsp	190
Organic Honey Sweetened Creamy	2 tbsp	190

FOOD	PORTION	CALS
Organic Natural Crunchy	2 tbsp	190
Barney Butter		
Crunchy	2 tbsp	180
Smooth	2 tbsp	180
Chet's		
Chocolate	2 tbsp	180
Roasted Nut	2 tbsp	180
Cream-Nut		
Natural	2 tbsp	190
Earth Balance		
Creamy or Chunky	1 tbsp	190
Estee		
Creamy Low Sodium	2 tbsp	180
Jif		
Creamy	2 tbsp	190
Creamy To Go	1 pkg (2.25 oz)	270
Extra Crunchy	2 tbsp	190
Peanut Butter & Honey	2 tbsp	190
Reduced Fat Creamy	2 tbsp	190
Reduced Fat Crunchy	2 tbsp	190
Simply	2 tbsp	190
Justin's		
Organic Cinnamon	2 tbsp (1.1 oz)	180
Organic Classic	2 tbsp (1.1 oz)	150
Kettle		
Organic Unsalted	2 tbsp	170
PB2		
Powdered Chocolate	2 tbsp	52
Powdered Chocolate Chip	2 tbsp	53
Peanut Better		
Cinnamon Currant	2 tbsp	180
Deep Chocolate	2 tbsp	170
Hickory Smoked	2 tbsp	190
Onion Parsley	2 tbsp	180
Peanut Praline	2 tbsp	180
Rosemary Garlic	2 tbsp	180
Spicy Southwestern	2 tbsp	190
Sweet Molasses	2 tbsp	180
Thai Ginger & Red Pepper	2 tbsp	180
Vanilla Cranberry	2 tbsp	170

FOOD	PORTION	CALS
Reese's		
Creamy	2 tbsp	200
Revolution Foods		
Organic Creamy or Crunchy	1 tbsp (1.1 oz)	200
Smart Balance		
Chunky Omega	2 tbsp	200
Smucker's		
Goober All Flavors	3 tbsp	240
Natural Chunky	2 tbsp	210
Natural Creamy	2 tbsp	210
Natural Honey	2 tbsp	200
Natural No Salt Added Creamy	2 tbsp	210
Natural Reduced Fat Creamy	2 tbsp	200
Teddies		
Old Fashioned	2 tbsp	190
Wonder		
Peanut Spread	2 tbsp	100
Peanut Spread Low Sodium	2 tbsp	100
PEANUT BUTTER SUBSTITUTES		
NoNuts		
Golden Peabutter	1 tbsp	93
PEANUTS		
chocolate coated	1	21
chocolate coated	¼ cup	193
cooked w/ salt	½ cup	286
dry roasted w/ salt	28 nuts (1 oz)	164
dry roasted w/o salt	28 (1 oz)	164
dry roasted w/o salt	¼ cup	214
honey roasted	¼ cup	191
sugar coated	¼ cup	203
yogurt coated	¼ cup	230
A Taste Of Thai		
Spicy Peanut Bake	¼ pkg	45
Brach's		
Double Dippers Chocolate Covered	15 pieces	210
Estee		
Chocolate Coated Fructose Sweetened	¼ cup	170
Frito Lay		
Salted	1 oz	160

FOOD	PORTION	CALS
Salted w/ Shells	½ cup	160
Lance		
Salted	1 pkg (1.1 oz)	200
Nuts Are Good		
Buffalo	1 oz	120
Pina Colada	1 oz	130
Raspberry	1 oz	130
Vanilla Rum	1 oz	130
Planters		
Cocktail	1 oz	170
Dry Roasted	1 oz	170
Sunfood		
Organic Wild Jungle	1 oz	174
True North		
Clusters	6 (1 oz)	170
PEAR		
CANNED		
halves in heavy syrup	1 (1.7 oz)	36
halves in heavy syrup	½ cup (3.5 oz)	74
halves in light syrup	1 (2.7 oz)	43
halves in light syrup	½ cup (4.4 oz)	72
halves juice pack	1 (2.7 oz)	38
halves juice pack	½ cup (4.4 oz)	62
halves water pack	1 (2.7 oz)	22
Del Monte		
Carb Clever Sliced	½ cup	40
Halves In 100% Juice	½ cup	60
Halves In Light Syrup	½ cup	60
Orchard Select Sliced Bartlett	½ cup	80
Liberty Gold		
Bartlett In Heavy Syrup	½ cup (4.5 oz)	90
S&W		
Halves In Lightly Sweetened Juice	½ cup	80
DRIED		
halves	1 (0.6 oz)	47
halves	5 (3 oz)	229
halves	½ cup (3.2 oz)	236
halves cooked w/o sugar	½ cup (4.5 oz)	162
Bare Fruit		
Organic	1 pkg (0.6 oz)	46

FOOD	PORTION	CALS
Brothers-All-Natural		
Crisps Asian Pear	1 pkg (0.35 oz)	40
FRESH		
asian	1 med (4.3 oz)	51
asian	1 lg (9.6 oz)	116
pear	1 sm (5.2 oz)	86
pear	1 med (6.2 oz)	103
pear	1 lg (8.1 oz)	133
sliced w/ skin	1 cup (4.9 oz)	81
PEAR JUICE		
nectar canned	1 cup (8.8 oz)	150
Froose		
Perfect Pear	1 box (4.2 oz)	80
Izze		
Sparkling Pear	8 oz	130
Langers		
Kid's 100% Juice	4 oz	60
PEAS		
CANNED		
green	½ cup	59
green low sodium	½ cup	59
Del Monte		
Sweet	½ cup	60
Sweet No Salt Added	½ cup	60
Sweet Very Young Small	½ cup	60
Green Giant		
50% Less Sodium Young Tender Sweet	½ cup	60
Young Tender Sweet	½ cup	60
Le Sueur		
50% Less Sodium Young Tender	½ cup	60
Libby's		
No Salt No Sugar Added	½ cup	70
Tillen Farms		
Crispy Snapper Pickled	¼ cup	15
DRIED		
split cooked	1 cup	231
Arrowhead Mills		
Organic Green Split not prep	¼ cup	160

FOOD	PORTION	CALS
HamPeas		
Green Split Peas as prep	½ cup	120
Snapea Crisps		
Baked Original	22 (1 oz)	70
Tree Of Life		
Wasabi Peas	¼ cup (1.1 oz)	120
FRESH		
green cooked	½ cup	67
green raw	½ cup	58
snap peas cooked	½ cup	34
snap peas raw	½ cup	30
Frieda's		
Snow Peas	1 cup	35
Sugar Snap	⅔ cup (3 oz)	35
Mann's		
Snow Peas	1 serv (3 oz)	35
River Ranch		
Sugar Snap	1½ cups	35
FROZEN		
green cooked	½ cup	63
snap peas cooked	½ cup	42
Birds Eye		
Steamfresh Garlic Baby Peas & Mushrooms	¾ cup	80
Steamfresh Singles Sweet Peas	1 pkg (3.2 oz)	70
C&W		
Alfredo	½ cup	110
Early Harvest Petite No Salt Added	⅔ cup	70
Sugar Snap	⅔ cup	40
Green Giant		
Early June No Sauce	⅔ cup	50
Pictsweet		
Green Peas	⅔ cup	70
SHELF-STABLE		
TastyBite		
Agra Peas & Greens	½ pkg (5 oz)	138
PECANS		
candied	1 oz	190
dry roasted	1 oz	187
dry roasted salted	1 oz	187
halves dried	1 cup	721

FOOD	PORTION	CALS
halves dry roasted w/ salt	20 (1 oz)	200
oil roasted	1 oz	195
oil roasted salted	1 oz	195
Emerald		
Glazed Pecan Pie	¼ cup	150
Emily's		
Roasted & Salted	¼ cup (1 oz)	210

PECTIN

| liquid | 1 oz | 3 |
| powder | 1 pkg (1.75 oz) | 162 |

PEPEAO

| dried | ¼ cup | 18 |
| raw sliced | 1 cup | 25 |

PEPPER

black	1 tsp	5
cayenne	1 tsp	6
white	1 tsp	7
McCormick		
Lemon & Pepper Seasoning Salt	¼ tsp	0

PEPPERMINT

| fresh chopped | 2 tbsp | 2 |

PEPPERS

CANNED

chili green	1 cup (5.5 oz)	29
chili green hot chopped	½ cup	17
chili pepper paste	1 tbsp	6
chili red hot	1 (2.6 oz)	18
chili red hot chopped	½ cup	17
green halves	½ cup	13
jalapeno chopped	½ cup	17
red halves	½ cup	13
B&G		
Cherry Hot	1 (1 oz)	10
Cherry Sweet	1 (1 oz)	10
Hot Pepper Rings	7 pieces (1 oz)	0
Pepperoncini	3 pieces (1 oz)	10
Roasted w/ Balsamic Vinegar	½ piece (1 oz)	10
Sweet Fried	1 oz	25

FOOD	PORTION	CALS
Gedney		
Hot & Sweet Jalapeno Peppers	¼ cup	30
Hot Banana Pepper Rings	¼ cup	10
Gertie's Finest		
Piquillo	1 oz	10
Las Palmas		
Diced Green Chiles	2 tbsp	5
Jalapenos Sliced	3 tbsp	10
Pace		
Green Chiles Diced	2 tbsp	10
Tillen Farms		
Bell Peppers Pickled Sweet	¼ cup	25
DRIED		
ancho	1 (0.6 oz)	48
ancho	1 tsp	3
casabel	1 tsp	3
chipotle smoked	1 tsp	3
green	1 tbsp	1
guajillo	1 tsp	3
mulato	1 tsp	3
pasilla	1 (7 g)	24
pasilla	1 tsp	3
red	1 tbsp	1
Frieda's		
California Chili	2 tbsp	15
FRESH		
banana	1 cup (4.4 oz)	33
banana	1 (4 in) 1.2 oz	9
chili green hot	1	18
chili green hot chopped	½ cup	30
chili red chopped	½ cup	30
chili red hot	1 (1.6 oz)	18
green	1 (2.6 oz)	20
green chopped	½ cup	13
green chopped cooked	½ cup	19
green cooked	1 (2.6 oz)	20
habanero	1 tsp	9
hungarian	1 (0.9 oz)	8
jalapeno	1 (0.5 oz)	4
jalapeno sliced	1 cup (3.2 oz)	27

FOOD	PORTION	CALS
red	1 (2.6 oz)	20
red chopped	½ cup	13
red chopped cooked	½ cup	19
red cooked	1 (2.6 oz)	20
serrano	1 (6 g)	2
serrano chopped	1 cup (3.7 oz)	34
yellow	10 strips	14
yellow	1 (6.5 oz)	50
Frieda's		
Peppadew	⅓ cup	40
FROZEN		
green chopped	1 oz	6
red chopped	1 oz	6
C&W		
Strips	¾ cup	25
Roast Works		
Flame Roasted Red	1 serv (3 oz)	45

PERCH
FRESH

cooked	3 oz	99
cooked	1 fillet (1.6 oz)	54
ocean perch atlantic cooked	3 oz	103
ocean perch atlantic cooked	1 fillet (1.8 oz)	60
ocean perch atlantic raw	3 oz	80
raw	3 oz	77
red raw	3.5 oz	114

PERSIMMONS

dried japanese	1 (1.2 oz)	93
fresh	1 (6 oz)	118
Frieda's		
Dried Fuyu	⅓ cup (1.4 oz)	140

PHEASANT

breast boneless cooked	½ (4.4 oz)	312
cooked diced	1 cup	332
drumstick & thigh cooked	1 (2.6 oz)	184

PHYLLO

sheet	1 (0.7 oz)	57

FOOD	PORTION	CALS
Ekizian		
Sheets	¼ lb	433
Fillo Factory		
Kataifi Shredded Fillo	1 (2 oz)	180
Organic	2 sheets (1.5 oz)	130
Organic Whole Wheat	2 sheets (1.8 oz)	140
Shells Large	1 (0.7 oz)	80

PICANTE (see SALSA)

PICKLES

FOOD	PORTION	CALS
bread & butter	6 slices	39
dill	1 lg (4.7 oz)	24
dill low sodium	1 med (2.3 oz)	12
dill sliced	6 slices	7
sweet gherkin	1 (1.2 oz)	41
tsukemono japanese pickles sliced	¼ cup	10
B&G		
Bread & Butter	3 slices (1 oz)	25
Kosher Dill	⅓ pickle (1 oz)	0
Kosher Dill No Salt	½ pickle (1 oz)	10
Sour	½ pickle (1 oz)	0
Sweet Gherkins	1 (1 oz)	35
Claussen		
Kosher Dills Whole	½ (1 oz)	5
Del Monte		
Dill Halves	1 piece (1 oz)	5
Hamburger Dill Chips	1 serv (1 oz)	0
Sweet	1 serv (1 oz)	40
Sweet Gherkins	1 serv (1 oz)	40
Tiny Kosher Dill	1 serv (1 oz)	5
Gedney		
Baby Dills	3 (1 oz)	5
Organic Baby Dills	2 (1 oz)	5
Hebrew National		
Dill	1	23
Texas Sassy		
Pickle Chips	1 tbsp (0.5 oz)	30
Tree Of Life		
Organic Sweet Bread & Butter Chips	4 (1 oz)	30

FOOD	PORTION	CALS

PIE (see also PIE CRUST, PIE FILLING)
FROZEN
Edwards

Pie Slices Chocolate Creme	1 slice (2.7 oz)	290
Pie Slices Key Lime	1 slice (3.2 oz)	330
Pie Slices Oreo Cream	1 slice (2.6 oz)	290

Mrs. Smith's

Bake & Serve No Sugar Added Apple	1 slice (4.6 oz)	310
Blueberry Crumb	1 slice (4.2 oz)	320
Cherry	1 slice (4.6 oz)	330
Cinnabon Apple Crumb	1 slice (4.6 oz)	350
Classic Cream Key Lime	1 slice (4.2 oz)	410
Coconut Custard	1 slice (4.4 oz)	300
Deep Dish Berry Burst	1 slice (4.2 oz)	340
Dutch Apple Crumb	1 slice (4.6 oz)	370
Pumpkin Custard	1 slice (4.6 oz)	300
Soda Shoppe Boston Cream	1 slice (2.7 oz)	220
Soda Shoppe Chocolate Cream	1 slice (4.6 oz)	350
Soda Shoppe Lemon Meringue	1 slice (4.2 oz)	300

Sara Lee

Apple	1 slice (4.6 oz)	340
Cherry	1 slice (4.6 oz)	320
Coconut Cream	1 slice (4.8 oz)	330
Dulce de Leche Caramel Swirl	1 slice (4.4 oz)	400
French Silk	1 slice (4.8 oz)	340
Key West Lime	1 slice (4.2 oz)	400
Lemon Meringue	1 slice (5 oz)	220
Mince	1 slice (4.6 oz)	370
Pumpkin	1 slice (4.6 oz)	260
Southern Pecan	1 slice (4.2 oz)	520
Southern Sweet Potato	1 slice (4.6 oz)	280

READY-TO-EAT
Entenmann's

Peach Raspberry Melba	⅛ pie (2.6 oz)	250

SNACK
Lance

Pecan	1 (3 oz)	350

Lifestream

Pie Oh-My Apple	1 (3.5 oz)	280
Pie Oh-My Pineapple	1 (3.5 oz)	280

FOOD	PORTION	CALS
TAKE-OUT		
apple one crust	1 slice (5.3 oz)	363
apple tart	1 (4.2 oz)	370
apple two crust	1 slice (5.3 oz)	356
apricot tart	1 (4.2 oz)	356
apricot two crust	1 slice (5.3 oz)	417
banana cream	1 slice (5.1 oz)	387
blackberry one crust	1 slice (4.4 oz)	341
blackberry two crust	1 slice (5.3 oz)	394
blueberry one crust	1 slice (4.8 oz)	292
blueberry tart	1 (4.2 oz)	346
blueberry two crust	1 slice (5.3 oz)	348
cherry one crust	1 slice (4.8 oz)	312
cherry two crust	1 slice (5.3 oz)	390
chess	1 slice (3 oz)	365
chocolate cream	1 slice (5 oz)	380
coconut creme	1 slice (5 oz)	429
custard	1 slice (4.8 oz)	286
grasshopper	1 slice (3.5 oz)	341
key lime	1 slice (5 oz)	420
lemon meringue	1 slice (4.8 oz)	367
lemon meringue tart	1 (4.1 oz)	298
mince two crust	1 slice (5.3 oz)	434
peach two crust	1 slice (5.3 oz)	334
pear two crust	1 slice (5.3 oz)	400
pecan	1 slice (4 oz)	456
pineapple two crust	1 slice (5.3 oz)	394
plum two crust	1 slice (5.3 oz)	441
prune one crust	1 slice (5.3 oz)	450
pumpkin	1 slice (5.4 oz)	323
raisin tart	1 (4.2 oz)	348
raisin two crust	1 slice (5.3 oz)	376
raspberry one crust	1 slice (4.8 oz)	330
raspberry two crust	1 slice (5.3 oz)	422
rhubarb two crust	1 slice (5.3 oz)	444
shoo-fly	1 slice (4 oz)	404
strawberry rhubarb two crust	1 slice (5.3 oz)	422
strawberry two crust	1 slice (6 oz)	386
sweet potato	1 piece (5.4 oz)	276

FOOD	PORTION	CALS
PIE CRUST		
baked	1/6 crust (1 oz)	147
chocolate wafer	1/8 crust (1.2 oz)	177
chocolate wafer tart shell	1 (0.8 oz)	111
deep dish frzn	1/8 crust (1.8 oz)	266
graham cracker	1/6 crust (1.2 oz)	172
graham cracker tart shell	1 (0.8 oz)	109
puff pastry shell	1 (1.4 oz)	223
tart shell	1 (1 oz)	149
Honey Maid		
Graham Cracker Crumbs as prep	1/8 pie	160
Jiffy		
Pie Crust Mix as prep	1/7 crust	180
Keebler		
Graham Reduced Fat	1/8 pie (0.7 oz)	100
Ready Crust Chocolate	1/8 pie (0.7 oz)	100
Ready Crust Graham	1/10 pie (0.9 oz)	130
Ready Crust Shortbread	1/8 pie (0.7 oz)	110
Mrs. Smith's		
Deep Dish Shell frzn	1 slice (1 oz)	130
Nilla Wafers		
Pie Crust	1/6 (1 oz)	140
Pepperidge Farm		
Puff Pastry Sheets frzn	1/6 sheet	170
Puff Pastry Shell frzn	1	190
Pillsbury		
Crusts Just Unroll	1/8 (1 oz)	110
Deep Dish frzn	1/8 (0.7 oz)	90
Pet Ritz frzn	1/8 (0.6 oz)	80
PIE FILLING		
apple	1 cup	155
blueberry	1 cup	474
cherry	1 cup	317
lemon	1 cup	923
pumpkin pie mix canned	1 cup	281
Chukar Cherries		
Triple Cherry	1/2 cup	190
Comstock		
Blueberry	1/3 cup	100
Country Cherry Original	1/3 cup (3.1 oz)	90

FOOD	PORTION	CALS
Light Cherry	⅓ cup	60
Farmer's Market		
Organic Pumpkin Pie Mix	½ cup	100
PIEROGI		
potato	1 (1.3 oz)	70
Mrs. T's		
Potato & 4 Cheese Blend	3 (4.2 oz)	230
Potato & Cheddar	3 (4.2 oz)	180
PIGEON PEAS		
dried cooked	½ cup	102
dried cooked	1 cup	204
PIGNOLIA (see PINE NUTS)		
PIG'S FEET		
cooked	1	201
pickled	1	177
Hormel		
Pigs Feet	2 oz	80
PIKE		
northern cooked	3 oz	96
northern cooked	½ fillet (5.4 oz)	176
northern raw	3 oz	75
roe raw	1 oz	37
walleye baked	3 oz	101
walleye fillet baked	4.4 oz	147
PILLNUTS		
canarytree dried	1 oz	204
PIMIENTOS		
canned	1 tbsp	3
canned	1 slice	0
PINE NUTS		
pignolia dried	1 tbsp	51
pignolia dried	1 oz	146
pinyon dried	1 oz	161
Frieda's		
Pine Nuts	¼ cup	150

FOOD	PORTION	CALS
Good Sense		
Pignolias	¼ cup	190
PINEAPPLE		
CANNED		
chunks in heavy syrup	1 cup	199
chunks juice pack	1 cup	150
crushed in heavy syrup	1 cup	199
slices in heavy syrup	1 slice	45
slices in light syrup	1 slice	30
slices juice pack	1 slice	35
slices water pack	1 slice	19
tidbits in heavy syrup	1 cup	199
tidbits in juice	1 cup	150
tidbits in water	1 cup	79
Del Monte		
Chunks In Heavy Syrup	½ cup	90
Chunks In Its Own Juice	½ cup	70
Crushed In Heavy Syrup	½ cup	90
Crushed In Its Own Juice	½ cup	70
Fruit Naturals Chunks	½ cup	70
Dole		
Chunks Juice Pack	½ cup	60
Gefen		
Chunks In Juice	½ cup (4.9 oz)	80
Liberty Gold		
Chunks In Natural Juice	½ cup (4.7 oz)	80
Crushed No Sugar Added	½ cup	80
Slices Natural Juice	½ cup	80
DRIED		
Brothers-All-Natural		
Crisps	1 pkg (0.53 oz)	60
Kopali		
Organic	1 pkg (1.7 oz)	170
Mrs. May's		
Fruit Chips	1 pkg	35
Sunsweet		
Pineapples	⅓ cup (1.4 oz)	130
FRESH		
diced	1 cup	77
sliced	1 slice	42

FOOD	PORTION	CALS
Cala Fruit		
Golden Sliced	1 serv (3.5 oz)	50
Frieda's		
Zululand Queen	1 cup (5 oz)	70
FROZEN		
chunks sweetened	½ cup	104
Europe's Best		
Aloha Gold	1 cup	70
Roast Works		
Flame Roasted	1 serv (3 oz)	80
PINEAPPLE JUICE		
canned	1 cup	139
frzn as prep	1 cup	129
frzn not prep	6 oz	387
Adina		
Pineapple Ginger Gin-Jah	8 oz	80
Langers		
100% Juice	8 oz	130
Sundia		
Purely	½ cup	60
Walnut Acres		
Organic	8 oz	130
PINK BEANS		
dried cooked	1 cup	252
PINTO BEANS		
dried cooked	1 cup	245
Arrowhead Mills		
Organic Dried not prep	¼ cup	150
Eden		
Organic Spicy	½ cup	120
Organic Spicy Refried	½ cup	90
HamBeens		
Dried as prep	½ cup	120
Tree Of Life		
Organic	½ cup (4.6 oz)	120
TAKE-OUT		
stewed w/ viandas	1 cup	222

FOOD	PORTION	CALS
PISTACHIOS		
dry roasted w/ salt	49 nuts (1 oz)	161
dry roasted w/o salt	49 nuts (1 oz)	162
in shells	½ cup	165
Love'n Bake		
Pistachio Paste	2 tbsp	160
True North		
Sea Salted In Shells	½ cup	170
Wonderful		
Roasted & Salted In Shells	½ cup	170
PITANGA		
fresh	1 cup	57
fresh	1	2
PIZZA (see also PIZZA CRUST)		
4Real		
Cheese	1 (4.2 oz)	220
Cheesy Pizza Quesadilla	1 (2.5 oz)	160
Turkey Pepperoni	1 (4.2 oz)	220
Alexia		
Pizza Snacks Pesto Chicken w/ Fresh Mozzarella	6 pieces (3 oz)	220
Pizza Snacks Sweet Italian Sausage Roasted Peppers & Parmesan	6 pieces (3 oz)	210
Boca		
Supreme w/ Rising Crust Sausage & Pepperoni	⅓ pkg (4.3 oz)	280
Cedarlane		
Zone Cheese	1 (6.5 oz)	380
Celeste		
4 Cheese	1 (5.7 oz)	360
Dr. Praeger's		
Bagel Pizza	1 (2 oz)	120
Ellio's		
All Cheesy	1 slice	160
Cheese	1 slice	150
Microwave Single Slice	1 slice	360
Pepperoni	1 slice	160
Farm Rich		
Slices Pepperoni	2 (3.5 oz)	280

FOOD	PORTION	CALS
Freschetta		
Pepperoni	½ pie (5.8 oz)	470
Glutino		
Gluten Free Duo Cheese	1 (6.1 oz)	420
Gluten Free Spinach & Feta	1 (6.1 oz)	430
Healthy Choice		
French Bread Cheese	1 pie	340
French Bread Pepperoni	1 pie	340
French Bread Supreme	1 pie	340
French Bread Vegetable	1 pie	320
Hot Pockets		
Croissant Five Cheese	1 (4.5 oz)	350
Croissant Pepperoni	1 (4.5 oz)	380
Sausage	1 (4.5 oz)	330
Ian's		
Cheese	1 slice (1.5 oz)	100
Jeno's		
Crisp 'N Tasty Cheese	1 pie (6.8 oz)	440
Crisp 'N Tasty Pepperoni	1 (6.7 oz)	490
Crisp 'N Tasty Supreme	1 (7.2 oz)	490
Kid Cuisine		
Cheese Pizza Painter	1 meal	320
Dip & Dunk Cheese Pizza Strips	1 meal	510
Primo Pepperoni Pizza	1 meal	400
Lean Cuisine		
Casual Eating Deluxe	1 pkg (6 oz)	370
Casual Eating Four Cheese	1 pkg (6 oz)	400
Casual Eating French Bread Cheese	1 serv (6 oz)	320
Casual Eating French Bread Deluxe	1 pkg (6.1 oz)	310
Casual Eating French Bread Pepperoni	1 pkg (5.25 oz)	300
Casual Eating Margherita	1 pkg (6 oz)	320
Casual Eating Pepperoni	1 pkg (6 oz)	380
Casual Eating Roasted Vegetable	1 pkg (6 oz)	330
Casual Eating Spinach & Mushroom	1 pkg (6.1 oz)	310
Casual Eating Three Meat	1 pkg (6.4 oz)	350
Lean Pockets		
Pepperoni	1 (4.5 oz)	260
Sausage & Pepperoni	1 (4.5 oz)	280
Lunchables		
Maxed Deep Dish	1 pkg	510

FOOD	PORTION	CALS
Mini Pizza	1 pkg	480
Pepperoni Sausage	1 pkg	440
Mr. P's		
Cheese	1 pie (6.5 oz)	410
Red Baron		
Classic Crust 4 Cheese	1 pie (8.6 oz)	740
Deep Dish Single Pepperoni	1 pizza	460
French Bread Supreme	1 pie (5.8 oz)	370
South Beach		
Deluxe w/ Wheat Crust	1 pie	340
Four Cheese w/ Wheat Crust	1 pie	340
Grilled Chicken & Vegetable w/ Wheat Crust	1 pie	330
Pepperoni w/ Wheat Crust	1 pie	350
Stouffer's		
Corner Bistro Flatbread Chicken Bacon & Spinach	1 pkg (9.13 oz)	640
Corner Bistro Flatbread Margherita	1 pkg (9.13 oz)	540
Corner Bistro Flatbread Shrimp & Roasted Garlic	1 pkg (9.33 oz)	600
French Bread Grilled Vegetable	1 pkg (11.63 oz)	340
French Bread Sausage	1 pkg (4.2 oz)	420
French Bread Sausage & Pepperoni	1 pkg (4.2 oz)	460
French Bread White Pizza	1 pkg (10.13 oz)	470
Tony's		
Pizza For One Cheese	1 (6.5 oz)	500
Totino's		
Crisp Crust Canadian Bacon	½ pie (5.1 oz)	320
Crisp Crust Combination	½ pie (5.3 oz)	380
Crisp Crust Pepperoni Trio	½ pie (5 oz)	370
Crisp Crust Three Meat	½ pie (5.2 oz)	350
Pizza Rolls Combination	6 (3 oz)	220
Pizza Rolls Supreme	6 (3 oz)	210
Pizza Rolls Mega Ultimate Combination	3 (3.3 oz)	200
TAKE-OUT		
cheese	⅛ of 16 in pie	423
cheese	16 in pie	3384
cheese & vegetables	⅛ of 16 in pie	428
cheese deep dish individual	1 (5.5 oz)	460
ground beef	16 in pie	3753
ham & pineapple	⅛ of 16 in pie	439

FOOD	PORTION	CALS
no cheese	⅛ of 16 in pie	262
pepperoni	⅛ of 16 in pie	469
white pizza	⅛ of 16 in pie	484

PIZZA CRUST
crust	1 slice (1.7 oz)	130
whole wheat	⅛ crust	140
Alvarado Street Bakery		
Sprouted Wheat California Style	⅛ pie	190
Carbsense		
Garlic & Herb as prep	1 slice	100
Jiffy		
Crust Mix as prep	⅕ crust	180
Keto		
Dough Mix as prep	1 slice	79
Martha White		
Mix not prep	¼ pkg	160
MiniCarb		
Parmesan Herb Mix as prep	1 slice	130
Pillsbury		
Classic	⅙ crust (2.3 oz)	160

PLANTAINS
cooked mashed	1 cup	232
sliced cooked	1 cup	179
Chester's		
Chips	1 oz	150
Grab Em Snacks		
Chips Black Pepper	1 oz	150
TAKE-OUT		
mofongo	1 serv	320
ripe fried	2.8 oz	214
sweet baked w/ ice cream	1 serv	285

PLUM JUICE
Nantucket Nectars		
Red Plum	8 oz	120
Sunsweet		
PlumSmart Light	8 oz	60

PLUMS
canned in heavy syrup	1 cup	163

FOOD	PORTION	CALS
canned purple juice pack	1 cup	146
canned purple water pack	1 cup	102
dried japanese	1	9
fresh	1	30
pickled	1	34
Eden		
Umeboshi Plum Paste	1 tsp	5
Umeboshi Plums	1 (8 g)	5
Oregon		
Whole In Heavy Syrup	½ cup (4.6 oz)	100

POI
poi	1 cup	240

POKEBERRY SHOOTS
cooked	½ cup	16
fresh	½ cup	18

POLENTA
Bob's Red Mill		
Corn Grits Polenta not prep	¼ cup	130
Frieda's		
Organic	2 slices (3.5 oz)	70

POLLACK
atlantic baked	3 oz	100
atlantic fillet baked	5.3 oz	178

POMEGRANATE
fresh	1 (5.4 oz)	105

POMEGRANATE JUICE
Apple & Eve		
Organic	8 oz	130
Arthur's		
Pom Plus	1 bottle (11 oz)	220
Frutzzo		
Organic 100% Juice	1 bottle (12 oz)	130
Izze		
Sparkling Pomegranate	8 oz	80
Langers		
100% Juice	8 oz	150

FOOD	PORTION	CALS
Naked Juice		
Pomegranate Passion	8 oz	150
Odwalla		
PomaGrand 100% Juice	8 oz	160
Old Orchard		
100% Pure	8 oz	140
POM		
100% Juice	8 oz	140
Pomegranate Blueberry	8 oz	140
Pomegranate Cherry	8 oz	140
Pomegranate Mango	8 oz	140
Pomegranate Tangerine	8 oz	150
Smart Juice		
Organic 100% Juice	8 oz	149
Tart Is Smart		
Concentrate	0.5 oz	37
POMPANO		
smoked	2 oz	109
steamed or poached	4 oz	156
TAKE-OUT		
battered & fried	4 oz	304
breaded & fried	4 oz	242
POPCORN (see also POPCORN CAKES)		
air popped	1 cup (0.3 oz)	31
caramel coated	1 cup (1.2 oz)	152
caramel coated w/ peanuts	⅔ cup (1 oz)	114
cheese	1 cup (0.4 oz)	58
oil popped	1 cup (0.4 oz)	55
Cape Cod		
White Cheddar	2⅓ cups	170
Chester's		
Microwave Butter	3 cups	170
Microwave Cheddar Cheese	3 cups	200
Cracker Jack		
Butter Toffee	¾ cup	140
Original	½ cup	120
Dale & Thomas		
Caramel	½ cup	75
Hall Of Fame Kettlecorn	½ cup	34

FOOD	PORTION	CALS
North Country Cheddar	½ cup	73
Peanut Butter & White Chocolate Drizzlecorn	½ cup	115
Purepopped Natural	½ cup	26
Sweet Georgia Pecan	½ cup	96
Toffee Crunch Drizzlecorn	½ cup	107
Divvies		
Caramel Corn Vegan	½ cup	80
Jay's		
Caramel	¾ cup	110
Ok-Ke-Doke Cheese	1 oz	160
Jolly Time		
American's Best White	5 cups	100
American's Best Yellow	5 cups	90
American's Best 94% Fat Free	5 cups	100
Blast O Butter Light	4 cups	120
Butter Licious Light	5 cups	130
Crispy'n White Light	5 cups	125
Healthy Pop 94% Fat Free	5 cups	100
Healthy Pop Caramel Apple	5 cups	110
Healthy Pop Kettle	4 cups	100
Healthy Pop Minis	4 cups	90
Mallow Magic	2.5 cups	180
The Big Cheez	3.5 cups	140
White	5 cups	100
Yellow	5 cups	100
Lance		
White Cheddar	1 pkg (0.7 oz)	100
LesserEvil		
Black&White	1 cup	120
KettleCorn	1 cup	120
MaplePecan	1 cup	120
PeanutButter & Choco	1 cup	120
SinNamon	1 cup	120
Mrs. Fields		
Clusters Butter Toffee Crunch	⅔ cup	170
Newman's Own		
Microwave 94% Fat Free	3½ cups	110
Microwave Butter	3½ cups	130
Microwave Butter Boom	3½ cups	130
Microwave Light Butter	3½ cups	120

FOOD	PORTION	CALS
Microwave Low Sodium Butter	3½ cups	130
Microwave Natural	3½ cups	130
Organic Pop's Corn Butter	3½ cups	160
Organic Pop's Corn No Butter No Salt 94% Fat Free	3½ cups	120
Oogie's		
Romano & Pesto	1 oz	138
Smoked Gouda	1 oz	132
Spicy Chipotle & Lime	1 oz	143
White Cheddar	1 oz	142
Orville Redenbacher's		
Hot Air	1 cup	15
Kernel Original	1 cup	15
Microwave Butter Light	1 cup	20
Microwave Kettle Korn Sweet	1 cup	35
Microwave Movie Theater Butter Light	1 cup	20
Microwave Movie Theater Extra Butter	1 cup	35
Microwave Natural Light	1 cup	20
Microwave Pour Over Butter	1 cup	40
Microwave Pour Over Cheddar	1 cup	50
Microwave Regular Butter	1 cup	35
Microwave Regular Corn On The Cob	1 cup	35
Microwave Regular Natural	1 cup	15
Microwave Regular Old Fashioned Butter	1 cup	35
Microwave Regular Tender White	1 cup	40
Microwave Smart Pop Butter	1 cup	15
Microwave Smart Pop Kettle Korn	1 cup	20
Microwave Smart Pop Movie Theater Butter	1 cup	20
Microwave Sweet Caramel	1 cup	90
Microwave Sweet Cinnabon	1 cup	50
Microwave Sweet Honey Butter	1 cup	35
Microwave Sweet 'N Buttery	1 cup	40
Microwave Ultimate Butter	1 cup	30
White	1 cup	15
Poppycock		
Cashew Lovers	½ cup (1.1 oz)	148
Original	½ cup (1.1 oz)	160
Pecan Delight	½ cup (1.1 oz)	150
Smart Balance		
Light as prep	4 cups	120

FOOD	PORTION	CALS
Low Fat as prep	5 cups	120
Movie Style as prep	3.5 cups	170
Smartfood		
Reduced Fat White Cheddar	3 cups	140
White Cheddar	1 pkg	160
Snyder's Of Hanover		
Butter	0.6 oz	100
Tree Of Life		
Organic Lightly Salted	4 cups	100
Utz		
Butter	2 cups	170
Cheese	2 cups	160
Puff'n Corn Original Hulless	2 cups	150
Wise		
Butter	1 pkg (0.5 oz)	80
Hot Cheese	1 oz	150

POPCORN CAKES (*see also* RICE CAKES)

FOOD	PORTION	CALS
Orville Redenbacher's		
Butter	2	60
Caramel	1	40
Chocolate	1	45
Mini Butter	8	60
Mini Caramel	7	50
Mini Peanut Caramel Crunch	6	60
Mini Peanut Crunch	6	60
Mini Sour Cream & Onion	8	60
White Cheddar	2	60

POPOVER

FOOD	PORTION	CALS
home recipe as prep w/ 2% milk	1 (1.4 oz)	87
home recipe as prep w/ whole milk	1 (1.4 oz)	90
mix as prep	1 (1.2 oz)	67

POPPY SEEDS

FOOD	PORTION	CALS
poppy seeds	1 tbsp	47
Bob's Red Mill		
Poppy Seeds	3 tbsp	170
Love'n Bake		
Poppy Seed Filling	2 tbsp	120

FOOD	PORTION	CALS
PORGY		
fresh	3 oz	77
PORK (see also HAM, JERKY, PORK DISHES)		
FRESH		
boneless loin lean & fat roasted	3.5 oz	195
center loin chop bone in broiled	1 (3 oz)	178
center rib chop lean & fat bone in broiled	1 (3 oz)	189
country style ribs bone in lean & fat braised	3.5 oz	288
dehydrated oriental style	1 cup (0.8 oz)	135
fresh ham rump half lean & fat roasted	4 oz	278
fresh ham shank half lean & fat roasted	4 oz	319
fresh ham whole lean & fat roasted	4 oz	302
ground cooked	4 oz	328
ham hock cooked	1	167
shoulder chop bone in braised	1 (3 oz)	229
sirloin roast lean & fat bone in roasted	4 oz	231
spareribs bone in roasted	3 oz	304
tail simmered	3 oz	336
tenderloin roast boneless lean & fat roasted	4 oz	145
top loin chop boneless lean & fat broiled	1 (3.5 oz)	195
Boar's Head		
Smoked Shoulder Butt Roast	3 oz	170
Hormel		
Extra Lean Boneless Tenderloin	4 oz	120
Organic Prairie		
Chop	1 (3.3 oz)	220
Ground	4 oz	300
Smithfield		
Boneless Smoked Pork Chop	3 oz	110
Smoked Pork Chop	3 oz	100
Tyson		
Baby Back Ribs Buffalo	4 oz	300
Ground Reduced Fat	4 oz	260
Half Loin Boneless	4 oz	190
Loin Chops Bone-In Center Cut	4 oz	190
Spareribs	4 oz	290
Stew Meat	4 oz	130
READY-TO-EAT		
Sara Lee		
Oven Roasted	2 oz	70

FOOD	PORTION	CALS
TAKE-OUT		
chicharrones pork cracklings fried	1 cup	492
chop breaded & fried	1 med (3.4 oz)	304
chop breaded & fried	1 lg (5 oz)	441
chop stewed	1 lg (4.6 oz)	315

PORK DISHES
A La Carte Gourmet
Pork Loin w/ Cream Spinach Feta Stuffing	1 serv (5 oz)	200

Hormel
Extra Lean Apple Bourbon	1 serv (4 oz)	140
Pork Roast Au Jus	1 serv (5 oz)	180

Morton's Of Omaha
Tender Pork Roast w/ Gravy & Vegetables	1 serv (5 oz)	210

Tyson
Roast Pork w/ Vegetables	1 serv (4 oz)	190

Wellshire
Baby Back Ribs w/ Sauce	2 ribs (5 oz)	260
Shredded Pork In BBQ Sauce	¼ cup	90

TAKE-OUT		
kalua pork	1 cup (7 oz)	497
pork satay w/ peanut sauce	5 sticks (3.5 oz)	214
spareribs barbecued w/ sauce	2 med (2.8 oz)	248
tourtiere	1 piece (4.9 oz)	451

PORK RINDS (*see* SNACKS)

POT PIE
Hot Pockets
Pot Pie Express Chicken	1 (4.5 oz)	330

Ian's
Chicken	1 pkg (9.4 oz)	510

Mon Cuisine
Vegan	1 pkg (9 oz)	650

Pepperidge Farm
Chili Beans & Cornbread	1 cup	360
Reduced Fat Roasted White Meat Chicken	1 cup	470
Roasted White Meat Chicken	1 cup	510

Stouffer's
Chicken White Meat	1 pkg (10 oz)	660

TAKE-OUT		
beef	1 (14.6 oz)	938

FOOD	PORTION	CALS
chicken	1 (14.6 oz)	897
ham	1 serv (11 oz)	752
oyster	1 serv (11.5 oz)	817
puerto rican pastelon de carne	1 piece (5 oz)	666
st. stephen's day pie	1 serv (16.7 oz)	549
tuna	1 (27 oz)	1715
vegetarian w/ meat substitute	1 (8 oz)	511

POTATO (see also CHIPS, KNISH, PANCAKES)
CANNED
potatoes	½ cup	54
Butterfield		
Whole White	3.5 pieces (5.8 oz)	90
Del Monte		
New Whole	2 med (5.5 oz)	60
Savory Sides Au Gratin	½ cup	80
Sunshine		
Whole White	3 pieces (5.9 oz)	90
FRESH		
baked skin only	1 skin (2 oz)	115
baked w/ skin	1 (6.5 oz)	220
baked w/o skin	1 (5 oz)	145
baked w/o skin	½ cup	57
boiled	½ cup	68
microwaved	1 (7 oz)	212
microwaved w/o skin	½ cup	78
raw w/o skin	1 (3.9 oz)	88
Frieda's		
Fingerling	4 (5 oz)	100
Green Giant		
Red Potatoes	1 med (5 oz)	100
Lucinda's		
Red "C"	1 med (5.2 oz)	100
SunLite		
SunLite	1 (5 oz)	87
FROZEN		
french fries	10	111
french fries thick cut	10	109
hash browns	½ cup	170
potato puffs	½ cup	138
potato puffs as prep	1	16

FOOD	PORTION	CALS
Alexia		
Hashed Browns	1 serv (3 oz)	80
Mashed Red w/ Garlic & Parmesan	½ cup	150
Mashed Yukon Gold & Sea Salt	½ cup	150
Oven Crinkles Classic	1 serv (3 oz)	120
Oven Crinkles Salt & Pepper	1 serv (3 oz)	120
Oven Fries Garlic	12 pieces	140
Oven Reds	1 serv (3 oz)	120
Waffle Fries	8 pieces	150
Yukon Gold Fries w/ Sea Salt	1 serv (3 oz)	130
Cascadian Farm		
Organic Country Style	¾ cup	50
Organic Hash Browns	1 cup	60
Funster		
BBQ Lite	14 pieces (3 oz)	140
Cheddar	14 pieces (3 oz)	135
Original	14 pieces (3 oz)	135
Green Giant		
Roasted Potatoes w/ Garlic & Herb Sauce as prep	½ cup	90
Healthy Choice		
Cheddar Broccoli Potatoes	1 pkg	270
Ian's		
Alphatots	1 serv (3.5 oz)	156
Inland Valley		
Crinkle Cuts	15 pieces (3 oz)	150
Crisscut Fries	13 pieces (3 oz)	160
Curly QQQ's	1⅓ cups (3 oz)	180
Fajita Fries	17 pieces (3 oz)	170
French Fries	15 pieces (3 oz)	130
Hash Browns	⅔ cup	70
Home Browns	1 patty (2.2 oz)	130
Mashed Homestyle	⅔ cup	160
Simply Shreds	1 cup	70
Stix	5 pieces (3 oz)	170
Stuffed Spudz w/ Cheese	5 pieces	210
Tater Babies	8 pieces (3 oz)	130
Tater Puffs	10 pieces	160
Twice Baked	1 (5.2 oz)	230
Twice Baked Sour Cream Bacon & Chives	1 (5.2 oz)	240

FOOD	PORTION	CALS
Twice Baked Triple Cheese	1 (5.2 oz)	250
Joy Of Cooking		
Elegant Scalloped	1 cup (8 oz)	300
Red Skin Mashed	1 cup (4.2 oz)	160
Larry's		
Mashed Broccoli & Cheddar Cheese	1 serv (5 oz)	180
Mashed Cheddar Cheese	1 serv (5 oz)	190
Mashed Old Fashioned Butter	1 serv (5 oz)	190
Mashed Sour Cream & Chives	1 serv (5 oz)	180
Mashed Sweet Potatoes	1 serv (4 oz)	140
Lean Cuisine		
One Dish Favorites Deluxe Cheddar	1 pkg (10.4 oz)	260
McCain		
French Fries Crinkle Cut	18 pieces (3 oz)	130
Mash-Bites	1 serv (3 oz)	50
Roasters All American	1 serv (3 oz)	120
Roasters Grilled Garlic & Onion	1 serv (3 oz)	120
Seasoned Wedges Skin On	1 serv (3 oz)	120
Shoestring French Fries	45 pieces (3 oz)	140
Smiles	6 pieces (3 oz)	160
Steak Fries	8 pieces (3 oz)	120
Tasti Tater	1 serv (3 oz)	160
Oh Boy!		
Stuffed w/ Onion Sour Cream & Chives	1 (5 oz)	110
Roast Works		
Roasted Seasoned Wedge	1 serv (3 oz)	100
Roasted Wedges Rosemary Redskin	1 serv (3 oz)	110
Roasted Wedges Yukon Gold	1 serv (3 oz)	110
MIX		
au gratin as prep	½ cup	160
instant mashed flakes as prep w/ whole milk & butter	½ cup	118
instant mashed flakes not prep	½ cup	78
instant mashed granules as prep w/ whole milk & butter	½ cup	114
instant mashed granules not prep	½ cup	372
scalloped	½ cup	105
Betty Crocker		
Au Gratin as prep	⅔ cup	150
Cheddar & Bacon as prep	⅔ cup	120

FOOD	PORTION	CALS
Cheesy Scalloped as prep	½ cup	120
Julienne as prep	⅔ cup	140
Mashed Butter & Herb	½ cup	160
Mashed Four Cheese as prep	½ cup	170
Mashed Sour Cream & Chives as prep	½ cup	170
Scalloped as prep	½ cup	130
Seasoned Skillets Hash Browns as prep	½ cup	120
Hungry Jack		
Casserole Potatoes Au Gratin as prep	½ cup	100
Casserole Potatoes Creamy Scalloped as prep	½ cup	150
Casserole Potatoes Four Cheese as prep	½ cup	150
Easy Mash'd Cheesy Homestyle not prep	¼ cup	150
Easy Mash'd Creamy Butter not prep	¼ cup	150
Easy Mash'd Premium Homestyle not prep	¼ cup	150
Original Mashed not prep	⅓ cup	80
REFRIGERATED		
Country Crock		
Garlic Mashed	⅔ cup	160
Homestyle Mashed	⅔ cup	190
Diner's Choice		
Mashed	⅔ cup	110
Reser's		
Potato Express Red Skinned Mashed	½ cup	140
Simply Potatoes		
Diced w/ Onion	⅔ cup	60
Homestyle Slices	⅔ cup	70
Mashed	⅔ cup	170
Mashed Sweet Potatoes	⅔ cup	160
Red Potato Wedges	½ cup	50
Shredded Hash Browns	½ cup	50
SHELF-STABLE		
TastyBite		
Bombay Potatoes	½ pkg (5 oz)	105
TAKE-OUT		
au gratin w/ cheese	½ cup	178
baked topped w/ cheese sauce	1	475
baked topped w/ cheese sauce & bacon	1	451
baked topped w/ cheese sauce & broccoli	1	402
baked topped w/ cheese sauce & chili	1	481
baked topped w/ sour cream & chives	1	394

FOOD	PORTION	CALS
cheese fries w/ ranch dressing	1 serv	3010
french fries	1 reg serv	235
hash browns	½ cup (2.5 oz)	151
indian yogurt potatoes	1 serv	315
mashed	½ cup	111
o'brien	1 cup	157
potato dumpling	3.5 oz	334
potato pancakes	1 (1.3 oz)	101
potato salad	½ cup	179
red new boiled	5 sm (5 oz)	120
scalloped	½ cup	127
twice baked w/ cheese	1 half (10 oz)	392

POTATO STARCH

potato starch	1 oz	96
Bob's Red Mill		
Potato Starch	1 tbsp	40

POUT

ocean baked	3 oz	86
ocean fillet baked	4.8 oz	139

PRETZELS

chocolate covered	1 (0.4 oz)	47
soft	1 lg (5 oz)	483
twists salted	10 (2.1 oz)	229
twists w/o salt	10 (2.1 oz)	229
whole wheat	2 sm (1 oz)	103
yogurt covered	1 cup (3 oz)	391
yogurt covered	1 (4 g)	19
Cape Cod		
Pretzels	25	130
Combos		
Cheddar Cheese Cracker	1 pkg (1.7 oz)	240
Nacho Cheese	1 pkg (1.7 oz)	230
Pizzeria Pretzel	1 pkg (1.7 oz)	230
Glenny's		
Organic Original Salted	8 (1 oz)	110
Organic Sourdough	6 (1 oz)	110
Glutino		
Gluten Free All Shapes	44 (1.4 oz)	190

FOOD	PORTION	CALS
Goodniks		
Yogurt Pretzels	15	180
Handi-Snack		
Mister Salty Pretzels 'N Cheese	1 pkg	90
Healthy Handfuls		
Python Pretzels	1 box (1.5 oz)	170
New York Style		
Pretzel Flatz Original Salt	12	110
Newman's Own		
Organic Bavarian Sour Dough	1	90
Organic Hi Protein	22	120
Organic Salt & Pepper Rounds	8	100
Organic Salt & Pepper Thins	10	120
Organic Salted Nuggets	20	120
Organic Salted Rods	4	120
Organic Salted Rounds	8	110
Organic Salted Sticks	13	110
Organic Salted Thins	10	110
Organic Spelt	20	120
Organic Unsalted Rounds	8	110
Quinlan		
Low Fat Mini	1 oz	110
Rold Gold		
Braided Twists	1 oz	110
Braided Twists Honey Wheat	1 oz	110
Dipped Twists Fudge Coated	1 oz	140
Mini Sticks Honey Mustard & Onion	1 oz	140
Pretzel Waves Cheddar	1 oz	130
Pretzel Waves Dark Chocolate Drizzle	1 oz	130
Pretzel Waves Vanilla Yogurt Drizzle	1 oz	130
Sourdough Hard	1	100
Sticks Classic	1 oz	100
Tiny Twists	1 oz	100
Salba Smart		
Omega-3 Enriched	1 oz	110
Snyder's Of Hanover		
100 Calorie Pack Snaps	1 pkg (0.9 oz)	100
100 Calorie Pack Stick	1 pkg (0.9 oz)	100
Dips Milk Chocolate	1 oz	140
Dips Special Dark Chocolate	1 oz	140

FOOD	PORTION	CALS
Mini Unsalted	1 oz	110
MultiGrain Sticks Lightly Salted	1 oz	120
MultiGrain Twists	1 oz	120
Nibblers Sourdough	1 oz	120
Old Tyme	1 oz	120
Organic Honey Wheat	1 oz	130
Organic Oat Bran	1 oz	120
Pieces Garlic Bread	1 oz	140
Pieces Honey Mustard & Onions	1 oz	140
Pieces Hot Buffalo Wing	1 oz	140
Pretzel Sandwich Peanut Butter	1 oz	140
Rods	1 oz	120
Snaps	1 oz	120
Sourdough Unsalted	1 oz	100
Sticks 12 MultiGrain	1 oz	130
Superpretzel		
Mozzarella	2 (1.8 oz)	130
Pretzelfils Pizza	2 (1.8 oz)	130
Soft	1 (2.25 oz)	160
Soft Bites	5 (1.9 oz)	150
Softstix	2 (1.8 oz)	130
Tom Sturgis		
Little Cheesers	17 (1 oz)	120
Little Ones	17 (1 oz)	110
Utz		
Braided Twists Baked Honey Wheat	1 oz	110
Chocolate Covered	6 (1.1 oz)	140
Hard	1	90
Special	1 oz	110
Special Multigrain	1 oz	110
Sticks Organic Whole Grain	1 oz	120
Wise		
Fat Free Sticks	1 oz	100
Low Fat Honey Wheat Braided Twists	1 oz	110
PRUNE JUICE		
jarred	1 cup	182
L&A		
100% Juice	8 oz	180
Lakewood		
Organic	8 oz	165

FOOD	PORTION	CALS
Langers		
Plus 100% Juice	8 oz	180
Old Orchard		
Healthy Balance	8 oz	70
Sunsweet		
100% Juice	8 oz	180
PlumSmart	8 oz	160
Tree Of Life		
Organic 100% Juice	8 oz	180
PRUNES		
cooked w/o sugar	½ cup	133
dried	1	20
Earthbound Farm		
Organic Dried Plums	5	110
Love'n Bake		
Prune Lekvar	2 tbsp	90
Newman's Own		
Organic	½ cup	110
Sunsweet		
Pitted Dried	5	100
PUDDING		
MIX		
Keto		
Banana not prep	½ scoop	62
Chocolate not prep	½ scoop	66
French Vanilla not prep	½ scoop	62
Uncle Ben's		
Rice Pudding Cinnamon & Raisins as prep	½ cup	160
Rice Pudding French Vanilla as prep	½ cup	120
READY-TO-EAT		
Hunt's		
Dessert Favorites Banana Cream Pie	1 serv (3.5 oz)	140
Dessert Favorites Chocolate Brownie	1 serv (3.5 oz)	190
Dessert Favorites Chocolate Mud Pie	1 serv (3.5 oz)	170
Dessert Favorites Chocolate Peanut Butter Pie	1 serv (3.5 oz)	190
Dessert Favorites Dulce De Leche Caramel Cream	1 serv (3.5 oz)	140
Dessert Favorites Lemon Meringue Pie	1 serv (3.5 oz)	130
Snack Pack Butterscotch	1 serv (3.5 oz)	130

FOOD	PORTION	CALS
Snack Pack Chocolate	1 serv (3.5 oz)	104
Snack Pack Chocolate Fudge	1 serv (3.5 oz)	150
Snack Pack Chocolate Marshmallow	1 serv (3.5 oz)	130
Snack Pack Fat Free Chocolate	1 serv (3.5 oz)	90
Snack Pack Fat Free Tapioca	1 serv (3.5 oz)	80
Snack Pack Fat Free Vanilla	1 serv (3.5 oz)	80
Snack Pack Lemon	1 serv (3.5 oz)	120
Snack Pack Swirl Chocolate Caramel	1 serv (3.5 oz)	140
Snack Pack Swirl S'mores	1 serv (3.5 oz)	140
Snack Pack Tapioca	1 serv (3.5 oz)	130
Snack Pack Vanilla	1 serv (3.5 oz)	130
Jell-O		
100 Calorie Pack Fat Free Chocolate Vanilla Swirl	1 pkg (4 oz)	100
100 Calorie Pack Fat Free Tapioca	1 pkg (4 oz)	100
Fat Free Vanilla Caramel	1 serv (4 oz)	100
Sugar Free Dulce De Leche	1 pkg (3.7 oz)	60
Tapioca	1 serv (4 oz)	110
Vanilla	1 serv (4 oz)	110
Kozy Shack		
Black Forest	1 pkg (4 oz)	120
Chocolate	1 pkg (4 oz)	139
Chocolate No Sugar Added	1 pkg (4 oz)	93
Rice	1 pkg (4 oz)	135
Tapioca	1 pkg (4 oz)	130
Tapioca No Sugar Added	1 pkg	90
Vanilla	1 pkg (4 oz)	130
Vanilla No Sugar Added	1 pkg (4 oz)	90
Lifeway		
Organic Chocolate	½ cup	170
Organic Rice	½ cup	140
Organic Vanilla	½ cup	150
Swiss Miss		
Chocolate	1 pkg	150
Low Fat Chocolate	1 pkg	130
Pie Lover's Banana Cream	1 pkg	130
Pie Lover's Lemon Meringue	1 pkg	140
Swirl Chocolate Vanilla	1 pkg	140
TAKE-OUT		
blancmange	1 serv (4.7 oz)	154
bread w/ raisins	1 cup	306

FOOD	PORTION	CALS
coconut	1 cup	291
corn	1 cup	328
indian pudding	½ cup	156
noodle pudding kugel	1 cup	297
plum pudding	1 slice (1.5 oz)	125
queen of puddings	1 serv (4.4 oz)	266
rice pudding	1 cup	302
sweet potato	½ cup	107
tapioca	1 cup	236
yorkshire	1 serv (3 oz)	177

PUFFERFISH
raw	3 oz	72

PUMMELO
fresh	1	228
sections	1 cup	71

Sunkist
Fresh	¼	90

PUMPKIN
butter	1 tbsp	32
canned	½ cup	41
cooked mashed	½ cup	24
flowers cooked	½ cup	10
flowers raw	1	0
leaves cooked	½ cup	7
leaves raw	½ cup	4
raw cubed	½ cup	15

Farmer's Market
Organic Puree	½ cup	50

Tree Of Life
Organic Puree	½ cup (4.3 oz)	50

TAKE-OUT
indian sago	1 serv (2.3 oz)	75

PUMPKIN SEEDS
dried	1 oz	154
roasted	¼ cup	296
salted & roasted	¼ cup	296
whole roasted	1 oz	127
whole roasted	¼ cup	71

FOOD	PORTION	CALS
whole salted roasted	¼ cup	71
David		
All Natural	¼ cup	160
Eden		
Dry Roasted & Salted	¼ cup	200
Good Sense		
Roasted & Salted	½ cup	160
Mrs. May's		
Pumpkin Crunch	1 oz	164
Tree Of Life		
Seeds Roasted & Salted	¼ cup (2 oz)	300
PURSLANE		
cooked	1 cup	21
fresh	1 cup	7
QUAIL		
cooked bone removed	1 (2.7 oz)	177
QUICHE		
Mrs. Smith's		
Pour-A-Quiche Bacon & Onion	1 serv (4.3 oz)	230
TAKE-OUT		
cheese	⅛ (9 in) pie	566
lorraine	⅛ (9 in) pie	568
mushroom	1 slice (3 oz)	256
spinach	⅛ (9 in) pie	342
QUINCE		
fresh	1	53
QUINOA		
cooked	1 cup (6.5 oz)	222
quinoa not prep	¼ cup (1.5 oz)	156
Alti Plano Gold		
Natural	1 pkg	170
Ancient Harvest Quinoa		
Flakes not prep	¼ cup	159
Organic Inca Red not prep	¼ cup	163
Organic Traditional not prep	¼ cup	172
Eden		
Quinoa not prep	¼ cup	180

FOOD	PORTION	CALS
Seeds Of Change		
French Herb Quinoa Blend as prep	1 cup	290
RABBIT		
domestic w/o bone roasted	3 oz	167
wild w/o bone stewed	3 oz	147
RACCOON		
roasted	3 oz	217
RADICCHIO		
raw shredded	½ cup	5
RADISHES		
chinese dried	½ cup	157
chinese raw	1 (12 oz)	62
chinese raw sliced	½ cup	8
chinese sliced cooked	½ cup	13
daikon dried	½ cup	157
daikon raw	1 (12 oz)	62
daikon raw sliced	½ cup	8
daikon sliced cooked	½ cup	13
red raw	10	7
red sliced	½ cup	10
white icicle raw	1 (0.5 oz)	2
white icicle raw sliced	½ cup	7
Cadis		
Fresh	6 (2.6 oz)	12
Eden		
Daikon Dried Shredded	2 tbsp	45
Daikon Pickled	2 slices (0.5 oz)	5
Frieda's		
Black	¾ cup	15
Chinese Lo Bok	⅔ cup	25
Daikon	½ cup	15
Korean Moo	⅔ cup	15
TAKE-OUT		
korean kimchee	½ cup	31
moo namul saengche korean salad	1 serv (3.7 oz)	34
RAISINS		
cinnamon coated	¼ cup	108
cooked	¼ cup	162

FOOD	PORTION	CALS
golden seedless	¼ cup	109
jumbo golden	¼ cup	130
milk chocolate coated	¼ cup	176
milk chocolate coated	28 (1 oz)	109
seedless	55 (1 oz)	86
sultanas	1 oz	88
Amazin' Raisin		
All Flavors	1 pkg (1 oz)	84
Bob's Red Mill		
Unsulfured	⅓ cup	130
Brach's		
California Chocolate Covered	35 pieces	170
Earthbound Farm		
Organic Jumbo Flame Seedless	¼ cup	120
Emily's		
Milk Chocolate Covered	29 (1.4 oz)	180
Estee		
Chocolate Covered Fructose Sweetened	¼ cup	180
Fool		
Cinnamon Raisin Spread	1 tbsp	20
Godiva		
Milk Chocolate Covered	1 pkg (1.2 oz)	150
Goodniks		
Yogurt Raisins	3 tbsp	145
Newman's Own		
Organic	¼ cup	130
Revolution Foods		
Organic	1 pkg (1.2 oz)	100
Sun-Maid		
California Golden	¼ cup	130
California Seedless	¼ cup	130
Sunsweet		
Red Flame	¼ cup	130
RAMBUTAN		
canned in syrup	1 (0.3 oz)	7
canned in syrup	1 cup (4.3 oz)	123
puerto rican fresh	5 (1.6 oz)	34
Polar		
In Syrup	½ cup	68

FOOD	PORTION	CALS
RASPBERRIES		
black fresh	1 cup	70
canned in heavy syrup	½ cup	116
canned water pack	1 cup	43
fresh	1 cup	64
fresh	1 pt	162
frzn sweetened	1 cup	129
frzn unsweetened	1 cup	65
C&W		
Ultimate Red	¾ cup	70
Cascadian Farm		
Organic frzn	1¼ cup	60
Europe's Best		
Raspberries frzn	¾ cup	60
Frieda's		
Dried	⅓ cup (1.4 oz)	145
Oregon		
In Heavy Syrup	½ cup	120
RASPBERRY JUICE		
Crystal Light		
Raspberry Ice Sugar Free	8 oz	5
Naked Juice		
Raspberry Ade	8 oz	90
Newman's Own		
Razz-Ma-Tazz Raspberry	8 oz	120
Old Orchard		
Organic 100% Juice	8 oz	120
RED BEANS		
CANNED		
Allens		
Red Beans	½ cup	100
RELISH		
hamburger	1 tbsp	19
hamburger	½ cup	158
hot dog	1 tbsp	14
hot dog	½ cup	111
piccalilli	1.4 oz	13
sweet	1 tbsp	19
sweet	½ cup	159

FOOD	PORTION	CALS
B&G		
India	1 tbsp	15
Piccalilli	1 tbsp	20
Sweet	1 tbsp	15
Cascadian Farm		
Organic Sweet Relish	1 tbsp (0.5 oz)	15
Del Monte		
Hamburger	1 tbsp	20
Hot Dog	1 tbsp	15
Sweet Pickle	1 tbsp	20
Frieda's		
Kim Chee	¼ cup	15
Gedney		
Hot Dog	1 tbsp	18
Organic Sweet	1 tbsp	15
Matouk's		
Hot Chow	2 tbsp	20
Kuchela	1 tsp	9
Patak's		
Brinjal Eggplant Sweet Spicy	1 tbsp	70
Garlic	1 tbsp	45
Lime Mild	1 tbsp	30
Mango Mild	1 tbsp	40
Peloponnese		
Sun Dried Tomato	1 tbsp	25
Texas Sassy		
Pickle Relish	1 tbsp (0.5 oz)	30
Tree Of Life		
Organic Sweet Pickle	1 tbsp (0.5)	15
RENNIN		
tablet	1 (0.9 g)	1
RHUBARB		
fresh	½ cup	13
frozen	½ cup	60
frzn as prep w/ sugar	½ cup	139
RICE (see also RICE CAKES, WILD RICE)		
arborio	½ cup	100
brown long grain cooked	1 cup (6.8 oz)	216
brown medium grain cooked	1 cup (6.8 oz)	218

FOOD	PORTION	CALS
glutinous cooked	1 cup (6.1 oz)	169
starch	1 oz	98
white long grain cooked	1 cup (5.5 oz)	205
white long grain instant cooked	1 cup (5.8 oz)	162
white medium grain cooked	1 cup (6.5 oz)	242
white short grain cooked	1 cup (6.5 oz)	242
A Taste Of Thai		
Coconut Garlic Basil as prep	¾ cup	160
Coconut Ginger as prep	¾ cup	190
Jasmine not prep	¼ cup	160
Yellow Curry as prep	¾ cup	180
Arrowhead Mills		
Organic Brown Basmati not prep	¼ cup	140
Organic Long Grain Brown not prep	¼ cup	160
Betty Crocker		
Bowl Appetit! Teriyaki Rice	1 bowl (2.5 oz)	260
Buitoni		
Risotto Garden Vegetable	1 serv	210
Risotto Portobello Mushrooms	1 serv	210
Risotto Rosemary & Potatoes	1 serv	210
Risotto Tomato Basil	1 serv	210
Carolina		
Saffron Yellow Mix not prep	1 serv	190
Country Crock		
Chicken Rice w/ Herbs	1 cup	210
Fantastic		
Arborio not prep	¼ cup	160
Basmati not prep	¼ cup	160
Jasmine not prep	¼ cup	160
Gourmet House		
Brown & White not prep	¼ cup	160
Green Giant		
Rice Pilaf	1 pkg (9.9 oz)	200
White & Wild & Green Beans	1 pkg (9.9 oz)	260
Knorr		
Asian Side Dish Chicken Fried Rice as prep	1 cup	240
Rice Sides Rice Medley as prep	1 cup	250
Rice Sides Sesame Chicken w/ Whole Grains as prep	⅔ cup	300

FOOD	PORTION	CALS
Lundberg		
Eco-Farmed Black Japonica not prep	¼ cup	170
Eco-Farmed California Brown Basmati not prep	¼ cup	160
Eco-Farmed White California Arborio not prep	¼ cup	10
Organic Brown Golden Rose not prep	¼ cup	160
Organic Rise Sensations Ginger Miso not prep	½ cup	116
Organic Risotto Porcini Mushroom not prep	½ cup	143
Organic White Sushi Rice not prep	¼ cup	150
Organic Wild Blend not prep	¼ cup	150
RiceXpress Chicken Herb	½ pkg (4.4 oz)	250
RiceXpress Santa Fe Grill	½ pkg (4.4 oz)	260
Risotto Butternut Squash not prep	½ cup	143
Marrakesh Express		
Pilaf Tomato & Basil as prep	1 cup	190
Risotto Parmesan as prep	1 cup	200
Minute		
Boil-In-Bag White as prep	1 cup	180
Brown as prep	1 cup	150
Ready To Serve Brown	1 pkg (4.4 oz)	170
Ready To Serve White	1 pkg (4.4 oz)	190
Ready To Serve Yellow	1 pkg (4.4 oz)	190
White as prep	1 cup	200
Near East		
Long Grain & Wild Original as prep	1 cup	220
Pilaf Curry as prep	1 cup	220
Pilaf Original as prep	1 cup	220
Pilaf Sesame Ginger as prep	1 cup	270
Pilaf Spanish Rice as prep	1 cup	310
Whole Grains Brown Rice as prep	1 cup	210
Nueva Cocina		
Arroz A La Mexicana	1 cup	190
Arroz Con Pollo	1 cup	150
Gallo Pinto	⅓ pkg	220
Moros Y Cristianos	⅓ pkg	220
Paella	⅕ pkg	160
Pacific Foods		
Ready-To-Serve Lemon & Herb	½ pkg	240
Ready-To-Serve Roasted Chicken	½ pkg	240

FOOD	PORTION	CALS
Ready-To-Serve Spanish Style	½ pkg	230
Ready-To-Serve Wild Rice & Mushroom	½ pkg	230
Patak's		
Basmati	1 pkg	430
Coconut	1 pkg	500
Yellow	1 pkg	440
Rice A Roni		
Beef as prep	1 cup	310
Chicken as prep	1 cup	310
Express Asian Fried	1 cup	280
Fried Rice as prep	1 cup	320
Garden Vegetable as prep	1 cup	270
Long Grain & Wild as prep	1 cup	250
Lower Sodium Chicken as prep	1 cup	270
Parmesan Chicken as prep	1 cup	370
Red Beans & Rice as prep	1 cup	290
Savory Whole Grain Blends Spanish as prep	1 cup	250
Spanish as prep	1 cup	260
Rice Select		
Jasmati	1 serv	150
Kasmati	1 serv	150
Risotto	1 serv	150
Royal Blend	1 serv	160
Royal Blend w/ Lentils	1 serv	130
Royal Blend w/ Red Beans	1 serv	130
Sushi Rice not prep	¼ cup	190
Teriyaki Fried Rice not prep	¼ cup	160
Texmati Brown	1 serv	170
Texmati Light Brown	1 serv	170
Texmati Royal Blend Brown & Wild	1 serv	160
Texmati White	1 serv	150
River Rice		
Brown Long Grain not prep	¼ cup	150
S&W		
Brown Long Grain not prep	¼ cup	150
Seeds Of Change		
Moroccan Lentil Rice Pilaf as prep	1 cup	180
Tuscan Rice & Beans as prep	1 cup	180
Success		
Boil-In-Bag Brown as prep	1 cup	150

FOOD	PORTION	CALS
Boil-In-Bag Jasmine as prep	¾ cup	150
Boil-In-Bag White as prep	1 cup	190
Ready To Serve Brown	1 cup	170
Ready To Serve White	1 pkg	190
Ready To Serve Yellow Rice Mix	1 pkg	190
Whole Grain Herb Roasted Chicken as prep	1 cup	290
Whole Grain Multigrain Pilaf as prep	1 cup	230
Whole Grain Portobello Mushroom as prep	1 cup	220
TastyBite		
Pilaf Multigrain	½ pkg (5 oz)	200
Pilaf Tandoori	½ pkg (5 oz)	183
Uncle Ben's		
Boil-In-Bag	1 cup	190
Brown Natural as prep	1 cup	170
Country Inn Chicken & Broccoli as prep	1 cup	190
Country Inn Chicken & Vegetables as prep	1 cup	200
Country Inn Mexican Fiesta as prep	1 cup	200
Country Inn Oriental Fried as prep	1 cup	200
Country Inn Three Cheese as prep	1 cup	200
Country Inn Wheat	1 cup	200
Fast & Natural	1 cup	190
Flavorful Four Cheese as prep	1 cup	190
Flavorful Garlic & Butter as prep	1 cup	200
Flavorful Lemon & Herb as prep	1 cup	200
Flavorful Spanish as prep	1 cup	200
Instant	1 cup	190
Long Grain & Wild Herb Roasted Chicken as prep	1 cup	190
Long Grain & Wild Original as prep	1 cup	200
Long Grain & Wild Roasted Garlic as prep	1 cup	200
Long Grain & Wild Sun-Dried Tomato Florentine as prep	1 cup	180
Ready Rice Long Grain & Wild as prep	1 cup	240
Ready Rice Original as prep	1 cup	230
Ready Rice Roasted Chicken as prep	1 cup	230
Ready Rice Teriyaki as prep	1 cup	190
Ready Rice Whole Grain Brown	1 cup	220
White Original as prep	1 cup	170
Water Maid		
White Medium Grain not prep	¼ cup	160

FOOD	PORTION	CALS
Zatarain's		
Black Beans & Rice as prep	1 cup	230
Caribbean Rice Mix as prep	1 cup	160
Yellow as prep	½ cup	110
TAKE-OUT		
coconut rice	1 serv	500
congee	½ cup (4.1 oz)	44
dirty rice w/ chicken giblets	1 cup (6.9 oz)	291
nasi goreng indonesian rice & vegetables	1 cup (4.9 oz)	130
pea palau rice & peas fried in ghee	1 serv	144
pilaf	½ cup	84
risotto	1 serv (6.6 oz)	426
spanish	¾ cup	363

RICE CAKES (see also POPCORN CAKES)

FOOD	PORTION	CALS
Hain		
Mini Munchies Apple Cinnamon	9 (0.5 oz)	60
Lundberg		
Eco-Farmed Apple Cinnamon	1 (0.7 oz)	80
Eco-Farmed Brown Rice Salt Free	1 (0.7 oz)	70
Eco-Farmed Toasted Sesame	1 (0.7 oz)	70
Organic Caramel Corn	1 (0.7 oz)	80
Organic Green Tea w/ Lemon	1 (0.7 oz)	80
Organic Mochi Sweet	1 (0.7 oz)	70
Mr. Krispers		
Baked Rice Krisps Barbecue	37	110
Baked Rice Krisps Nacho	37	120
Baked Rice Krisps Sea Salt & Pepper	37	110
Baked Rice Krisps Sour Cream & Onion	37	110
Quaker		
Mini Delights Chocolatey Drizzle	1 pkg (0.7 oz)	90
Riceworks		
Sweet Chili	10 (1 oz)	140
Wasabi	10 (1 oz)	140

ROCKFISH

FOOD	PORTION	CALS
pacific cooked	3 oz	103
pacific cooked	1 fillet (5.2 oz)	180
pacific raw	3 oz	80

ROE (see also individual fish names)

FOOD	PORTION	CALS
fresh baked	1 oz	58

FOOD	PORTION	CALS
ROLL		
FROZEN		
Alexia		
Ciabatta	1 (1.5 oz)	100
French	1 (1.5 oz)	100
Three Cheese Focaccia	1 (1.5 oz)	110
Whole Grain	1 (1.5 oz)	90
Eggo		
Toaster Swirlz Cinnamon Roll Minis	4 (1.6 oz)	120
Joy Of Cooking		
Ciabatta Olive Oil Rosemary	1 (1.7 oz)	120
French Baguettes Mini	1 (1.6 oz)	100
Pillsbury		
Dinner Rolls Crusty French	1 (1.2 oz)	90
Dinner Rolls Crusty Sourdough	1 (1.2 oz)	90
Dinner Rolls Whole Wheat	1 (1.2 oz)	90
Sara Lee		
Deluxe Cinnamon Rolls w/ Icing	1 (2.7 oz)	320
READY-TO-EAT		
bialy	1 (2.2 oz)	138
brioche sweet roll	1 (3.5 oz)	410
brown & serve	1 (1 oz)	85
cheese	1 (2.3 oz)	238
cinnamon raisin	1 (2¾ in)	223
dinner	1 (1 oz)	85
egg	1 (2½ in)	107
french	1 (1.3 oz)	105
hamburger	1 (1.5 oz)	123
hamburger multigrain	1 (1.5 oz)	113
hamburger reduced calorie	1 (1.5 oz)	84
hard	1 (3½ in)	167
hot cross bun	1	202
hot dog	1 (1.5 oz)	123
hot dog reduced calorie	1 (1.5 oz)	84
hot dog whole wheat	1 (1.5 oz)	110
kaiser	1 (3½ in)	167
oat bran	1 (1.2 oz)	78
rye	1 (1 oz)	81
submarine	1 (4.7 oz)	155
wheat	1 (1 oz)	77

FOOD	PORTION	CALS
whole wheat	1 (1 oz)	75
Ecce Panis		
Focaccia	1 (3.2 oz)	260
Natural Ovens		
Better Wheat Buns	1 (2.2 oz)	170
Nature's Own		
100% Whole Grain Sugar Free	1 (1.9 oz)	110
Butter Buns	1 (1.7 oz)	120
Pepperidge Farm		
Hamburger 100% Whole Wheat	1	120
Hoagie Soft w/ Sesame Seeds	1	210
Hot & Crusty Sourdough	1	100
Hot Dog	1	140
Hot Dog Whole Grain White	1	110
Parker House Dinner	1	80
Premium Wheat	1	220
Sandwich Buns Sesame Seeds	1 (1.6 oz)	130
Rudi's Organic Bakery		
100% Whole Wheat	1 (2.3 oz)	160
Hot Dog Spelt	1 (2 oz)	140
Hot Dog Wheat	1 (2 oz)	150
Hot Dog White	1 (2 oz)	150
S. Rosen's		
Brat & Sausage Rolls	1 (2.1 oz)	160
Klassic Kaiser	1 (2.6 oz)	230
Sara Lee		
Hamburger Bun Classic	1 (2.6 oz)	200
Hamburger Bun Classic Wheat	1 (2.6 oz)	200
Heart Healthy Hamburger Bun Wheat	1 (2.6 oz)	190
Hot Dog Gourmet	1 (1.5 oz)	120
Stroehmann		
Hot Dog Wheat	1 (1.8 oz)	140
Super Bakery		
Daily Donut Reduced Fat	1 (2.2 oz)	200
Organic Sandwich Bun	1 (3.6 oz)	250
Sub Roll	1 (3.6 oz)	250
Weight Watchers		
Sandwich Wheat	1 (2 oz)	140
REFRIGERATED		
cinnamon w/ frosting	1	109

FOOD	PORTION	CALS
crescent	1 (1 oz)	98
Pillsbury		
Crescent Big & Buttery	1 (1.7 oz)	170
Crescent Butter Flake	1 (1 oz)	110
Crescent Original	1 (1 oz)	110
Crescent Reduced Fat	1 (1 oz)	90

ROSE APPLE

fresh	3.5 oz	32

ROSE HIP

fresh	1 oz	26

ROSELLE

fresh	1 cup	28

ROSEMARY

dried	1 tsp	4
fresh	1 tbsp	1

ROUGHY

orange baked	3 oz	75

RUBS (see HERBS/SPICES)

RUTABAGA

cooked mashed	1 cup	94
cubed cooked	1 cup	66
Glory		
Cut Fresh	1 cup	50
Sunshine		
Diced	½ cup	30

SABLEFISH

baked	3 oz	213
fillet baked	5.3 oz	378
smoked	1 oz	72
smoked	3 oz	218

SAFFLOWER

seeds dried	1 oz	147

SAFFRON

dried	1 tsp	2

FOOD	PORTION	CALS
SAGE		
ground	1 tsp	2
SALAD (*see also* SALAD DRESSINGS, SALAD TOPPINGS)		
Dole		
American Blend	1½ cups	15
Baby Spinach Salad	1½ cups (3 oz)	20
Butter & Red Leaf	1½ cups (3 oz)	10
Classic Iceberg	1½ cups (3 oz)	15
Classic Romaine	1½ cups (3 oz)	15
European Blend	1½ cups (3 oz)	15
Field Greens	1½ cups (3 oz)	15
French Blend	1½ cups (3 oz)	15
Greener Selection	1½ cups (3 oz)	15
Hearts Delight	1½ cups (3 oz)	15
Italian Blend	1½ cups (3 oz)	15
Kits Asian Crunch	1½ cups (3.5 oz)	120
Kits Bacon Lettuce Toss	1½ cups (3.5 oz)	130
Kits Caesar	1½ cups (3 oz)	170
Kits Caesar Light	1½ cups (3 oz)	100
Kits Fall Harvest	1½ cups (3.5 oz)	150
Kits Romano	1½ cups (3 oz)	150
Kits Spring Garden	1½ cups (3.5 oz)	140
Kits Sunflower Ranch	1½ cups (3 oz)	160
Mediterranean Blend	1½ cups	15
Very Veggie Blend	1½ cups (3 oz)	20
Earthbound Farm		
Organic Baby Arugula Salad	2 cups	20
Organic Baby Lettuce Salad	2 cups	15
Organic Baby Spinach Salad	2 cups	10
Organic Fresh Herb Salad	2 cups	15
Organic Mixed Baby Greens	2 cups	15
Fresh Express		
50/50 Mix	3 cups	10
Caesar Lite w/ Dressing as prep	2½ cups	100
Caesar w/ Dressing as prep	2½ cups	150
Fancy Field Greens	3 cups	20
Gourmet Cafe Caribbean Chicken as prep	1 pkg (3.5 oz)	120
Gourmet Cafe Chicken Caesar w/ Crostini as prep	1 pkg (3.5 oz)	150
Gourmet Cafe Chopped Turkey Chef as prep	1 pkg (3.5 oz)	120

FOOD	PORTION	CALS
Gourmet Cafe Orchard Harvest as prep	1 pkg (3.5 oz)	230
Gourmet Cafe Tuscan Pesto Chicken as prep	1 pkg (3.5 oz)	130
Gourmet Cafe Waldorf Chicken as prep	1 pkg (3.5 oz)	190
More Carrots American	1½ cups	15
Organic Italian	2½ cups	15
Original Iceberg Garden With Zip	1½ cups	15
Pacifica! Veggie Supreme w/ Dressing as prep	3 cups	220
Spring Mix	3 cups	15
Sweet Baby Greens	3 cups	10
Veggie Lover's	2 cups	20
Mann's		
Rainbow	3 oz	25
River Ranch		
American Blend	1½ cups	15
Caesar Kit	1½ cups	110
European Blend	1¾ cups	10
Garden	1½ cups	15
Garden Supreme	1½ cups	15
Italian Blend	1¾ cups	15
Raspberry Vinaigrette Kit	1¾ cups	130
Riviera Blend	1½ cups	10
TAKE-OUT		
7-layer salad	2 cups	557
caesar	4 cups	734
chef salad w/o dressing	3 cups	535
cobb w/ dressing	4 cups	645
greek w/ dressing	4 cups	424
mixed salad greens shredded	1 cup	9
somen w/ lettuce egg fish pork	2 cups	550
spinach w/o dressing	4 cups	429
tossed w/ avocado w/o dressing	2 cups	90
tossed w/ chicken w/o dressing	3 cups	194
tossed w/ egg w/o dressing	2 cups	93
tossed w/ seafood w/o dressing	3 cups	120
tossed w/ shrimp & egg w/o dressing	3 cups	185
tossed w/o dressing	2 cups	22
waldorf	1 cup	242
wilted lettuce w/ bacon dressing	1 cup	99

FOOD	PORTION	CALS

SALAD DRESSING (see also SALAD TOPPINGS)
MIX
A Taste Of Thai

Peanut Dressing as prep	2 tbsp	40

Good Seasons

Italian as prep	2 tbsp	130

READY-TO-EAT

blue cheese	1 tbsp	77
french	1 tbsp	67
french reduced calorie	1 tbsp	22
italian	1 tbsp	69
italian reduced calorie	1 tbsp	16
japanese ginger salad dressing	2 tbsp	90
russian	1 tbsp	76
russian reduced calorie	1 tbsp	23
sesame seed	1 tbsp	68
thousand island	1 tbsp	59
thousand island reduced calorie	1 tbsp	24

Annie's Naturals

Cilantro & Lime	2 tbsp	100
French	2 tbsp	90
Goddess Dressing	2 tbsp	130
Low Fat Mustard Vinaigrette	2 tbsp	45
Organic Buttermilk	2 tbsp	70
Organic No Fat Yogurt w/ Dill	2 tbsp	20
Organic Papaya Poppy Seed	2 tbsp	120
Organic Red Wine	2 tbsp	160
Sea Veggie & Sesame	2 tbsp	110
Tuscany Italian	2 tbsp	80

Bernstein's

Chunky Blue Cheese	2 tbsp	120
Creamy Caesar	2 tbsp	120
Italian Restaurant Recipe	2 tbsp	120
Light Fantastic Roasted Garlic Balsamic	2 tbsp	45
Red Wine & Garlic Italian	2 tbsp	110

Bragg

Ginger & Sesame	2 tbsp	150
Organic Vinaigrette	2 tbsp	150

Cains

Caesar Creamy	2 tbsp	170

FOOD	PORTION	CALS
Caesar Fat Free	2 tbsp	30
Caesar Light	2 tbsp	70
Chianti Vinaigrette	2 tbsp	130
Creamy Dill Cucumber Fat Free	2 tbsp	35
French	2 tbsp	120
French Light	2 tbsp	80
Greek	2 tbsp	160
Italian Fat Free	2 tbsp	15
Ranch	2 tbsp	180
Ranch Light	2 tbsp	80
Carb Options		
Italian	2 tbsp	70
Ranch	2 tbsp	150
Consorzio		
Balsamic Vinaigrette	2 tbsp	60
Caesar Parmesan & Romano	2 tbsp	120
Honey Mustard	2 tbsp	100
Italian	2 tbsp	60
Mango	1 tbsp	15
Raspberry & Balsamic	1 tbsp	15
Strawberry Balsamic	1 tbsp	10
David Burke		
Flavor Spray Ranch	2 sprays	0
Emeril's		
Bleu Cheese	2 tbsp	110
Honey Mustard	2 tbsp	100
House Herb Vinaigrette	2 tbsp	100
Kicked Up French	2 tbsp	80
Follow Your Heart		
Lemon Herb	2 tbsp (1 oz)	100
Sesame Miso	2 tbsp (1 oz)	64
Thousand Island	2 tbsp (1 oz)	80
Girard's		
White Balsamic Vinaigrette	2 tbsp	140
Gotta Luv It		
Chipotle Lime	2 tbsp	110
Raspberry Balsamic Vinaigrette	2 tbsp	150
Sweet & Tangy Italian	2 tbsp	140
Ken's		
Bacon Ranch	2 tbsp	140

FOOD	PORTION	CALS
Caesar	2 tbsp	170
Country French w/ Vermont Honey	2 tbsp	150
Fat Free Italian	2 tbsp	25
Fat Free Raspberry Pecan	2 tbsp	50
Honey Mustard	2 tbsp	130
Italian w/ Aged Romano	2 tbsp	110
Lite Chunky Blue Cheese	2 tbsp	80
Lite Italian	2 tbsp	50
Lite Ranch	2 tbsp	80
Lite Red Wine Vinegar & Olive Oil	2 tbsp	50
Lite Vinaigrette Balsamic & Basil	2 tbsp	50
Red Wine Vinegar & Olive Oil	2 tbsp	120
Russian	2 tbsp	140
Thousand Island	2 tbsp	140
Kraft		
Free French	2 tbsp	50
Free Ranch	2 tbsp	50
Free Thousand Island	2 tbsp	45
Honey Dijon	2 tbsp	100
Italian Creamy	2 tbsp	100
Light Done Right Caesar	2 tbsp	60
Light Done Right Red Wine Vinaigrette	2 tbsp	45
Ranch Garlic	2 tbsp	120
Special Collection Classic Italian Vinaigrette	2 tbsp	60
Special Collection Parmesan Romano	2 tbsp	140
Special Collection Tangy Tomato Bacon	2 tbsp	100
Thousand Island w/ Bacon	2 tbsp	100
LiteHouse		
Bleu Cheese Bacon	2 tbsp	150
Organic Vinaigrette Raspberry Lime	2 tbsp	40
Ranch Homestyle	2 tbsp	120
Ranch Lite	2 tbsp	70
Sesame Ginger	2 tbsp	35
Spinach Salad	2 tbsp	50
Vinaigrette Huckleberry	2 tbsp	20
Vinaigrette Lite Honey Dijon	2 tbsp	130
Lucini		
Delicate Cucumber & Shallots	2 tbsp (1 oz)	120
Fig & Walnut Savory Balsamic	2 tbsp (1 oz)	110
Roasted Hazelnut & Extra Virgin Olive Oil	2 tbsp (1 oz)	120

FOOD	PORTION	CALS
Marie's		
Blue Cheese Lite Chunky	2 tbsp	80
Blue Cheese Vinaigrette	2 tbsp	120
Caesar	2 tbsp	170
Coleslaw	2 tbsp	120
Creamy Ranch	2 tbsp	170
Red Wine Vinaigrette	2 tbsp	60
Sesame Ginger	2 tbsp	70
Milo's		
Gorgonzola Pear Riesling	2 tbsp	70
Pomegranate Port	2 tbsp	90
Nasoya		
Creamy Dill	1 tbsp	30
Creamy Italian	2 tbsp	70
Garden Herb	2 tbsp	60
Sesame Garlic	2 tbsp	60
Naturally Fresh		
Balsamic Vinaigrette	2 tbsp	10
Bleu Cheese	2 tbsp	170
Bleu Cheese Bacon	2 tbsp	170
Bleu Cheese Lite	2 tbsp	100
Buffalo Ranch	2 tbsp	110
Classic Oriental	2 tbsp	100
Ginger	2 tbsp	70
Greek Feta	2 tbsp	100
Honey French	2 tbsp	100
Honey Mustard	2 tbsp	140
Orange Miso	2 tbsp	100
Ranch Classic	2 tbsp	150
Ranch Lite	2 tbsp	80
Slaw	2 tbsp	90
Newman's Own		
Balsamic Vinaigrette	2 tbsp	90
Caesar	2 tbsp	150
Creamy Caesar	2 tbsp	150
Family Recipe Italian	2 tbsp	120
Lighten Up Balsamic Vinaigrette	2 tbsp	45
Lighten Up Caesar	2 tbsp	70
Lighten Up Honey Mustard	2 tbsp	70
Lighten Up Italian	2 tbsp	60

FOOD	PORTION	CALS
Lighten Up Low Fat Sesame Ginger	2 tbsp	35
Lighten Up Raspberry & Walnut	2 tbsp	70
Lighten Up Red Wine Vinegar & Olive Oil	2 tbsp	110
Olive Oil & Vinegar	2 tbsp	150
Parmesan & Roasted Garlic	2 tbsp	110
Ranch	2 tbsp	140
Two Thousand Island	2 tbsp	140
San-J		
Tamari Mustard	2 tbsp	25
Tamari Peanut	2 tbsp	60
Tamari Sesame	2 tbsp	45
School House Kitchen		
Balsamic Vinaigrette Basico	2 tbsp	160
Seeds Of Change		
Vinaigrette Balsamic	2 tbsp	60
Vinaigrette Greek Feta	2 tbsp	60
Vinaigrette Roasted Garlic	2 tbsp	60
Vinaigrette Sweet Basil	2 tbsp	60
Sonoma		
Creamy Tomato Bacon	2 tbsp	150
South Beach		
Balsamic Vinaigrette	2 tbsp	50
Italian	2 tbsp	60
Ranch	2 tbsp	70
Soy Vay		
Cha-Cha Chinese Chicken	3 tbsp	190
Spectrum		
Honey Dijon	2 tbsp	35
Organic Creamy Dill	2 tbsp	25
Organic Creamy Garlic	2 tbsp	20
Organic Greek Goddess	2 tbsp	110
Organic Porcini Mushroom Vinaigrette	2 tbsp	70
Organic Rocky Mountain Ranch	2 tbsp	130
Organic Sweet Onion & Garlic	2 tbsp	15
Organic Toasted Sesame	2 tbsp	15
Organic Omega 3 Balsamic Vinaigrette	2 tbsp	80
Organic Omega 3 Ginger Garlic Vinaigrette	2 tbsp	80
Organic Omega 3 Raspberry Vinaigrette	2 tbsp	80
Provencal Garlic Lover's	2 tbsp	50
Zesty Italian	2 tbsp	30

FOOD	PORTION	CALS
Steel's		
Honey Mustard	1 tbsp	90
Texas Sassy		
Vinaigrette	2 tbsp (1 oz)	80
Three Acre Kitchen		
Balsamic Vinaigrette	2 tbsp (1.1 oz)	130
Vino De Milo		
Gorgonzola Pear Riesling	2 tbsp	80
Pomegranate Port	2 tbsp	90
Wild Thymes Farm		
Salad Refreshers Black Currant	1 tbsp	36
Salad Refreshers Meyer Lemon	1 tbsp	35
Salad Refreshers Morello Cherry	1 tbsp	34
Salad Refreshers Pomegranate	1 tbsp	33
Vinaigrette Mandarin Orange Basil	1 tbsp	43
Vinaigrette Raspberry Pear	1 tbsp	43
Vinaigrette Roasted Apple Shallot	1 tbsp	42
Vinaigrette Toasted Sesame Wasabi	1 tbsp	42
Wishbone		
Blue Cheese w/ Gorgonzola	2 tbsp	140
Bountifuls Berry Delight	2 tbsp	35
Bountifuls Tuscan Romano Basil	2 tbsp	25
Caesar w/ Aged Romano	2 tbsp	80
Classic Ranch Extra Thick	2 tbsp	140
Creamy Caesar	2 tbsp	170
Creamy Italian	2 tbsp	110
Deluxe French	2 tbsp	50
Fat Free Chunky Blue Cheese	2 tbsp	35
Fat Free Italian	2 tbsp	20
Fat Free Ranch	2 tbsp	30
Fat Free Western	2 tbsp	45
Five Cheese Italian	2 tbsp	120
Italian	2 tbsp	90
Just 2 Good Blue Cheese	2 tbsp	45
Just 2 Good Creamy Caesar	2 tbsp	50
Just 2 Good Deluxe French	2 tbsp	50
Just 2 Good Italian	2 tbsp	35
Just 2 Good Ranch	2 tbsp	40
Just 2 Good Thousand Island	2 tbsp	50
Just 2 Good Western	2 tbsp	70

FOOD	PORTION	CALS
Light Ranch Extra Thick	2 tbsp	70
Light Vinaigrette Asian Sesame	2 tbsp	70
Light Vinaigrette Raspberry Walnut	2 tbsp	80
Ranch	2 tbsp	160
Russian	2 tbsp	110
Salad Spritzers Balsamic Breeze	10 sprays	10
Salad Spritzers Italian	10 sprays	10
Salad Spritzers Red Wine Mist	10 sprays	10
Thousand Island	2 tbsp	130
Vinaigrette Berry	2 tbsp	50
Vinaigrette Lemon Garlic & Herb	2 tbsp	70
Vinaigrette Olive Oil	2 tbsp	60
Western	2 tbsp	160
TAKE-OUT		
vinegar & oil	1 tbsp	72

SALAD TOPPINGS
Fresh Gourmet

FOOD	PORTION	CALS
Crispy Onions Garlic Pepper	1½ tbsp	35
Tortilla Strips Lightly Salted	2 tbsp	35
Wonton Strips Wasabi Ranch	2 tbsp	35
Naturally Fresh		
Fruit & Nut Mix	½ tbsp	45
Glazed Almond & Pecan Pieces	½ tbsp	40
Salad Pizazz!		
Asian Medley	1 tbsp	40
Cherry Cranberry Pecano	1 tbsp	35
Honey Toasted Delites	1 tbsp	40
Orange Cranberry Almondine	1 tbsp	35
Raspberry Cranberry Walnut Frisco	1 tbsp	30
Tomato 'N Bacon Parmesano	1 tbsp	30
Tomato Pinenut Tuscano	1 tbsp	130

SALBA
Salba Smart

FOOD	PORTION	CALS
Ground	2 tbsp	65
Whole Grain	1 tbsp	65

SALMON
CANNED

FOOD	PORTION	CALS
w/ bone	½ cup	106

FOOD	PORTION	CALS
Bumble Bee		
Blueback	¼ cup	110
Keta	¼ cup	90
Pink	¼ cup	90
Red	¼ cup	110
Skinless & Boneless	¼ cup	50
Smoked Fillets In Oil	⅓ cup	150
Chicken Of The Sea		
Pink	1 pkg (3 oz)	90
Red	¼ cup	110
Smoked Pacific	1 pkg (3 oz)	120
Libby's		
Red	¼ cup	110
Polar		
Pink	¼ cup	90
Sockeye Red	¼ cup	110
FRESH		
atlantic farmed baked	4 oz	233
cloudberry native alaska	3.5 oz	51
coho wild poached	4 oz	209
pink baked	4 oz	169
roe raw	1 oz	59
sockeye baked	4 oz	245
FROZEN		
Dr. Praeger's		
Salmon Cakes	1 (2.9 oz)	190
Gorton's		
Fillets Classic Grilled	1 (3 oz)	100
Phillips Seafood		
Salmon Cakes	1 (3 oz)	180
SMOKED		
lox	1 oz	33
TAKE-OUT		
guisado salmon stew	1 serv (7.4 oz)	320
roulette w/ spinach stuffing	1 serv (4 oz)	160
salmon cake	1 (4.2 oz)	264
salmon loaf	1 slice (3.7 oz)	206
SALSA		
black bean & corn	2 tbsp	15
citrus	2 tbsp (1 oz)	10

FOOD	PORTION	CALS
peach	2 tbsp	15
tomatoless corn & chile	2 tbsp	45
Bone Suckin'		
Fat Free Gluten Free	2 tbsp	40
Cape Cod		
Medium & Mild	2 tbsp	15
Chi-Chi's		
Fiesta Mild	2 tbsp	10
Chukar Cherries		
Peach Cherry	1 tbsp	13
Dei Fratelli		
Casera Mild	2 tbsp (1.1 oz)	5
Emeril's		
Original Recipe	2 tbsp	10
Muir Glen		
Organic Medium	2 tbsp	10
Newman's Own		
Bandito Mild	2 tbsp	10
Bandito Peach	2 tbsp	25
Bandito Pineapple	2 tbsp	15
Bandito Roasted Garlic	2 tbsp	10
Bandito Tequila Lime	2 tbsp	15
Ortega		
Garden Style Mild	2 tbsp	10
Picante Mild	2 tbsp	10
Pace		
Black Bean & Corn	2 tbsp	25
Organic Picante	2 tbsp	10
Thick & Chunky	2 tbsp	10
Robert Rothschild Farm		
Tomatillo & Pepper	2 tbsp	20
Salba Smart		
Organic Omega-3 Enriched	2 tbsp	12
Seeds Of Change		
Black Bean & Tomato Mild	2 tbsp	15
Garlic & Cilantro Mild	2 tbsp	15
Snyder's Of Hanover		
Sweet	2 tbsp	20
Tostitos		
All Natural	2 tbsp	15

FOOD	PORTION	CALS
Con Queso	2 tbsp	40
Monterey Jack Queso	2 tbsp	40
Restaurant Style	2 tbsp	15
Utz		
Sweet	2 tbsp	10
Walnut Acres		
Organic Fiesta Cilantro	2 tbsp	10
Organic Sweet Southwestern Peach	2 tbsp	20
SALSIFY		
fresh sliced cooked	½ cup	46
Frieda's		
Salsify	¾ cup	70
SALT SUBSTITUTES		
gomasio sesame salt	2 tsp	34
AlsoSalt		
Butter Flavored	¼ tsp	1
Garlic Flavored	¼ tsp	1
Original	¼ tsp	1
Chef Paul Prudhomme's		
Magic Salt Free Seasoning	¼ tsp	0
Eden		
Organic Gomasio Sesame Salt	1 tsp	15
Organic Seaweed Gomasio Sesame Salt	1 tsp	15
French's		
No Salt	¼ cup	0
Nu-Salt		
Salt Substitute	1 pkg (1 g)	0
SALT/SEASONED SALT		
kosher	¼ tsp	0
salt	1 tbsp (0.6 oz)	0
salt	1 dash (0.4 g)	0
salt	1 tsp (6 g)	0
sea salt coarse	1 tsp	0
sea salt fine	¼ tsp	0
BaconSalt		
Original	¼ tsp	0
Peppered	¼ tsp	0
Bob's Red Mill		
Garlic Salt Blend	¼ tsp	0

FOOD	PORTION	CALS
Sea Salt	¼ tsp	0
Eden		
French Celtic Salt	¼ tsp	0
Portuguese Coast Salt	¼ tsp	0
Maine Coast		
Sea Salt w/ Sea Veg	¼ tsp	0
McCormick		
Celery Salt	¼ tsp	0
Morton		
Iodized	¼ tsp	0
Ocean's Flavor		
Natural Sea Salt	¼ tsp	0
Spice Hunter		
Celery Salt	¼ tsp	0
Garlic Salt	¼ tsp	0

SANDWICHES
Alexia

FOOD	PORTION	CALS
Panini Tuscan Four Cheese w/ Roasted Tomato & Basil	1 pkg (6 oz)	380
Panini Tuscan Grilled Chicken w/ Mozzarella	1 pkg (6 oz)	400
Panini Tuscan Grilled Steak w/ Mushrooms & Onions	1 pkg (6 oz)	370
Panini Tuscan Smoked Chicken w/ Fire Roasted Vegetables & Parmesan	1 pkg (6 oz)	410
Aunt Jemima		
Biscuit Sausage Egg & Cheese	1 (4 oz)	340
Croissant Sausage Egg & Cheese	1 (4 oz)	350
Griddlecake Sausage Egg & Cheese	1 (4.4 oz)	350
Aunt Trudy's		
Fillo Pocket Cheese & Tomato	1 (5 oz)	320
Fillo Pocket Classic Samosa	1 (5 oz)	280
Fillo Pocket Mediterranean Olive & Veggies	1 (5 oz)	270
Organic Fillo Pocket Roasted Sweet Potato	1 (5 oz)	310
Cedarlane		
Wrap Low Fat Couscous & Vegetable Veggie	1 (6 oz)	220
Fillo Factory		
Organic Fillo Pocket Asian Vegetable	1 (5 oz)	240
Gardenburger		
100% Meatless Margherita Pizza Wrap	1 (4.7 oz)	240
Wrap Black Bean Chipotle	1 (4.7 oz)	240

FOOD	PORTION	CALS
Guiltless Gourmet		
Wrap Black Bean Chipotle	1 (5.7 oz)	270
Wrap California Veggie	1 (5.7 oz)	300
Wrap Mediterranean Spinach	1 (5.7 oz)	270
Hot Pockets		
Bacon Egg & Cheese	1 (2.2 oz)	160
Barbecue Beef	1 (4.5 oz)	310
Biscuit Sausage Egg & Cheese	1 (4.5 oz)	270
Calzone Four Meat & Four Cheese	½ (4.2 oz)	300
Calzone Pepperoni & Three Cheese	½ (4.2 oz)	330
Chicken Melt	1 (4.5 oz)	300
Croissant Chicken Parmesan	1 (4.5 oz)	340
Croissant Turkey Bacon Club	1 (4.5 oz)	320
Ham & Cheese	1 (4.5 oz)	290
Meatballs & Mozzarella	1 (4.5 oz)	300
Philly Steak & Cheese	1 (4.5 oz)	270
Steak Fajita	1 (4.5 oz)	280
Turkey & Ham w/ Cheese	1 (4.5 oz)	280
Ian's		
Mini Chicken Patty	2 (5.3 oz)	368
Jimmy Dean		
Bagel Sausage Egg & Cheese	1 (4.8 oz)	380
Biscuit Sausage Egg & Cheese	1 (4.5 oz)	440
Croissant Sausage Egg & Cheese	1 (4.5 oz)	430
D-Lights Croissants Turkey Sausage Egg White & Cheese	1 (4.8 oz)	300
D-Lights Honey Wheat Muffin Canadian Bacon Egg White & Cheese	1 (4.5 oz)	230
Muffin Sausage Egg & Cheese	1 (4.6 oz)	350
Lean Pockets		
Bacon Egg & Cheese	1 (2.2 oz)	150
Barbecue Beef	1 (4.5 oz)	290
Chicken Cheddar & Broccoli	1 (4.5 oz)	260
Chicken Fajita	1 (4.5 oz)	240
Chicken Parmesan	1 (4.5 oz)	290
Ham & Cheese	1 (4.5 oz)	270
Meatballs & Mozzarella	1 (4.5 oz)	260
Philly Steak & Cheese	1 (4.5 oz)	270
Sausage Egg & Cheese	1 (2.2 oz)	140
Steak Fajita	1 (4.5 oz)	250

FOOD	PORTION	CALS
Three Cheese & Chicken Quesadilla	1 (4.5 oz)	260
Turkey & Ham w/ Cheddar	1 (4.5 oz)	280
Turkey Broccoli & Cheese	1 (4.5 oz)	270
Lunchables		
Chicken Dunks	1 pkg	310
Stackers Ham & American	1 pkg	430
Stackers Turkey & American	1 pkg	420
Madalena's Masterpiece		
Calzone Artichoke Parmesan	1 (10 oz)	570
Calzone Grilled Chicken	1 (10 oz)	520
Calzone Sausage Pepperoni	1 (10 oz)	640
Panini Garlic Chicken	1 (8 oz)	450
Panini Honey Ham	1 (8 oz)	520
Panini Turkey Pesto	1 (8 oz)	500
Panini Veggie	1 (8 oz)	480
Quesabake Mexican Sausage	1 (7 oz)	510
Quesabake Roasted Veggie	1 (7 oz)	460
Oscar Mayer		
Deli Creations Honey Ham & Swiss	1 pkg (6.8 oz)	440
Deli Creations Steakhouse Cheddar	1 pkg (7.1 oz)	450
Deli Creations Turkey & Cheddar Dijon	1 pkg (6.7 oz)	430
PBJammerz		
Peanut Butter & Jelly All Flavors	1 (2 oz)	220
Pillsbury		
Toaster Scrambles Cheese Egg & Bacon	1 (1.6 oz)	180
Toaster Scrambles Cheese Egg & Sausage	1 (1.6 oz)	180
Smucker's		
Uncrustables Grilled Cheese	1 (1.8 oz)	150
Uncrustables Peanut Butter & Grape Jelly	1 (2 oz)	210
Uncrustables Peanut Butter & Strawberry Jam	1 (2 oz)	210
South Beach		
Breakfast Wraps All American	1 serv (4.6 oz)	200
Breakfast Wraps Denver	1 serv (4.6 oz)	180
Wrap Kit Deli Ham & Turkey	1 pkg	220
Wrap Kit Grilled Chicken Caesar	1 pkg	230
Wrap Kit Southwestern Style Chicken	1 pkg	250
Wrap Kit Turkey & Bacon Club	1 pkg	250
Stouffer's		
Corner Bistro Panini Philly Style Steak & Cheese	1 pkg (6 oz)	340

FOOD	PORTION	CALS
Corner Bistro Panini Southwestern Chicken	1 pkg (6 oz)	360
Van's		
Breakfast In A Pocket Sandwich Ham Egg & Cheese	1 (4.5 oz)	370
Breakfast In A Pocket Sandwich Veggie Egg & Cheese	1 (4.5 oz)	340
Breakfast Panini Huevos Rancheros	1 (4.5 oz)	270
Breakfast Panini Sausage Egg & Cheese	1 (4.5 oz)	290
TAKE-OUT		
bacon & egg	1 (6.2 oz)	388
bacon lettuce & tomato w/ mayo	1 (5.8 oz)	344
beef barbecue w/ bun	1 (6.7 oz)	417
calzone beef & cheese	1 (14 oz)	1476
calzone cheese	1 (15 oz)	1632
chicken fillet	1 (6.4 oz)	515
chicken fillet w/ cheese	1 (8 oz)	632
chicken salad	1 (5 oz)	333
crab cake w/ bun	1	308
crispy chicken fillet w/ lettuce tomato & mayo	1 (7.7 oz)	537
croque monsieur	1 (12.4 oz)	765
egg salad	1 (5.6 oz)	485
french dip w/ roll	1 (6.8 oz)	357
fried egg	1 (3.4 oz)	226
grilled cheese	1 (2.9 oz)	290
gyro	1 (13.7 oz)	593
ham & egg	1 (4.4 oz)	272
ham w/ cheese lettuce & mayo	1 (5.4 oz)	369
hot turkey w/ gravy	1	389
peanut butter & banana	1	617
peanut butter & jelly	1 (3.3 oz)	327
reuben w/ sauerkraut & cheese	1 (6.4 oz)	463
roast beef w/ gravy	1 (7.8 oz)	386
sloppy joe pork on bun	1 (6.5 oz)	318
tuna melt	1 (5.3 oz)	350
tuna salad w/ lettuce	1 (5.9 oz)	289
turkey w/ mayo	1 (5 oz)	329

SAPODILLA

fresh	1	140
fresh cut up	1 cup	199

FOOD	PORTION	CALS
SAPOTES		
fresh	1	301
SARDINES		
CANNED		
atlantic in oil w/ bone	2	50
atlantic in oil w/ bone	1 can (3.2 oz)	192
pacific in tomato sauce w/ bone	1	68
pacific in tomato sauce w/ bone	1 can (13 oz)	658
Beach Cliff		
In Louisiana Hot Sauce	1 can (3.7 oz)	150
In Mustard Sauce	1 can (3.7 oz)	150
In Olive Oil	1 can (3.7 oz)	200
In Tomato Sauce	1 can (3.7 oz)	140
In Water	1 can (3.7 oz)	150
Small In Soybean Oil	1 can (3.7 oz)	200
W/ Hot Green Chilies	1 can (3.7 oz)	180
Brunswick		
In Louisiana Hot Sauce	1 can (3.7 oz)	150
In Mustard Sauce	1 can (3.7 oz)	150
In Soybean Oil	1 can (3.7 oz)	110
In Spring Water	1 can (3.7 oz)	150
In Tomato Sauce	1 can (3.7 oz)	150
W/ Hot Tabasco Peppers	1 can (3.7 oz)	110
Bumble Bee		
In Hot Sauce	¼ cup	90
In Mustard	¼ cup	70
In Oil	1 can (3.7 oz)	130
In Water	1 can (3.7 oz)	120
Chicken Of The Sea		
In Hot Sauce	1 can (3.75 oz)	130
In Mustard Sauce	1 can (3.75 oz)	150
In Oil	1 can (3.75 oz)	190
In Tomato Sauce	1 can (3.75 oz)	130
In Water	1 can (3.75 oz)	100
Goya		
In Tomato Sauce	2 pieces (2.2 oz)	50
King Oscar		
In Olive Oil	1 can (3.75 oz)	150
Skinless Boneless In Soya Oil	3 pieces (1.9 oz)	120

FOOD	PORTION	CALS
Polar		
In Mustard	1 can (4.5 oz)	170
In Tomato Sauce	1 can (4.5 oz)	120
In Water	1 can (3 oz)	100
FRESH		
raw	3.5 oz	135
SAUCE (*see also* BARBECUE SAUCE, GRAVY, SPAGHETTI SAUCE)		
adobo fresco	2 tbsp	81
bearnaise	1 oz	177
cheese mix as prep w/ milk	1 cup	307
curry mix as prep	1 cup	120
curry mix as prep w/ milk	1 cup	270
enchilada sauce green	¼ cup	46
enchilada sauce red	¼ cup	79
fish sauce chinese	1 tbsp	9
fish sauce vietnamese nuoc mam	1 tbsp	6
hoisin	1 tbsp	35
moroccan tagine	½ cup (4 oz)	70
mushroom mix as prep w/ milk	1 cup	228
oyster	1 tbsp	8
plum sauce	0.5 oz	42
satay peanut sauce	1 oz	77
sour cream mix as prep w/ milk	1 cup	509
stroganoff mix as prep	1 cup	271
sweet & sour mix as prep	1 cup	294
teriyaki	1 tbsp	15
teriyaki mix as prep	1 cup	131
white sauce mix as prep w/ milk	1 cup	241
A Taste Of Thai		
Chili Sauce Garlic Pepper	1 tsp	10
Chili Sauce Sweet Red	1 tsp	10
Fish Sauce	1 tbsp	15
Pad Thai Sauce Mix	2 tbsp	90
Peanut Satay	2 tbsp	80
Peanut Sauce Mix	¼ pkg	45
Ahh!Gourmet		
Perky Savory Coffee Sauce	4 tbsp	71
Ritzy Kumquat Plum Sauce	4 tbsp	98
Spicy Garlicky Sweet Sauce Paste	4 tbsp	101
Spiky Ginger Soy Sauce Paste	4 tbsp	137

FOOD	PORTION	CALS
Annie Chun's		
Marinade & Dressing Lemongrass Herb	1 tbsp	25
Noodle Sauce & Dressing Sesame Cilantro	1 tbsp	60
Shiitake Mushroom	1 tbsp	15
Annie's Naturals		
Marinade Organic Spicy Ginger	2 tbsp	35
Marinade Organic Teriyaki	1 tbsp	30
Organic Worcestershire	1 tbsp	20
Asian Creations		
Marvelous Mango	¼ cup	20
Pad Thai Pizzazz	2 oz	110
Peanut Passion	¼ cup	130
Asian Gourmet		
Duck Sauce Peking Style	2 tbsp	40
Bear-Man		
Sap-Happy Golden Bear	2 tbsp	60
Boar's Head		
Ham Glaze Sugar & Spice	2 tbsp	120
Bone Suckin'		
Hiccuppin' Hot	1 tsp	10
Yaki Stir Fry	1 tbsp	30
Burbon Chicken		
Marinade Original	1 tbsp (0.6 oz)	5
Cains		
Tartar	2 tbsp	160
Carb Options		
Alfredo	¼ cup	110
Asian Teriyaki Marinade	1 tbsp	5
Steak Sauce	1 tbsp	5
China Pride		
Duck Sauce Sweet & Pungent	2 tbsp	80
Consorzio		
Marinade Baja Lime	1 tbsp	60
Marinade California Teriyaki	1 tbsp	40
Marinade Dijon Peppercorn	1 tbsp	15
Marinade Jamaican Jerk	1 tbsp	10
Marinade Lemon Pepper	1 tbsp	60
Marinade Roasted Garlic	1 tbsp	35
Marinade Sesame Ginger	1 tbsp	25
Marinade Southwestern Chipotle	1 tbsp	30

FOOD	PORTION	CALS
Marinade Tropical Grill	1 tbsp	40
Dei Fratelli		
Sloppy Joe Sauce	¼ cup (2.2 oz)	35
Del Monte		
Seafood Cocktail	¼ cup	100
Sloppy Joe Hickory Flavor	¼ cup	60
Sloppy Joe Original	¼ cup	50
D'Oni		
Happy Together Orange Chili Garlic	2 tbsp	50
Moondance Marinade	1 tbsp	10
Eden		
Ponzu Sauce	1 tbsp	5
Emeril's		
Kicked Up Red Sauce	1 tsp	0
Marinade Hickory Maple Chipotle	1 tbsp	35
Marinade Lemon Rosemary Gaaahlic	1 tbsp	70
Marinade Orange Herb Poppyseed	1 tbsp	150
Steak Sauce	1 tbsp	20
Fage		
Tzatziki	2 tbsp	30
Frank's		
Buffalo Wing Sauce	1 tbsp	5
RedHot Chile & Lime Sauce	1 tsp	0
RedHot Original Cayenne Pepper Sauce	1 tsp	0
RedHot X-tra Hot	1 tsp	0
French's		
Worcestershire	1 tsp	0
Good Clean Food		
Simmer Sauce Balsamic Mushroom	⅜ cup (3 oz)	100
Simmer Sauce Cacciatore	⅜ cup (3 oz)	70
Simmer Sauce Creole	⅜ cup (3 oz)	45
Simmer Sauce Dill	⅜ cup (3 oz)	60
Simmer Sauce French Tarragon	⅜ cup (3 oz)	90
Simmer Sauce Mediterranean	⅜ cup (3 oz)	50
House Of Tsang		
General Tsao	1 tsp	45
Hoisin	1 tsp	15
Kobe Steak Grill	1 tbsp	50
Korean Teriyaki Stir Fry	1 tbsp	35
Peanut Sauce Bangkok Padang	1 tbsp	45

FOOD	PORTION	CALS
Spicy Brown Bean	1 tbsp	15
Sweet & Sour	1 tbsp	35
Sweet Ginger Sesame	1 tbsp	40
Thai Peanut	1 tbsp	50
Ken's		
Marinade Herb & Garlic	1 tbsp	20
Marinade Lemon & Pepper	1 tbsp	10
Marinade Teriyaki	1 tbsp	20
Knorr		
Alfredo Mix as prep	2 oz	60
Bearnaise Mix as prep	2 oz	35
Curry Indian Madras	1 oz	30
Curry Thai	1 oz	35
Demi-Glace Mix as prep	2 oz	30
Green Peppercorn Mix as prep	2 oz	35
Hollandaise Mix as prep	2 oz	35
Mango Habanero	1 oz	20
Sweet Red Chili	1 oz	80
White Mix as prep	2 oz	20
La Choy		
Sweet & Sour	2 tbsp (1.2 oz)	60
Teriyaki	1 tbsp (0.6 oz)	40
Las Palmas		
Enchilada Green	¼ cup	25
Enchilada Mild	¼ cup	20
Red Chili	¼ cup	20
Latino Chef		
Chimichurri Sun Dried Tomato	2 tbsp	120
Sofrito	2 tbsp	20
Lea & Perrins		
Worcestershire	1 tsp	5
Lee Kum Kee		
Plum Sauce	2 tbsp	100
Lollipop Tree		
Grilling & Glazing Chipotle	1 tbsp	50
Grilling & Glazing Mango Garlic	2 tbsp	60
Manwich		
Sloppy Joe Original	¼ cup (2.2 oz)	30
Matouk's		
Calypso	1 tsp	0

FOOD	PORTION	CALS
Milo's		
Simmer Sauce Bombay Cabernet	3 oz	35
Mrs. Dash		
10 Minute Marinade Lemon Herb Peppercorn	1 tbsp	25
10 Minute Marinade Mesquite Grille	1 tbsp	25
10 Minute Marinade Southwestern Chipotle	1 tbsp	20
10 Minute Marinade Zesty Garlic Herb	1 tbsp	25
Nando's		
Curry Coconut	¼ cup	71
Fresh Lemon	¼ cup	61
Marinade Lime & Cilantro	1 tbsp	27
Marinade Sundried Tomato	1 tbsp	15
Peri-Peri Pepper Extra Hot	1 oz	17
Peri-Peri Pepper Garlic	1 oz	12
Peri-Peri Pepper Hot	1 oz	16
Peri-Peri Pepper Wild Herb	1 oz	14
Roasted Red	¼ cup	70
Sweet Apricot	¼ cup	51
Naturally Fresh		
Seafood Cocktail	2 tbsp	25
Tartar Sauce	2 tbsp	130
Newman's Own		
Fra Diavolo	½ cup	70
Steak Sauce	1 tbsp	20
Old El Paso		
Enchilada Mild	¼ cup	25
Ortega		
Enchilada	¼ cup	15
Taco	1 tbsp	10
Pace		
Taco Sauce Green	1 tbsp	5
Taco Sauce Red	2 tbsp	10
Patak's		
Jalfrezi Sweet Peppers & Coconut	½ cup	140
Korma Rich Creamy Coconut	½ cup	240
Rogan Josh Spicy Tomato & Cardamom	½ cup	90
Tikka Masala Tangy Lemon & Cilantro	½ cup	120
Road's End Organics		
Alfredo Style Dairy Free Gluten Free	⅓ pkg	35
Cheddar Style Dairy Free	⅓ pkg	35

FOOD	PORTION	CALS
Robert Rothschild Farm		
Anne Mae's Smoky Sweet Chipotle	2 tbsp	35
San-J		
Japanese Steak	1 tbsp	13
Sweet & Tangy	1 tbsp	50
Szechuan	1 tsp	5
Teriyaki	1 tbsp	10
Thai Peanut	2 tbsp	70
Simply Boulder		
Coconut Peanut	2 tbsp (1 oz)	90
Lemon Pesto	2 tbsp (1 oz)	50
Zesty Pineapple	2 tbsp (1 oz)	45
South Beach		
Steak Sauce	1 tbsp	5
Soy Vay		
Hoisin Garlic Asian Glaze & Marinade	1 tbsp	40
Veri Veri Teriyaki	1 tbsp	35
Steel's		
Sugar Free Cocktail w/ Dill & Lemon	¼ cup	36
Sugar Free Hoisin	2 tbsp	15
Sugar Free Sweet & Sour	2 tbsp	10
Tabasco		
Pepper Sauce	1 tsp	0
Texas Sassy		
Marinade Salsa	1 tbsp (0.5 oz)	15
Pickle Sauce	1 tbsp (0.5 oz)	30
The Wizard's		
Organic Worcestershire Vegetarian Wheat Free	1 tsp	0
Three Acre Kitchen		
Marinade Balsamic w/ Juniper & Rosemary	1 tbsp (0.5 oz)	50
Ty Ling		
Duck	2 tbsp	70
Walden Farms		
Calorie Free Scampi Sauce	2 tbsp	0
Wild Thymes Farm		
Marinade Hawaiian Teriyaki	1 tbsp	19
Marinade Korean Ginger Scallion	1 tbsp	20
Marinade New Orleans Creole	1 tbsp	11

FOOD	PORTION	CALS
WildWood		
Aioli	1 tbsp	80
Pesto Basil & Pine Nuts	¼ cup	230
Wingers		
Hotter Than Hot	1 tsp	0
Zatarain's		
Cocktail	¼ cup	70
Etouffee Base as prep	½ cup	35
TAKE-OUT		
cucumber yogurt sauce	1½ tbsp	20
SAUERKRAUT		
canned	½ cup	22
Boar's Head		
Sauerkraut	2 tbsp (1 oz)	5
Dei Fratelli		
Sauerkraut	2 tbsp (1 oz)	5
Del Monte		
Bavarian Style	2 tbsp	15
Sauerkraut	2 tbsp	0
Eden		
Organic	½ cup	25
Gedney		
Sauerkraut	½ cup	15
Hebrew National		
Sauerkraut	2 tbsp	5
Tree Of Life		
Organic	½ cup (3.6 oz)	15
SAUSAGE		
beef & pork	1 link (2.3 oz)	196
beef & pork w/ cheddar cheese	1 link (2.7 oz)	228
bierschinken	3.5 oz	174
bierwurst	3.5 oz	258
blutwurst uncooked	3.5 oz	424
bockwurst	3.5 oz	276
bratwurst chicken cooked	1 (3 oz)	148
bratwurst pork cooked	1 link (2.5 oz)	226
brotwurst pork & beef	1 link (2.5 oz)	226
chipolata	3.5 oz	342
chorizo	1 link (2.1 oz)	273

FOOD	PORTION	CALS
fleischwurst	3.5 oz	305
free range chicken breakfast	2 links (2.7 oz)	110
gelbwurst uncooked	3.5 oz	363
italian pork cooked	1 (2.4 oz)	230
jagdwurst	3.5 oz	211
knockwurst pork & beef	1 (2.5 oz)	221
mettwurst uncooked	3.5 oz	483
plockwurst uncooked	3.5 oz	312
polish kielbasa	2 oz	127
pork cooked	2 links (1.7 oz)	163
regensburger uncooked	3.5 oz	354
turkey italian smoked	1 (2 oz)	88
vienna canned	1 link (0.5 oz)	37
vienna canned	1 can (4 oz)	260
weisswurst uncooked	3.5 oz	305
zungenwurst (tongue)	3.5 oz	285
Al Fresco		
Apple Maple	1 (1.2 oz)	70
Buffalo Style	1 (3 oz)	160
Country Style	1 (1.2 oz)	60
Italian Sweet	1 (3 oz)	170
Roasted Garlic	1 (3 oz)	170
Spicy Jalapeno	1 (3 oz)	120
Sundried Tomato & Basil	1 (3 oz)	180
Sweet Apple	1 (3 oz)	160
Teriyaki Ginger	1 (3 oz)	180
Wild Blueberry	1 (1.2 oz)	90
Applegate Farms		
Organic Andouille	1 (3 oz)	120
Organic Spinach & Feta	1 (3 oz)	120
Armour		
Brown'N Serve Lite Original	3	120
Brown'N Serve Turkey	3	120
Sizzle & Serve Turkey	3 (1.8 oz)	130
Banquet		
Brown 'N Serve Lite Maple	3 (2 oz)	130
Brown 'N Serve Lite Original	3 (2.1 oz)	120
Boar's Head		
Bratwurst	1 (4 oz)	300
Hot Smoked	1 (3.2 oz)	250

FOOD	PORTION	CALS
Kielbasa	2 oz	120
Knockwurst Beef	1 (4 oz)	310
Butterball		
Bratwurst Turkey	1 (3.2 oz)	140
Breakfast Turkey	3 (3 oz)	130
Polska Kielbasa Turkey	2 oz	100
Sweet Italian Turkey	1 (3.2 oz)	140
Healthy Ones		
Smoked	2 oz	80
Hebrew National		
Knockwurst Beef	1 (3 oz)	260
Honeysuckle White		
Turkey Roll Mild Italian	2.5 oz	100
Jennie-O		
Italian Hot	1 (3.9 oz)	160
Turkey Italian Sweet	1 link (3.9 oz)	160
Jimmy Dean		
Fully Cooked Original Links	3 (2.4 oz)	240
Fully Cooked Original Patties	2 (2.4 oz)	240
Fully Cooked Turkey Links	3 (2.4 oz)	120
Fully Cooked Turkey Patties	2 (2.4 oz)	120
Original Links	3 (2 oz)	170
Original Patties cooked	2 (2.4 oz)	240
Pork All Natural cooked	2 oz	190
Pork Light cooked	2 oz	140
Johnsonville		
Bratwurst Original	1 (3 oz)	270
Breakfast Patty Original	2 (2 oz)	180
Grilling Chorizo	1 (3 oz)	280
Italian Mild	1 (3 oz)	270
Original Summer	1 (2 oz)	170
Polish	1 (2.7 oz)	240
Pork	2 oz	180
Smoked Turkey	1 (3 oz)	110
Jones		
Light 50% Less Fat	2 (1.6 oz)	110
Little Pork	3	190
Libby's		
Vienna Sausage BBQ	3	140

FOOD	PORTION	CALS
Murray's		
Chicken Sun Dried Tomato	3 oz	110
Chicken Sweet Italian	3 oz	130
Organic Prairie		
Bratwurst Pork	1 (3 oz)	210
Shady Brook		
Turkey Bratwurst	3 oz	160
Turkey Breakfast	1 (2.3 oz)	80
Turkey Sweet Italian	1 (2.5 oz)	110
Soy Lean		
Pork Breakfast Patty	1 (2 oz)	75
Wampler		
Bratwurst as prep	1 (2.5 oz)	230
Breakfast Links as prep	2 (1.2 oz)	130
Breakfast Patties as prep	1 (1.1 oz)	120
Italian as prep	1 (2.5 oz)	230
Wellshire		
Andouille	1 link (3 oz)	197
Andouille Turkey	2 oz	59
Chorizo	1 piece (2 oz)	130
Chorizo Dried	1 oz	100
Italian Turkey Mild	1 link (2 oz)	70
Kielbasa Polska	1 piece (2 oz)	130
Kielbasa Turkey	1 piece (2 oz)	59
Turkey Maple Breakfast	1 link (2 oz)	70

SAUSAGE DISHES
TAKE-OUT

italian sausage w/ peppers & onions	1 cup	210
sausage roll	1 (2.3 oz)	311

SAUSAGE SUBSTITUTES

meatless	1 link (0.9 oz)	64
meatless	1 patty (1.3 oz)	98
Boca		
Bratwurst	1 (2.5 oz)	140
Breakfast Links	2 (1.6 oz)	70
Breakfast Patties	1 (1.3 oz)	60
Italian	1 (2.5 oz)	130
Gardenburger		
Veggie Breakfast	1 (1.5 oz)	45

FOOD	PORTION	CALS
Veggie Breakfast	1 patty (1.5 oz)	45
Lightlife		
Gimme Lean	2 oz	50
Smart Brats	1 (2 oz)	120
Smart Links Breakfast	2 (2 oz)	100
Smart Links Italian	1 (2 oz)	120
Smart Menu Breakfast Patty	1	45
Morningstar Farms		
Breakfast Patties	1 (1.3 oz)	80
Quorn		
Links	2 (1.6 oz)	70
Tofurky		
Turkey Beerbrats	1 (3.5 oz)	280
Turkey Breakfast Links	1 (1.6 oz)	130
Turkey Italian Sweet	1 (3.5 oz)	280
Turkey Kielbasa	1 (3.5 oz)	240
Worthington		
Saucettes Breakfast Links	1 (1.3 oz)	90
Yves		
Veggie Brats Classic	1 (3.3 oz)	160
SAVORY		
ground	1 tsp	4
SCALLOP		
raw	3 oz	75
Mrs. Paul's		
Fried	13 (3.7 oz)	260
TAKE-OUT		
breaded & fried	2 lg	67
SCONE		
King Arthur		
English Cream Tea Scone not prep	⅓ cup	180
TAKE-OUT		
apricot	1	232
blueberry	1 (3 oz)	270
cheese	1 (3.5 oz)	364
orange poppy	1 (3 oz)	260
plain	1 (3.5 oz)	362
raisin	1 (3 oz)	270

FOOD	PORTION	CALS
SCUP		
fresh baked	3 oz	115
SEA BASS (see BASS)		
SEA CUCUMBER		
dried	1 oz	74
fresh	1 oz	20
SEA URCHIN		
canned	1 oz	39
fresh	1 oz	36
roe paste	1 tbsp	19
SEATROUT (see TROUT)		
SEAWEED		
agar dried	1 oz	87
agar fresh	1 oz	tr
hijiki dried	1 tbsp	9
irish moss fresh	1 oz	14
kelp fresh	1 oz	12
kombu fresh	1 oz	12
laver fresh	1 oz	10
nori fresh	1 oz	10
nori sheet dried	1 (8 x 8 in)	5
seahair dried	1 tbsp	13
spirulina dried	1 oz	83
spirulina fresh	1 oz	7
tangle fresh	1 oz	12
wakame fresh	1 oz	13
Eden		
Agar Agar Bars	1 bar (7 g)	25
Agar Agar Flakes	1 tbsp	0
Arame Wild	½ cup	30
Hiziki Wild	½ cup	30
Kombu Wild	½ piece (3.3 g)	5
Nori Sheets	1 (2.5 g)	10
Organic Dulse Flakes	1 tsp	3
Maine Coast		
Organic Alaria Whole Leaf	⅓ cup	18
Organic Dulse Granules	1 tsp	6

FOOD	PORTION	CALS
Organic Dulse Whole Leaf	½ cup	19
Organic Kelp Granules	½ tsp	5
Organic Kelp Whole Leaf	⅓ cup	17
Organic Laver Whole Leaf	⅓ cup	22

SEITAN (see WHEAT)

SEMOLINA

dry	1 cup (5.9 oz)	601

SESAME

seeds	1 tsp	16
sesame butter	1 tbsp	95
sesame crunch candy	1 oz	146
sesame crunch candy	20 pieces (1.2 oz)	181
tahini from roasted & toasted kernels	1 tbsp	89
tahini from stone ground kernels	1 tbsp	86
tahini from unroasted kernels	1 tbsp	85
Arrowhead Mills		
Organic Seeds	¼ cup	210
Organic Tahini	2 tbsp	190
Mrs. May's		
Black Sesame Crunch	1 oz	165
Peloponnese		
Tahini	1 tbsp	100
Sabra		
Tahini Sauce Taratore	1 oz	80
Tree Of Life		
Organic Sesame Tahini	2 tbsp	108
Seeds	¼ cup (1.3 oz)	210

SESBANIA

flower	1	1
flowers	1 cup	5
flowers cooked	1 cup	23

SHAD

american baked	3 oz	214
cooked	1 oz	55
roe baked w/ butter & lemon	1 oz	36

SHALLOTS (see ONION)

FOOD	PORTION	CALS
SHARK		
fin dried	1 oz	32
raw	3 oz	111
TAKE-OUT		
batter-dipped & fried	3 oz	194
SHEEPSHEAD FISH		
cooked	3 oz	107
cooked	1 fillet (6.5 oz)	234
raw	3 oz	92
SHELLFISH (see individual names, SHELLFISH SUBSTITUTES)		
SHELLFISH SUBSTITUTES		
crab imitation	1 cup (4.4 oz)	144
scallop imitation	3 oz	84
shrimp imitation	3 oz	86
surimi	1 oz	28
surimi	3 oz	84
Chicken Of The Sea		
Imitation Crab	1 pkg (2.5 oz)	40
Louis Kemp		
Crab Delights	½ cup (3 oz)	80
Crab Delights Chunk Style	½ cup (3 oz)	80
Crab Delights Easy Shred	½ cup (3 oz)	80
Crab Delights Leg Style	½ cup (3 oz)	80
Lobster Delights Chunk or Salad Style	½ cup (3 oz)	80
Scallop Delights Bay Style	½ cup (3 oz)	80
TAKE-OUT		
crab salad	1 cup	395
SHELLIE BEANS		
canned	½ cup	37
SHERBET		
orange	½ cup (4 oz)	132
orange	½ gal	2158
orange	1 bar (2.75 oz)	91
Blue Bunny		
Cool Tubes Orange Sherbet	1 (3 oz)	110
Lime	½ cup	110
Rainbow	½ cup	110

FOOD	PORTION	CALS
Raspberry	½ cup	110
Ciao Bella		
Lemon	1 pkg (3.5 oz)	120
Mango	1 pkg (3.5 oz)	100
Raspberry	1 pkg (3.5 oz)	110
Dippin' Dots		
Lemon Lime	½ cup	97
Hola Fruta		
Bar Pomegranate & Blueberry	1 (2.5 oz)	100
Mango	½ cup	130
Margarita	½ cup	140
Peach	½ cup	130
Pomegranate	½ cup	140
Hood		
Orange Burst	½ cup	120
Land O Lakes		
Orange	½ cup (3.2 oz)	130
Turkey Hill		
Fruit Rainbow	½ cup	120
Orange Grove	½ cup	120
SHRIMP		
CANNED		
canned	1 can (6 oz)	136
chinese shrimp paste	1 tbsp	46
Bumble Bee		
Broken Shrimp	¼ cup	40
Small or Medium	¼ cup	40
Tiny	¼ cup	40
Chicken Of The Sea		
Tiny or Small or Medium	½ can (2 oz)	45
Polar		
Tiny Peeled	¼ cup (2 oz)	44
DRIED		
dried	10	15
FRESH		
broiled	6 med	46
steamed	6 med	41
FROZEN		
Blue Horizon Organic		
Garlic Shrimp	1 serv (3.5 oz)	160

FOOD	PORTION	CALS
Panko Shrimp	1 serv (3.5 oz)	160
Popcorn Shrimp	1 serv (3.5 oz)	160
Tempura Shrimp	1 serv (3.5 oz)	160
Chicken Of The Sea		
Cooked Large Peeled Deveined Tail On	3 oz	80
Large Raw Cleaned Tail Off	4 oz	120
Contessa		
Orange Shrimp	11–13 (6 oz)	250
Ragin' Cajun	8–10 (4 oz)	170
Shrimp Scampi	8–10 (4 oz)	290
Gorton's		
Popcorn Crunchy Golden	20 (3.2 oz)	240
Temptations Breaded Butterfly	5 (3.5 oz)	250
Temptations Scampi Sauced	1 serv (4 oz)	120
Margaritaville		
Calypso Coconut + Sauce	5 pieces	350
Island Lime	6 pieces	130
Jammin' Jerk	7 pieces	140
Paradise Cocktail + Sauce	5 pieces	85
Sunset Scampi	1 serv (½ pkg)	270
Surfside Skewers + Sauce	2 skewers	105
Mrs. Paul's		
Butterfly	7 (4 oz)	250
Phillips Seafood		
Breaded Shrimp	5 pieces	230
Buffalo Shrimp	5 pieces	260
Coconut Shrimp	5 pieces	330
Crab Stuffed Shrimp	3 pieces	160
Van de Kamp's		
Battered	6 (4 oz)	200
Breaded Popcorn	20 (4 oz)	260
TAKE-OUT		
breaded & fried	6 med (2.3 oz)	162
cocktail w/ sauce	4	87
curried	1 cup	295
gingered	4	80
jambalaya	1 cup	309
shrimp newburg	1 serv (6.4 oz)	456
shrimp salad	¾ cup	212
shrimp scampi	1 cup	310

FOOD	PORTION	CALS
shrimp w/ crab stuffing	5	158

SMELT
rainbow cooked	3 oz	106
rainbow raw	3 oz	83

SMOOTHIES (see also FRUIT DRINKS, YOGURT DRINKS)
8th Continent
Refresher Orange Pineapple Banana	8 oz	150
Refresher Strawberry Banana	8 oz	150

Arthur's
Carrot Energizer	1 bottle (11 oz)	200
Green Energy	1 bottle (11 oz)	230

Bolthouse Farms
Green Goodness	8 oz	140
Mango Lemonade	8 oz	120
Passion Fruit Apple Carrot Juice	8 oz	120
Strawberry Banana Fruit	8 oz	124

C&W
Berry Blend	½ cup	90
Peach	½ cup	80

E4B
100% Fruit Puree Blueberry Raspberry	4 oz	70
100% Fruit Puree Kiwi	4 oz	70
100% Fruit Puree Mango	4 oz	70
100% Fruit Puree Pear Caramel	4 oz	70
100% Fruit Puree Strawberry Banana	4 oz	70

Horizon Organic
Tropical Punch	1 bottle (6.2 oz)	120

Jammin' Juice
Mambo Mango	6 oz	92

Jammin' Nectars
C-Beta Carrot	6 oz	96
Ginger Party	6 oz	6
Guanabana Limbo	6 oz	78
Pure Passion	6 oz	78
Razz-Ade	6 oz	89

Kidz Dream
Orange Cream	1 box	120

LightFull
Satiety Smoothie Cafe Latte	1 (11 oz)	90

FOOD	PORTION	CALS
Satiety Smoothie Chocolate Fudge	1 (11 oz)	90
Satiety Smoothie Peaches & Cream	1 (11 oz)	100
Satiety Smoothie Strawberries & Cream	1 (11 oz)	90
Luna		
Berry Pomegranate	1 pkg	140
Orange Blossom	1 pkg	130
Vanilla Macadamia	1 pkg	150
Naked Juice		
Chocolate Karma	8 oz	190
Vanilla Chai	8 oz	170
Nutiva		
Organic HempShake Amazon Acai not prep	4 tbsp	100
Organic HempShake Chocolate not prep	4 tbsp	80
Odwalla		
Bluberry B Monster	8 oz	140
Citrus C Monster	8 oz	150
Mango Tango	8 oz	150
Sambazon		
Acai Amazon Cherry	8 oz	156
Acai Mango Banana	8 oz	190
Acai Mango Uprising	8 oz	190
Acai Protein Warrior Chocolate	8 oz	215
Acai Protein Warrior Vanilla	8 oz	215
Acai Shaman's Immunity	8 oz	90
Acai Soy Energy	8 oz	210
Acai Strawberry Sensation	8 oz	210
Acai Supergreens Revolution	8 oz	200
Organic Acai	1 bottle	155
Smooze		
Mango + Coconut	1 box (8.5 oz)	250
Passion Fruit + Coconut	1 box (8.5 oz)	225
Pineapple + Coconut	1 box (8.5 oz)	200
Soy Blendz		
Mango Orange Dream	1 bottle (10 oz)	220
Mixed Berry Medley	1 bottle (10 oz)	210
Orange Citrus Splash	1 bottle (10 oz)	220
Strawberry Banana Blast	1 bottle (10 oz)	230
Soy Fusion		
Berry	1 box (8.45 oz)	120
Matcha Green Tea	1 box (8.45 oz)	110

FOOD	PORTION	CALS
Tropicana		
Fruit Smoothie Mixed Berry	1 bottle (11 oz)	220
Fruit Smoothie Tropical Fruit	1 bottle (11 oz)	220
V8		
Splash Tropical Colada	8 oz	100
WholeSoy & Co.		
Organic Soy Peach	8 oz	210
Organic Soy Raspberry	8 oz	210
Organic Soy Strawberry	8 oz	210
SNACKS		
cheese puffs	1 oz	122
oriental mix	1 oz	155
pork skins	1 oz	154
pork skins barbecue	1 oz	152
Baken-ets		
Fried Pork Skins	9 pieces	80
Fried Pork Skins Hot'n Spicy	9 pieces	80
Fried Pork Skins Sweet & Tangy BBQ	9 pieces	80
Pork Cracklins	8 pieces	90
Pork Cracklins Hot'n Spicy	8 pieces	80
Barbara's Bakery		
Cheese Puffs Bakes Original	¾ cup	160
Cheese Puffs Original	¾ cup (1 oz)	150
Carole's		
Soycrunch Cinnamon & Raisins	½ cup	110
Soycrunch Original	½ cup	120
Soycrunch Toffee	½ cup	110
Cheetos		
Asteriods Go Snack	¾ cup (1 oz)	160
Baked Crunchy	34 pieces (1 oz)	130
Crunchy	1 pkg (1.25 oz)	200
Natural White Cheddar	32 pieces (1 oz)	150
Puffs	13 pieces (1 oz)	160
Twisted	7 pieces (1 oz)	160
Cheez It		
Right Bites Party Mix	1 pkg (0.74 oz)	100
Chester's		
Puffcorn Butter	3 cups	160
Puffcorn Cheese	3 cups	160

FOOD	PORTION	CALS
Funyuns		
Mini Onion Rings Go Snacks	1 pkg	260
Onion Rings	13 pieces	140
Garden Of Eatin'		
Organic Baked Cheese Puffs	32 pieces	150
Organic Baked Chunchitos	35 pieces	140
Good Sense		
Snack Mix Cajun Corn 'N Sesame	¼ cup	150
Kangaroo		
Pita Snackers Crispy Cinnamon	10 pieces (1 oz)	90
Pita Snackers Sea Salt	10 pieces (1 oz)	90
Lance		
Cheese Puffs	9 (1 oz)	170
Gold-N-Chees	1 oz	150
Michael Season's		
Cheese Puffs & Curls	1½ cups	180
Munchies		
Snack Mix Flamin' Hot	1 oz	140
Snack Mix Kids	1 oz	130
Robert's American Gourmet		
Booty Barbeque	1 oz	130
Booty Pirate's	1 oz	130
Booty Veggie	1 oz	130
Smart Puffs	1 oz	130
Tings	1 oz	160
Sabritones		
Chile & Lime	23 pieces	150
Snikiddy		
Puffs Grilled Cheese	1 pkg (0.6 oz)	80
Puffs Rockin' Ranch	1 pkg (0.6 oz)	83
Snyder's Of Hanover		
CheddAirs	1 oz	130
MultiGrain Cheese Puffs	1 oz	130
Tumaro's		
Organic Krispy Crunchy Puffs Cheddar	22	120
Organic Krispy Crunchy Puffs Natural Corn	22	120
Organic Krispy Crunchy Puffs Ranch & Herb	22	130
Organic Krispy Crunchy Puffs Tangy BBQ	22	120
Utz		
Cheese Balls	50 (1 oz)	150

FOOD	PORTION	CALS
Cheese Curls	18 (1 oz)	150
Onion Rings	41 (1 oz)	130
Party Mix	1 oz	150
Pork Cracklins	0.5 oz	90
Pork Rinds Original	0.5 oz	80
Wise		
Cheez Doodles Crunchy	1 pkg (1 oz)	150
Cheez Doodles Crunchy Reduced Fat	1 oz	130
Cheez Doodles Puffed	1 pkg (0.7 oz)	110
Doodle O's	1 oz	160
Onion Rings	1 oz	140
Pork Rinds Original	1 oz	90
SNAIL		
cooked	3 oz	233
raw	3 oz	117
TAKE-OUT		
escargot cooked	5	25
SNAKE		
fresh	3 oz	78
SNAPPER		
cooked	3 oz	109
cooked	1 fillet (6 oz)	217
raw	3 oz	85
SODA		
club	12 oz	0
cola	12 oz	151
cream	12 oz	191
diet cola	12 oz	2
ginger ale	12 oz can	124
grape	12 oz	161
lemon lime	12 oz	149
orange	12 oz	177
pepper type	12 oz	151
quinine	12 oz	125
root beer	12 oz	152
shirley temple	1 serv	159
tonic water	12 oz	125

FOOD	PORTION	CALS
7 Up		
Diet	8 oz	0
Original	8 oz	100
Plus	1 can (12 oz)	10
AJ Stephans		
Birch Beer	1 bottle	170
Black Cherry	1 bottle	180
Cream	1 bottle	170
Jamaican Style Ginger Beer	1 bottle	170
Lemon & Lime	1 bottle	190
Olde Style Root Beer	1 bottle	170
Ale 8 One		
Soft Drink	1 bottle (12 oz)	120
Barq's		
Diet French Vanilla Creme	8 oz	1
Diet Red Creme	8 oz	4
Diet Root Beer	8 oz	1
Floatz	8 oz	127
French Vanilla Creme	8 oz	112
Red Creme	8 oz	115
Root Beer	8 oz	111
Big Red		
Vanilla Float	1 can	180
Blumers		
Black Cherry	1 bottle (12 oz)	138
Blueberry Cream	1 bottle (12 oz)	190
Cream	1 bottle (12 oz)	181
Orange Cream	1 bottle (12 oz)	187
Root Beer	1 bottle (12 oz)	190
Bubble Yum		
All Flavors	8 oz	110
Cape Cod Dry		
Cranberry	8 oz	120
Diet Cranberry	8 oz	10
Carver's		
Ginger Ale	8 oz	94
Celsius		
Cola	1 bottle (12 oz)	5
Chronic 187		
Orange	1 bottle (12 oz)	300

FOOD	PORTION	CALS
Coca-Cola		
Blak	8 oz	46
C2	8 oz	45
Classic	8 oz	97
W/ Lime	8 oz	98
Coke		
Cherry	8 oz	104
Diet	8 oz	1
Diet Cherry	8 oz	1
Diet Plus	8 oz	0
Diet Vanilla	8 oz	1
Diet w/ Lime	8 oz	2
Vanilla	8 oz	100
Dr Pepper		
Original	1 can (12 oz)	150
DRY		
Juniper Berry	1 bottle (12 oz)	55
Lavender	1 bottle (12 oz)	70
Lemongrass	1 bottle (12 oz)	50
Vanilla Bean	1 bottle (12 oz)	60
Fanta		
Apple	8 oz	121
Citrus	8 oz	91
Orange	8 oz	111
Firefighter		
Backdraft Root Beer	8 oz	90
Courageous Cola	8 oz	90
Flashover Orange	8 oz	20
Incendiary Citrus	8 oz	90
Rolling Code Black Cherry	8 oz	90
Fresca		
Soda	8 oz	2
Frostie		
Diet Cherry Limeade	1 bottle (12 oz)	0
Diet Root Beer	1 bottle (12 oz)	0
Vanilla Root Beer	1 bottle (12 oz)	180
GuS		
Dry Cola	1 bottle (12 oz)	95
Dry Crimson Grape	1 bottle (12 oz)	90
Dry Pomegranate	1 bottle (12 oz)	98

FOOD	PORTION	CALS
Star Ruby Grapefruit	1 bottle (12 oz)	90
Hansen's		
Natural Creamy Root Beer	1 can (12 oz)	160
Health Cola		
Soda	1 bottle (12 oz)	140
Hiball		
Club	1 bottle (10 oz)	5
Tonic Water	1 bottle (10 oz)	120
IBC		
Cream	1 bottle (12 oz)	180
Inca Kola		
Diet	8 oz	1
Soda	8 oz	96
Jolt		
Blue	8 oz	120
Cherry Bomb	8 oz	90
Cola	8 oz	100
Red	8 oz	120
Ultra	8 oz	0
Jones Soda		
Blue Bubble Gum	1 bottle (12 oz)	190
Cream	1 bottle (12 oz)	190
Crushed Melon	1 bottle (12 oz)	190
FuFu Berry	1 bottle (12 oz)	190
Green Apple	1 bottle (12 oz)	180
Orange Cream	1 bottle (12 oz)	180
Lucozade		
Soda	7 oz	136
Maine Root		
All Flavors	1 bottle (12 oz)	165
Manzana Mia		
Soda	8 oz	99
Mello Yellow		
Diet	8 oz	3
Soda	8 oz	118
Mountain Dew		
Pitch Black	8 oz	110
Mr. Pibb		
Diet	8 oz	1

FOOD	PORTION	CALS
Nesbitt's		
Orange	1 bottle (12 oz)	190
Northern Neck		
Diet Ginger Ale	8 oz	4
Ginger Ale	8 oz	94
Nuky		
Rose Soda	8 oz	120
Nutrisoda		
Calm Sparkling Wild Berry & Citron	1 can (8.7 oz)	0
Flex Sparkling Black Cherry & Apple	1 can (8.7 oz)	5
Immune Sparkling Tangerine & Lime	1 can (8.7 oz)	15
Slender Sparkling Guava & Grapefruit	1 can (8.7 oz)	10
Olde Brooklyn		
Coney Island Cream	8 oz	130
Williamsburg Root Beer	8 oz	120
Oogave Natural		
All Flavors	8 oz	68
Pibb		
Zero	8 oz	2
Polar		
Birch Beer	8 oz	110
Bitter Lemon Mixer	8 oz	120
Collins Mixer	8 oz	90
Cream	8 oz	120
Diet Pomegranate Dry	8 oz	10
Orange	8 oz	130
Pomegranate Dry	8 oz	120
Seltzer All Flavors	8 oz	0
Strawberry	8 oz	120
Tonic Water	8 oz	90
Vichy Water	8 oz	0
Red Flash		
Soda	8 oz	105
Reed's		
Ginger Brew Original	1 bottle (12 oz)	145
Santa Cruz		
Organic Cherry	1 can	140
Organic Concord Grape	1 can	150
Organic Ginger Ale	1 can	150
Organic Lemon Lime	1 can	130

FOOD	PORTION	CALS
Organic Orange Mango	1 can	130
Organic Root Beer	1 can	150
Organic Vanilla Creme	1 can	160
Schweppes		
Ginger Ale	8 oz	120
Sex Kola		
Diet All Flavors	1 bottle (12 oz)	0
Sierra Mist		
Lemon Lime	1 can (12 oz)	140
Sioux City		
Cream	1 bottle (12 oz)	180
Orange Cream	1 bottle (12 oz)	200
Root Beer	1 bottle (12 oz)	170
Sarsaparilla	1 bottle (12 oz)	170
Snow		
Sparkling Mint	8 oz	75
Sprite		
Diet Zero	8 oz	0
ReMix Aruba Jam	8 oz	97
Soda	8 oz	96
Steaz		
Organic Green Tea Soda Cola	8 oz	90
Organic Green Tea Soda Diet Black Cherry	8 oz	20
Organic Green Tea Soda Ginger Ale	8 oz	90
Organic Green Tea Soda Lemon	8 oz	90
Stirrings		
Club	1 bottle (6.3 oz)	0
Ginger Ale	8 oz	120
Tonic Water	1 bottle (6.3 oz)	85
Sunkist		
Diet Orange	8 oz	0
Orange	8 oz	130
Tab		
Soda	8 oz	1
Tava		
Sparkling Brazilian Samba	8 oz	0
Sparkling Mediterranean Fiesta	8 oz	0
Thomas Kemper		
Black Cherry	1 bottle (12 oz)	170
Ginger Ale	1 bottle (12 oz)	150

FOOD	PORTION	CALS
Orange Cream	1 bottle (12 oz)	170
Root Beer	1 bottle (12 oz)	160
Root Beer Low Calorie	1 bottle (12 oz)	20
Vanilla Cream	1 bottle (12 oz)	150
Tommyknocker		
Almond Creme	1 bottle (12 oz)	150
Key Lime Creme	1 bottle (12 oz)	180
Orange Creme	1 bottle (12 oz)	180
Root Beer	1 bottle (12 oz)	150
Root Beer Float	1 bottle (12 oz)	110
Strawberry Creme	1 bottle (12 oz)	150
Tropicana		
Twister Orange	1 can (12 oz)	180
Uno Mas		
All Flavors	1 can (12 oz)	130
Vignette		
Wine Country Soda Chardonnay	1 bottle (12 oz)	130
Wine Country Soda Pinot Noir	1 bottle (12 oz)	130
Virgil's		
Micro Brewed Root Beer	1 bottle (12 oz)	160
White Rock		
Organics Raspberry Creme	1 can (12.4 oz)	120
Organics Red Peach	1 can (12.4 oz)	120
Windy City		
Root Beer	1 bottle (12 oz)	170
Z Cola		
No Artificial Sweeteners	8 oz	0

SOLE
cooked	3 oz	99
cooked	1 fillet (4.5 oz)	148
lemon raw	3.5 oz	85
TAKE-OUT		
breaded & fried	3.2 oz	211

SORGHUM
sorghum	1 cup (6.7 oz)	651

SOUFFLE
Heavenly Souffle
Chocolate	1 (2.6 oz)	262

FOOD	PORTION	CALS
TAKE-OUT		
cheese	1 cup	194
chicken	1 cup (5.6 oz)	278
corn	1 cup	257
lime chilled	1 cup	388
seafood	1 cup	245
spinach	1 cup	124
SOUP		
CANNED		
Allens		
Chicken Broth	1 cup	10
Butterball		
Chicken Broth 99% Fat Free	1 cup	10
Campbell's		
25% Less Sodium Chicken Noodle as prep	1 cup	60
25% Less Sodium Cream of Mushroom as prep	1 cup	110
98% Fat Free Cream Of Broccoli as prep	1 cup	70
98% Fat Free Cream Of Celery as prep	1 cup	60
98% Fat Free Cream Of Chicken as prep	1 cup	70
Cheddar Cheese as prep	1 cup	110
Chicken & Stars as prep	1 cup	70
Chicken Alphabet as prep	1 cup	70
Chicken Noodle O's as prep	1 cup	90
Chunky Beef and Country Vegetables	1 cup	150
Chunky Chicken Mushroom Chowder	1 cup	210
Chunky Grilled Chicken w/ Vegetables & Pasta	1 cup	100
Chunky Hearty Vegetable w/ Pasta	1 cup	120
Chunky New England Clam Chowder	1 cup	210
Chunky Roadhouse Beef & Bean Chili	1 cup	230
Chunky Sirloin Burger w/ Country Vegetables	1 cup	180
Curly Noodle as prep	1 cup	80
Double Noodle Chicken as prep	1 cup	110
Goldfish Pasta Meatball as prep	1 cup	90
Healthy Request Chicken Noodle as prep	1 cup	60
Healthy Request Chicken Rice as prep	1 cup	70
Healthy Request Cream Of Chicken as prep	1 cup	80
Healthy Request Italian Style Wedding	1 cup	120
Healthy Request Minestrone as prep	1 cup	80
Healthy Request Tomato as prep	1 cup	90

FOOD	PORTION	CALS
Low Sodium Chicken Broth	1 can	25
Mega Noodle as prep	1 cup	90
Microwavable Bowl Chicken Noodle	1 cup	70
Microwavable Bowl Vegetable	1 cup	110
Select Beef w/ Roasted Barley	1 cup	130
Select Blended Red Pepper Black Bean	1 cup	110
Select Chicken w/ Egg Noodles	1 cup	90
Select Honey Roasted Chicken w/ Golden Potatoes	1 cup	110
Select Italian Sausage w/ Pasta & Pepperoni	1 cup	150
Select Italian Style Wedding	1 cup	110
Select Mexican Chicken Tortilla	1 cup	130
Select Potato Broccoli Cheese	1 cup	120
Select Savory Chicken & Long Grain Rice	1 cup	90
Select Split Pea w/ Roasted Ham	1 cup	160
Select Vegetable Beef	1 cup	110
Select Harvest Chicken w/ Egg Noodles	1 cup	120
Select Harvest Tomato w/ Basil	1 cup	80
Select Harvest Light Savory Chicken w/ Vegetables	1 cup	80
Select Harvest Light Southwestern Style Vegetable	1 cup	50
Soup At Hand 25% Less Sodium Chicken w/ Mini Noodles	1 pkg (10.75 oz)	80
Soup At Hand Creamy Chicken	1 pkg (10.75 oz)	130
Soup At Hand Italian Style Wedding	1 pkg	90
Soup At Hand Vegetable Medley	1 pkg (10.75 oz)	100
Soup At Hand Velvety Potato	1 pkg (10.75 oz)	160
V8 Garden Broccoli	1 cup	80
V8 Golden Butternut Squash	1 cup	140
V8 Sweet Red Pepper	1 cup	120
V8 Tomato Herb	1 cup	90
College Inn		
Beef Broth Fat Free Lower Sodium	1 cup	15
Chicken Broth Light & Fat Free	1 cup	5
Comfort Care		
Hearty Beef Barley	1 cup (8 oz)	190
Savory Chicken	1 cup (8 oz)	200
Tomato Cheddar Jack	1 cup (8 oz)	90

FOOD	PORTION	CALS
Gold's		
Borscht Low Calorie	1 cup	20
Borscht Unsalted	1 cup	70
Hungarian Cabbage	6 oz	70
Schav	1 cup	15
Health Valley		
Beef Broth Fat Free	1 cup	10
Chicken Broth Fat Free	1 cup	20
Chicken Broth Fat Free No Salt Added	1 cup	35
Chicken Broth Low Fat	1 cup	35
Clam Chowder Manhattan	1 cup	90
Clam Chowder New England	1 cup	110
Corn & Vegetable Fat Free	1 cup	70
Garden Vegetable Fat Free	1 cup	80
Lentil & Carrot Fat Free	1 cup	100
Organic Black Bean	1 cup	130
Organic Cream Of Mushroom	1 cup	90
Organic Minestrone	1 cup	100
Organic Minestrone No Salt Added	1 cup	70
Organic Mushroom Barley	1 cup	70
Organic Mushroom Barley No Salt Added	1 cup	70
Organic Split Pea No Salt Added	1 cup	110
Organic Tomato	1 cup	80
Organic Tomato No Salt Added	1 cup	80
Tomato Vegetable Fat Free	1 cup	80
Vegetable Broth Fat Free	1 cup	20
Healthy Choice		
Bean & Ham	1 cup	180
Beef & Potato	1 cup	110
Chicken & Dumplings	1 cup	140
Chicken & Pasta	1 cup	110
Chicken Corn Chowder	1 cup	140
Chicken Fiesta	1 cup	100
Chicken w/ Rice	1 cup	90
Chicken w/ Roasted Garlic	1 cup	120
Chili Beef	1 cup	170
Clam Chowder	1 cup	110
Country Vegetable	1 cup (8.6 oz)	110
Creamy Tomato	1 cup	100
Garden Vegetable	1 cup	120

FOOD	PORTION	CALS
Hearty Chicken	1 cup	120
Italian Bean & Pasta	1 cup	100
Old Fashioned Chicken Noodle	1 cup	100
Roasted Italian Style Chicken	1 cup	120
Split Pea w/ Ham	1 cup	170
Turkey w/ Rice	1 cup	90
Vegetable Beef	1 cup	130
Vegetable Clam Chowder	1 cup	230
Zesty Gumbo	1 cup	100
Imagine		
Lobster Bisque	1 cup	130
Organic Creamy Butternut Squash	1 cup	90
Organic Creamy Chicken	1 cup	70
Organic Creamy Sweet Corn	1 cup	120
Organic Sweet Potato	1 cup	110
Organic Bistro Cuban Black Bean Bisque	1 cup	170
Organic Broth Beef	1 cup	20
Organic Broth Free Range Chicken	1 cup	10
Organic Broth Vegetable	8 oz	20
Lucini		
Roman Tomato Cream	1 cup (8.6 oz)	170
Umbrian Lentil	1 cup (8.6 oz)	160
Manischewitz		
Clear Chicken Condensed	½ cup	15
Muir Glen		
Organic Garden Vegetable	1 cup	80
Organic Southwest Black Bean	1 cup	140
Original SoupMan		
Italian Wedding	1 cup	120
New England Clam Chowder	1 cup	290
Organic Butternut Squash	1 cup	250
Tomato Basil	1 cup	140
Turkey Chili	1 cup	210
Pacific Foods		
Beef Broth	1 cup	20
Creamy Butternut Squash	1 cup	90
Creamy Roasted Carrot	1 cup	100
Creamy Roasted Red Pepper & Tomato	1 cup	100
Hearty Beef Barley	1 cup	110
Hearty Chicken Noodle	1 cup	80

FOOD	PORTION	CALS
Hearty Chicken Tortilla	1 cup	130
Hearty Roasted Red Pepper & Corn Chowder	1 cup	210
Organic Creamy Tomato	1 cup	100
Organic Free Range Chicken Broth	1 cup	10
Organic French Onion	1 cup	35
Organic Low Sodium Chicken Broth	1 cup	10
Organic Mushroom Broth	1 cup	5
Organic Vegetarian Broth	1 cup	15
Progresso		
40% Less Sodium Italian Style Wedding	1 cup (8.7 oz)	90
50% Less Sodium Garden Vegetable	1 cup (8.8 oz)	100
50% Less Sodium Zesty Chicken Gumbo	1 cup (8.7 oz)	110
Light Beef Pot Roast	1 cup (8.4 oz)	80
Light Chicken Vegetable Rotini	1 cup (8.3 oz)	70
Light Italian Style Vegetable	1 cup (8.6 oz)	60
Light Savory Vegetable Barley	1 cup (8.5 oz)	60
Light Vegetable	1 cup (8.4 oz)	60
Light Vegetable & Noodle	1 cup (8.7 oz)	60
Reduced Sodium Chicken Broth	1 cup (8.4 oz)	20
Rich & Hearty Beef Pot Roast	1 cup (8.7 oz)	120
Rich & Hearty Chicken & Homestyle Noodles	1 cup (8.6 oz)	100
Rich & Hearty Chicken Pot Pie	1 cup (8.6 oz)	170
Rich & Hearty Savory Beef Barley Vegetable	1 cup (8.6 oz)	130
Rich & Hearty Sirloin Steak & Vegetables	1 cup	130
Rich & Hearty Slow Cooked Vegetable Beef	1 cup (8.6 oz)	120
Rich & Hearty Steak & Roasted Russet Potatoes	1 cup (8.6 oz)	140
Traditional Beef & Vegetable	1 cup (8.7 oz)	120
Traditional Beef Barley	1 cup (8.5 oz)	120
Traditional Chickarina	1 cup (8.3 oz)	120
Traditional Chicken & Sausage Gumbo	1 cup (8.7 oz)	130
Traditional Chicken & Wild Rice	1 cup (8.4 oz)	100
Traditional Chicken Noodle	1 cup (8.3 oz)	100
Traditional Homestyle Chicken	1 cup (8.4 oz)	100
Traditional Italian Style Wedding	1 cup (8.4 oz)	100
Traditional Manhattan Clam Chowder	1 cup (8.4 oz)	100
Traditional New England Clam Chowder	1 cup (8.4 oz)	110
Traditional Potato Broccoli & Cheese	1 cup (8.8 oz)	180
Traditional Split Pea w/ Ham	1 cup (8.5 oz)	140
Traditional Turkey Noodle	1 cup (8.4 oz)	80
Vegetable Classics Creamy Mushroom	1 cup (8.1 oz)	130

FOOD	PORTION	CALS
Vegetable Classics French Onion	1 cup (8 oz)	50
Vegetable Classics Hearty Black Bean w/ Bacon	1 cup (8.5 oz)	160
Vegetable Classics Hearty Tomato	1 cup (8.6 oz)	110
Vegetable Classics Lentil	1 cup (8.5 oz)	150
Vegetable Classics Vegetable	1 cup (8.4 oz)	80
Rienzi		
Chicken & Rice	1 cup	110
Italian Wedding Bell	1 cup	130
Snow's		
Clam Chowder	1 cup (8.4 oz)	200
Swanson		
100% Fat Free Lower Sodium Beef Broth	1 cup	15
99% Fat Free 33% Less Sodium Chicken Broth	1 cup	15
Organic Beef Broth	1 cup	15
Organic Chicken Broth	1 cup	15
Organic Vegetable Broth	1 cup	15
Valley Fresh		
Chicken Broth	1 cup	30
Chicken Broth 40% Less Sodium	1 cup	15
Wolfgang Puck		
Chicken Parmesan w/ Pasta	1 cup	300
Hearty Lentil & Vegetable	1 cup	170
FROZEN		
Kettle Cuisine		
Angus Beef Steak Chili w/ Beans Gluten Free Dairy Free	1 pkg (10 oz)	250
Chicken w/ Rice Noodles Gluten Free	1 pkg (10 oz)	140
New England Clam Chowder Gluten Free	1 pkg (10 oz)	330
Roasted Vegetable Gluten Free Dairy Free	1 pkg (10 oz)	140
Phillips Seafood		
Cream Of Crab	1 cup	310
Shrimp Bisque	1 cup	280
Tabatchnick		
Barley Mushroom	1 serv (7.5 oz)	80
Chicken w/ Dumplings	1 serv (7.5 oz)	150
Cream Of Broccoli	1 serv (7.5 oz)	130
Macaroni & Cheese	1 serv (7.5 oz)	250
Minestrone	1 serv (7.5 oz)	100
No Salt Pea	1 serv (7.5 oz)	140

FOOD	PORTION	CALS
Old Fashioned Potato	1 serv (7.5 oz)	100
Southwest Bean	1 serv (7.5 oz)	220
Split Pea	1 serv (7.5 oz)	140
Vegetable	1 serv (7.5 oz)	90
Vegetarian Chili	1 serv (7.5 oz)	180
Wild Rice	1 serv (7.5 oz)	80
MIX		
beef broth cube	1 cube	6
chicken broth cube	1 cube (4.8 g)	9
A Taste Of Thai		
Coconut Ginger	2 tsp	15
Annie Chun's		
Noodle Bowl Chicken Noodle	1 pkg	260
Noodle Bowl Hot & Sour	1 pkg	280
Noodle Bowl Korean Kimchi	½ pkg	140
Noodle Bowl Miso	1 pkg	230
Noodle Bowl Thai Tom Yum	½ pkg	150
Noodle Bowl Udon	1 pkg	220
Azumaya		
Asian Style Thin Noodle	1 cup	120
Asian Style Wide Noodle	1 cup	120
Edward & Sons		
Bouillon Cubes Not-Beef	½ cube	20
Bouillon Cubes Not-Chicken	½ cube	15
Veggie Low Sodium	½ cup	20
Fantastic		
Noodle Bowl Hot & Sour as prep	2 cups	138
Noodle Bowl Miso w/ Tofu as prep	1 cup	100
Noodle Bowl Sesame Miso as prep	2 cups	90
Noodle Bowl Spring Vegetable as prep	2 cups	90
Noodle Soup Cup Vegetarian Chicken as prep	1 cup	90
Noodle Soup Spicy Thai as prep	2 cups	110
Soup Cup Italian Tomato as prep	2 cups	130
Soup Cup Mandarin Broccoli as prep	2 cups	110
HamBeens		
15 Bean as prep	½ cup	120
15 Bean Beef as prep	½ cup	120
15 Bean Cajun as prep	½ cup	120
15 Bean Chicken as prep	½ cup	120
Spanish American Black Bean as prep	½ cup	120

FOOD	PORTION	CALS
Health Valley		
Chicken Noodles w/ Vegetables	1 cup	110
Creamy Potato w/ Broccoli Fat Free	1 cup	80
Leahey Gardens		
No Beef Noodle	1½ cups	89
No Chicken Noodle	1½ cups	94
Manischewitz		
Matzo Ball Soup	1 cup	40
Southwestern Black Bean as prep	1 cup	90
Vegetable & Pasta as prep	1 cup	90
MiniCarb		
Miso w/ Tofu & Shiitake	1 pkg	33
Miso-Cup		
Golden Vegetable as prep	1 cup	30
Japanese Restaurant Style as prep	1 cup	60
Organic Traditional w/ Tofu as prep	1 cup	35
Reduced Sodium as prep	1 cup	25
Savory Seaweed as prep	1 cup	30
Nissin		
Chicken Vegetable as prep	1 pkg	290
White Cheddar as prep	1 pkg	290
Nueva Cocina		
Frijoles Negros Con Chipotle Chile	1 cup	140
Sopa De Calabaza	1 cup	180
Sopa De Frijoles Colorados	1 cup	140
Sopa De Frijoles Negros	1 cup	140
Sopa De Maiz	1 cup	150
Sopa De Tortilla	1 cup	140
San-J		
Miso Dark	1 pkg	40
Miso Mild	1 pkg	45
Simply Asia		
Soy Noodle Bowl	1 pkg	70
Streit's		
Matzo Ball as prep	1 cup	50
Uncle Ben's		
Black Bean & Rice as prep	1 cup	150
Broccoli Cheese & Rice as prep	1 cup	110

FOOD	PORTION	CALS
REFRIGERATED		
Moosewood		
Organic Creamy Potato & Corn Chowder	1 cup (8.4 oz)	170
Organic Hungarian Vegetable Noodle	1 cup (8.4 oz)	80
Organic Savannah Sweet Potato Bisque	1 cup (8.4 oz)	200
Organic Texas Two Bean Chili	1 cup (8.4 oz)	200
Organic Tuscan White Bean & Vegetable	1 cup (8.4 oz)	130
Organic Classics		
French Onion w/ Croutons	1 cup	140
Seafood Chowder	1 cup	160
TAKE-OUT		
ban mien fish head	1 serv (10 oz)	277
beef stew soup	1 cup (8.8 oz)	221
bird's nest	1 cup (8.6 oz)	112
black bean turtle soup	1 cup	241
broccoli cheese	1 cup	165
brunswick stew soup	1 cup (8.5 oz)	232
caldo de res beef soup	1 cup	143
chinese velvet corn	1¼ cups	135
corn & cheese chowder	¾ cup	215
duck soup	1 cup (8.6 oz)	412
egg drop	1 cup	73
gazpacho	1 cup	46
greek lemon	¾ cup	63
hot & sour	1 serv (14 oz)	173
matzo ball soup	1 cup	118
minestrone	1 cup	233
miso w/ tofu	1 cup	84
onion soup gratinee	1 serv	492
oxtail	1 cup	68
pasta e fagioli	1 cup (8.8 oz)	194
ratatouille	1 cup (7.5 oz)	266
shark fin	1 bowl (10 oz)	164
shrimp bisque	1 cup	263
sopa de albondigas	1 cup	171
thai lemon grass	1 bowl	100
vietnamese pho beef noodle	1 serv (7.8 oz)	480
wonton soup	1 cup	183
zupa koprowa polish dill soup	1 bowl	54

FOOD	PORTION	CALS
SOUR CREAM		
sour cream	1 tbsp (0.4 oz)	26
sour cream	1 cup (8 oz)	493
Cabot		
Light	2 tbsp	35
No Fat	2 tbsp	20
Sour Cream	2 tbsp	50
Daisy		
No Fat	2 tbsp	20
Sour Cream	2 tbsp	60
Friendship		
All Natural	2 tbsp (1 oz)	60
Light	1 tbsp (1 oz)	40
Nonfat	2 tbsp (1 oz)	25
Hood		
Fat Free	2 tbsp	20
Low Fat	2 tbsp	35
Sour Cream	2 tbsp	60
Horizon Organic		
Lowfat	2 tbsp	35
Sour Cream	2 tbsp	60
Land O Lakes		
Fat Free	2 tbsp (1.1 oz)	20
Light	2 tbsp (1.1 oz)	40
Sour Cream	2 tbsp (1.1 oz)	60
Nancy's		
Organic	2 tbsp	60
Organic Valley		
Lowfat	2 tbsp	40
SOUR CREAM SUBSTITUTES		
nondairy	1 oz	59
nondairy	1 cup	479
Vegan Gourmet		
Alternative Sour Cream	2 tbsp (1 oz)	50
SOURSOP		
fresh	1	416
fresh cut up	1 cup	150

FOOD	PORTION	CALS

SOY (see also CHEESE SUBSTITUTES, ICE CREAM AND FROZEN DESSERTS, MILK SUBSTITUTES, MISO, SMOOTHIES, SOY SAUCE, SOYBEANS, TEMPEH, TOFU, YOGURT FROZEN)

FOOD	PORTION	CALS
soya cheese	1.4 oz	128
Bob's Red Mill		
Protein Powder	1 tbsp	20
Good Sense		
Soynuts Honey Roasted	⅓ cup	140
Soynuts Roasted & Salted	⅓ cup	140
Soynuts Roasted w/o Salt	⅓ cup	140
Simple Food		
Soynut Butter Chocolate	2 tbsp	190
Soynut Butter No Sugar No Salt	2 tbsp	200
South Beach		
Soy Nuts Dark Chocolate	1 pkg (0.7 oz)	100
Soy Wonder		
Creamy Spread	2 tbsp	170

SOY DRINKS (see MILK SUBSTITUTES, SMOOTHIES)

SOY SAUCE

FOOD	PORTION	CALS
shoyu	1 tbsp	9
soy sauce	1 tbsp	7
tamari	1 tbsp	11
Eden		
Organic Shoyu	1 tbsp	15
Organic Shoyu Reduced Sodium	1 tbsp	10
Organic Tamari	1 tbsp	15
House Of Tsang		
Ginger Soy Sauce	1 tbsp	20
Less Sodium	1 tbsp	5
La Choy		
Lite	1 tbsp (0.5 oz)	15
San-J		
Shoyu Organic	1 tbsp	15
Tamari	1 tbsp	15
Tamari Organic Wheat Free	1 tbsp	15
Tamari Organic Wheat Free Reduced Sodium	1 tbsp	20
Tamari Reduced Sodium	1 tbsp	20
Soy Vay		
Wasablyaki	1 tbsp	35

FOOD	PORTION	CALS
Tree Of Life		
Organic Shoyu	1 tbsp (0.5 oz)	15
Organic Tamari Wheat Free	1 tbsp (0.5 oz)	15

SOYBEANS

FOOD	PORTION	CALS
dried cooked	1 cup	298
dry roasted	½ cup	387
green cooked	½ cup	127
roasted	½ cup	405
roasted & toasted	1 cup	490
roasted & toasted salted	1 cup	490
sprouts raw	½ cup	43
sprouts steamed	½ cup	38
sprouts stir fried	1 cup	125
Arrowhead Mills		
Organic Dried not prep	¼ cup	160
C&W		
In the Pod	½ cup	110
Eden		
Organic Blacksoy	½ cup	120
Frieda's		
Edamame	½ cup (2.6 oz)	100
Seapoint Farms		
Edamame Dry Roasted Goji Blend	¼ cup	120
Edamame Dry Roasted Lightly Salted	¼ cup	130
Edamame Dry Roasted Wasabi	¼ cup	130
Edamame In Pods frzn	½ cup	100
Edamame In Pods Lightly Salted	½ cup	100
Edamame Shelled	½ cup	100
Organic Edamame In Pods	½ cup	100
Organic Edamame Shelled	½ cup	100
Soyafarm		
Edamame Yuba Sticks	7 (2.5 oz)	123

SPAGHETTI (see PASTA, PASTA DINNERS, PASTA SALAD, SPAGHETTI SAUCE)

SPAGHETTI SAUCE
JARRED

FOOD	PORTION	CALS
marinara sauce	1 cup	171
spaghetti sauce	1 cup	272
Barilla		
Arrabbiata Tomato & Spicy Pepper	½ cup	90

FOOD	PORTION	CALS
Basilico Tomato & Basil	½ cup	70
Campagnola Roasted Garlic & Onion	½ cup	60
Garden Vegetable	½ cup	70
Green & Black Olive	½ cup	80
Mushroom & Garlic	½ cup	70
Rustica Sweet Peppers & Garlic	½ cup	70
Catelli		
Garden Select Country Mushroom	½ cup	80
Garden Select Diced Tomatoes & Basil	½ cup	80
Garden Select Fine Herbs	½ cup	80
Garden Select Garlic & Onion	½ cup	80
Garden Select Parmesan & Romano	½ cup	80
Garden Select Zucchini Primavera	½ cup	80
Classico		
Tomato & Basil	½ cup	60
Dei Fratelli		
Arrabbiata	½ cup (4.2 oz)	50
Pizza Sauce	¼ cup (2.2 oz)	30
Del Monte		
Chunky Garlic & Herb	½ cup	60
Chunky Italian Herb	½ cup	60
Garlic & Onion	½ cup	80
Tomato & Basil	½ cup	70
W/ Four Cheese	½ cup	70
W/ Green Peppers & Mushrooms	½ cup	80
W/ Meat	½ cup	60
W/ Mushrooms	½ cup	60
DelGrosso		
Aunt Linda's Arrabbiata Memories	½ cup	80
Uncle Bo's Roasted Red Pepper Tour	½ cup	80
Uncle Fred's Fireworks	½ cup	90
Uncle Jim's Late Night Puttanesca	½ cup	70
Eden		
Organic	½ cup	80
Organic No Salt	½ cup	80
Organic Pizza Pasta Sauce	½ cup	65
Emeril's		
Homestyle Marinara	½ cup	90
Roasted Gaaahlic	½ cup	70
Sicilian Gravy	½ cup	90

FOOD	PORTION	CALS
Vodka	½ cup	130
Francesco Rinaldi		
Chunky Garden Tomato Garlic & Onion	½ cup	70
Hearty Mushroom Pepper & Onion	½ cup	70
Three Cheese	½ cup	80
Traditional No Salt Added	½ cup	70
Hunt's		
Basil Garlic & Oregano	¼ cup	15
Cheese & Garlic	½ cup	50
Chunky Vegetable	½ cup	50
Family Favorites Lasagna	¼ cup	30
Family Favorites Pizza Sauce	¼ cup	25
Four Cheese	½ cup	50
Italian Sausage	½ cup	60
Light	½ cup	45
Meat	½ cup	60
No Added Sugar	½ cup	45
Roasted Garlic & Onion	½ cup	50
Traditional	½ cup	50
W/ Mushrooms	½ cup	45
Joey Pots & Pans		
Arrabbiata	½ cup	100
Marinara	½ cup	50
Vodka Sauce	½ cup	110
Knorr		
W/ Meat	4 oz	110
Lucini		
Rustic Tomato Basil	½ cup (4.4 oz)	80
Spicy Tuscan	½ cup (4.4 oz)	80
Milo's		
Portobello Shiraz	4 oz	40
Muir Glen		
Organic Chunky Tomato	¼ cup	15
Organic Garlic Roasted Garlic	½ cup	60
Organic Pizza Sauce	¼ cup	40
Organic Tomato Sauce No Salt Added	¼ cup	25
Newman's Own		
Bambolina	½ cup	90
Cabernet Marinara	½ cup	70
Five Cheese	½ cup	80

FOOD	PORTION	CALS
Italian Sausage & Peppers	½ cup	90
Marinara	½ cup	70
Marinara w/ Mushrooms	½ cup	70
Pesto & Tomato Sauce	½ cup	80
Roasted Garlic & Green Peppers	½ cup	70
Sockarooni	½ cup	70
Tomato & Roasted Garlic	½ cup	70
Vodka Sauce	½ cup	110
Pomi		
Marinara	½ cup	80
Prego		
100% Natural Roasted Garlic Parmesan	½ cup	100
Heart Smart Traditional Italian	½ cup	100
Italian	½ cup	70
Italian Marinara	½ cup	100
Italian Meat	½ cup	130
Italian Roasted Red Pepper & Garlic	½ cup	90
Italian Three Cheese	½ cup	80
Italian Tomato Basil & Garlic	½ cup	80
Organic Mushroom	½ cup	90
Progresso		
Lobster Sauce	½ cup (4.3 oz)	100
Red Clam w/ Tomato & Basil	½ cup (4.4 oz)	60
White Clam w/ Garlic & Herb	½ cup (4.4 oz)	120
Ragu		
Chunky Garden Style Tomato Garlic & Onion	½ cup (4.5 oz)	110
Fresh Italian	4 oz	110
Marinara	4 oz	100
Pizza Quick Fresh Italian	2 oz	35
Robert Rothschild Farm		
Artichoke	½ cup	80
Seeds Of Change		
Balsamic Olive & Onion	½ cup	80
Garden Vegetable	½ cup	70
Mushroom & Onion	½ cup	70
Three Cheese Marinara	½ cup	70
Traditional Herb	½ cup	70
Tuttorosso		
Pasta Sauce Meat	½ cup	90

FOOD	PORTION	CALS
Vino De Milo		
Mediterranean Pinot Grigio	½ cup	90
Portobello Shiraz	½ cup	40
Tuscan Merlot	½ cup	80
Walden Farms		
Alfredo Sauce Calorie Free	¼ cup	0
Marinara Calorie Free	⅓ cup	0
Walnut Acres		
Organic Garlic Garlic	½ cup	125
Organic Marinara & Zinfandel	½ cup	125
Organic Roasted Garlic	½ cup	125
Organic Tomato & Basil	½ cup	125
REFRIGERATED		
Buitoni		
Alfredo	¼ cup	140
Alfredo Light	¼ cup	80
Alfredo Portabello Mushroom	¼ cup	100
Marinara	½ cup	80
Marinara Roasted Garlic	½ cup	60
Pesto	¼ cup	330
Pesto w/ Basil	¼ cup	300
Pesto w/ Basil Reduced Fat	¼ cup	230
Pesto w/ Sun Dried Tomatoes	¼ cup	210
Tomato Herb Parmesan	½ cup	120
TAKE-OUT		
bolognese	5 oz	195
SPANISH FOOD		
FROZEN		
Cedarlane		
Organic Burrito Low Fat Rice & Cheese	1 (6 oz)	260
Organic Enchilada Low Fat Black Bean & Tofu	1 (9 oz)	220
Roasted Chile Relleno	1 pkg (10 oz)	400
Zone Burrito Beans & Cheese	1 (6 oz)	350
Contessa		
Fajitas Shrimp	2 (8 oz)	230
Paella w/ Chicken & Seafood	1½ cups	200
Seafood Veracruz not prep	1¾ cups	180
El Monterey		
Burrito Bean & Cheese	1 (5 oz)	280
Burrito Beef & Bean	1 (5 oz)	370

FOOD	PORTION	CALS
Burrito Half Pound Spicy Red Hot Beef & Bean	1 (8 oz)	600
Burrito Supreme Breakfast Egg Cheese & Sausage	1 (4.5 oz)	300
Burrito Supreme Shredded Steak & Cheese	1 (5 oz)	290
Burrito XX Large Bean & Cheese	1 (10 oz)	590
Burrito XX Large Beef & Bean	1 (10 oz)	730
Cruncheros Cheese & Beef	3 (4.5 oz)	330
Cruncheros Taco Beef & Cheese	4 (5.6 oz)	460
Enchiladas Cheese w/ Sauce	1 serv (8 oz)	250
Enchiladas Shredded Beef w/ Sauce	1 serv (4 oz)	140
Quesadillas Chicken & Cheese	2 (6 oz)	380
Quesadillas Steak & Cheese	2 (6 oz)	400
Tamales Chicken	1 (4.5 oz)	240
Tamales Shredded Beef	1 (4.5 oz)	310
Taquitos Corn Shredded Beef	3 (4.5 oz)	300
Taquitos Flour Char-Broiled Chicken Breast	3 (5 oz)	380
Taquitos Flour Chicken & Cheese	3 (4.5 oz)	350
Taquitos Southwest Chicken In A Seasoned Batter	2 (2.8 oz)	175
Tornados Apple Cinnamon	1 (3 oz)	180
Tornados Sausage Egg & Cheese	1 (3 oz)	230
Tornados Shredded Beef	1 (3 oz)	210
Tornados Steak Egg & Cheese	1 (3 oz)	170
Tornados Xxl Southwest Chicken	1 (4.2 oz)	210
Healthy Choice		
Enchilada Chicken	1 pkg	300
Helen's Kitchen		
Cheese Enchiladas w/ Tofu Steaks In Spicy Red Sauce	½ pkg (5 oz)	150
Jose Ole		
Burrito Beef & Cheese	1 (5 oz)	300
Burrito Chicken	1 (5 oz)	270
Chimichanga Chicken & Cheese	1 (5 oz)	330
Chimichanga Shredded Beef	1 (5 oz)	350
Mini Burrito Chicken & Cheese	3	200
Mini Chimichanga Beef & Cheddar	3	240
Mini Quesadilla Grilled Chicken	3	220
Mini Tacos Beef & Cheese	4	200
Mini Taquitos Beef & Cheese	4	180
Soft Taco Beef & Cheese	1 (5 oz)	280

FOOD	PORTION	CALS
Taquitos Beef & Cheese Flour Tortilla	2	220
Taquitos Buffalo Chicken Flour Tortilla	2	200
Taquitos Chicken Flour Tortilla	3	180
Taquitos Chicken & Cheese Flour Tortilla	2	220
Taquitos Pepperoni Pizza Flour Tortilla	2	240
Taquitos Shredded Beef Corn Tortilla	3	180
Lean Cuisine		
One Dish Favorites Chicken Enchilada	1 pkg (9 oz)	280
Patio		
Burrito Bean & Cheese	1 (5 oz)	280
Burrito Beef & Bean Medium	1 (5 oz)	300
Burrito Chicken	1 (5 oz)	280
Stouffer's		
Chicken Enchilada w/ Cheese Sauce & Rice	1 pkg (7.13 oz)	280
Tyson		
Meal Kit Chicken Fajita	1 (3.8 oz)	130
Meal Kit Quesadilla Chicken	1 (4 oz)	250
READY-TO-EAT		
taco shell corn	1 (6.5 inch)	98
taco shell flour	1 (7 inch)	173
Ortega		
Tostada Shells	2 (1 oz)	140
SHELF-STABLE		
Fantastic		
Spanish Paella	1 pkg (8 oz)	280
TAKE-OUT		
arroz con coco	1 cup	532
burrito w/ beans	1 med (5 oz)	295
burrito w/ beans & rice	1 (3.5 oz)	221
burrito w/ beef	1 sm (3.4 oz)	297
burrito w/ beef & beans	1 med (5 oz)	331
burrito w/ beef beans & cheese	1 med (5 oz)	379
burrito w/ chicken & beans	1 med (5 oz)	295
burrito w/ pork & beans	1 med (5 oz)	320
chiles rellenos meat & cheese filled	1 (5 oz)	213
chimichanga w/ bean cheese lettuce & tomato	1 (4.1 oz)	271
chimichanga w/ beef & rice	1 (10 oz)	634
chimichanga w/ beef beans lettuce & tomato	1 (4.1 oz)	254
chimichanga w/ beef cheese lettuce & tomato	1 (4.1 oz)	337

FOOD	PORTION	CALS
chimichanga w/ chicken sour cream lettuce & tomato	1 (4 oz)	277
empanada sweet potato	1 (7.8 oz)	546
enchilada w/ beans	1 (4.1 oz)	179
enchilada w/ beans & cheese	1 (4.6 oz)	233
enchilada w/ beef	1 (4 oz)	214
enchilada w/ beef & beans	1 (4 oz)	195
frijoles	1 cup	278
frijoles w/ cheese	1 cup	225
nachos w/ beans & cheese	1 serv (9.4 oz)	616
nachos w/ beef beans cheese & sour cream	1 serv (19 oz)	1620
paella	1 serv (7 oz)	308
pupusa meat filled	1 (3.6 oz)	187
quesadilla w/ cheese	1 (5 oz)	498
quesadilla w/ meat & cheese	1 (6.5 oz)	605
taco de jueye w/ crab meat	1 (4.2 oz)	266
taco w/ beans lettuce tomato & salsa	1 (2.8 oz)	117
taco w/ chicken lettuce tomato & salsa	1 (2.5 oz)	114
taco w/ fish lettuce tomato & salsa	1 (2.7 oz)	101
tostada w/ beef lettuce tomato & salsa	1 (2.7 oz)	143

SPICES (see individual names, HERBS/SPICES)

SPINACH
CANNED

drained	1 cup	49
Del Monte		
Whole Leaf	½ cup	30
Freshlike		
Cut Leaf	½ cup	45
Popeye		
Leaf Spinach	½ cup	30
Leaf Spinach No Salt Added	½ cup	40
FRESH		
baby raw	2 cups	20
cooked	1 cup	41
malabar cooked	1 cup	10
mustard cooked	1 cup	29
new zealand cooked	1 cup	22
raw	1 cup	7

FOOD	PORTION	CALS
Fresh Express		
Baby Spinach	3 cups	20
Organic Baby Spinach	3 cups	35
FROZEN		
chopped cooked	1 cup	30
Birds Eye		
Chopped	⅓ cup	20
C&W		
Baby Chopped	1 cup	30
Creamed	½ cup	100
Cascadian Farm		
Organic Cut	⅓ cup	25
Cedarlane		
Organic Spanakopita Spinach & Feta Pie	½ pkg (5 oz)	260
Dr. Praeger's		
Spinach Bites	2 (2 oz)	110
Fillo Factory		
Spanakopita Spinach & Cheese Fillo Appetizers	3 (3 oz)	190
Green Giant		
No Sauce	½ cup	25
Stouffer's		
Creamed	½ pkg (4.5 oz)	200
Taverna		
Spinach Pie	1 piece (4.8 oz)	190
TAKE-OUT		
indian saag	1 serv	28
spanakopita spinach pie	1 serv (3 oz)	148
SPINACH JUICE		
juice	7 oz	14
SPORTS DRINKS (see ENERGY DRINKS)		
SPOT		
baked	3 oz	134
SPROUTS		
kidney bean	½ cup	27
lentil sprouts	½ cup	40
mung bean	½ cup	16
mung bean canned	½ cup	8

FOOD	PORTION	CALS
mung bean cooked	½ cup	13
pea	½ cup	77
radish	½ cup	8
Brassica		
Broccoli Sprouts	½ cup (1 oz)	16
La Choy		
Bean Sprouts	⅔ cup	15
TAKE-OUT		
mung bean stir fried	½ cup	31

SQUAB

boneless baked	1 (4 oz)	242

SQUASH (*see also* SQUASH SEEDS, ZUCCHINI)

CANNED		
crookneck sliced	½ cup	14
Farmer's Market		
Organic Butternut	½ cup	50
Sunshine		
Slice Yellow	½ cup	25
FRESH		
acorn cooked mashed	½ cup	41
acorn cubed baked	½ cup	57
butternut baked	½ cup	41
crookneck sliced cooked	½ cup	18
hubbard baked	½ cup	51
hubbard cooked mashed	½ cup	35
scallop sliced cooked	½ cup	14
spaghetti cooked	½ cup	23
Frieda's		
Acorn	¾ cup (3 oz)	35
Baby Crookneck	⅔ cup (3 oz)	15
Baby Scallop	⅔ cup (3 oz)	15
Eight Ball	2 (4.4 oz)	18
Hubbard	¾ cup (3 oz)	35
Mini Pumpkin	¾ cup (3 oz)	20
Spaghetti	¾ cup (3 oz)	30
Star Spangled	⅔ cup (3 oz)	20
Turban	¾ cup (3 oz)	30
Glory		
Yellow Sliced	¾ cup	20

FOOD	PORTION	CALS
FROZEN		
butternut cooked mashed	½ cup	47
crookneck sliced cooked	½ cup	24
C&W		
Butternut	½ cup	45
McKenzie's		
Southland Butternut	½ cup	70
TAKE-OUT		
fritter	1 (0.8 oz)	81
squash pie	1 slice (5.4 oz)	291
SQUASH SEEDS		
dried	1 oz	154
roasted	1 oz	148
salted & roasted	1 oz	148
whole roasted	1 oz	127
SQUID		
baked	1 cup	192
canned in its own ink	1 can (4 oz)	122
dried	1 sm (1.5 oz)	147
pickled	1 oz	26
steamed	1 cup	147
Contessa		
Calamari + Sauce	13 pieces + 2 tbsp sauce	160
Margaritaville		
Captain's Calamari Strips + Sauce	⅓ pkg	330
Van de Kamp's		
Fried Calamari	15 pieces (4 oz)	270
TAKE-OUT		
arroz con calamares	1 cup	400
calamari breaded & fried	1 cup	296
SQUIRREL		
roasted	3 oz	147
STARFRUIT		
fresh	1	42
Frieda's		
Dried	⅓ cup (1.4 oz)	120

FOOD	PORTION	CALS
STRAWBERRIES		
canned in heavy syrup	½ cup	117
fresh halves	1 cup	49
fresh whole	1 cup	46
fresh whole	1 pint	114
frzn sweetened sliced	½ cup	122
frzn whole unsweetened	1 cup	77
organic fresh whole	8 med	45
whole sweetened frzn	1 cup	199
C&W		
Ultimate Sliced frzn	⅔ cup	50
Chukar Cherries		
Dried	¼ cup	120
Emily's		
Dark Chocolate Covered	6 (1.4 oz)	170
Europe's Best		
Sliced frzn	¾ cup	40
Frieda's		
Dried	½ cup (1.4 oz)	150
LiteHouse		
Glaze Sugar Free	3 tbsp	35
Marie's		
Glaze	2 tbsp	40
Polar		
Strawberries In Syrup	½ cup	90
STRAWBERRY JUICE		
Adina		
California Kiss Hibiscus Strawberry	8 oz	80
Giant Berry Farms		
Just Strawberries	1 bottle (12 oz)	140
Nesquik		
Strawberry Powder no prep	2 tbsp (0.6 oz)	60
STUFFING/DRESSING		
Fresh Gourmet		
All Natural Multi-Grain w/ Cranberries not prep	⅓ cup (1 oz)	110
Organic Seasoned not prep	⅓ cup (1 oz)	110
Kellogg's		
Stuffing Mix as prep	1 cup	240

FOOD	PORTION	CALS
Pepperidge Farm		
Corn Bread	¾ cup	170
Cube	¾ cup	140
Herb Seasoned	¾ cup	170
One Step Turkey	½ cup	170
Tofurky		
Wild Rice & Mushroom	½ cup	110
Zatarain's		
Creole Chicken as prep	½ cup	100
French Bread as prep	½ cup	100
TAKE-OUT		
bread	1 cup	352
cornbread	½ cup	179
kishke stuffed derma	1 piece (1.3 oz)	166
oyster	1 cup	304
sausage	½ cup	292
STURGEON		
broiled	3 oz	115
roe raw	1 oz	59
smoked	1 oz	49
TAKE-OUT		
breaded & fried	4 oz	252
SUCKER		
white baked	3 oz	101
SUGAR (*see also* FRUCTOSE, SYRUP)		
brown organic	1 tsp	17
brown packed	1 cup (7.7 oz)	828
brown unpacked	1 cup (5.1 oz)	547
cinnamon sugar	1 tsp	16
cube	1 (2 g)	9
maple	1 piece (1 oz)	99
powdered	1 tbsp (0.3 oz)	31
powdered unsifted	1 cup (4.2 oz)	467
raw	1 pkg (5 g)	19
sugarcane stem	3 oz	54
white	1 packet (3 g)	12
white	1 tsp (4 g)	15
white	1 tbsp (0.4 oz)	49
white	1 cup (7 oz)	773

FOOD	PORTION	CALS
Bob's Red Mill		
Date Sugar	1 tsp	11
Turbinado	1 tsp	10
Domino		
Dark Brown	1 tsp	15
Demerara Raw Cane	1 tsp	15
Organic Cane Sugar	1 tsp	15
White	1 tsp	15
Equinox		
Organic Maple Flakes	2 tsp	15
Gluco Burst		
Arctic Cherry	1 pkg (1.3 oz)	70
Sugar In The Raw		
Turbinado Sugar	1 pkg (5 g)	20
Tree Of Life		
Date Sugar	1 tsp (4 g)	10
Organic Cane Juice Dehydrated	1 tsp (3.5 g)	15
Turbinado	1 tsp (4 g)	15
Wholesome Sweeteners		
Organic Fair Trade Dark Brown	1 tsp	15
Organic Fair Trade Powdered	¼ cup	120
Organic Fair Trade Sucanat	1 tsp	15
Organic Turbinado	1 tsp	15
SUGAR SUBSTITUTES		
Equal		
Flavor Sticks	1 pkg	0
Packet	1 pkg	0
Spoonful	1 tsp	0
Sugar Lite	1 tsp	8
Fructevia		
All Natural	1 tsp (4 g)	5
Nature's Family		
Sun Crystals	1 pkg (4.5 g)	4
Nevella		
Mo Calorie Sweetener	1 tsp	0
Neway		
Sweet Sensation	¼ tsp	0
Splenda		
Flavor Blends All Flavors	1 pkg	0
No Calorie Granules	1 tsp	0

FOOD	PORTION	CALS
Sugar Blend For Baking	½ tsp	10
Sweetener	1 pkg	0
Stevia In The Raw		
100% Natural Sweetener	1 pkg (1 g)	0
Steviva		
Blend	1 tbsp (0.4 oz)	2
Sun Crystals		
Natural Sweetener	1 pkg (5 g)	4
Sweet Fiber		
All Natural	1 pkg	0
Sweet Simplicity		
Sweetener	1 pkg	0
Sweete		
Sugar Free	1 pkg	0
SweetLeaf		
SteviaPlus	1 pkg	0
Truvia		
Calorie Free Sweetener	1 pkg (3.5 g)	0
Whey Low		
Gold	1 tsp	4
Granular	1 tsp	4
Maple Buzz	¼ cup	57
Powder	1 tsp	4
Wholesome Sweeteners		
Organic Zero	1 pkg (6 g)	0
ZSweet		
All Natural	1 pkg (1 g)	0
SUGAR-APPLE		
fresh	1	146
fresh cut up	1 cup	236
SUNCHOKE		
fresh raw sliced	½ cup	57
Frieda's		
Sunchoke	½ cup (3 oz)	70
SUNFISH		
pumpkinseed baked	3 oz	97
SUNFLOWER		
seeds dry roasted w/ salt	¼ cup	186

FOOD	PORTION	CALS
seeds dry roasted w/o salt	¼ cup	186
seeds w/ hulls dried	¼ cup	66
Arrowhead Mills		
Organic Seeds	¼ cup	170
Bob's Red Mill		
Seeds Roasted & Salted	3 tbsp	186
Dakota Gourmet		
Seeds Honey Roasted	¼ cup (1 oz)	170
David		
Kernels Original	¼ cup	200
Seeds BBQ	¼ cup	190
Seeds BBQ Sizzlin	¼ cup	190
Seeds Jalapeno	¼ cup	190
Seeds Nacho Cheese	¼ cup	180
Seeds Original	¼ cup	190
Seeds Ranch	¼ cup	190
Seeds Reduced Sodium	¼ cup	190
Frito Lay		
Seeds	3 tbsp	180
Good Sense		
Nuts Honey Roasted	¼ cup	190
Nuts Raw	¼ cup	170
Nuts Roasted & Salted	¼ cup	190
Seeds In Shell Roasted & Salted	½ cup	150
Sunflower Nuts Roasted w/o Salt	¼ cup	190
Lance		
Shelled Seeds	1 pkg (1.8 oz)	300
SunButter		
Creamy	2 tbsp	200
Organic	2 tbsp	203
SunGold		
Seeds Roasted Salted	1 oz	172
Tree Of Life		
Seeds Kernels Raw	¼ cup (1.3 oz)	210
SUSHI		
TAKE-OUT		
cucumber roll	1 (1.1 oz)	43
inari	1 sm	46
prawn cooked	1 (1.1 oz)	36
roll california	1 (1.2 oz)	48

FOOD	PORTION	CALS
roll fresh salmon	4 pieces	250
roll preserved radish	3 (1 oz)	27
roll seaweed	1 (1.1 oz)	43
roll tuna	1 (1.1 oz)	37
roll vegetable	1 (1.2 oz)	27
roll yellowtain	1 (0.6 oz)	25
saba	1 (0.8 oz)	33
sashimi	1 serv (6 oz)	198
scallop cooked	1 (1 oz)	43
seasoned jellyfish	1 (1.2 oz)	58
sweet beancurd	1 (1.2 oz)	64
unagi	1 (1 oz)	540
vinegared ginger	⅓ cup (1.6 oz)	48
wasabi	2 tsp (0.3 oz)	5

SWAMP CABBAGE
chopped cooked w/o salt	1 cup	20

SWEET POTATO (see also YAM)
baked w/ skin w/o salt	1 med (4 oz)	103
baked w/ skin w/o salt	1 lg (6.3 oz)	162
canned in syrup	½ cup	106
canned mashed	½ cup	129
leaves cooked w/o salt	1 cup	22
paste dulce de calabaza	1 oz	82
Diner's Choice		
Mashed	⅔ cup	160
Dr. Praeger's		
Sweet Potato Bites	2 (2 oz)	110
Farmer's Market		
Organic Puree	½ cup	96
Glory		
Casserole	½ cup	180
Cut Fresh	1 serv (5 oz)	140
Sweet Potatoes	⅔ cup	160
Green Giant		
Candied	¾ cup	240
Ian's		
Fries	7 (2.5 oz)	70
Mann's		
Fresh Cubes	1 serv (3 oz)	60

FOOD	PORTION	CALS
Mrs. Paul's		
Candied	1 serv (5 oz)	300
Princella		
In Light Syrup	⅔ cup	160
Mashed	⅔ cup	120
Royal Prince		
Candied	½ cup	210
Trappey's		
Sugary Sam Cut Sweet	⅔ cup	160
Tree Of Life		
Organic Puree	½ cup (4.5 oz)	130
TAKE-OUT		
candied	1 serv (3.7 oz)	151
white fried batata blanca frita	1 serv (8 oz)	792
SWEETBREAD (PANCREAS)		
beef braised	3 oz	230
lamb braised	3 oz	199
pork braised	3 oz	186
veal braised	3 oz	218
Rumba		
Beef	4 oz	260
SWISS CHARD		
cooked	½ cup	18
raw chopped	½ cup	3
Frieda's		
Bright Lights	1 cup (3 oz)	15
SWORDFISH		
cooked	3 oz	132
raw	3 oz	103
SYRUP		
corn dark & light	¼ cup	240
date	1 tbsp	63
maple	1 cup (11.1 oz)	824
maple	1 tbsp	52
raspberry	1 oz	76
rose hip	1 oz	9
sorghum	1 tbsp (0.7 oz)	61
sorghum	1 cup (11.6 oz)	957

FOOD	PORTION	CALS
sugar syrup	¼ cup	76
Cary's		
Maple	¼ cup	210
Sugar Free	¼ cup	30
Eden		
Organic Barley Malt	1 tbsp	60
Estee		
Blueberry	¼ cup	30
Karo		
Corn Syrup Dark	2 tbsp	120
Corn Syrup Light	2 tbsp	120
Lundberg		
Organic Sweet Dreams Brown Rice	2 tbsp	110
Navitas Naturals		
Yacon	2 tbsp	90
Nesquik		
Strawberry Calcium Fortified	2 tbsp (1.4 oz)	110
Neway		
Sweet Sensation Luo Han Guo Syrup	1 tsp	8
Pacifica Culinaria		
Pomegranate	1 tbsp	60
Watermelon	1 tbsp	60
Smucker's		
Blackberry	¼ cup	210
Blueberry	¼ cup	210
Boysenberry	¼ cup	210
Red Raspberry	¼ cup	210
Strawberry	¼ cup	210
Sundae Syrup 3 Musketeers	2 tbsp	110
Sundae Syrup Butterscotch	2 tbsp	100
Sundae Syrup Caramel	2 tbsp	100
Sundae Syrup Strawberry	2 tbsp	110
Spectrum		
Balsamic Organic	1 tbsp	35
Tree Of Life		
Maple Grade A	¼ cup	200
Wholesome Sweeteners		
Organic Blue Agave	1 tbsp	60
Organic Corn Syrup	2 tbsp	120

TAHINI (see SESAME)

FOOD	PORTION	CALS
TAMARILLOS		
Frieda's		
Gold or Red	2 (4.2 oz)	40
TAMARIND		
dried sweetened pulpitas	½ cup	279
dried sweetened pulpitas	1 piece (0.8 oz)	56
fresh	1 (2 g)	5
fresh cut up	1 cup	143
TAMARIND JUICE		
nectar	1 cup	143
TANGERINE		
CANNED		
in light syrup	1 cup	154
juice pack	1 cup	92
FRESH		
fresh	1 sm (2.7 oz)	40
fresh	1 med (3.1 oz)	47
fresh	1 lg (4.2 oz)	64
sections	1 cup	103
River Pride		
Sweet	1 (3.8 oz)	50
Sunkist		
Fresh	1 (3.8 oz)	50
TANGERINE JUICE		
canned sweetened	1 cup	124
fresh	1 cup	106
Italian Volcano		
Organic	1 serv (6.75 oz)	94
Naked Juice		
Tangerine Scream	8 oz	110
Odwalla		
100% Juice	8 oz	110
Ssips		
Drink	1 box (7 oz)	120
TAPIOCA		
pearl dry	¼ cup (1.3 oz)	136
starch	1 oz	98

FOOD	PORTION	CALS
Let's Do Organic		
Granulated	1 tbsp	35
Starch	1 tbsp	0
TARO		
chips	10 (0.8 oz)	115
leaves cooked	½ cup	18
raw sliced	½ cup	56
shoots sliced cooked	½ cup	10
sliced cooked	½ cup (2.3 oz)	94
tahitian sliced cooked	½ cup	30
Frieda's		
Taro Root	⅔ cup (3 oz)	90
TARPON		
fresh	3 oz	87
TARRAGON		
dried crumbled	1 tsp	2
ground	1 tsp	5
TEA/HERBAL TEA (*see also* ICED TEA)		
HERBAL		
chamomile brewed	1 cup	2
Celestial Seasonings		
Chamomile	1 cup	0
Dessert Tea English Toffee	1 cup	0
Moroccan Pomegranate Red	1 cup	0
Peppermint	1 cup	0
Red Safari Spice	1 cup	0
Roastaroma Herb	1 cup	0
Wellness Tea Ginseng Energy	1 tea bag	0
Zinger Acai Mango	1 cup	0
Zinger Lemon	1 cup	0
Eden		
Organic Genmaicha Tea	1 tea bag	0
Organic Kukicha Tea	1 tea bag	0
Lipton		
Cinnamon Apple	1 tea bag	0
Ginger Twist	1 tea bag	0
Honey Lemon	1 tea bag	0
Lemon	1 tea bag	0

FOOD	PORTION	CALS
Mango	1 tea bag	0
Orange	1 tea bag	0
Peach	1 tea bag	0
Peppermint	1 tea bag	0
Quietly Chamomile	1 tea bag	0
Raspberry	1 tea bag	0
Tetley		
Chamomile	1 cup	0
Orange & Peach	1 cup	0
Peppermint	1 cup	0
REGULAR		
brewed tea	6 oz	2
Celestial Seasonings		
Black Decaf Victorian Earl Grey	1 cup	0
Black Fast Lane	1 cup	0
Chai White Honey Vanilla	1 tea bag	0
Green	1 cup	0
Green Antioxidant	1 cup	0
Green Tropical Acai	1 cup	0
Morning Thunder	1 cup	0
TeaHouse Chai Cinnamon Spice as prep	1 serv	110
White Tea Antioxidant Plum	1 tea bag	0
Daily Detox		
Original	1 tea bag	0
Eden		
Organic Bancha Green Tea	1 tea bag	0
Organic Hojicha Tea	1 tea bag	0
General Foods		
International Tea Chai Latte	1 serv	70
Lipton		
Black Tea as prep	1 tea bag	0
Black Tea French Vanilla	1 tea bag	0
Black Tea Honey & Lemon	1 tea bag	0
Black Tea Mint	1 tea bag	0
Black Tea Orange & Spice	1 tea bag	0
Black Tea Spiced Chai	1 tea bag	0
Decaffeinated Black Tea as prep	1 serv	0
Earl Grey	1 tea bag	0
English Breakfast	1 tea bag	0
English Estate	1 tea bag	0

FOOD	PORTION	CALS
Green Tea as prep	1 tea bag	0
Green Tea Citrus Blossom	1 tea bag	5
Green Tea Decaffeinated	1 tea bag	0
Green Tea Lemon Ginseng	1 tea bag	0
Green Tea Mint	1 tea bag	0
Raspberry Truffle	1 tea bag	0
Vanilla Hazelnut	1 tea bag	0
Oregon Chai		
Chai Tea Latte Original Caffeine Free Concentrate	½ cup	78
Chai Tea Latte Original Concentrate	½ cup	78
Chai Tea Latte Spiced Original Mix	1 pkg	100
Chai Tea Latte Vanilla Mix	1 pkg	120
Organic Chai Cider Concentrate	½ cup	110
Organic Chai Nog Concentrate	½ cup	90
Red Rose		
Black Tea Tea Bag	1	0
Decaffeinated	1 cup	0
English Breakfast Tea Bag	1 cup	0
Salada		
Original Blend Black Tea	1 tea bag	0
Tea Tech		
Instant Green Tea All Flavors	1 tube	0
XtraGreen Tea Mix All Flavors	1 tube	0
Tetley		
Chai Black Tea	1 cup	0
Earl Grey	1 cup	0
English Breakfast	1 cup	0
Honey Lemon Green Tea	1 cup	0
TEMPEH		
tempeh	½ cup	165
Lightlife		
Garden Veggie	1 serv (4 oz)	230
Organic Flax	1 serv (4 oz)	230
Organic Grilles Lemon	1 patty (2.7 oz)	140
Organic Grilles Tamari	1 patty (2.7 oz)	130
Organic Soy	1 serv (4 oz)	210
Organic Three Grain	1 serv (4 oz)	240
Organic Wild Rice	1 serv (4 oz)	280

FOOD	PORTION	CALS
Tofurky		
Edamame Veggie	3 oz	145
Five Grain	3 oz	190
Soy	3 oz	160
WildWood		
Organic Nori Seaweed	3 oz	170
TESTICLES		
prairie oysters cooked	1 pair (6.8 oz)	241
THYME		
dried crumbled	1 tsp	3
fresh	1 tsp	1
ground	1 tsp	4
TILAPIA		
Beacon Light		
Farm Raised Fillets	3 oz	85
Gorton's		
Fillets Crunchy Breaded frzn	1 (3 oz)	80
Van de Kamp's		
Lightly Breaded Fillets	1 (4 oz)	240
TAKE-OUT		
battered & fried	1 fillet (4 oz)	206
breaded & fried	1 fillet (4 oz)	300
broiled w/o fat	1 fillet (3.5 oz)	128
TILEFISH		
cooked	3 oz	125
cooked	½ fillet (5.3 oz)	220
raw	3 oz	81
TOFU		
firm	¼ block (3 oz)	118
firm	½ cup	183
fresh fried	1 piece (0.5 oz)	35
fuyu salted & fermented	1 block (⅓ oz)	13
koyadofu dried frozen	1 piece (½ oz)	82
okara	½ cup	47
regular	¼ block (4 oz)	88
regular	½ cup	94
Azumaya		
Extra Firm	1 serv (2.8 oz)	70

FOOD	PORTION	CALS
Firm	1 serv (2.8 oz)	70
Lite Extra Firm	1 serv (2.8 oz)	60
Lite Silken	1 serv (3.2 oz)	40
Seasoned Oriental Spice	1 serv (3 oz)	90
Seasoned Zesty Garlic & Onion	1 serv (3 oz)	90
Silken	1 serv (3.2 oz)	40
Eden		
Dried	1 piece (0.4 oz)	50
House		
Atsu-Age Cutlet	1 (2.5 oz)	100
Cut-Age Shredded Fried	1 serv (0.5 oz)	50
Ganmodoki Fritter Small	3 (1.6 oz)	120
Medium Firm	3 oz	60
Organic Extra Firm	3 oz	90
Organic Firm	3 oz	60
Soft Silken	3 oz	50
Steak Cajun	1 (3 oz)	40
Steak Grilled	1 (3 oz)	90
Sukui	3 oz	45
Tokusen Kinugoshi	1 piece (5 oz)	90
Yaki Broiled	3 oz	90
Nasoya		
Chinese Spice	¼ pkg (3 oz)	90
Extra Firm	⅕ pkg (2.8 oz)	80
Firm	⅕ pkg (2.8 oz)	70
Garlic & Onion	¼ pkg (3 oz)	90
Lite Firm	⅕ pkg (2.8 oz)	40
Lite Silken	⅕ pkg (3.2 oz)	30
Seasoned Ginger Sesame	½ pkg (5.5 oz)	210
Seasoned Sweet & Sour	½ pkg (5.5 oz)	190
Seasoned Teriyaki	½ pkg (5.5 oz)	190
Seasoned Thai Peanut	½ pkg (5.5 oz)	240
Silken	⅕ pkg (3.2 oz)	45
Soft	⅕ pkg (2.8 oz)	60
TofuMate Breakfast Scramble	¼ pkg	15
TofuMate Eggless Salad	¼ pkg	15
TofuMate Mandarin Stirfry	¼ pkg	25
TofuMate Mediterranean Herb	¼ pkg	15
TofuMate Szechwan Stirfry	¼ pkg	25
TofuMate Texas Taco	¼ pkg	15

FOOD	PORTION	CALS
Soyafarm		
Baked Tofu	10 pieces (3.5 oz)	147
Nuggets	4 (3.5 oz)	162
Tofu & Yuba Patties	1 (3.5 oz)	243
Tree Of Life		
Organic Firm	½ block (3.2 oz)	110
WildWood		
Organic Baked Aloha	1 piece (3.5 oz)	180
Organic Calcium Rich Medium	3 oz	70
Organic Golden Pineapple Teriyaki	3 oz	160
Organic High Protein Super Firm	3 oz	100
Organic Smoked Mild Szechuan	3 oz	150
TAKE-OUT		
breaded deep fried w/ soy sauce japanese style	1 piece (0.4 oz)	15
soy sauce marinated & grilled	1 serv (4 oz)	181
TOMATILLO		
fresh	1 (1.2 oz)	11
fresh chopped	½ cup	21
Las Palmas		
Tomatillos Crushed	½ cup	45
TOMATO		
CANNED		
paste	½ cup	110
puree	1 cup	102
puree w/o salt	1 cup	102
red whole	½ cup	24
sauce	½ cup	37
sauce spanish style	½ cup	40
sauce w/ mushrooms	½ cup	42
sauce w/ onion	½ cup	52
stewed	½ cup	34
w/ green chiles	½ cup	18
wedges in tomato juice	½ cup	34
Cento		
Crushed	¼ cup	35
Paste	2 tbsp (1.2 oz)	30
Puree	¼ cup	25

FOOD	PORTION	CALS
Contadina		
Crushed w/ Italian Herbs	¼ cup	20
Paste Italian Herbs	2 tbsp	35
Petite Cut Diced	½ cup	25
Dei Fratelli		
Chopped Italian Tomatoes	½ cup (4.3 oz)	40
Del Monte		
Chunky Pasta Style	½ cup	45
Diced No Salt Added	½ cup	25
Diced w/ Garlic & Onion	½ cup	40
Diced w/ Green Pepper & Onion	½ cup	40
Diced Zesty Chili Style	½ cup	30
Diced Zesty w/ Mild Green Chilies	½ cup	30
Garden Select Petite Diced	½ cup	15
Organic Diced	½ cup	25
Organic Diced w/ Basil Garlic & Oregano	½ cup	50
Organic Tomato Paste	2 tbsp	30
Petite Cut	½ cup	25
Petite Cut Garlic & Olive Oil	½ cup	45
Sauce	¼ cup	20
Stewed Cajun Recipe	½ cup	35
Stewed Italian Recipe	½ cup	30
Stewed Mexican Recipe	½ cup	35
Stewed No Salt Added	½ cup	35
Stewed Original	½ cup	35
Wedges	½ cup	35
Eden		
Organic Crushed	¼ cup	20
Organic Diced	½ cup	30
Organic Whole Roma	½ cup	30
Hunt's		
Crushed	½ cup	30
Diced In Tomato Sauce	½ cup	30
Diced Original	½ cup	20
Diced w/ Basil Garlic & Oregano	½ cup	35
Diced w/ Green Pepper Celery & Onions	½ cup	45
Diced w/ Mild Green Chilies	½ cup	30
Diced w/ Roasted Garlic	½ cup	30
Diced w/ Sweet Onion	½ cup	45
Family Favorites Meatloaf	¼ cup	30

FOOD	PORTION	CALS
Paste	2 tbsp	25
Paste No Salt Added	2 tbsp	30
Paste w/ Basil Garlic & Oregano	2 tbsp	25
Petite Diced w/ Mushrooms	½ cup	40
Puree	½ cup	30
Sauce	¼ cup	15
Sauce Garlic & Herb	½ cup	40
Sauce No Salt Added	2 tbsp	30
Sauce Roasted Garlic	¼ cup	15
Stewed	½ cup	35
Stewed No Salt Added	½ cup	40
Whole No Salt Added	¼ cup	20
Muir Glen		
Organic Chunky Tomato & Herb	½ cup	60
Organic Diced Fire Roasted	½ cup	30
Organic Diced w/ Basil & Garlic	½ cup	30
Polar		
Grape	½ cup	50
Pomi		
Chopped	½ cup	20
Progresso		
Crushed w/ Added Puree	¼ cup (2.1 oz)	20
Diced	½ cup (4.4 oz)	25
Puree	¼ cup (2.2 oz)	25
Whole Peeled w/ Basil	½ cup (4.2 oz)	20
Redpack		
Crushed In Puree	¼ cup	20
Diced In Juice	½ cup	25
Paste	2 tbsp	0
Petite Diced Onion Celery & Green Pepper	½ cup	45
Rienzi		
Paste	2 tbsp	25
Ro-Tel		
Diced In Sauce	½ cup	40
Mexican Festival	½ cup	30
Original	½ cup	20
Tillen Farms		
Sunnyside Tomatoes	3 pieces (1 oz)	40
Tuttorosso		
Puree	¼ cup	20

FOOD	PORTION	CALS
DRIED		
sun dried	1 piece	5
sun dried	1 cup	140
sun dried in oil	1 cup (4 oz)	235
sun dried in oil	1 piece (3 g)	6
Frieda's		
Red Chopped	⅓ cup (1.1 oz)	100
FRESH		
bruschetta	¼ cup	50
cooked	½ cup	32
grape tomatoes	20	30
green	1	30
red	1 (4.5 oz)	26
red chopped	1 cup	35
Earthbound Farm		
Organic Roma	1 med (5.2 oz)	35
Eurofresh		
Tomatoes On The Vine	1 med (5.2 oz)	35
Foxy		
Roma	1 med (5 oz)	35
Frieda's		
Baby Roma	⅔ cup (3 oz)	120
Tear Drop	⅔ cup (3 oz)	20
TAKE-OUT		
bruschetta on toasted italian bread	1 slice	106
stewed	1 cup	80
TOMATO JUICE		
beef broth & tomato	1 can (5.5 oz)	62
clam & tomato	1 can (5.5 oz)	77
tomato juice	6 oz	32
tomato juice	½ cup	21
Campbell's		
Healthy Request	8 oz	50
Low Sodium	8 oz	50
Organic	8 oz	50
Dei Fratelli		
Tomato Juice	8 oz	40
Del Monte		
Juice	8 oz	50

FOOD	PORTION	CALS
Kagome		
Sweet Summer	8 oz	50
Lakewood		
Organic	8 oz	35
Luvli Juices		
Smashing Tomato	1 bottle (10 oz)	125
Spicy Tomato	1 bottle (10 oz)	125
Tree Of Life		
Organic 100% Juice	8 oz	50
TONGUE		
beef simmered	3 oz	241
lamb braised	3 oz	234
pork braised	3 oz	230
veal braised	3 oz	172
Rumba		
Beef	4 oz	250
TORTILLA		
corn	1 (6 in diam)	56
corn w/o salt	1 (6 in diam)	56
flour w/o salt	1 (8 in diam)	114
Alvarado Street Bakery		
Sprouted Wheat Burrito Size	1 (2.2 oz)	170
Food For Life		
Sprouted Corn	2 (1.7 oz)	120
French Meadow Bakery		
Organic Fat Flush	1 (1 oz)	100
La Tortilla Factory		
Carb Cutting Original	1 (1.3 oz)	60
Organic Yellow Corn	2 (2.4 oz)	120
Smart & Delicious Low Fat Low Sodium	1 (2.5 oz)	150
Manny's		
Burrito Tortilla	1 (2.1 oz)	180
Fajita Tortilla	1 (2 oz)	170
Fat Free	1 (1 oz)	65
Low Carb	1 (1.7 oz)	140
Soft Taco Tortilla	1 (1 oz)	80
Tortilla Wrap Tomato Basil	1 (1.4 oz)	100
White Corn Gluten Free	1 (2 oz)	60
Whole Wheat	1 (2 oz)	170

FOOD	PORTION	CALS
Rudi's Organic Bakery		
Spelt	1 (2 oz)	140
Salba Smart		
Whole Wheat Omega-3 Enriched	1 (1.5 oz)	120
Super Bakery		
Organic	1 (2.5 oz)	210
Tumaro's		
Honey Wheat	1 (8 in)	110
Low In Carbs Garden Vegetable	1 (8 in)	100
Low In Carbs Green Onion	1 (8 in)	100
Low In Carbs Multi Grain	1 (8 in)	100
Low In Carbs Salsa	1 (8 in)	100
Pesto & Garlic	1 (8 in)	110
Premium White	1 (8 in)	120
Soy-full Heart 8 Grain 'N Soy	1 (1.4 oz)	100
Soy-full Heart Apple 'N Cinnamon	1 (1.4 oz)	90
Soy-full Heart Wheat Soy & Flax	1 (1.4 oz)	90
Spinach & Vegetables	1 (8 in)	110

TORTILLA CHIPS *(see CHIPS)*

TRAIL MIX
FOOD	PORTION	CALS
Enjoy Life		
Gluten Free Not Nuts! Beach Bash	1 oz	130
Gluten Free Not Nuts! Mountain Mambo	1 oz	140
Good Sense		
Dietary Snack Mix	¼ cup	130
Organic Tropical	⅓ cup	160
Kopali		
Organic Mix	½ pkg (1 oz)	130
Mrs. May's		
Coconut Almond Crunch	1 oz	183
Navitas Naturals		
3 Berry Cacao Nibs & Cashews	1 oz	110
Goji Cacao Nibs & Cashews	1 oz	120
Goji Golden Berry & Mulberry	1 oz	90
Organic Trails		
Summit Blend	¼ cup	150
Planters		
Berry Nut & Chocolate	3 tbsp (1 oz)	120

FOOD	PORTION	CALS
SunRise		
Honey Coated	3 tbsp (1 oz)	137
W/ Fruit	3 tbsp (1 oz)	130
TREE FERN		
chopped cooked	½ cup	28
TRIPE		
beef simmered	3 oz	80
Rumba		
Beef Tripe	4 oz	110
TAKE-OUT		
mondongo w/ potatoes	1 cup	300
TRITICALE		
dry	½ cup (3.4 oz)	323
TROUT		
baked	3 oz	162
rainbow cooked	3 oz	129
seatrout baked	3 oz	113
TRUFFLES		
fresh	0.5 oz	4
TUNA		
CANNED		
light in oil	3 oz	169
light in oil	1 can (6 oz)	399
light in water	3 oz	99
light in water	1 can (5.8 oz)	192
white in oil	3 oz	158
white in oil	1 can (6.2 oz)	331
white in water	3 oz	116
white in water	1 can (6 oz)	234
Bumble Bee		
Chunk Light In Oil	¼ cup	110
Chunk Light In Water	2 oz	60
Chunk Light Touch Of Lemon In Water	¼ cup	60
Chunk White In Oil	¼ cup	100
Chunk White In Water	¼ cup	60
Chunk White In Water Very Low Sodium	¼ cup	70
Light In Oil	¼ cup	110

FOOD	PORTION	CALS
Sensations Lemon & Pepper w/ Crackers	1 pkg (3.6 oz)	200
Solid White In Oil	¼ cup	90
Solid White In Water	2 oz	70
Tonno In Olive Oil	¼ cup	120
Chicken Of The Sea		
Albacore Solid In Water	2 oz	70
Chunk Light In Oil	2 oz	110
Chunk White Low Sodium In Spring Water	1 can (3 oz)	80
Chunk White In Spring Water	½ can	60
Premium Albacore Pouch	2 oz	60
Coral		
Light In Water	¼ cup	60
Polar		
Albacore Solid White In Water	2 oz	70
Chunk Light In Water	2 oz	60
Progresso		
Albacore Solid White Olive Oil	¼ cup (2 oz)	90
Solid Light Olive Oil drained	¼ cup (2 oz)	120
StarKist		
Chunk Light In Water	¼ cup (2 oz)	60
Chunk Light In Water Flavor Pouch	1 pkg (3 oz)	90
Low Sodium Chunk White In Water	¼ cup (2 oz)	60
Solid Light In Water	2 oz	60
Solid White Albacore In Water	2 oz	70
Tuna Creations Hickory Smoked Flavor Pouch	2 oz	60
Tree Of Life		
Wild Light Tongol Chunk In Spring Water No Salt Added	¼ cup (2.4 oz)	50
FRESH		
bluefin cooked	3 oz	157
bluefin raw	3 oz	122
skipjack baked	3 oz	112
yellowfin baked	3 oz	118
MIX		
Chicken Of The Sea		
Salad Kit	1 serv (3.5 oz)	380
Tuna Salad Kit Single Mayo & Onion	1 pkg	380
StarKist		
Lunch To-Go Chunk Light	1 pkg	310

FOOD	PORTION	CALS
Tuna Helper		
Creamy Broccoli as prep	1 cup	310
Creamy Pasta as prep	1 cup	320
Tetrazzini as prep	1 cup	290
SHELF-STABLE		
Bumble Bee		
Steak Entrees Ginger & Soy	1 pkg (4 oz)	170
Steak Entrees Lemon & Cracked Pepper	1 pkg (4 oz)	160
Steak Entrees Mesquite Grilled	1 pkg (4 oz)	150
TAKE-OUT		
tuna salad	1 cup	383

TURBOT

FOOD	PORTION	CALS
european baked	3 oz	104

TURKEY (see also JERKY, TURKEY DISHES, TURKEY SUBSTITUTES)

FOOD	PORTION	CALS
CANNED		
w/ broth	1 cup	220
Valley Fresh		
Chunk White	2 oz	80
FRESH		
breast pre-basted w/ skin roasted	3.5 oz	126
breast w/ skin roasted	4 oz	212
dark meat w/o skin roasted	3 oz	170
dark meat w/o skin roasted	1 cup (5 oz)	262
ground cooked	3 oz	193
leg w/ skin roasted	1 (19 oz)	1136
light meat w/ skin roasted half turkey	2.3 lbs	2069
light meat w/o skin roasted	4 oz	183
neck simmered	1 (5.3 oz)	274
skin roasted	1 oz	141
skin roasted from half turkey	8.7 oz	1096
tail cooked	1 (2 oz)	197
w/ skin roasted	1 serv (8.4 oz)	498
w/ skin roasted	½ turkey (4 lbs)	3857
w/o skin roasted	1 cup (5 oz)	238
w/o skin roasted	1 serv (7.3 oz)	354
wing w/ skin roasted	1 (6.5 oz)	426
wing w/o skin roasted	1	237
Butterball		
Burger Patties	1 (4 oz)	150

FOOD	PORTION	CALS
Cutlets	4 oz	120
Drumstick	4 oz	170
Ground 7% Fat	4 oz	150
Ground White	4 oz	130
Strips	4 oz	120
Thighs	4 oz	170
Wings	1 (6.3 oz)	380
Honeysuckle White		
85% Lean Ground	4 oz	240
93% Lean Patties	1 (4 oz)	160
97% Lean Ground White	4 oz	130
99% Fat Free Breast Cutlets	4 oz	120
99% Fat Free Breast Tenderloin	4 oz	120
Drumettes	4 oz	180
Marinated Strips Asian Grill	4 oz	160
Necks	4 oz	150
Tenderloins Creamy Dijon Mustard	4 oz	140
Tenderloins Homestyle	4 oz	130
Tenderloins Teriyaki	4 oz	140
Thighs	4 oz	190
Whole Honey Roasted	4 oz	180
Wings	4 oz	220
Jennie-O		
Ground	4 oz	160
Shady Brook		
Breast Cutlets	4 oz	110
Breast Tenderloin	4 oz	130
Breast Tenderloin Creamy Dijon Mustard	4 oz	140
Breast Tenderloin Teriyaki	4 oz	140
Ground 85% Lean	4 oz	220
Ground 93% Lean	4 oz	160
Ground 99% Lean	4 oz	120
Marinated Strips Asian Grill	4 oz	160
Marinated Strips Mild Herb	4 oz	130
Necks	4 oz	150
Tenderloins Turkey Breast Homestyle	4 oz	130
Thigh	4 oz	145
Whole Turkey	4 oz	180
Wing	4 oz	210

FOOD	PORTION	CALS
FROZEN		
roast boneless seasoned light & dark meat roasted	3.5 oz	155
sticks breaded fried	1 (2.2 oz)	179
Butterball		
Boneless Roast	4 oz	130
Breast Boneless Roast	4 oz	110
Breast Tenderloin Teriyaki	4 oz	110
Breast Whole	4 oz	110
Breast Whole Smoked Cooked	3 oz	120
Whole Turkey	1 serv (4 oz)	170
Whole Turkey Baked	3 oz	130
Honeysuckle White		
Breast Boneless Roast	4 oz	170
Jennie-O		
Burger	1 (4 oz)	160
Organic Prairie		
Whole Young	4 oz	190
READY-TO-EAT		
bologna	1 slice (1 oz)	59
breast	1 slice (0.7 oz)	22
ham	1 slice (1 oz)	35
pastrami	2 oz	70
salami	1 slice (1 oz)	48
Applegate Farms		
Organic Herb	2 oz	50
Boar's Head		
Breast 50% Lower Sodium Skin On	2 oz	60
Breast Cracked Pepper Smoked	2 oz	60
Breast Hickory Smoked Black Forest	2 oz	60
Breast Maple Glazed Honey Coat	2 oz	70
Breast Ovengold	2 oz	60
Breast Ovengold Skinless	2 oz	60
Breast Roasted Mesquite Smoked Skinless	2 oz	60
Breast Roasted Salsalito	2 oz	60
Butterball		
Breast Honey Roasted Thick Sliced	1 slice (1 oz)	35
Breast Oven Roasted Extra Thin Sliced	7 slices (2 oz)	70
Breast Smoked Thin Sliced	4 slices (1.9 oz)	70
Breast Strips Oven Roasted	½ pkg (3 oz)	90

FOOD	PORTION	CALS
Deep Fried Original Thick Sliced	1 slice (1 oz)	30
Carl Buddig		
Honey Roasted Sliced	2 oz	90
Turkey Sliced	2 oz	90
Healthy Choice		
Smoked Breast	4 slices (1.8 oz)	60
Healthy Ones		
Oven Roasted 97% Fat Free	7 slices (2 oz)	60
Hebrew National		
98% Fat Free Oven Roasted	5 slices (2 oz)	50
98% Fat Free Smoked Breast	5 slices (2 oz)	60
Honeysuckle White		
Simply Done Whole Breast	4 oz	160
Jordan's		
Fat Free Turkey Breast	1 slice (1 oz)	25
Organic Prairie		
Roasted Breast Slices	2 oz	60
Oscar Mayer		
Breast Smoked Shaved	2 oz	50
Russer		
Turkey Breast Honey Roasted	1 slice (1 oz)	25
Sara Lee		
Breast Cracked Pepper	4 slices (1.8 oz)	50
Breast Hardwood Smoked	4 slices (1.8 oz)	50
Shady Brook		
Breast Bone-In Oven Roasted	3 oz	160
Hickory Smoked Breast Fat Free	2 oz	50
Turkey Ham Smoked	2 oz	60
Whole Oven Roasted	3 oz	160
Tyson		
Breast Oven Roasted	2 slices (1.6 oz)	40

TURKEY DISHES
FROZEN

gravy & turkey	1 cup (8.4 oz)	160

READY-TO-EAT
Jennie-O

Stuffed Breast Cheddar Cheese & Broccoli	1 serv (6 oz)	240

FOOD	PORTION	CALS
READY-TO-EAT		
Perdue		
Meal Time Starters Turkey Breast Roast w/ Homestyle Gravy	½ cup (4.6 oz)	144
TAKE-OUT		
a la king	1 cup (8.5 oz)	465
boneless breast w/ cranberry apple stuffing	1 serv (5 oz)	260
creole w/o rice	1 cup	189
croquette	1 (2 oz)	158
divan	1 cup	321
fricassee	1 cup	322
meatloaf	1 lg slice (5 oz)	243
salad	1 cup	417
tetrazzini	1 cup	369

TURKEY SUBSTITUTES
Lightlife

FOOD	PORTION	CALS
Smart Deli Roast Turkey	4 slices (2 oz)	80
Tofurky		
Deli Slices Cranberry	3 slices (1.8 oz)	98
Deli Slices Hickory Smoked	3 slices (1.8 oz)	100
Deli Slices Italian	3 slices (1.8 oz)	103
Deli Slices Original	3 slices (1.8 oz)	103
Deli Slices Peppered	3 slices (1.8 oz)	103
Deli Slices Philly Steak	3 slices (1.8 oz)	110
Roast	1 serv (4 oz)	190
Worthington		
Turkee Slices	3 slices (3.3 oz)	180
Yves		
Meatless Deli Turkey Slices	4 slices	100
Meatless Ground Turkey	⅓ cup	60

TURMERIC

FOOD	PORTION	CALS
ground	1 tsp	8

TURNIPS

FOOD	PORTION	CALS
canned greens	½ cup	17
cooked mashed	½ cup (4.2 oz)	47
cubed cooked	½ cup (3 oz)	33
frzn greens cooked	½ cup	24
greens chopped cooked	½ cup	15
greens raw chopped	½ cup	7

FOOD	PORTION	CALS
raw cubed	½ cup (2.4 oz)	25
Allens		
Seasoned	½ cup	35
Glory		
Greens Fresh	2 cups	20
Greens Seasoned canned	½ cup	35
Root Cut Fresh	½ cup	20
Sensibly Seasoned Greens	½ cup	20
TURTLE		
raw	3.5 oz	85
TUSK FISH		
raw	3.5 oz	79
VANILLA		
vanilla extract	1 tsp (4.2 g)	12
vanilla extract	1 tbsp (0.5 oz)	37
vanilla extract alcohol free	1 tsp (4.2 g)	2
Bob's Red Mill		
Organic Extract	1 tsp	0
Virginia Dare		
Extract	1 tsp	10
VEAL (see also VEAL DISHES)		
breast braised	3 oz	226
chop breaded fried	1 med (6.5 oz)	290
chop cooked	1 med (6.5 oz)	230
cubed braised	3 oz	160
cutlet cooked	3 oz	141
ground broiled	3 oz	146
leg roasted	3 oz	136
loin roasted	3 oz	184
patty breaded fried	1 (2.8 oz)	211
shank braised	3 oz	162
VEAL DISHES		
TAKE-OUT		
cordon bleu	1 serv (8 oz)	490
parmigiana	1 serv (6.4 oz)	362
scallopini	1 slice + sauce (3.4 oz)	238
stew	1 serv (8.8 oz)	192

FOOD	PORTION	CALS
veal marengo	1 serv (8.8 oz)	274
veal marsala	1 slice + sauce (3.4 oz)	268
veal paprikash	1 serv (8.6 oz)	280
veal picatta	1 piece + sauce (3.5 oz)	154

VEGETABLE JUICE

FOOD	PORTION	CALS
low sodium tomato & vegetable juice	1 cup	53
vegetable juice cocktail	8 oz	46
Bolthouse Farms		
Vedge Tomato Carrot Celery	8 oz	60
Dei Fratelli		
Vegetable Juice	8 oz	45
Green To Go		
100% Natural Organic as prep	1 pkg (0.3 oz)	32
Lakewood		
Super Veggie	6 oz	40
V8		
100% Vegetable Essential Antioxidants	8 oz	50
Calcium Enriched	8 oz	50
High Fiber	8 oz	60
Low Sodium	8 oz	50
Organic	8 oz	50
V-Fusion Acai Mixed Berry	8 oz	110
Walnut Acres		
Organic Incredible Vegetable	8 oz	50

VEGETABLES MIXED

CANNED

FOOD	PORTION	CALS
mixed vegetables	½ cup	39
peas & carrots	½ cup	48
peas & onions	½ cup	30
succotash	½ cup	102
Del Monte		
Mixed	½ cup	40
Mixed Vegetables w/ Potatoes	½ cup	45
Peas And Carrots	½ cup	60
Savory Sides Homestyle Vegetable Medley	½ cup	70
Savory Sides Rio Grande Vegetables	½ cup	70

FOOD	PORTION	CALS
Veg-All		
Original Mixed	½ cup	40
DRIED		
Fun-Yums		
Fresh Crispy Mixed Veggies	1 serv (0.9 oz)	114
FRESH		
Mann's		
Broccoli & Cauliflower	1 serv (3 oz)	25
California Stir Fry	1 serv (3 oz)	30
Medley	1 serv (3 oz)	25
Veggies On The Go w/ Dip	1 cup + 1 tbsp dip	100
River Ranch		
Broccoli & Carrots	1 cup	25
Broccoli & Cauliflower	1 cup	25
Stir Fry Blend	1 cup	30
Vegetable Medley	1 cup	25
FROZEN		
mixed vegetables cooked	½ cup	54
peas & carrots cooked	½ cup	38
peas & onions cooked	½ cup	40
succotash cooked	½ cup	79
Birds Eye		
Asparagus Gold & White Corn & Baby Carrots	⅔ cup	70
Italian Herb Harvest Vegetables	1¼ cups	90
Spring Vegetables In Citrus Sauce	1¼ cups	70
Steamfresh Asian Medley	1 cup (3.3 oz)	50
Steamfresh Broccoli Carrots Sugar Snap Peas & Water Chestnuts	¾ cup (2.9 oz)	35
Steamfresh Broccoli & Cauliflower	1 cup	30
Steamfresh Broccoli Cauliflower & Carrots	¾ cup	30
Steamfresh Mixed Vegetables	⅔ cup (3.2 oz)	40
C&W		
Early Harvest Peas & Baby Carrots	⅔ cup	60
Petite Peas & Pearl Onions	⅔ cup	60
Cascadian Farm		
Organic Mixed Vegetables	⅔ cup	60
Organic Peas & Carrots	⅔ cup	50
Europe's Best		
Zen Garden	¾ cup	60

FOOD	PORTION	CALS
Green Giant		
Broccoli & Carrots w/ Garlic & Herbs as prep	½ cup	40
Garden Vegetable Medley as prep	½ cup	70
Mixed Vegetables as prep	½ cup	50
Southwestern Style as prep	½ cup	90
Szechuan Vegetables as prep	½ cup	50
La Choy		
Chop Suey Vegetables	½ cup (2.2 oz)	15
Fancy Chinese Mixed Vegetables	½ cup (2.9 oz)	15
Stir Fry Vegetables	½ cup	15
Lean Cuisine		
Cafe Classics Roasted Potatoes w/ Broccoli & Cheddar Cheese Sauce	1 pkg (10.25 oz)	230
McKenzie's		
Gumbo Mixture	1 serv (2.9 oz)	35
Okra Tomatoes w/ Onions	1 serv (2.8 oz)	20
Melrose Made Gourmet		
Vegetable Souffle Fat Free	1 serv (4 oz)	70
Pictsweet		
Peas & Carrots	⅔ cup	50
Roast Works		
Flame Roasted Redskins & Vegetables	1 serv (3 oz)	90
Seapoint Farms		
Organic Veggie Blends w/ Edamame Eat Your Greens	¾ cup	60
Veggie Blends w/ Edamame Garden	¾ cup	60
Veggie Blends w/ Edamame Oriental	¾ cup	60
TAKE-OUT		
buddha's delight	1 serv (16 oz)	174
pakoras	4 (1.7 oz)	57
ratatouille	1 serv (3.5 oz)	96
samosa	1 (2.4 oz)	206
stir fry mixed vegetables	1 serv (4 oz)	66
succotash	½ cup	111
tapenade grilled vegetables	¼ cup	40

VENISON (see also JERKY)

roasted	4 oz	215

VINEGAR

balsamic	1 tbsp	14

FOOD	PORTION	CALS
cider	1 tbsp	3
red wine	1 tbsp	3
vinegar	1 tbsp	3
Carapelli		
Balsamic	1 tbsp	15
Red Wine	1 tbsp	5
White Wine	1 tbsp	5
Eden		
Organic Apple Cider	1 tbsp	0
Organic Brown Rice	1 tbsp	2
Red Wine	1 tbsp	0
Ume Plum	1 tsp	0
Gedney		
Apple Cider	1 tbsp	3
Distilled White	1 tbsp	3
Latino Chef		
Lulo	1 tbsp	35
Passion Fruit	1 tbsp	40
Lucini		
Balsamic 10 Year Gran Reserve	1 tbsp (0.5 oz)	20
Balsamic Dark Cherry Infused	1 tbsp	30
Italian Wine Pinot Noir	1 tbsp (0.5 oz)	tr
Newman's Own		
Organic Balsamic	1 tbsp	20
Pacifica Culinaria		
Balsamic Dark Sweet Cherry	1 tbsp	15
Pear Pomegranate	1 tbsp	10
Progresso		
Balsamic	2 tbsp (0.5 oz)	10
Regina		
Red Wine	1 tbsp	0
Spectrum		
Apple Cider Organic	1 tbsp	7
Balsamic Organic	1 tbsp	6
Brown Rice Organic	1 tbsp	10
Golden Balsamic Organic	1 tbsp	6
Red Wine Organic	1 tbsp	0
White Organic	1 tbsp	2
White Wine Organic	1 tbsp	0

FOOD	PORTION	CALS
Tree Of Life		
Organic Apple Cider Raw Unfiltered	1 tbsp	0
WAFFLES		
FROZEN		
Aunt Jemima		
Blueberry	2 (2.5 oz)	190
Low Fat	2 (2.5 oz)	160
Eggo		
Buttermilk	2	180
Homestyle	2	190
Homestyle Minis	12	250
Nutri-Grain Low Fat Whole Wheat	2	140
Special K	3	190
Waf-Fulls Strawberry	1	150
EnviroKidz		
Organic Gorilla Banana	2 (2.7 oz)	230
Kashi		
Heart To Heart Honey Oat	2 (3 oz)	160
Lifestream		
Organic Fig + Flax	2 (2.8 oz)	210
Organic Pomegran Plus	2 (2.8 oz)	190
Van's		
Belgian Multigrain	2 (2.7 oz)	190
Homestyle Mini	4 (2.8 oz)	210
Organic Flax	2 (2.7 oz)	190
Organic Homestyle	2 (2.7 oz)	200
Original 97% Fat Free	2 (2.7 oz)	140
Original Buttermilk	2 (2.7 oz)	220
Wheat Free Buckwheat	2 (3 oz)	230
Wheat Free Flax	2 (3 oz)	210
MIX		
plain 7 in diam as prep	1 (2.6 oz)	218
READY-TO-EAT		
Kashi		
GoLean Blueberry	2 (3 oz)	170
GoLean Original	2 (3 oz)	170
TAKE-OUT		
belgian	1 (4.7 oz)	412
blueberry 9 in sq	1 (7 oz)	556
round 10 in diam	1 (6.8 oz)	598

FOOD	PORTION	CALS
square 9 in	1 (7 oz)	620
whole wheat 9 in sq	1 (7 oz)	534

WALNUTS
black chopped	¼ cup	193
english chopped	¼ cup	191
english ground	¼ cup	131
english halves	14 (1 oz)	185
english in shell	7 (1 oz)	183
honey roasted	¼ cup	172

Diamond
Chopped	¼ cup	200

Emerald
Glazed	¼ cup	140

Good Sense
Organic Raw Walnuts	¼ cup	210

WASABI (see HORSERADISH)

WATER
ice cubes	3	0
tap water	8 oz	0

Adironack
Sparkling All Flavors	8 oz	0

Aloe Breeze
Organic All Flavors	8 oz	0

Aloe Splash
All Flavors	8 oz	0

Apple & Eve
Water Fruits All Flavors	1 bottle (10 oz)	90

Aqua Pacific
Water	1 liter	0

Aquafina
Alive Wellness Berry Pomegranate	8 oz	10
Sparkling Citrus Twist	8 oz	0

Aroma Water
All Flavors	8 oz	0

Ayala's
Herbal All Flavors	1 bottle	0

Base Energy + Water
All Flavors	8 oz	28

FOOD	PORTION	CALS
Blu Italy		
Sparkling Lemon	8 oz	0
Bot		
Fortified All Flavors	1 bottle (12 oz)	40
Carpe Diem		
Botanic Water All Flavors	8 oz	35
Clearly Canadian		
Sparkling Blackberry	8 oz	90
Sparkling Cherry	8 oz	85
Sparkling Raspberry	8 oz	75
Sparkling Strawberry	8 oz	85
Zero Sparkling All Flavors	8 oz	0
Crystal Geyser		
Spring Water	8 oz	0
Dasani		
Purified Water	8 oz	0
W/ Lemon	8 oz	2
W/ Raspberry	8 oz	1
Eden		
Springs Artesian	8 oz	0
Evian		
Spring Water	1 liter	0
Fiji		
Natural Artesian	1 liter	0
FlavH2O		
All Flavors	1 can (12.3 oz)	80
Fruit 2 O		
Grape	8 oz	0
Natural Berry	8 oz	0
Watermelon Kiwi	8 oz	0
Fruit Refreshers		
Lemonade	8 oz	0
Gerolsteiner		
Sparkling Mineral	8 oz	0
H2Odwalla		
Enhanced Tropical Orange	1 bottle (20 oz)	120
Organic Enhanced Blueberry Tea	1 bottle (20 oz)	120
Organic Enhanced Jasmine Lime	1 bottle (20 oz)	120
Hawaiian Springs		
Naturally Pure	1 liter	0

FOOD	PORTION	CALS
Highland Spring		
Spring Water	1 liter	0
Hint		
All Flavors	1 bottle (15 oz)	0
IQ		
H2O Orange Mango	8 oz	40
Island Chill		
Artesian Water	1 liter	0
Jana		
Natural European Artesian	1 liter	0
Jones Soda		
24C Multi Vitamin Enhanced All Flavors	1 bottle	100
Klear Splash		
Mini Sip	1 pkg (4 oz)	0
Life Water		
B-Strong	1 bottle (20 oz)	100
Enlighten	1 bottle (20 oz)	100
Zingseng	1 bottle (20 oz)	100
Liquid Salvation		
Ultra Hydrating	1 bottle	0
Multi Vitamin Enhanced Water		
All Flavors	8 oz	50
No Carb All Flavors	8 oz	0
Nestle		
Pure Life Splash All Flavors	8 oz	0
Nui		
All Natural Kid Water	10 oz	90
O Water		
Hydrate Black Raspberry	8 oz	25
Replenish Lemon Lime	8 oz	25
Vitalize Peach Mango	8 oz	25
Pellegrino		
Mineral Water	8 oz	0
Pink2O		
Fortified	1 bottle (20 oz)	0
Propel		
Fitness Water All Flavors	1 bottle (23.7 oz)	30
Rapid		
Hydra-Cell Water	1 bottle (16.9 oz)	0

FOOD	PORTION	CALS
San Benedetto		
Sparkling Mineral Water	1 liter	0
Skinny Water		
Hi-Energy Acai Grape Blueberry	8 oz	0
Total-V Passionfruit Lemonade	8 oz	0
SoBe		
All Flavors	8 oz	50
SoNu		
Water All Flavors	8 oz	45
Special K2O		
Protein Water All Flavors	1 bottle (16.6 oz)	50
Splash		
All Flavors	8 oz	0
Stacker 2		
Protein Water All Flavors	1 bottle (19.44 oz)	80
Sulinka		
Sparkling Mineral	8 oz	0
TalkingRain		
Ice All Flavors	8 oz	5
Tao Tea		
Lychee Water	8 oz	67
Thorpedo		
Ultra Low GI Energy Water	8 oz	45
Tipperary		
Mineral Water	1 liter	0
Trim Water		
Purified	1 bottle (20 oz)	10
Trinity		
Energize	8 oz	50
Multi-Essential	8 oz	50
Revive	8 oz	50
Strength	8 oz	50
Think	8 oz	50
Twist		
Organics All Flavors	8 oz	10
Vasa		
Natural Spring	8 oz	0
Vitamin + Fiber Water		
All Fruit Flavors	8 oz	50

FOOD	PORTION	CALS
VitaminWater		
XXX Acai Blueberry Pomegranate	8 oz	50
Volvic		
Mineral Water	1 liter	0
Natural Lemon	8 oz	0
Natural Orange	8 oz	30
Voss		
Artesian	8 oz	0
W2O For Women		
All Flavors	8 oz	40
WaterPlus		
Antioxidants Acai Berry	8 oz	50
Electrolytes Fruit Punch	8 oz	50
Extra-C Orange Tangerine	8 oz	50
Vitamins Dragonfruit Kiwi	8 oz	50
Wateroos		
All Flavors	1 box (8 oz)	0
Wild Waters		
All Flavors	8 oz	50
WATER CHESTNUTS		
chinese sliced canned	½ cup	35
fresh sliced	½ cup	66
La Choy		
Sliced	½ cup	25
Polar		
Sliced	2 tbsp	10
WATERCRESS		
cooked w/o fat	1 cup	15
raw chopped	1 cup	4
Frieda's		
Watercress	1 cup	10
WATERMELON		
cut up	1 cup	46
seeds dried	¼ cup	150
wedge	1 sm (2.5 oz)	21
wedge	1 med (10 oz)	86
wedge	1 lg (20 oz)	172
whole melon	1 (9 lb)	1227

FOOD	PORTION	CALS
Dulcinea		
Fresh Mini Seedless	2 cups	88
Frieda's		
Yellow Seedless	½ cup (3 oz)	25
Sundia		
Fresh	2 cups	80
WATERMELON JUICE		
juice	8 oz	71
Sundia		
100% Natural	8 oz	110
Tang		
Watermelon Wallop	1 box (7 oz)	90
WHALE		
beluga	3.5 oz	97
beluga dried	1 oz	92
WHEAT		
sprouted	1 cup (3.8 oz)	214
starch	3.5 oz	348
Arrowhead Mills		
Whole Grain Wheat	¼ cup (1.6 oz)	150
Bob's Red Mill		
Vital Wheat Gluten	¼ cup	120
Hodgson Mill		
Vital Wheat Gluten	4 tsp	40
Near East		
Taboule Wheat Salad as prep	⅔ cup (3.5 oz)	120
WHEAT GERM		
plain	¼ cup	108
Bob's Red Mill		
Wheat Germ	2 tbsp	59
Hodgson Mill		
Untoasted	2 tbsp	55
Kretschmer		
Original Toasted	¼ cup (0.6 oz)	35
Tree Of Life		
Toasted	3 tbsp (0.8 oz)	100
WHEY		
acid dry	1 tbsp	10

FOOD	PORTION	CALS
sweet dry	1 tbsp	26
sweet fluid	½ cup	33
whey cheese	1 oz	126
Bob's Red Mill		
Protein Concentrate	¼ cup	80
Sweet Dairy	1 tbsp	30
Wellements		
Whey Protein Chocolate	1 scoop (1 oz)	120
Whey Protein Vanilla	1 scoop (1 oz)	120

WHIPPED TOPPINGS

cream pressurized	1 tbsp (3 g)	8
cream pressurized	1 cup (2.1 oz)	154
nondairy frzn	1 tbsp	13
nondairy powdered as prep w/ whole milk	1 cup	151
nondairy pressurized	1 tbsp (4 g)	11
nondairy pressurized	1 cup	184
Estee		
Whipped Topping as prep	1 serv	10
Hood		
Light Sugar Free Whipped Cream	2 tbsp	10
Whipped Light Cream	2 tbsp	20
Reddiwip		
Chocolate	2 tbsp	15
Extra Creamy	2 tbsp	15
Fat Free	2 tbsp	5
Original	2 tbsp	15
Soyatoo		
Soy Whip	2 tbsp	10
TruWhip		
Whipped Topping	2 tbsp (0.4 oz)	130

WHITE BEANS

canned	1 cup	306
dried regular cooked	1 cup	249
dried small cooked	1 cup	253

WHITEFISH

baked	3 oz	146
smoked	1 oz	39
smoked	3 oz	92

FOOD	PORTION	CALS
WHITING		
broiled w/o fat	3 oz	99
fillet broiled w/o fat	1 (2.5 oz)	84
fillet steamed w/o fat	1 (2.6 oz)	84
hake raw	3.5 oz	84
TAKE-OUT		
fillet battered & fried	1 (3.1 oz)	157
fillet breaded & fried	1 (3.1 oz)	191
WILD RICE		
cooked	1 cup (5.8 oz)	166
Gourmet House		
White & Wild not prep	¼ cup	170
Lundberg		
Organic Quick not prep	¼ cup	150
WINE		
chianti	1 serv (5 oz)	125
chinese cooking	1 bottle (15 oz)	559
cooking	¼ cup (2 oz)	29
haiku	1 serv	93
japanese plum	3 oz	139
japanese sake	2 oz	78
kir	1 serv	78
liebfraumilch	4 oz	86
madeira	3.5 oz	169
marsala	4 oz	80
merlot	4 oz	95
muscat	1 serv (5 oz)	123
nonalcoholic	1 serv (5 oz)	9
port	1 serv (3.5 oz)	165
red barbera	1 serv (5 oz)	125
red burgundy	1 serv (5 oz)	127
red cabernet franc	1 serv (5 oz)	122
red claret	1 serv (5 oz)	122
red gamay	1 serv (5 oz)	115
red mouvedre	1 serv (5 oz)	129
red pinot noir	1 serv (5 oz)	121
red syrah	1 serv (5 oz)	122
red zinfandel	1 serv (5 oz)	129
sake screwdriver	1 serv	175

FOOD	PORTION	CALS
sangria	1 serv	88
sangria blanco	1 serv	155
sherry	2 oz	84
vermouth dry	3.5 oz	105
vermouth sweet	3.5 oz	167
wassail wine	1 serv	142
white	1 serv (5 oz)	121
white fume blanc	1 serv (5 oz)	121
white pinot blanc	1 serv (5 oz)	119
white pinot grigio	1 serv (5 oz)	122
white riesling	1 serv (5 oz)	118
white sauvignon blanc	1 serv (5 oz)	119
wine cooler	1 (7 oz)	116
wine spritzer	1 serv (7 oz)	73
Almanden		
Merlot	5 oz	115
Bartles & Jaymes		
Wine Cooler Classic Original	1 bottle (12 oz)	190
Beringer		
Chardonnay	5 oz	125
Carlo Rossi		
Cabernet Sauvignon	5 oz	125
Eden		
Mirin Rice Cooking Wine	1 tbsp	25
Franzia Vinter		
Select Merlot	5 oz	105
Twin Valley		
Cabernet Sauvignon	5 oz	120

WINGED BEANS
dried cooked w/o salt	1 cup	253

WRAPS (see BREAD, SANDWICHES)

YACON
Navitas Naturals

Slices Dried	1 oz	90

YAM (see also SWEET POTATO)
CANNED
Bruce's

In Syrup	⅔ cup	150

FOOD	PORTION	CALS
Glory		
Candied	½ cup	210
FRESH		
mountain yam hawaii cooked w/o salt	1 cup	119
yam cooked w/o salt	1 cup	158
Earthbound Farm		
Organic	1 med (4.6 oz)	130
Frieda's		
Name	¾ cup	100
House		
Black Ita Konnyaku Yam Cake	1 serv (2 oz)	5
YARDLONG BEANS		
sliced cooked w/o salt	1 cup	49
YAUTIA (*see* MALANGA)		
YEAST		
baker's compressed	1 cake (0.6 oz)	18
baker's dry	1 pkg (7 g)	21
baker's dry	1 tbsp	35
brewer's dry	1 tbsp	35
Bob's Red Mill		
Active Dry	1 tbsp	25
Hodgson Mill		
Active Dry	1 tsp	30
Fast Rise	1 tsp (9 g)	25
YELLOW BEANS		
fresh cooked w/o salt	1 cup	44
fresh raw	1 cup	34
YELLOWTAIL		
baked	4 oz	199
YOGURT (*see also* YOGURT DRINKS, YOGURT FROZEN)		
plain low fat	8 oz	143
plain nonfat	8 oz	127
plain whole milk	8 oz	138
tofu yogurt	1 cup	246
Axelrod		
Fat Free Lemon	1 pkg (6 oz)	90

FOOD	PORTION	CALS
Better Whey		
All Fruit Flavors	1 pkg (6 oz)	145
Plain	1 pkg (6 oz)	130
Breyers		
Creme Savers Orange & Creme	1 pkg (8 oz)	240
Creme Savers Raspberries & Creme	1 pkg (8 oz)	240
Light! Probiotic Plus Apple Cinnamon	1 pkg (8 oz)	100
Light! Probiotic Plus Blueberries 'N Cream	1 pkg (8 oz)	110
Light! Probiotic Plus Lemon Chiffon	1 pkg (8 oz)	100
Light! Probiotic Plus Peaches 'N Cream	1 pkg (8 oz)	100
Light! Probiotic Plus Strawberry Banana	1 pkg (8 oz)	110
Light! Probiotic Plus Strawberry Cheesecake	1 pkg (8 oz)	110
Smart! w/ DHA Black Cherry	1 pkg (6 oz)	170
Smart! w/ DHA Mixed Berry	1 pkg (6 oz)	170
Smart! w/ DHA Peach	1 pkg (6 oz)	170
Smart! w/ DHA Pineapple	1 pkg (6 oz)	170
Smart! w/ DHA Strawberry	1 pkg (6 oz)	170
Smart! w/ DHA Strawberry Banana	1 pkg (6 oz)	170
Smooth & Creamy Peaches 'N Cream	1 pkg (8 oz)	240
Smooth & Creamy Strawberry	1 pkg (8 oz)	230
Smooth & Creamy Vanilla Cream	1 pkg (8 oz)	240
YoCrunch Blueberry w/ Granola	1 pkg	240
YoCrunch Cookie N' Cream w/ Oreo	1 pkg	240
YoCrunch Naturals Strawberry Banana w/ Granola	1 pkg	245
YoCrunch Naturals Strawberry w/ Dark Chocolate Chips	1 pkg	280
YoCrunch Raspberry w/ Granola	1 pkg	240
YoCrunch Strawberry w/ Granola	1 pkg	240
YoCrunch Vanilla Nestle	1 pkg	260
YoCrunch Vanilla w/ Butterfinger	1 pkg	260
YoCrunch Light Cookies N' Cream w/ Oreo	1 pkg	170
YoCrunch Light Strawberry w/ Granola	1 pkg	170
Cabot		
Greek	1 pkg (6 oz)	210
Greek 2%	1 pkg (6 oz)	160
Non Fat Berry Banana	1 cup	130
Non Fat Black Cherry	1 cup	130
Non Fat French Vanilla	1 cup	130
Non Fat Plain	1 cup	100

FOOD	PORTION	CALS
Non Fat Raspberry	1 cup	130
Chobani		
Greek Yogurt Lowfat Plain	1 pkg (6 oz)	130
Greek Yogurt Nonfat Peach	1 pkg (6 oz)	140
Greek Yogurt Nonfat Plain	1 pkg (6 oz)	100
Greek Yogurt Original Plain	1 pkg (6 oz)	240
Dannon		
Activia Blueberry	1 pkg (4 oz)	110
Activia Mixed Berry	1 pkg (4 oz)	110
Activia Peach	1 pkg (4 oz)	110
Activia Prune	1 pkg (4 oz)	110
Activia Strawberry	1 pkg (4 oz)	110
Activia Vanilla	1 pkg (4 oz)	110
Activia Vanilla Light Fat Free	4 oz	70
All Natural Blended Mini Blueberry	1 (3.3 oz)	110
All Natural Blended Mini Strawberry	1 (3.3 oz)	110
Creamy Fruit Blends Raspberry	6 oz	170
Fruit On The Bottom Apple Cinnamon	6 oz	150
Fruit On The Bottom Peach	6 oz	150
Fruit On The Bottom Pineapple	6 oz	150
Fruit On The Bottom Raspberry	6 oz	150
La Creme Mousse French Vanilla	1 (2.6 oz)	110
La Creme Vanilla	4 oz	140
Light & Fit 0% Fat Plus Vanilla	4 oz	50
Light & Fit Carb & Sugar Control Blueberries 'N Cream	4 oz	60
Light & Fit Nonfat Cherry Vanilla	6 oz	60
Light & Fit Nonfat Lemon Chiffon	6 oz	60
Light & Fit Nonfat Raspberry	6 oz	60
Light & Fit Nonfat White Chocolate Raspberry	6 oz	90
Fage		
Sheep & Goat's Milk	1 pkg (7 oz)	190
Friendship		
Plain	1 cup	150
Horizon Organic		
Fat Free Peach	1 pkg (6 oz)	140
Fat Free Vanilla	1 cup	180
Kids Strawberry	1 pkg (4 oz)	110
Lowfat Blended Blueberry	1 pkg (6 oz)	160
Tube Lowfat Blueberry	1 (2 oz)	70

FOOD	PORTION	CALS
Whole Milk Plain	1 cup	160
La Yogurt		
Lowfat Blueberries 'N' Cream	1 pkg (6 oz)	200
Lowfat Fruit On The Bottom Cherry	1 pkg (8 oz)	230
Lowfat Fruit On The Bottom Probiotic Peach	1 pkg (6 oz)	160
Lowfat Fruit On The Bottom Strawberry	1 pkg (8 oz)	220
Lowfat Peaches 'N' Cream	1 pkg (6 oz)	200
Lowfat Pina Colada	1 pkg (6 oz)	160
Lowfat Probiotic Pina Colada	1 pkg (6 oz)	160
Lowfat Probiotic Plain	1 pkg (6 oz)	100
Lowfat Probiotic Vanilla	1 pkg (6 oz)	150
Lowfat Vanilla 'N' Cream	1 pkg (6 oz)	200
Nonfat Banana Cream	1 pkg (6 oz)	100
Nonfat Probiotic Cherry	1 pkg (6 oz)	100
Nonfat Probiotic Peach	1 pkg (6 oz)	90
Nonfat Probiotic Raspberry	1 pkg (6 oz)	90
Nonfat Probiotic Vanilla	1 pkg (6 oz)	90
Sabor Latino Lowfat Dulce De Leche	1 pkg (6 oz)	190
Sabor Latino Lowfat Guava	1 pkg (6 oz)	190
Sabor Latino Lowfat Horchata	1 pkg (6 oz)	210
Sabor Latino Lowfat Papaya	1 pkg (6 oz)	190
Land O Lakes		
Strawberry Light	1 pkg (8 oz)	80
Strawberry Lowfat	1 pkg (8 oz)	190
Nancy's		
Lowfat Maple	1 pkg (8 oz)	180
Lowfat Plain	1 pkg (8 oz)	150
Lowfat Vanilla	1 pkg (8 oz)	140
Nonfat Fruit On The Top Cherry	1 pkg (8 oz)	140
Nonfat Plain	1 pkg (8 oz)	120
Nonfat Vanilla	1 pkg (8 oz)	220
Organic Soy Kiwi Lime	1 pkg (8 oz)	160
Organic Soy Plain	1 pkg (8 oz)	150
Organic Soy Vanilla	1 pkg (8 oz)	120
Whole Milk Fruit On The Top Peach	1 pkg (8 oz)	220
Whole Milk Honey	1 pkg (8 oz)	170
Oikos		
Organic Greek Vanilla	1 pkg (5.3 oz)	110
Organic Honey	1 pkg (5.3 oz)	120
Organic Plain	1 pkg (5.3 oz)	90

FOOD	PORTION	CALS
Rachel's		
Essence Berry Jasmine w/ Zinc	1 pkg (6 oz)	160
Essence Plum Honey Lavender	1 pkg (6 oz)	160
Essence Pomegrante Acai	1 pkg (6 oz)	170
Exotic Kiwi Passion Fruit Lime	1 pkg (6 oz)	160
Exotic Orange Strawberry Mango	1 pkg (6 oz)	160
Exotic Pomegranate Blueberry	1 pkg (6 oz)	170
Redwood Hill Farm		
Goat Milk Apricot Mango	1 cup	180
Goat Milk Cranberry Orange	1 cup	180
Goat Milk Plain	1 cup	130
Goat Milk Strawberry	1 cup	180
Goat Milk Vanilla	1 cup	190
SoDelicious		
Coconut Milk Plain	1 pkg (6 oz)	130
Coconut Milk Vanilla	1 pkg (6 oz)	150
Dairy Free Cinnamon Bun	1 pkg (6 oz)	160
Dairy Free Raspberry	1 pkg (6 oz)	150
Stonyfield Farm		
Kids' Lowfat BaNilla	1 pkg (4 oz)	110
Light Black Cherry	1 pkg (6 oz)	100
Light Blueberry	1 pkg (4 oz)	100
Light Peach	1 pkg (6 oz)	100
Light Strawberry	1 pkg (4 oz)	100
Nonfat French Vanilla	1 pkg	90
Nonfat Strawberry	1 pkg	140
O'Soy Chocolate	1 pkg (6 oz)	160
O'Soy Peach	1 pkg (4 oz)	100
Squeezers Lowfat Strawberry	1 tube (2 oz)	60
Whole Milk French Vanilla	1 pkg (6 oz)	190
Straus		
Organic Maple Nonfat	1 pkg (8 oz)	170
Organic Maple Whole Milk	1 pkg (8 oz)	210
Organic Plain Lowfat	1 pkg (8 oz)	150
Organic Plain Nonfat	1 pkg (8 oz)	110
Organic Plain Whole Milk	1 pkg (8 oz)	160
Total		
Greek Yogurt 0% Fat	1 pkg (5.3 oz)	80
Greek Yogurt 2% Fat	1 pkg (7 oz)	130
Greek Yogurt Classic	1 pkg (7 oz)	180

FOOD	PORTION	CALS
Greek Yogurt Light	1 pkg (5.3 oz)	130
Honey	1 pkg (3.5 oz)	250
Wallaby		
Organic Banana Vanilla	1 pkg (6 oz)	150
Organic Lemon	1 pkg (6 oz)	150
Organic Maple	1 pkg (6 oz)	150
Organic Plain	1 cup	150
Organic Raspberry	1 pkg (6 oz)	150
Organic Vanilla	1 pkg (6 oz)	150
Organic Nonfat Mango Lime	1 pkg (6 oz)	140
Organic Nonfat Plain	1 cup	130
Organic Nonfat Vanilla Bean	1 pkg (6 oz)	140
WholeSoy & Co.		
Organic Soy Apricot Mango	1 pkg (6 oz)	160
Organic Soy Lemon	1 pkg (6 oz)	160
Organic Soy Plain	1 pkg (6 oz)	150
Organic Soy Raspberry	1 pkg (6 oz)	170
Organic Soy Vanilla	1 pkg (6 oz)	150
WildWood		
Organic Soyogurt Low Fat Peach	1 pkg (6 oz)	160
Organic Soyogurt Low Fat Vanilla	1 pkg (6 oz)	160
Organic Soyogurt Plain Unsweetened	1 pkg (6 oz)	110
Yofarm		
YoSmooth Apricot	1 pkg	220
YoSmooth Peach	1 pkg	220
YoSmooth Raspberry	1 pkg	230
Yoplait		
Go-Gurt All Fruit Flavors	1 pkg (2.25 oz)	80
Grande 99% Fat Free All Flavors	1 cup	250
Grande Fat Free Plain	1 cup	90
Kids Banana Vanilla	1 pkg (4 oz)	100
Kids Strawberry Vanilla	1 pkg (4 oz)	100
Light All Fruit Flavors	1 pkg (6 oz)	180
Light Indulgent All Flavors	1 pkg (6 oz)	110
Light Thick & Creamy All Fruit Flavors	1 pkg (6 oz)	100
Original All Fruit Flavors	1 pkg (6 oz)	170
Original Coconut Cream	1 pkg (6 oz)	190
Original Lemon Burst	1 pkg (6 oz)	180
Original Pina Colada	1 pkg (6 oz)	170
Trix All Fruit Flavors	1 pkg (4 oz)	120

FOOD	PORTION	CALS
Yo Plus All Flavors	1 pkg (4 oz)	110

YOGURT DRINKS (*see also* SMOOTHIES)

FOOD	PORTION	CALS
lassi	7 oz	78
Dahlicious		
Lassi Green Tea	1 bottle	110
Lassi Mango	1 bottle	130
Lassi Plain	1 bottle	110
Dannon		
DanActive Plain	1 bottle (3.3 oz)	90
DanActive Vanilla	1 bottle (3.3 oz)	90
Danimals Rockin' Raspberry	1 bottle (3.1 oz)	70
Danimals Strawberry Explosion	1 bottle (3.1 oz)	70
Danimals Strikin' Strawberry Kiwi	1 bottle (3.1 oz)	70
Frusion Cherry Berry Blend	1 bottle (10 oz)	260
Frusion Pina Colada	1 bottle (10 oz)	260
Frusion Strawberry Blend	1 bottle (10 oz)	260
Light & Fit Carb & Sugar Control Berries 'N Cream	1 bottle (7 oz)	60
Light & Fit Smoothie Peach Passion	1 bottle (7 oz)	70
Light & Fit Smoothie Strawberry Banana	1 bottle (7 oz)	70
Lifeway		
Lassi Lowfat All Flavors	8 oz	174
Promise		
Activ All Flavors	1 bottle (3.5 oz)	70
Stonyfield Farm		
Kids' Juice Smoothie Orange Strawberry Banana Wave	1 bottle (6 oz)	160
Smoothie Light Strawberry	1 bottle (10 oz)	130
Smoothie Lowfat Strawberry	1 bottle (10 oz)	250
Yo On The Go		
All Flavors	1 box (8 oz)	180
Yoplait		
Go-Gurt All Fruit Flavors	1 bottle (5 oz)	120
Light All Flavors	1 bottle (8.3 oz)	90
Nouriche All Fruit Flavors	1 bottle (11 oz)	260
Smoothie All Flavors	1 bottle (8.3 oz)	220

YOGURT FROZEN

FOOD	PORTION	CALS
chocolate soft serve	1 cup	230
vanilla soft serve	1 cup	236

FOOD	PORTION	CALS
Dippin' Dots		
Strawberry Cheesecake	½ cup	100
Edy's		
Black Cherry Vanilla Swirl	½ cup	90
Caramel Praline Crunch	½ cup	100
Chocolate	½ cup	90
Strawberry	½ cup	100
Vanilla	½ cup	90
Vanilla Chocolate Swirl	½ cup	90
Hood		
Fat Free Old Fashioned Vanilla	½ cup	110
Fat Free Strawberry	½ cup	100
Vanilla Swiss Almond	½ cup	150
Turkey Hill		
Fudge Ripple	½ cup	100
Neapolitan	½ cup	90
Smoothie Orange Cream Swirl	½ cup	100
Smoothie Peach Mango	½ cup	90
Vanilla Bean	½ cup	100
WholeSoy & Co.		
Organic All Flavors	½ cup	120
ZUCCHINI		
baby raw	1 (0.5 oz)	3
canned italian style	1 cup	66
fresh	1 sm (4.1 oz)	19
pickled	¼ cup	16
raw sliced	1 cup	19
sliced cooked w/o salt	1 cup	29
C&W		
Yellow & Green	⅔ cup	20
Frieda's		
Baby	⅔ cup (3 oz)	20
TAKE-OUT		
breaded & fried	6 slices (3 oz)	141
indian pakora	1 serv	46
sticks breaded & fried	6 (2 oz)	90

PART TWO

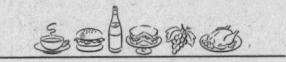

Restaurant Chains

> *The larger the portion size you are served, and the more variety you are offered, the more likely you are to overeat. Go easy on super-sizes and choose wisely at buffets.*

FOOD	PORTION	CALS
A&W		
BEVERAGES		
Coke	1 sm (11 oz)	145
Diet Coke	1 sm (11 oz)	0
Diet Root Beer	1 sm (15 oz)	0
Float Diet Root Beer	1 sm (14 oz)	170
Float Root Beer	1 sm (14 oz)	330
Milkshake Chocolate	1 med	700
Milkshake Strawberry	1 med	670
Milkshake Vanilla	1 med	720
Root Beer	1 sm (15 oz)	220
DESSERTS		
Cone Vanilla	1 med	260
Freeze A&W Root Beer	1 med	480
Polar Swirl M&M	1 med	710
Polar Swirl Oreo	1 med	690
Polar Swirl Reese's	1 med	740
Sundae Caramel	1 med	340
Sundae Chocolate	1 med	320
Sundae Hot Fudge	1 med	350
Sundae Strawberry	1 med	300
Sundae Vanilla	1 med	310
MAIN MENU SELECTIONS		
Cheese Curds	1 serv	570
Cheese Dog	1	320
Cheeseburger Original Bacon	1	570
Cheeseburger Original Bacon Double	1	800
Cheeseburger Original Double	1	720
Chicken Strips	3	500
Chili Bowl	1 serv	190
Coney Chili Dog	1	310
Coney Chili Dog Cheese	1	350
Fries	1 lg	430
Fries Cheese	1 serv	380
Fries Chili	1 serv	370
Fries Chili & Cheese	1 serv	400
Hot Dog Plain	1	280
Onion Rings	1 serv	350
Papa Burger	1	720
Sandwich Crispy Chicken	1	590

FOOD	PORTION	CALS
Sandwich Grilled Chicken	1	440
SAUCES		
Dipping Sauce BBQ	1 serv (1 oz)	40
Dipping Sauce Honey Mustard	1 serv (1 oz)	100
Dipping Sauce Ranch	1 serv (1 oz)	160
Dipping Sauce Sweet & Sour	1 serv (1 oz)	45

ARBY'S
BEVERAGES

FOOD	PORTION	CALS
Dr Pepper	1 (16 oz)	180
Jamocha Shake	1 reg	498
Pepsi	1 (16 oz)	130
Shake Chocolate	1 reg	507
Shake Orange Cream	1 (17 oz)	637
Shake Strawberry	1 reg	498
Shake Strawberry Banana Swirl	1 (17 oz)	567
Sierra Mist	1 (16 oz)	100
Vanilla Shake	1 reg	437
BREAKFAST SELECTIONS		
Biscuit	1	273
Biscuit Bacon Egg & Cheese	1	461
Biscuit Chicken	1	417
Biscuit Ham Egg & Cheese	1	437
Biscuit Sausage Egg & Cheese	1	557
Biscuit Sausage Gravy	1	961
Biscuit w/ Bacon	1	340
Biscuit w/ Ham	1	316
Biscuit w/ Sausage	1	436
Breakfast Syrup	1 serv (1 oz)	78
Cinnamon Roll Original Gourmet	1	507
Croissant	1	190
Croissant Bacon & Egg	1	337
Croissant Bacon Egg & Cheese	1	378
Croissant Ham & Cheese	1	274
Croissant Ham Egg & Cheese	1	434
Croissant Sausage & Egg	1	433
Croissant Sausage Egg & Cheese	1	475
French Toastix	1 serv	312
Muffin Blueberry	1	320
Pecan Sticky Bun	1	688
Sourdough Bacon Egg & Cheese	1	437

FOOD	PORTION	CALS
Sourdough Egg & Cheese	1	392
Sourdough Ham Egg & Cheese	1	679
Sourdough Sausage Egg & Cheese	1	514
Twist Chocolate	1	250
Twist Cinnamon	1	260
Wrap Bacon Egg & Cheese	1	515
Wrap Ham Egg & Cheese	1	568
Wrap Sausage Egg & Cheese	1	689
CHILDREN'S MENU SELECTIONS		
Kids Meal Chicken Tenders	1 serv	289
Kids Meal Junior Roast Beef Sandwich	1	272
Market Fresh Mini Ham & Cheese Sandwich	1	228
Market Fresh Mini Turkey & Cheese Sandwich	1	235
DESSERTS		
Cookie Chocolate Chip	1 (1.6 oz)	202
Turnover Apple	1	377
Turnover Cherry	1	377
SALAD DRESSINGS AND SAUCES		
Arby's Sauce	1 serv (0.5 oz)	15
Dipping Sauce BBQ	1 pkg (1 oz)	40
Dipping Sauce Bronco Berry	1 serv (2 oz)	122
Dipping Sauce Buffalo	1 serv (1 oz)	10
Dipping Sauce Cool Ranch Sour Cream	1 serv (1.5 oz)	158
Dipping Sauce Honey Mustard	1 serv (1 oz)	129
Dressing Buttermilk Ranch	1 serv (2.2 oz)	325
Dressing Buttermilk Ranch Light	1 serv (2 oz)	112
Dressing Sante Fe Ranch	1 pkg (2.2 oz)	296
Horsey Sauce	1 pkg (0.5 oz)	62
Ketchup	1 pkg	13
Sauce Cheddar Cheese	1 serv (0.7 oz)	30
Sauce Spicy Three Pepper	1 serv (0.5 oz)	22
Sauce Tangy Southwest	1 serv (2 oz)	333
SALADS		
Chicken Club	1 serv	487
Martha's Vineyard	1 serv	277
Santa Fe	1 serv	477
SANDWICHES		
Arby's Melt	1	302
Beef'N Cheddar	1	445
Chicken Bacon & Swiss Crispy	1	624

FOOD	PORTION	CALS
Chicken Bacon & Swiss Grilled	1	462
Chicken Cordon Bleu Crispy	1	650
Chicken Cordon Bleu Grilled	1	488
Chicken Fillet Crispy	1	576
Chicken Fillet Grilled	1	414
Chicken Salad w/ Pecans	1	769
Corned Beef Reuben	1	606
Fish	1	543
French Dip	1	391
French Dip & Swiss	1	473
Ham & Swiss Melt	1	275
Roast Beef Regular	1	320
Roast Beef Super	1	398
Roast Beef & Swiss	1	777
Roast Beef 'N Cheddar	1	521
Roast Ham & Swiss	1	705
Roast Turkey & Swiss	1	725
Roast Turkey Ranch & Bacon	1	834
Roast Turkey Reuben	1	611
Sourdough Melt Beef	1	355
Sourdough Melt Ham	1	380
Spicy Cajun Fish	1	603
Sub Toasted Classic Italian	1	828
Sub Toasted French Dip & Swiss	1	622
Sub Toasted Philly Beef	1	739
Sub Toasted Turkey Bacon Club	1	619
Swiss Melt	1	303
Ultimate BLT	1	779
Wrap Chicken Salad w/ Pecans	1	638
Wrap Corned Beef Reuben	1	577
Wrap Roast Turkey Ranch & Bacon	1	700
Wrap Roast Turkey Reuben	1	581
Wrap Southwest Chicken	1	567
Wrap Ultimate BLT	1	648
SIDES		
Bites Jalapeno	5	305
Bites Loaded Potato	5	353
Cheddar Fries	1 med	465
Chicken Tenders	3 pieces	379
Croutons Cheese & Garlic	1 pkg	77

FOOD	PORTION	CALS
Curly Fries	1 sm	338
Curly Fries	1 lg	631
Fruit Cup	1 serv	35
Homestyle Fries	1 sm	302
Homestyle Fries	1 lg	566
Mozzarella Sticks	8 pieces	849
Onion Petals	1 reg	331
Popcorn Chicken	1 reg	365
Potato Cakes	2	246
Seasoned Tortilla Strips	1 serv	71

AU BON PAIN
BAKED SELECTIONS

FOOD	PORTION	CALS
Bagel Asiago Cheese	1	360
Bagel Cinnamon Raisin	1	320
Bagel Everything	1	350
Bagel Honey 9 Grain	1	330
Bagel Jalapeno Double Cheddar	1	350
Bagel Onion Dill	1	350
Bagel Plain	1	290
Bagel Poppy Seed	1	290
Bagel Sesame Seed	1	330
Baguette Artisan Honey Multigrain Salad Size	1 (3.5 oz)	240
Baguette Artisan Honey Multigrain Sandwich Size	1 (4.7 oz)	310
Baguette Artisan Salad Size	1 (3.5 oz)	210
Baguette Artisan Sandwich Size	1 (4.7 oz)	290
Blondie	1	330
Bread Artisan Multigrain	1 serv (4 oz)	260
Bread Artisan Sundried Tomato	1 serv (4 oz)	240
Bread Cheese	1 serv (4.8 oz)	290
Bread Country White	1 serv (4 oz)	240
Bread Bowl	1 (9.24 oz)	640
Bread Stick Rosemary Garlic	1 (2.3 oz)	200
Brownie Chocolate Chip	1	380
Brownie Hazelnut Mocha	1	430
Brownie Rocky Road	1	410
Ciabatta	1 sm	180
Cinnamon Roll	1	350
Cookie Chocolate Chip	1 (2 oz)	260
Cookie Confetti	1 (2.4 oz)	310

FOOD	PORTION	CALS
Cookie English Toffee	1 (2 oz)	210
Cookie Gingerbread	1 (2.7 oz)	300
Cookie Hazelnut Fudge	1 (2.25 oz)	290
Cookie Oatmeal Raisin	1 (2 oz)	230
Cookie Shortbread	1 (2.3 oz)	310
Creme De Fleur	1 serv	550
Croissant Almond	1	560
Croissant Apple	1	230
Croissant Chocolate	1	330
Croissant Plain	1 (2.8 oz)	260
Croissant Raspberry Cheese	1	330
Croissant Sweet Cheese	1	320
Danish Cherry	1	370
Danish Sweet Cheese	1	380
Focaccia	1 piece (4.4 oz)	310
Lahvash	1 (4 oz)	320
Macaroon Chocolate Dipped Cranberry Almond	1	320
Mini Loaf Bacon & Cheese	1 (4.8 oz)	540
Muffin Blueberry	1	510
Muffin Carrot Walnut	1	520
Muffin Corn	1	460
Muffin Cranberry Walnut	1	500
Muffin Double Chocolate Chunk	1	590
Muffin Low Fat Triple Berry	1	290
Muffin Pumpkin	1	490
Muffin Raisin Bran	1	410
Pastry Hazelnut Creme	1	540
Poundcake Cappuccino	1 slice (5.2 oz)	530
Poundcake Chocolate	1 slice (4.7 oz)	500
Poundcake Lemon	1 slice (4.9 oz)	520
Poundcake Marble	1 slice (4.7 oz)	490
Roll Soft	1 (4.7 oz)	410
Roll Pecan	1	630
Scone Cinnamon	1	430
Scone Orange	1	410
Shortbread Chocolate Dipped	1	350
Toasts Basil Pesto Cheese	3 pieces (2 oz)	140
Tulip Blueberry	1	370
Tulip Chocolate Raspberry	1	430

FOOD	PORTION	CALS
Tulip Key Lime	1	440
BEVERAGES		
Blast Caramel	1 med (16 oz)	540
Blast Coffee	1 med (16 oz)	440
Blast Mocha	1 med (16 oz)	440
Blast Vanilla	1 med (12 oz)	540
Caffe Americano	1 sm (12 oz)	5
Caffe Latte	1 sm (12 oz)	200
Cappuccino	1 sm (12 oz)	120
Caramel Macchiato	1 sm (12 oz)	350
Chai Latte	1 sm (12 oz)	290
Chocolate Milk	1 (12 oz)	320
Hot Chocolate	1 sm (12 oz)	350
Iced Caffe Latte	1 sm (12 oz)	110
Iced Caramel Macchiato	1 sm (12 oz)	290
Iced Chai Latte	1 sm (12 oz)	190
Iced Mocha Latte	1 sm (12 oz)	210
Iced Tea Peach	1 med (22 oz)	120
Iced Vanilla Latte	1 sm (12 oz)	240
Iced White Chocolate Latte	1 sm (12 oz)	250
Lemonade	1 med (22 oz)	300
Mocha Latte	1 sm (12 oz)	300
Orange Juice	1 (8 oz)	110
Smoothie Peach	1 med (16 oz)	310
Smoothie Strawberry	1 med (16 oz)	310
Vanilla Latte	1 sm (12 oz)	320
White Chocolate Latte	1 sm (12 oz)	310
MAIN MENU SELECTIONS		
Fruit Cup	1 sm (6 oz)	70
Harvest Rice Bowl Cajun Shrimp	1 (20 oz)	520
Harvest Rice Bowl Cajun Shrimp w/ Brown Rice	1 (20 oz)	56
Harvest Rice Bowl Mayan Chicken	1 (19.25 oz)	490
Harvest Rice Bowl Mayan Chicken w/ Brown Rice	1 (19.25 oz)	540
Harvest Rice Bowl Steak Teriyaki	1 (19.25 oz)	530
Harvest Rice Bowl Steak Teriyaki w/ Brown Rice	1 (19.25 oz)	570
Macaroni & Cheese	1 med (12 oz)	440
Stew Beef	1 med (12 oz)	300

FOOD	PORTION	CALS
Stew Chicken Vegetable	1 med (12 oz)	290
SALAD DRESSINGS AND SPREADS		
Artichoke Aioli	1 serv (1 oz)	130
Basil Pesto	1 serv (1 oz)	140
Chili Dijon	1 serv (1 oz)	120
Cream Cheese Honey Pecan	1 serv (2 oz)	120
Cream Cheese Honey Walnut	1 serv (2 oz)	140
Cream Cheese Lite	1 serv (2 oz)	120
Cream Cheese Plain	1 serv (2 oz)	170
Cream Cheese Strawberry	1 serv (2 oz)	180
Cream Cheese Sundried Tomato	1 serv (2 oz)	120
Cream Cheese Vegetable	1 serv (2 oz)	170
Dressing Balsamic Vinaigrette	1 serv (2.25 oz)	190
Dressing Blue Cheese	1 serv (1.75 oz)	230
Dressing Caesar	1 serv (2 oz)	280
Dressing Fat Free Raspberry Vinaigrette	1 serv (2.25 oz)	70
Dressing Light Honey Mustard	1 serv (2.25 oz)	180
Dressing Light Olive Oil Vinaigrette	1 serv (2.25 oz)	130
Dressing Light Ranch	1 serv (2.25 oz)	150
Dressing Thai Peanut	1 serv (2.25 oz)	230
Guacamole	1 serv (1 oz)	60
Honey Mustard	1 serv (2.5 oz)	210
Hummus Roasted Red Pepper	1 serv (2 oz)	80
Mayonnaise	1 serv (1 oz)	200
Mayonnaise Herb	1 serv (1 oz)	210
Mayonnaise Jalapeno	1 serv (1 oz)	140
Mayonnaise Tarragon Sauce	1 serv (2 oz)	420
Mustard	1 tsp	0
Spread Herb	1 serv (2 oz)	130
Spread Sundried Tomato	1 serv (0.53 oz)	70
SALADS		
Caesar Asiago	1 serv	210
Caesar Asiago Grilled Chicken	1 (8.5 oz)	340
Caesar Asiago Side	1 (3.2 oz)	120
Chef's	1 serv	230
Garden	1 (7 oz)	80
Garden Side	1 (3.6 oz)	50
Mediterranean Chicken	1 (9.75 oz)	330
Riviera	1 (9.5 oz)	260
Thai Peanut Chicken	1 (11 oz)	250

FOOD	PORTION	CALS
Tuna Garden	1 (10.5 oz)	350
Turkey Medallion Cobb	1 (11 oz)	340
Turkey Spinach Sonoma	1 (12.3 oz)	310
SANDWICHES		
Arizona Chicken	1 (12 oz)	750
Baguette Turkey & Swiss	1 (12.3 oz)	770
Baja Turkey	1 (13 oz)	700
Breakfast Asiago Bagel Prosciutto & Egg	1 (9.6 oz)	660
Breakfast Asiago Bagel Sausage Egg & Cheddar	1 (10.2 oz)	770
Breakfast Bagel & Bacon	1 (4.2 oz)	340
Breakfast Egg On A Bagel	1 (6.8 oz)	370
Breakfast Egg On A Bagel w/ Bacon	1 (7.2 oz)	410
Breakfast Egg On A Bagel w/ Bacon Cheese	1 (7.9 oz)	500
Breakfast Egg On A Bagel w/ Cheese	1 (7.6 oz)	450
Breakfast Onion Dill Bagel Smoked Salmon & Wasabi	1 (7.1 oz)	490
Caprese	1 (11.8 oz)	700
Chicken Mozzarella	1 (14.5 oz)	800
Chicken Pesto	1 (12.5 oz)	700
Chicken Tarragon	1 (11 oz)	720
Ciabatta Bacon & Egg Melt	1 (7 oz)	400
Ciabatta Ham & Cheddar	1 (12 oz)	650
Club Smoked Turkey	1 (11.6 oz)	780
Croissant Ham & Cheese	1 (4.2 oz)	350
Croissant Spinach & Cheese	1	250
Hot BBQ Chicken On Farmhouse Roll	1 (14.3 oz)	970
Hot Eggplant & Mozzarella	1 (12.4 oz)	710
Hot Steakhouse On Ciabatta	1 (13 oz)	800
Melt Tuna	1 (12.5 oz)	760
Melt Turkey	1 (12.2 oz)	890
Portobello & Goat Cheese	1 (10 oz)	610
Portobello Egg & Cheddar	1 (8.5 oz)	590
Prosciutto Mozzarella	1 (12.7 oz)	880
Spicy Tuna	1 (10.3 oz)	640
The Montana	1 (12.5 oz)	560
Turkey & Cranberry Chutney	1 (10.9 oz)	680
Wrap Chicken Caesar Asiago	1	700
Wrap Chopped Turkey Club	1 (12 oz)	660
Wrap Mediterranean	1 (12.8 oz)	670

FOOD	PORTION	CALS
Wrap Southwest Tuna	1 (14 oz)	900
Wrap Thai Peanut Chicken	1 (14.5 oz)	660
Wrap Turkey Spinach Sonoma	1 (12 oz)	630
Wrap Hot Cajun Shrimp	1 (14.9 oz)	700
Wrap Hot Mayan Chicken	1 (13.5 oz)	630
Wrap Hot Steak Teriyaki	1 (13.5 oz)	660
SOUPS		
Baked Stuffed Potato	1 med (12 oz)	350
Broccoli Cheddar	1 med (12 oz)	310
Carrot Ginger	1 med (12 oz)	130
Chicken & Dumplings	1 med (12 oz)	210
Chicken Florentine	1 med (12 oz)	240
Chicken Noodle	1 med (12 oz)	130
Clam Chowder	1 med (12 oz)	320
Corn & Green Chili Bisque	1 med (12 oz)	250
Corn Chowder	1 med (12 oz)	350
Curried Rice & Lentil	1 med (12 oz)	150
French Moroccan Tomato Lentil	1 med (12 oz)	180
French Onion	1 med (12 oz)	130
Garden Vegetable	1 med (12 oz)	80
Harvest Pumpkin	1 med (12 oz)	190
Hearty Cabbage	1 med (12 oz)	110
Italian Wedding	1 med (12 oz)	170
Jamaican Black Bean	1 med (12 oz)	180
Mediterranean Pepper	1 med (12 oz)	100
Old Fashioned Tomato Rice	1 med (12 oz)	120
Pasta E Fagioli	1 med (12 oz)	240
Portuguese Kale	1 med (12 oz)	120
Potato Cheese	1 med (12 oz)	250
Potato Leek	1 med (12 oz)	300
Red Beans Italian Sausage & Rice	1 med (12 oz)	200
Southern Black Eyed Pea	1 med (12 oz)	180
Southwest Tortilla	1 med (12 oz)	200
Southwest Vegetable	1 med (12 oz)	160
Split Pea	1 med (12 oz)	210
Thai Coconut Curry	1 med (12 oz)	150
Tomato Basil Bisque	1 med (12 oz)	210
Tomato Cheddar	1 med (12 oz)	240
Tomato Florentine	1 med (12 oz)	120
Tuscan Vegetable	1 med (12 oz)	170

FOOD	PORTION	CALS
Vegetable Beef Barley	1 med (12 oz)	140
Vegetarian Chili	1 med (12 oz)	230
Vegetarian Lentil	1 med (12 oz)	140
Vegetarian Minestrone	1 med (12 oz)	120
Wild Mushroom Bisque	1 med (12 oz)	190
YOGURT		
Blueberry w/ Fruit	1 sm (7.5 oz)	220
Blueberry w/ Granola & Fruit	1 sm (8.5 oz)	310
Strawberry w/ Blueberries	1 sm (7.5 oz)	220
Strawberry w/ Granola & Blueberries	1 sm (8.5 oz)	310
Vanilla w/ Blueberries	1 sm (7.5 oz)	190
Vanilla w/ Granola & Blueberries	1 sm (8.5 oz)	310

AUNTIE ANNE'S
BEVERAGES

FOOD	PORTION	CALS
Dutch Ice Blue Raspberry	1 (14 oz)	165
Dutch Ice Grape	1 (14 oz)	180
Dutch Ice Kiwi Banana	1 (14 oz)	190
Dutch Ice Lemonade	1 (14 oz)	315
Dutch Ice Lemonade Strawberry	1 (14 oz)	330
Dutch Ice Mocha	1 (14 oz)	400
Dutch Ice Orange Creme	1 (14 oz)	280
Dutch Ice Pina Colada	1 (14 oz)	220
Dutch Ice Strawberry	1 (14 oz)	220
Dutch Ice Watermelon	1 (14 oz)	200
Dutch Ice Wild Cherry	1 (14 oz)	210
Dutch Latte Caramel	1 (14 oz)	350
Dutch Latte Coffee	1 (14 oz)	290
Dutch Latte Mocha	1 (14 oz)	160
Dutch Shake Chocolate	1 (14 oz)	580
Dutch Shake Coffee	1 (14 oz)	590
Dutch Shake Strawberry	1 (14 oz)	610
Dutch Shake Vanilla	1 (14 oz)	510
Dutch Smoothie Blue Raspberry	1 (14 oz)	230
Dutch Smoothie Grape	1 (14 oz)	230
Dutch Smoothie Kiwi Banana	1 (14 oz)	240
Dutch Smoothie Lemonade	1 (14 oz)	300
Dutch Smoothie Mocha	1 (14 oz)	330
Dutch Smoothie Orange Creme	1 (14 oz)	280
Dutch Smoothie Pina Colada	1 (14 oz)	260
Dutch Smoothie Strawberry	1 (14 oz)	250

FOOD	PORTION	CALS
Dutch Smoothie Wild Cherry	1 (14 oz)	250
Lemonade	1 (22 oz)	180
Lemonade Strawberry	1 (22 oz)	190
DIPPING SAUCES		
Caramel Dip	1 serv (1.5 oz)	135
Cheese Sauce	1 serv (1.25 oz)	100
Cream Cheese Light	1 serv (1.25 oz)	70
Hot Salsa Cheese	1 serv (1.25 oz)	100
Marinara Sauce	1 serv (1.25 oz)	10
Sweet	1 serv (1.4 oz)	40
Sweet Mustard	1 serv (1.25 oz)	60
PRETZELS		
Almond	1	400
Almond w/o Butter	1	350
Cinnamon Raisin w/o Butter	1	350
Cinnamon Sugar	1	450
Garlic	1	350
Garlic w/o Butter	1	320
Glazin' Raisin	1	510
Glazin' Raisin w/o Butter	1	470
Jalapeno	1	310
Jalapeno w/o Butter	1	270
Original	1	370
Original w/o Butter	1	340
Pretzel Dog	1	290
Sesame	1	410
Sesame w/o Butter	1	350
Sour Cream & Onion	1	340
Sour Cream & Onion w/o Butter	1	310
Stix	6	370
Stix w/o Butter	6	340
Whole Wheat	1	370
Whole Wheat w/o Butter	1	350

BABS DELI
BAGELS

FOOD	PORTION	CALS
Apple Cinnamon	1	332
Banana Nut	1	340
Blueberry	1	330
Blueberry Cobbler	1	392
Cheddar Herb	1	352

FOOD	PORTION	CALS
Cheddar Nacho	1	352
Chocolate Chip	1	348
Cinnamon Apple Pie	1	386
Cinnamon Bun	1	400
Cinnamon Danish	1	396
Cinnamon Raisin	1	336
Cinnamon Sugar	1	350
Cranberry Walnut	1	352
Egg	1	328
Everything	1	336
French Toast	1	372
Garlic	1	330
Honey Oat	1	320
Jalapeno	1	350
Onion	1	336
Plain	1	334
Poppy	1	344
Pumpernickel	1	332
Quiche Lorraine	1	354
Salt	1	324
Sesame	1	358
Spinach	1	356
Strawberry	1	342
Strawberry White Chocolate	1	364
Swiss Melt	1	368
Tomato Basil	1	322
Vegetable	1	318
Wheat	1	330
White Chocolate Swirl	1	396
BEVERAGES		
Americano	1 (16 oz)	12
Cafe Caramello	1 (16 oz)	212
Cappuccino 2% Milk	1 (16 oz)	195
Cappuccino Fat Free Milk	1 (16 oz)	133
Coffee Black Forest	1 (16 oz)	198
Icepresso Caramel Decadence	1 (16 oz)	300
Icepresso Classic	1 (16 oz)	300
Icepresso Java Chip	1 (16 oz)	360
Icepresso Latte	1 (16 oz)	300
Icepresso Mocha	1 (16 oz)	300

FOOD	PORTION	CALS
Icepresso Strawberry	1 (16 oz)	340
Italiano 2% Milk	1 (16 oz)	131
Italiano Fat Free Milk	1 (16 oz)	89
Jittery Monkey 2% Milk	1 (16 oz)	482
Jittery Monkey Fat Free Milk	1 (16 oz)	429
Latte 2% Milk	1 (16 oz)	212
Latte Cinnamon Toast 2% Milk	1 (16 oz)	299
Latte Cinnamon Toast Fat Free Milk	1 (16 oz)	240
Latte Creme Caramel 2% Milk	1 (16 oz)	303
Latte Creme Caramel Fat Free Milk	1 (16 oz)	244
Latte Fat Free Milk	1 (16 oz)	145
Latte Oregon Chai Tea 2% Milk	1 (16 oz)	274
Latte Oregon Chai Tea Fat Free Milk	1 (16 oz)	231
Latte Raspberry Cheesecake 2% Milk	1 (16 oz)	319
Latte Raspberry Cheesecake Fat Free Milk	1 (16 oz)	259
Latte Vanilla Creme 2% Milk	1 (16 oz)	275
Mocha Whipped Cream 2% Milk	1 (16 oz)	454
Mocha Whipped Cream Fat Free Milk	1 (16 oz)	392
Turtle Mocha Fat Free Milk	1 (16 oz)	522
MUFFINS		
My Favorite Banana Nut	2 mini	195
My Favorite Blueberry	2 mini	168
My Favorite Blueberry Cheesecake	2 mini	199
My Favorite Boston Cream Pie	2 mini	176
My Favorite Cherry Cheesecake	2 mini	170
My Favorite Chocolate Cheesecake	2 mini	202
My Favorite Chocolate Chip	2 mini	211
My Favorite Cinnamon Crumb Cake	2 mini	212
My Favorite Cinnamon Swirl Cheesecake	2 mini	214
My Favorite Deep Dish Apple	2 mini	177
My Favorite Double Chocolate	2 mini	210
My Favorite Fat Free Blueberry	2 mini	108
My Favorite Fat Free Cherry Pie	2 mini	109
My Favorite Fat Free Chocolate Marble	2 mini	125
My Favorite Fat Free Cinnamon Bun	2 mini	168
My Favorite Fat Free Raspberry Amaretto	2 mini	127
My Favorite Golden Corn Bread	2 mini	197
My Favorite Lemon Poppyseed	2 mini	201
My Favorite Pumpkin Spice	2 mini	181

FOOD	PORTION	CALS
SALADS		
Calypso Chicken	1 (13.6 oz)	637
Calypso Chicken w/ Lite Italian	1 (13.6 oz)	317
Chicken Caesar	1 (11.5 oz)	524
Chicken Caesar w/ Lite Italian	1 (11.5 oz)	268
Classic Caesar	1 (8.4 oz)	414
Classic Caesar Cafe	1 (4.3 oz)	225
Classic Caesar w/ Lite Italian	1 (8.4 oz)	158
Garden Mix	1 (12.4 oz)	197
Garden Mix Cafe	1 (6.5 oz)	100
Grilled Chicken Club	1 (17.9 oz)	820
Grilled Chicken Club w/ Lite Italian	1 (17.9 oz)	500
Low Carb Tuna Salad Plate	1 serv (8.9 oz)	356
Mediterranean Bread	1 (18.8 oz)	973
Mediterranean Bread w/ Lite Italian	1 (18.8 oz)	626
SANDWICHES		
Breakfast BLT	1	704
Breakfast Lox & Cream Cheese	1	602
Breakfast Morning Classic	1	486
Breakfast Northern Omelet	1	699
Breakfast Southern Tradition w/ Bacon	1	566
Breakfast Southern Tradition w/ Ham	1	547
Breakfast Southern Tradition w/ Sausage	1	696
Build Your Own Ham	1	495
Build Your Own Roast Beef	1	480
Build Your Own Tuna	1	547
Build Your Own Turkey	1	465
Enchilada Bagellata	1	522
Gourmet Classic Turkey	1	552
Gourmet Holey Guacamole	1	476
Gourmet Kick-N Roast Beef	1	579
Gourmet Mediterranean Veg-Out	1	506
Overstuffed Classic Reuben	1	962
Overstuffed Corned Beef	1	661
Overstuffed Ham & Cheese	1	889
Overstuffed Manhattan Club	1	1122
Overstuffed Pastrami	1	661
Overstuffed TD Classic California	1	759
Overstuffed TD Classic Club	1	1110
Overstuffed TD Clubhouse	1	1079

FOOD	PORTION	CALS
Pizzaah Bruschetta	1 piece	162
Pizzaah Cheese	1 piece	189
Pizzaah Grilled Chicken Bruschetta	1 piece	343
Pizzaah Sausage	1 piece	211
Pizzaah Veggie	1 piece	238
Specialty All American Duo	1	752
Specialty Big Apple Club	1	797
Specialty Chicken Caesar	1	611
Specialty Roma Italian	1	764
Specialty Turkey Club	1	782
Toasted Cafe Chicken Melt	1	815
Toasted Deli Style Turkey	1	732
Toasted Roast Beef Parmesan Grinder	1	583
Toasted Spicy Italian Sub	1	770
Toasted Tuna Melt	1	641
SOUPS		
Beef Barley Mushroom	1 serv (8 oz)	100
Boston Clam Chowder	1 serv (8 oz)	210
Chicken & Wild Rice	1 serv (8 oz)	190
Chicken Gumbo	1 serv (8 oz)	130
Cream Of Potato	1 serv (8 oz)	240
Hearty Vegetable Beef	1 serv (8 oz)	100
New England Clam Chowder	1 serv (8 oz)	220
Split Pea w/ Ham	1 serv (8 oz)	90
Wisconsin Cheese	1 serv (8 oz)	210
SPREADS		
Cream Cheese	2 tbsp	90
Cream Cheese Cheddar Jalapeno	2 tbsp	90
Cream Cheese Garden Vegetable	2 tbsp	90
Cream Cheese Lite	2 tbsp	60
Cream Cheese Onion Chive	2 tbsp	80
Cream Cheese Strawberry	2 tbsp	90
Cream Cheese Whipped	2 tbsp	70
Cream Cheese Whipped Brown Sugar Cinnamon	2 tbsp	70
Cream Cheese Whipped Reduced Fat Spring Veggie	2 tbsp	60

BAJA FRESH
CHILDREN'S MENU SELECTIONS

Kid's Mini Burrito Bean & Cheese	1 serv	540

FOOD	PORTION	CALS
Kid's Mini Burrito Bean & Cheese w/ Chicken	1 serv	590
Kid's Mini Quesadilla Cheese	1 serv	610
Kid's Mini Quesadilla Cheese w/ Chicken	1 serv	650
Kid's Taquitos Chicken	1 serv	630
MAIN MENU SELECTIONS		
Black Beans	1 serv	360
Burrito Baja Breaded Fish	1 serv	850
Burrito Baja Carnitas	1 serv	830
Burrito Baja Chicken	1 serv	790
Burrito Baja Mahi Mahi	1 serv	780
Burrito Baja Shrimp	1 serv	760
Burrito Baja Steak	1 serv	850
Burrito Bare Carnitas	1 serv	600
Burrito Bare Chicken	1 serv	640
Burrito Bare Steak	1 serv	700
Burrito Bare Veggie & Cheese	1 serv	580
Burrito Bean & Cheese Breaded Fish	1 serv	1030
Burrito Bean & Cheese Carnitas	1 serv	1010
Burrito Bean & Cheese Chicken	1 serv	970
Burrito Bean & Cheese Mahi Mahi	1 serv	960
Burrito Bean & Cheese No Meat	1 serv	840
Burrito Bean & Cheese Shrimp	1 serv	950
Burrito Bean & Cheese Steak	1 serv	1030
Burrito Dos Manos Breaded Fish	1 serv	890
Burrito Dos Manos Carnitas	1 serv	780
Burrito Dos Manos Chicken	½ serv	760
Burrito Dos Manos Mahi Mahi	1 serv	780
Burrito Dos Manos Shrimp	1 serv	780
Burrito Dos Manos Steak	½ serv	795
Burrito Grilled Veggie	1 serv	506
Burrito Mexicano Breaded Fish	1 serv	850
Burrito Mexicano Carnitas	1 serv	830
Burrito Mexicano Chicken	1 serv	790
Burrito Mexicano Mahi Mahi	1 serv	790
Burrito Mexicano Shrimp	1 serv	770
Burrito Mexicano Steak	1 serv	860
Burrito Ultimo Breaded Fish	1 serv	940
Burrito Ultimo Carnitas	1 serv	920
Burrito Ultimo Chicken	1 serv	880
Burrito Ultimo Mahi Mahi	1 serv	880

FOOD	PORTION	CALS
Burrito Ultimo Shrimp	1 serv	860
Burrito Ultimo Steak	1 serv	950
Chips & Guacamole	1 serv	1340
Chips & Salsa Baja	1 serv	810
Fajitas Corn Tortillas Breaded Fish	1 serv	1060
Fajitas Corn Tortillas Carnitas	1 serv	920
Fajitas Corn Tortillas Chicken	1 serv	860
Fajitas Corn Tortillas Mahi Mahi	1 serv	840
Fajitas Corn Tortillas Shrimp	1 serv	840
Fajitas Corn Tortillas Steak	1 serv	960
Fajitas Flour Tortillas Breaded Fish	1 serv	1340
Fajitas Flour Tortillas Carnitas	1 serv	1190
Fajitas Flour Tortillas Chicken	1 serv	1140
Fajitas Flour Tortillas Mahi Mahi	1 serv	1120
Fajitas Flour Tortillas Shrimp	1 serv	1120
Fajitas Flour Tortillas Steak	1 serv	960
Guacamole Side	1 (3 oz)	110
Nachos Breaded Fish	1 serv	2090
Nachos Carnitas	1 serv	2060
Nachos Cheese	1 serv	1890
Nachos Chicken	1 serv	2020
Nachos Mahi Mahi	1 serv	2020
Nachos Shrimp	1 serv	2000
Nachos Steak	1 serv	2120
Pico De Gallo Side	1 serv (8 oz)	50
Pinto Beans	1 serv	320
Pronto Guacamole Side	1 serv (6 oz)	560
Quesadilla Breaded Fish	1 serv	1400
Quesadilla Carnitas	1 serv	1370
Quesadilla Cheese	1 serv	1200
Quesadilla Chicken	1 serv	1330
Quesadilla Mahi Mahi	1 serv	1330
Quesadilla Shrimp	1 serv	1310
Quesadilla Steak	1 serv	1430
Quesadilla Veggie	1 serv	1260
Rice	1 serv	280
Rice & Beans Plate	1 serv	420
Salsa Baja Side	1 serv (8 oz)	70
Salsa Roja Side	1 serv (8 oz)	70
Salsa Verde Side	1 serv (8 oz)	50

FOOD	PORTION	CALS
Soup Tortilla w/ Chicken	1 serv (13.6 oz)	320
Soup Tortilla w/o Chicken	1 serv (12.4 oz)	270
Taco Grilled Mahi Mahi	1 serv	230
Taco Baja Breaded Fish	1 serv	250
Taco Baja Chicken	1 serv	210
Taco Baja Shrimp	1 serv	200
Taco Baja Steak	1 serv	230
Taco Soft Breaded Fish	1 serv	240
Taco Soft Carnitas	1 serv	250
Taco Soft Chicken	1 serv	230
Taco Soft Mahi Mahi	1 serv	240
Taco Soft Shrimp	1 serv	230
Taco Soft Steak	1 serv	260
Taquitos Chicken w/ Beans	3	780
Taquitos Chicken w/ Rice	3	740
Veggie Mix	1 serv	110
SALAD DRESSINGS		
Chipotle Vinaigrette	1 serv (2.5 oz)	110
Fat Free Salsa Verde	1 serv (2.5 oz)	15
Olive Oil Vinaigrette	1 serv (2.5 oz)	290
Ranch	1 serv (2.5 oz)	260
SALADS		
Baja Ensalada Chicken	1 serv	310
Baja Ensalada Shrimp	1 serv	230
Baja Ensalada Steak	1 serv	450
Chipotle w/ Carnitas	1 serv	640
Chipotle w/ Chicken	1 serv	590
Chipotle w/ Steak	1 serv	700
Side By Side Carnitas	1 serv	570
Side By Side Chicken	1 serv	500
Side By Side Steak	1 serv	620
Side Salad	1 (6.5 oz)	130
Tostada Breaded Fish	1 serv	1200
Tostada Carnitas	1 serv	1180
Tostada Chicken	1 serv	1140
Tostada Mahi Mahi	1 serv	1130
Tostada No Meat	1 serv	1010
Tostada Shrimp	1 serv	1120
Tostada Steak	1 serv	1230

FOOD	PORTION	CALS
BEAR ROCK CAFE		
SANDWICHES		
Colorado Turkey Club	1	855
Coop's Chicken Salad Croissant	1	439
Garden Grill Ciabatta	1	406
Giant Panda Wrap	1	556
Hoot Owl	1	641
Rising Sunflower	1	596
Roast Turkey & Bacon	1	522
Rockslide Focaccia	1	958
The Moose	1	976
BEN & JERRY'S		
FROZEN YOGURT		
Low Fat Cherry Garcia	½ cup	170
Low Fat Chocolate Fudge Brownie	½ cup	190
Low Fat Half Baked	½ cup	190
Phish Food	½ cup	220
ICE CREAM		
Bar Cherry Garcia	1	270
Bar Half Baked	1	340
Bar Vanilla	1	300
Bar Vanilla Almond	1	340
Black & Tan	½ cup	230
Brownie Batter	½ cup	310
Butter Pecan	½ cup	280
Cherry Garcia	½ cup	250
Chocolate	½ cup	260
Chocolate Chip Cookie Dough	½ cup	270
Chocolate Fudge Brownie	½ cup	260
Chubby Hubby	½ cup	330
Chunky Monkey	½ cup	300
Coffee	½ cup	240
Coffee Heath Bar Crunch	½ cup	290
Dave Matthews Band Magic Brownies	½ cup	250
Dublin Mudslide	½ cup	270
Everything But The	½ cup	310
Fossil Fuel	½ cup	280
Fudge Central	½ cup	300
Half Baked	½ cup	280
In A Crunch	½ cup	350

FOOD	PORTION	CALS
Karamel Sutra	½ cup	280
Marsha Marsha Marshmallow	½ cup	300
Mint Chocolate Cookie	½ cup	260
Neapolitan Dynamite	½ cup	250
New York Super Fudge Chunk	½ cup	310
Oatmeal Cookie Chunk	½ cup	270
Organic Chocolate Fudge Brownie	½ cup	270
Organic Strawberry	½ cup	210
Organic Sweet Cream & Cookies	½ cup	250
Organic Vanilla	½ cup	220
Peanut Butter Cup	½ cup	360
Phish Food	½ cup	280
Pistachio Pistachio	½ cup	260
Sandwich Wich Ice Cream Cookie	1	350
Strawberry	½ cup	230
The Godfather	½ cup	270
Turtle Soup	½ cup	280
Uncanny Cashew	½ cup	290
Vanilla Caramel Fudge	½ cup	280
Vanilla Heath Bar Crunch	½ cup	290
Vermonty Python	½ cup	310
SORBETS		
Berried Treasure	½ cup	110
Jamaican Me Crazy	½ cup	130
Strawberry Kiwi Swirl	½ cup	110

BILLY'S BURGER HUT
BEVERAGES

Shake Chocolate	1 (20 oz)	420
Shake Vanilla	1 (20 oz)	320
MAIN MENU SELECTIONS		
Big Billy's Roast Beef Sub	1	843
Billyburger	1	426
Billyburger w/ Cheese	1	498
Billy's Best Red Potato Salad	1 serv	190
Billy's Biggest Burger ½ Pounder w/ Everything	1	852
Billy's Famous 7 Layer Salad	1 serv	558
Billy's Seafood Sandwich	1	399
Caesar Side Salad	1 serv	360
Chili w/ Cheese & Onion	1 serv	380

FOOD	PORTION	CALS
Cowboy Cobb Salad	1 serv	735
Cowboy Coleslaw	1 serv	180
French Fries	1 reg	230
Onion Rings	1 serv	250
Super Billy Burger w/ Bacon	1	663

BOB EVANS
BAKED SELECTIONS

FOOD	PORTION	CALS
Biscuit	1	277
Bread Apple Walnut	1 slice	142
Bread Banana Nut	1 slice	186
Bread Garlic	1 slice	218
Bread Sourdough	1	130
Bun Kaiser	1	167
Bun Mini	1	105
English Muffin	1	139
Roll Cinnamon Swirl Frosted	1	607
Roll Cinnamon Swirl Unfrosted	1	510
Roll Dinner	1	201
Texas Toast	1 slice	120

BEVERAGES

FOOD	PORTION	CALS
Coca-Cola	12.5 oz	145
Coffee Decafe	7 oz	5
Coffee Regular	7 oz	2
Creamer Half & Half	0.5 oz	40
Creamer Non-Dairy	0.5 oz	19
Diet Coke	12.5 oz	4
Dr Pepper	12.5 oz	145
Hot Chocolate	1 serv (8.8 oz)	142
Hot Tea	7 oz	2
Iced Tea	9.4 oz	3
Iced Tea Blackberry	9.4 oz	92
Iced Tea Strawberry	9.4 oz	120
Kool Aid Ice Blue Raspberry Lemonade	1 kids cup (8 oz)	70
Lemonade	12 oz	136
Lemonade Blackberry	12 oz	214
Lemonade Strawberry	12 oz	242
Root Beer	12.5 oz	145
Sprite	12.5 oz	142
Strawberry Splash	12.5 oz	218

FOOD	PORTION	CALS
BREAKFAST SELECTIONS		
Bacon	1 piece	36
Benedict Ham & Cheese	1 serv	826
Country Benedict Sausage	1 serv	936
Country Benedict Spinach Bacon & Tomato	1 serv	729
Country Biscuit Breakfast	1 serv	659
Egg Hardcooked	1	60
Egg Over Easy	1	101
Egg Beaters	1 serv	173
Eggs Scrambled	1 serv	255
French Toast	1 slice	131
French Toast Stuffed Plain	1 serv	599
Fruit & Yogurt Plate	1 serv	403
Grits	1 serv	178
Ham Smoked	1 slice	87
Hotcake Blueberry	1	328
Hotcake Buttermilk	1	318
Hotcake Cinnamon	1	417
Hotcake Multigrain	1	322
Mush	1 serv	79
Oatmeal	1 serv	172
Omelet Bacon & Cheese	1 serv	825
Omelet Border Scramble	1	756
Omelet Egg Beaters Bacon & Cheese	1 serv	615
Omelet Egg Beaters Border Scramble	1 serv	517
Omelet Egg Beaters Farmer's Market	1 serv	569
Omelet Egg Beaters Garden Harvest	1 serv	444
Omelet Egg Beaters Ham & Cheddar	1 serv	426
Omelet Egg Beaters Sausage & Cheddar	1 serv	502
Omelet Egg Beaters Three Cheese	1 serv	435
Omelet Farmer's Market	1	778
Omelet Garden Harvest	1 serv	654
Omelet Ham & Cheddar	1 serv	634
Omelet Sausage & Cheddar	1 serv	741
Omelet Three Cheese	1 serv	645
Omelet Western	1 serv	654
Pot Roast Hash	1 serv	652
Sausage Gravy Bowl	1 serv	268
Sausage Link	1	125
Skillet Sunshine	1 serv	842

FOOD	PORTION	CALS
Waffles Sweet Cream	1 serv	598
CHILDREN'S MENU SELECTIONS		
Fruit & Yogurt Dippers	1 serv	275
Hotcakes	1 serv	501
Kids' Macaroni & Cheese	1 serv	320
Kids' Pasta	1 serv	113
Mini Cheeseburgers	1 serv	306
Smiley Face Potatoes	1 serv	524
Sundae Fudge Blast	1 serv	244
Sundae Reese's I'm Smiling	1 serv	330
DESSERTS		
A La Mode Vanilla Ice Cream	1 serv	159
Cake Hershey's Hot Fudge	1 slice	688
Cake Pineapple Upside Down	1 slice	500
Oreo Cheesecake	1 slice	625
Peach Cobbler	1 serv	499
Pie Apple Dumpling	1 slice	682
Pie Banana Cream	1 slice	456
Pie Coconut Cream	1 slice	461
Pie French Silk	1 slice	653
Pie Lemon Meringue	1 slice	536
Pie No Sugar Added Apple	1 slice	483
Pie Reese's Peanut Butter Cup	1 slice	1130
Pie Strawberry Supreme	1 slice	589
Sundae Fudge	1	501
Sundae Reese's	1 serv	769
MAIN MENU SELECTIONS		
Applesauce	1 serv	101
Baked Potato Loaded	1	427
Baked Potato Plain	1	207
Broccoli Florets	1 serv	156
Broccoli Florets Cheddar	1 serv	230
Carrots Glazed	1 serv	188
Catfish Grilled New Orleans	1 piece	255
Cheeseburger Bacon Plain	1	1005
Cheeseburger Plain	1	691
Chicken & Broccoli Alfredo	1 serv	826
Chicken Fried	1 piece	291
Chicken Grilled	1 piece	229
Chicken Pot Pie	1 serv	758

FOOD	PORTION	CALS
Chicken Quesadilla	1 serv	502
Chicken Tenders Grilled	1 piece	103
Chicken-N-Noodle	1 serv	407
Coleslaw	1 serv	198
Corn Buttered	1 serv	225
Cottage Cheese	1 serv	122
Country Fried Steak w/ Gravy	1 serv	535
Country Fried Steak w/o Gravy	1 serv	481
Dressing Bread & Celery	1 serv	362
Fish Market Halibut	1 piece	209
French Fries	1 serv	217
Green Beans w/ Ham	1 serv	83
Grilled Garden Vegetables	1 serv	290
Hamburger Patty	1	388
Hamburger Plain	1	585
Hamburger Shroomin' Onion Plain	1	695
Home Fries	1 serv	193
Mashed Potatoes	1 serv	171
Meat Loaf	1 serv	626
Mushrooms Grilled	1 serv	152
Onion Rings	1 serv	460
Open Faced Roast Beef Dinner	1 serv	633
Pork Chop Dinner	1 serv	466
Pork Chop Dinner w/ Garlic Herb Butter	1 serv	624
Pork Chop Dinner w/ Wildfire Barbecue Sauce	1 serv	645
Rice Pilaf	1 serv	163
Salmon	1 serv	334
Salmon w/ Garlic Herb Butter	1 serv	491
Salmon w/ Wildfire Barbecue Sauce	1 serv	512
Sandwich Bob's BLT	1	795
Sandwich Chicken Salad	1	694
Sandwich Fish Market Haddock	1	570
Sandwich Fried Chicken	1	508
Sandwich Fried Chicken Club	1	994
Sandwich Grilled Cheese	1	391
Sandwich Grilled Chicken	1	447
Sandwich Grilled Chicken Club	1	993
Sandwich Pot Roast	1	728
Sandwich Turkey Bacon Melt	1	872
Seniors Chicken Parmesan	1 serv	522

FOOD	PORTION	CALS
Seniors Garden Vegetable Alfredo	1 serv	363
Seniors Garden Vegetable Alfredo Chicken	1 serv	452
Seniors Steak Tips & Noodles	1 serv	422
Seniors Stir-Fry Chicken	1 serv	368
Spaghetti & Marinara Sauce	1 serv	619
Spaghetti w/ Meatballs	1 serv	1087
Steak Monterey	1 serv	584
Steak Tips & Noodles	1 serv	985
Stir-Fry Grilled Chicken	1 serv	728
Stir-Fry Grilled Shrimp	1 serv	713
Stir-Fry Vegetable	1 serv	497
T-Bone Steak Plain	1 serv	1335
T-Bone Steak w/ Garlic Herb Butter	1 serv	1492
Turkey & Dressing	1 serv	542
SALAD DRESSINGS AND TOPPINGS		
Dressing Bleu Cheese	1 serv (1.5 oz)	220
Dressing Colonial	1 serv (1.5 oz)	232
Dressing French	1 serv (1.5 oz)	219
Dressing Honey Mustard	1 serv (1.5 oz)	192
Dressing Hot Bacon	1 serv (1.5 oz)	106
Dressing Lite Italian	1 serv (1.5 oz)	82
Dressing Oriental	1 serv (1.5 oz)	194
Dressing Ranch	1 serv (1.5 oz)	156
Dressing Ranch Lite	1 serv (1.5 oz)	103
Dressing Raspberry Vinaigrette	1 serv (1.5 oz)	155
Dressing Thousand Island	1 serv (1.5 oz)	212
Dressing Wildfire Ranch	1 serv (1.5 oz)	212
Gravy Chicken	1 serv (3 oz)	29
Gravy Country	1 serv (3 oz)	54
Gravy Sausage	1 serv (7 oz)	244
Syrup	1 serv (3 oz)	213
Syrup Sugar Free	1 serv (3 oz)	47
Topping Oregon Berry	1 serv (3 oz)	49
Topping Strawberry	1 serv (3 oz)	50
Whipped Topping	1 serv	69
SALADS		
Chicken Salad Plate	1 serv	789
Cobb Salad w/ Grilled Chicken	1 serv	778
Country Spinach w/ Grilled Chicken	1 serv	532
Frisco Salad w/ Fried Chicken	1 serv	672

FOOD	PORTION	CALS
Frisco Salad w/ Grilled Chicken	1 serv	599
Fruit & Yogurt	1 serv	414
Raspberry Grilled Chicken	1 serv	637
Speciality Side	1 serv	174
Wildfire Fried Chicken Salad	1 serv	806
Wildfire Grilled Chicken Salad	1 serv	733
SOUPS		
Bean	1 cup	144
Cheddar Baked Potato	1 cup	294
Sausage Chili	1 cup	268
Vegetable Beef	1 cup	135

BOJANGLES

FOOD	PORTION	CALS
Biscuit	1	243
Biscuit Sandwich Bacon	1	290
Biscuit Sandwich Bacon Egg Cheese	1	550
Biscuit Sandwich Cajun Filet	1	454
Biscuit Sandwich Country Ham	1	270
Biscuit Sandwich Egg	1	400
Biscuit Sandwich Sausage	1	350
Biscuit Sandwich Smoked Sausage	1	380
Biscuit Sandwich Steak	1	649
Botato Rounds	1 serv	235
Buffalo Bites	1 serv	180
Cajun Pintos	1 serv	110
Cajun Spiced Breast	1 serv	278
Cajun Spiced Leg	1 serv	264
Cajun Spiced Thigh	1 serv	310
Cajun Spiced Wing	1 serv	355
Chicken Supremes	1 serv	337
Corn On The Cob	1 serv	140
Dirty Rice	1 serv	166
Green Beans	1 serv	25
Macaroni & Cheese	1 serv	198
Marinated Cole Slaw	1 serv	136
Potatoes w/o Gravy	1 serv	80
Sandwich Cajun Filet w/ Mayo	1	437
Sandwich Cajun Filet w/o Mayo	1	337
Sandwich Grilled Filet w/ Mayo	1	335
Sandwich Grilled Filet w/o Mayo	1	235
Seasoned Fries	1 serv	344

FOOD	PORTION	CALS
Southern Style Breast	1 serv	261
Southern Style Leg	1 serv	254
Southern Style Thigh	1 serv	308
Southern Style Wing	1 serv	337
Sweet Biscuit Bo Berry	1	320
Sweet Biscuit Cinnamon	1	320

BOSTON MARKET
DESSERTS
Apple Pie	1 slice	420
Brownie Chocolate Chip Fudge	1	580
Chocolate Cake	1 serv	600
Cookie Chocolate Chip	1	370
Cornbread	1 piece	180

MAIN MENU SELECTIONS
Broccoli w/ Garlic Butter	1 serv	80
Butternut Squash	1 serv	140
Carver Boston Chicken	1	700
Carver Boston Meatloaf	1	940
Carver Boston Sirloin Dip	1	1000
Carver Boston Turkey	1	770
Carver Boston Turkey Dip	1	770
Carver Half Boston Chicken	1	340
Carver Half Boston Sirloin Dip	1	500
Carver Half Boston Turkey	1	390
Cinnamon Apples	1 serv	210
Cranberry Walnut Relish	1 serv	140
Creamed Spinach	1 serv	280
Dip Spinach Artichoke	1 serv	100
Family Meals Boneless Turkey Breast	1 serv (5 oz)	180
Family Meals Roasted Turkey	1 serv (5 oz)	180
Family Meals Rotisserie Chicken	1 serv (6 oz)	290
Family Meals Spiral Sliced Ham	1 serv (8 oz)	450
Family Meals Whole Turkey	1 serv (6.7 oz)	310
Fresh Vegetable Stuffing	1 serv	190
Garden Fresh Coleslaw	1 serv	170
Garlic Dill New Potatoes	1 serv	140
Green Bean Casserole	1 serv	60
Green Beans	1 serv	60
Individual Meal ¼ White Rotisserie Chicken	1 serv	290

FOOD	PORTION	CALS
Individual Meals Award Winning Roasted Sirloin	1 serv	290
Individual Meals 1 Thigh & 1 Drumstick	1 serv	300
Individual Meals ¼ White Rotisserie Chicken No Skin	1 serv	210
Individual Meals 3 Piece Dark	1 serv	380
Individual Meals 3 Piece Dark Skinless	1 serv	240
Individual Meals Meatloaf	1	480
Individual Meals Roasted Turkey	1 serv	180
Macaroni & Cheese	1 serv	330
Mashed Potatoes	1 serv	210
Pot Pie Pastry Topped Chicken	1	780
Poultry Gravy	1 serv (4 oz)	15
Seasonal Fresh Fruit Salad	1 serv	60
Spinach w/ Garlic Butter Sauce	1 serv	130
Squash Casserole	1 serv	320
Steamed Fresh Vegetables	1 serv	60
Sweet Corn	1 serv	170
Sweet Potato Casserole	1 serv	460
SALADS		
Entree Caesar	1	500
Entree Caesar w/o Dressing	1	140
Entree Market Chopped	1	580
Entree Market Chopped w/o Dressing	1	210
Side Caesar	1	400
Side Caesar w/o Dressing	1 serv	40
Side Market Chopped	1	440
Side Market Chopped w/o Dressing	1	80
SOUPS		
Chicken Noodle	1 serv	170
Chicken Tortilla w/ Toppings	1 serv	340
Tortilla Soup w/o Toppings	1 serv	80

BOSTON PIZZA
CHILDREN'S MENU SELECTIONS

Baked Salmon w/ Caesar Salad	1 serv	330
Bug N' Cheese	1 serv	500
Chicken Fingers w/ Fries	1 serv	390
Pizza Pint Size	1	390
Quesadilla Bacon Double Cheeseburger w/ Caesar Salad	1 serv	540

FOOD	PORTION	CALS
Reduced Size Fruit Cup	1 serv	80
Sandwich Grilled Chicken w/ Garden Greens	1 serv	600
Super Spaghetti	1 serv	440
Wrap Ham & Cheese w/ Fries	1 serv	550
DESSERTS		
Blondie Maple	1	850
Blondie Maple Bite Size	1	430
Brownie Chocolate Addiction	1	490
Brownie Chocolate Addiction Bite Size	1	200
Cheesecake New York	1 slice	620
Cheesecake Vanilla Bean	1 slice	770
Chocolate Explosion	1 serv	890
Tarte Au Sucre	1 serv	310
MAIN MENU SELECTIONS		
Angus Beef Sirloin Steak w/ Spaghetti	1 serv	1260
Baked 3 Cheese Penne	1 half order	460
Baked Seven Cheese Ravioli	1 half order	310
Baked Shrimp & Feta Penne	1 half order	480
Boston's Lasagna	1 half order	340
Boston's Smokey Mountain Spaghetti	1 order	1290
Chicken & Mushroom Fettuccini	1 half order	710
Chicken Parmesan w/ Seasonal Vegetables	1 serv	1060
Fries	1 serv	430
Garlic Mashed Potatoes	1 serv	730
Garlic Toast	1 slice	150
Homestyle Lasagna	1 order	590
Jambalaya Fettuccini	1 half order	860
Lemon Baked Salmon w/ Fries	1 serv	1150
Mama Meata Penne	1 half order	940
Mushroom Chicken w/ Garlic Mashed Potatoes	1 serv	1030
Pad Thai w/ Chicken	1 serv	2110
Pad Thai w/ Shrimp	1 serv	2090
Pollo Pomodoro Spaghetti	1 serv	520
Salmon Filet Lemon Baked	1 serv	430
Scallop & Prawn Fettuccini	1 half order	710
Seasoned Vegetables	1 serv	70
Shrimp Skewers Lime & Parmesan	1 serv	190
Sicilian Penne	1 half order	720
Sirloin Steak w/ Prawns & Fries	1 serv	1480

FOOD	PORTION	CALS
Slow Roasted Pork Back Ribs w/ Fries	1 serv	1680
Spaghetti w/ Alfredo Sauce	1 half order	440
Spaghetti w/ Bolognese	1 half order	400
Spaghetti w/ Creamy Tomato Sauce	1 half order	410
Spaghetti w/ Pomodoro Sauce	1 half order	450
Spicy Italian Penne	1 half order	980
Starter Baked Ravioli Bites	1 serv	450
Starter Basket Garlic Twist	1 serv	1140
Starter Basket Three Cheese Toast	1 serv	730
Starter Boston's Poutine	1 serv	740
Starter Bruschetta Sun Dried Tomato	1 serv	470
Starter Cactus Cuts Potatoes & Dip	1 serv	1150
Starter Chicken Fingers	1 serv	360
Starter Chicken Fingers Buffalo Style	1 serv	370
Starter Cracked Pepper Dry Ribs	1 serv	380
Starter Nachos Cactus w/ Cactus Dip	1 serv	1830
Starter Nachos Spicy Chicken w/ Sour Cream & Salsa	1 serv	1430
Starter Nachos Taco Beef w/ Sour Cream & Salsa	1 serv	1560
Starter Nachos w/ Sour Cream & Salsa	1 serv	1320
Starter Panzerotti Roll	1	820
Starter Pizza Bread Bandera w/ Santa Fe Ranch Dip	1 serv	960
Starter Pizza Bread w/o Sauce	1 serv	500
Starter Potato Skins	1 serv	650
Starter Quesadilla Oven Roasted Chicken	1 serv	900
Starter Quesadilla Southwest w/ Sour Cream & Salsa	1 serv	770
Starter Shrimp Stuffed Mushroom Caps	1 serv	490
Starter Team Platter w/ Dips & Sauces	1 serv	3030
Starter Thai Chicken Bites	1 serv	540
Starter Wings Breaded BBQ	1 serv	930
Starter Wings Breaded Honey Garlic	1 serv	940
Starter Wings Breaded Mild	1 serv	880
Starter Wings Breaded Teriyaki	1 serv	940
Starter Wings Breaded Thai	1 serv	1110
Starter Wings Oven Roasted BBQ	1 serv	670
Starter Wings Oven Roasted Honey Garlic	1 serv	700
Starter Wings Oven Roasted Hot	1 serv	620

FOOD	PORTION	CALS
Starter Wings Oven Roasted Teriyaki	1 serv	670
Starter Wings Oven Roasted Thai Chili	1 serv	770
The Ribber w/ Spaghetti	1 serv	970
Tortellini w/ Alfredo Sauce	1 half order	340
Tortellini w/ Bolognese	1 half order	300
Tortellini w/ Creamy Tomato Sauce	1 half order	310
Tortellini w/ Pomodoro Sauce	1 half order	340
Veal Parmesan w/ Spaghetti	1 serv	1020
PIZZA		
Bacon Double Cheeseburger Individual	1 pie	1140
Bacon Double Cheeseburger Slice	1 med	280
BBQ Chicken Individual	1 pie	730
BBQ Chicken Slice	1 med	190
Boston Royal Individual	1 pie	840
Boston Royal Slice	1 med	210
Californian Slice	1 med	280
Clubhouse Individual	1 pie	1040
Deluxe Individual	1 pie	850
Deluxe Slice	1 med	220
Great White North Individual	1 pie	960
Great White North Slice	1 med	240
Hawaiian Individual	1 pie	780
Hawaiian Slice	1 med	210
Indy California	1 (11.3 oz)	440
La Quebecoise Individual	1 pie	770
La Quebecoise Slice	1 med	200
Meateor Individual	1 pie	950
Meateor Slice	1 med	260
Pepperoni Individual	1 pie	750
Pepperoni Slice	1 med	200
Pepperoni & Mushroom Individual	1 pie	750
Pepperoni & Mushroom Slice	1 med	200
Popeye Individual	1 pie	720
Popeye Slice	1 med	200
Rustic Italian Individual	1 pie	950
Rustic Italian Slice	1 med	260
Spicy Perogy Individual	1 pie	980
Spicy Perogy Slice	1 med	280
Szechuan Individual	1 pie	750
Szechuan Slice	1 med	200

FOOD	PORTION	CALS
Tandoori Individual	1 med	730
Tandoori Slice	1 med	200
Thai Chicken Individual	1 pie	840
Thai Chicken Slice	1 med	240
The Basic Individual	1 pie	620
The Basic Slice	1 med	160
Tropical Chicken Individual	1 pie	970
Tropical Chicken Slice	1 med	260
Tuscan Individual	1 pie	940
Tuscan Slice	1 med	250
Ultimate Pepperoni Individual	1 pie	870
Ultimate Pepperoni Slice	1 med	230
Vegetarian Individual	1 pie	680
Vegetarian Slice	1 med	180
Zorba The Greek Individual	1 pie	800
Zorba The Greek Slice	1 med	210
SALAD DRESSINGS AND TOPPINGS		
House Dressing	1 serv (2 oz)	270
Ketchup	1 serv (2 oz)	60
Salsa	1 serv (2 oz)	20
Sour Cream	1 serv (2 oz)	100
SALADS		
Chipotle Chicken & Bacon	1 serv	630
Crispy Chicken Pecan	1 serv	1100
Entree Caesar	1 serv	500
Entree Spinach	1 serv	450
Garden Greens w/ House Dressing	1 serv	310
Garden Greens w/ Low Fat Raspberry Vinaigrette	1 serv	130
Side Caesar	1 serv	170
Starter Spinach	1 serv	250
Taco Salad Beef w/o Sour Cream & Salsa	1 serv	610
Taco Salad Chicken w/o Sour Cream & Salsa	1 serv	480
Thai Chicken Salad	1 serv	1060
SANDWICHES		
Beef Dip w/ Fries & Au Jus	1 serv	1340
Boston Brute w/ Caesar Salad & Au Jus	1 serv	820
Boston Cheesesteak w/ Caesar Salad & Au Jus	1 serv	1300
Buffalo Chicken w/ Fries	1 serv	1220
Chicken Parmesan w/ Fries	1 serv	1370

FOOD	PORTION	CALS
Ciabatta Chicken w/ Caesar Salad	1 serv	920
New York Steak w/ Garden Greens & Au Jus	1 serv	660
Stromboli Bacon Double Cheeseburger w/ Caesar Salad	1 serv	910
Stromboli Chicken Santa Fe w/ Caesar Salad	1 serv	750
Stromboli Smoked Ham & Chicken w/ Caesar Salad	1 serv	880
Wrap Thai Chicken	1	570
SOUPS		
Baked French Onion	1 serv	330
Clam Chowder	1 serv	260

BROWN'S CHICKEN & PASTA

Breadsticks Garlic	1	50
Breast	3 oz	284
Cheezy Potatoes	1 serv (12 oz)	188
Coleslaw	3 oz	131
Corn Fritters	3 oz	415
Corn On Cob	1 ear (3 inch)	126
French Fries	3 oz	503
Gizzard	3 oz	387
Leg	3 oz	287
Liver	3 oz	341
Mostaccioli Meatless Sauce	1 serv (12 oz)	792
Mostaccioli w/ Meat Sauce	1 serv (12 oz)	835
Mushrooms	3 oz	289
Potato Salad	3 oz	94
Ravioli w/ Meat Sauce	1 serv (12 oz)	865
Ravioli w/ Meatless Sauce	1 serv (12 oz)	822
Shrimp	3 oz	277
Spaghetti w/ Meat Sauce	1 serv (12 oz)	835
Spaghetti w/ Meatless Sauce	1 serv (12 oz)	792
Thigh	3 oz	355
Wing	3 oz	385

BRUEGGER'S BAGELS
BAGELS

Asiago Parmesan	1	330
Baked Apple	1	370
Blueberry	1	330
Chocolate Chip	1	350

FOOD	PORTION	CALS
Cinnamon Sugar	1	330
Cranberry Orange	1	330
Everything	1	320
Garlic	1	320
Honey Grain	1	330
Jalapeno Bagel	1	320
Multi-Grain	1	350
Onion	1	320
Plain	1	320
Poppy	1	320
Pumpernickel	1	330
Pumpkin	1	330
Rosemary Olive Oil	1	350
Salt	1	320
Sesame	1	360
Sourdough	1	340
Square Asiago Parmesan	1	360
Square Everything	1	320
Square Plain	1	350
Square Sesame	1	360
Sun Dried Tomato	1	320
Whole Wheat	1	390
DESSERTS		
Brownie Chocolate Chunk	1	330
Cake Lemon Pound	1 slice	320
Cookie Chocolate Chip	1	500
Cookie Oatmeal Raisin	1	460
Cookie Peanut Butter	1	480
Cookie Triple Chocolate Chunk	1	560
Cookie White Chocolate Macadamia	1	580
Luscious Lemon Bar	1	300
Marshmallow Chew	1	280
Muffin Blueberry	1	450
Muffin Chocolate	1	460
Oreo Dream Bar	1	470
Pecan Chocolate Chunk	1 slice	310
Raspberry Sammies	1 slice	340
Seven Layer Bar	1	650
Toffee Almond Bar	1	400

FOOD	PORTION	CALS
SALADS		
Caesar w/ Dressing	1 serv	270
Tossed Chicken Caesar w/ Dressing	1 serv	370
Tossed Mandarin Medley	1 serv	340
Tossed Sesame Chicken	1 serv	480
SANDWICHES		
BLT w/ Mayo	1	570
Chicken Breast	1	660
Chicken Fajita	1	530
Chicken Salad w/ Mayo	1	630
Cranberry Gobbler	1	620
Cuban Chicken	1	680
Denver Egg	1	460
Egg Cheese	1	420
Egg Cheese Bacon	1	460
Egg Cheese Ham	1	460
Egg Cheese Sausage	1	640
Ham	1	460
Herby Turkey	1	560
Leonardo Da Veggie	1	480
Radishy Roast Beef	1	560
Roadhouse Chicken	1	710
Roast Beef	1	730
Santa Fe Turkey	1	490
Smoked Salmon	1	490
Softwich BLT w/ Mayo	1	600
Softwich Chicken Breast	1	630
Softwich Chicken Fajita	1	570
Softwich Chicken Salad	1	670
Softwich Cranberry Gobbler	1	730
Softwich Cuban Chicken	1	810
Softwich Garden Veggie	1	380
Softwich Ham	1	510
Softwich Herby Turkey	1	580
Softwich Hummus	1	540
Softwich Leonardo De Veggie	1	550
Softwich Mediterranean	1	790
Softwich Peanut Chicken	1	590
Softwich Radishy Roast Beef	1	670
Softwich Roadhouse Chicken	1	670

FOOD	PORTION	CALS
Softwich Roast Beef	1	750
Softwich Roasted Turkey	1	550
Softwich Smoked Salmon	1	520
Softwich Supreme Club w/o Mayo	1	880
Softwich Tuna Salad	1	720
Softwich Western Wheat	1	820
Supreme Club w/o Mayo	1	470
Tuna Salad	1	620
Turkey	1	510
Wrap Classic w/ Bacon	1	520
Wrap Classic w/ Ham	1	510
Wrap Classic w/ Sausage	1	660
Wrap Rio Grande Bacon	1	560
Wrap Rio Grande Ham	1	630
Wrap Rio Grande Sausage	1	510
Wrap Sesame Chicken Salad	1	770
Wrap Tossed Chicken Caesar	1	660
Wrap Tossed Mandarin Medley Salad	1	630
SOUPS		
Chicken Pot Pie	1 cup	250
Chicken Spaetzle	1 cup	120
Chicken Wild Rice	1 cup	260
Creamy Tomato	1 cup	150
Hearty Mushroom Barley	1 cup	110
Italian Wedding	1 cup	160
Minestrone	1 cup	120
Moroccan Stew	1 cup	140
New England Clam	1 cup	300
Sweet Potato Cheddar	1 cup	200
SPREADS		
Cream Cheese Bacon Scallion	1 scoop (1.5 oz)	140
Cream Cheese Cucumber Dill	1 scoop (1.5 oz)	140
Cream Cheese Garden Veggie	1 scoop (1.5 oz)	130
Cream Cheese Honey Walnut	1 scoop (1.5 oz)	150
Cream Cheese Jalapeno	1 scoop (1.5 oz)	140
Cream Cheese Light Garden Veggie	1 scoop (1.5 oz)	90
Cream Cheese Light Herb Garlic	1 scoop (1.5 oz)	100
Cream Cheese Light Plain	1 scoop (1.5 oz)	100
Cream Cheese Olive Pimento	1 scoop (1.5 oz)	140
Cream Cheese Onion & Chive	1 scoop (1.5 oz)	140

FOOD	PORTION	CALS
Cream Cheese Plain	1 scoop (1.5 oz)	130
Cream Cheese Pumpkin	1 scoop (1.5 oz)	120
Cream Cheese Strawberry	1 scoop (1.5 oz)	140
Cream Cheese Wildberry	1 scoop (1.5 oz)	140
Hummus	1 scoop (2 oz)	110

BURGER KING
BEVERAGES

FOOD	PORTION	CALS
Apple Juice	1 (6.67 oz)	90
BK Joe Regular	1 sm	5
BK Joe Turbo	1 sm (12 oz)	10
Chocolate Milk 1% Low Fat	1 (9 oz)	180
Coke Classic	1 sm (16 oz)	140
Diet Coke	1 sm (16 oz)	0
Dr Pepper	1 sm (16 oz)	140
Iced Coffee Mocha BK Joe	1 (16 oz)	380
Icee Coca-Cola	1 sm (16 oz)	110
Icee Minute Maid Cherry	1 sm (16 oz)	110
Milk 1% Low Fat	1	110
Minute Maid Orange Juice	8 oz	140
Shake Chocolate	1 sm (16 oz)	470
Shake Oreo Sundae Chocolate	1 sm (16 oz)	680
Shake Oreo Sundae Strawberry	1 sm (16 oz)	660
Shake Oreo Sundae Vanilla	1 sm (16 oz)	610
Shake Strawberry	1 sm (16 oz)	460
Shake Vanilla	1 sm (16 oz)	400
Sprite	1 sm (16 oz)	140
Water Nestle Pure Life	1 bottle (16 oz)	0

BREAKFAST SELECTIONS

FOOD	PORTION	CALS
Biscuit Bacon Egg & Cheese	1	410
Biscuit Ham Egg & Cheese	1	390
Biscuit Sausage	1	390
Biscuit Sausage Egg & Cheese	1	530
Croissan'wich Bacon Egg & Cheese	1	340
Croissan'wich Double w/ Bacon Egg & Cheese	1	430
Croissan'wich Double w/ Ham Bacon Egg & Cheese	1	420
Croissan'wich Double w/ Ham Egg & Cheese	1	420
Croissan'wich Double w/ Ham Sausage Egg & Cheese	1	550

FOOD	PORTION	CALS
Croissan'wich Double w/ Sausage Bacon Egg & Cheese	1	550
Croissan'wich Double w/ Sausage Egg & Cheese	1	680
Croissan'wich Egg & Cheese	1	300
Croissan'wich Ham Egg & Cheese	1	340
Croissan'wich Sausage & Cheese	1	370
Croissan'wich Sausage Egg & Cheese	1	470
French Toast Sticks	3 pieces	240
Hash Browns	1 sm	260
Hash Browns	1 lg	620
Omelet Sandwich Enormous	1	730
Omelet Sandwich Ham	1	290
DESSERTS		
Cini-minis	1 serv	390
Dutch Apple Pie	1 serv	300
Hershey Sundae Pie	1	310
MAIN MENU SELECTIONS		
BK Chicken Fries	6 pieces	260
BK Stacker Double	1	610
BK Stacker Quad	1	1000
BK Stacker Triple	1	800
BK Veggie Burger	1	420
Cheeseburger	1	330
Cheeseburger Double	1	500
Chicken Sandwich Original	1	660
Chicken Sandwich Tendercrisp	1	790
Chicken Sandwich Tendergrill	1	510
Chicken Tenders	5 pieces	210
Chick'n Crisp Spicy Sandwich	1	480
Double Cheeseburger	1	410
French Fries No Salt Added	1 sm	230
French Fries Salted	1 sm	230
French Fries Salted	1 lg	500
Hamburger	1	290
Onion Rings	1 sm	140
Onion Rings	1 lg	440
Sandwich BK Big Fish	1	640
The Angus Steak Burger	1	640
Whopper	1	670

FOOD	PORTION	CALS
Whopper w/ Cheese	1	760
Whopper Double	1	900
Whopper Double w/ Cheese	1	990
Whopper Jr.	1	370
Whopper Jr. w/ Cheese	1	410
Whopper Triple	1	1130
Whopper Triple w/ Cheese	1	1230
SALAD DRESSINGS AND TOPPINGS		
Breakfast Syrup	1 serv (1 oz)	80
Croutons Garlic Parmesan	1 serv	60
Dipping Sauce Barbecue	1 serv (1 oz)	40
Dipping Sauce Honey Mustard	1 serv (1 oz)	90
Dipping Sauce Ranch	1 serv (1 oz)	140
Dipping Sauce Sweet And Sour	1 serv (1 oz)	40
Dressing Ken's Creamy Caesar	1 serv (2 oz)	210
Dressing Ken's Fat Free Ranch	1 serv (2 oz)	60
Dressing Ken's Honey Mustard	1 serv (2 oz)	270
Dressing Ken's Ranch	1 serv (2 oz)	190
Jam Grape	1 serv	30
Jam Strawberry	1 serv	30
Ketchup	1 pkg	10
Mayonnaise	1 pkg	80
SALADS		
Chicken Garden Tendercrisp	1	410
Chicken Garden Tendergrill w/o Dressing or Croutons	1	240
Side Garden w/o Dressing	1	15

BURGERVILLE
BEVERAGES

FOOD	PORTION	CALS
Barq's Root Beer	1 (20 oz)	180
Coca-Cola	1 (20 oz)	161
Diet Coke	1 (20 oz)	0
Hot Chocolate Ghirardelli	1 (12 oz)	230
House Coffee	1 (10 oz)	5
Iced Tea	1 (20 oz)	0
Iced Tea Nestea Raspberry	1 (20 oz)	127
Lemonade Odwalla	1 (20 oz)	240
Milk 2%	1 (8 oz)	121
Orange Juice Odwalla	1 (10 oz)	138
Pibb Xtra	1 (20 oz)	163

FOOD	PORTION	CALS
Sprite	1 (20 oz)	158
BREAKFAST SELECTIONS		
Bagel	1	310
Bagel Bacon And Egg	1	490
Bagel Ham And Egg	1	490
Bagel Sausage And Egg	1	640
Breakfast Platter w/ Bacon	1 serv	730
Breakfast Platter w/ Ham	1 serv	725
Breakfast Platter w/ Sausage	1 serv	880
Hash Browns	1 serv	230
Toaster Biscuit	1	320
Toaster Biscuit Bacon And Egg	1	450
Toaster Biscuit Ham And Egg	1	440
Toaster Biscuit Sausage And Egg	1	600
DESSERTS		
Cone Vanilla	1	250
Cone YoCream Frozen Yogurt	1	190
Cookie Chocolate Chunk	1	320
Cookie Oatmeal Raisin	1	290
Cookie Sugar	1	305
Cookie White Chocolate Macadamia	1	340
Strawberry Shortcake	1 serv	440
Sundae Caramel	1	380
Sundae Fresh Strawberry	1	340
Sundae Hot Fudge	1	380
Sundae Triple Berry	1	340
Sundae YoCream Caramel	1	260
Sundae YoCream Hot Fudge	1	260
Sundae YoCream Strawberry	1	220
Sundae YoCream Triple Berry	1	200
MAIN MENU SELECTIONS		
Apple Slices	1 serv	29
Cheeseburger	1	350
Cheeseburger Colossal	1	520
Cheeseburger Double Beef	1	430
Cheeseburger Tillamook	1	630
Cheeseburger Tillamook Pepper Bacon	1	690
Chicken Strips	5	320
French Fries	1 serv	410
Gardenburger Spicy Black Bean	1	550

FOOD	PORTION	CALS
Gardenburger The Original	1	450
Halibut	3 pieces	320
Hamburger	1	300
Hamburger Burgerville Classic	1	510
Onion Rings Walla Walla	1 serv	810
Sandwich Crispy Chicken	1	490
Sandwich Deluxe Crispy Chicken	1	590
Sandwich Halibut	1	480
Sandwich Low Fat Grilled Chicken	1	320
Sandwich Nine Grain Turkey Club	1	550
Sweet Potato Fries	1 serv	530
Turkey Burger Seasoned	1	540
Yukon Golds	1 serv	450
SALAD DRESSINGS AND TOPPINGS		
Burgerville Spread Cups	1	280
Cream Cheese	1 serv	100
Cream Cheese Light	1 serv	70
Dip BBQ Sauce	1 serv	60
Dressing Blue Cheese	1 serv	240
Dressing Caesar	1 serv	220
Dressing Honey Mustard	1 serv	210
Dressing Ranch	1 serv	195
Sauce Sweet And Sour	1 serv	90
Tartar Cups	1	260
Vinaigrette Honey Lime	1 serv	250
Vinaigrette Raspberry	1 serv	45
SALADS		
Grilled Chicken	1	430
Rogue River Smokey Blue	1	290
Side Salad	1	50
Wild Smoked Salmon & Hazelnuts	1	440

CAPTAIN D'S SEAFOOD

FOOD	PORTION	CALS
Baked Chicken Dinner	1 serv	350
Baked Fish Dinner	1 serv	390
Baked Potato	1 serv	190
Baked Salmon Dinner	1 serv	470
Carb Counter Chicken Dinner	1 serv	320
Carb Counter Fish Dinner	1 serv	350
Cole Slaw	1 serv	150
Corn On The Cob	1 serv	150

FOOD	PORTION	CALS
Fresh Steamed Broccoli	1 serv	25
Green Beans	1 serv	90
Rice Pilaf	1 serv	160
Shrimp Scampi Dinner	1 serv	370
Side Salad w/o Dressing	1	30
Tuscan Style Vegetables	1 serv	30

CARIBOU COFFEE

FOOD	PORTION	CALS
Black Forest Mocha	1 med	553
Black Forest Wild Drink	1 med	553
Cappuccino	1 med (16 oz)	113
Cappuccino 2%	1 med (16 oz)	162
Caramel Hirise	1 med (16 oz)	414
Chai Latte 2%	1 med (16 oz)	286
Chai Skim	1 med (16 oz)	236
Cooler Caramel	1 med (12 oz)	450
Cooler Chocolate	1 med (12 oz)	257
Cooler Coffee	1 med (16 oz)	230
Cooler Espresso	1 med (16 oz)	193
Cooler Mint Oreo	1 med (12 oz)	614
Cooler Vanilla	1 med (16 oz)	257
Glacier Gum	2 pieces	5
Hot Apple Blast	1 med	379
Latte 2%	1 med (16 oz)	171
Latte Skim	1 med (16 oz)	121
Latte Skinny Bou Low Cal	1 med	120
Lite White Berry	1 med (16 oz)	311
Mint Condition	1 med (16 oz)	520
Mints All Flavors	3 pieces	5
Mocha 2%	1 med (16 oz)	347
Mocha Skim	1 med (16 oz)	302
Mocha Turtle	1 med (16 oz)	559
Smoothie Passion Green Tea	1 med (16 oz)	252
Smoothie Raspberry	1 med (12 oz)	293
Smoothie Strawberry Banana	1 med (16 oz)	253
Smoothie Wild Berry	1 med (16 oz)	235

CARL'S JR.
BEVERAGES

FOOD	PORTION	CALS
Malt Chocolate	1 (15 oz)	780
Malt Oreo Cookie	1 (15 oz)	790

FOOD	PORTION	CALS
Malt Strawberry	1 (15 oz)	770
Malt Vanilla	1 (15 oz)	760
Shake Chocolate	1 (14 oz)	710
Shake Oreo Cookie	1 (14 oz)	720
Shake Strawberry	1 (14 oz)	700
Shake Vanilla	1 (14 oz)	710
BREAKFAST SELECTIONS		
Breakfast Burger	1	830
Burrito Bacon & Egg	1	570
Burrito Loaded Breakfast	1	820
Burrito Steak & Egg	1	660
French Toast Dips w/o Syrup	5	430
Hash Brown Nuggets	1 serv	330
Sandwich Sourdough Breakfast	1 serv	460
Sunrise Croissant Sandwich	1	560
DESSERTS		
Cheesecake Strawberry Swirl	1 serv	290
Chocolate Cake	1 serv	300
Cookie Chocolate Chip	1	350
MAIN MENU SELECTIONS		
Burger Jalapeno	1	720
Burger Teriyaki	1	660
Cheeseburger Double Western Bacon	1	970
Cheeseburger Western Bacon	1	710
Chicken Breast Strips	3	420
Chicken Stars	4	170
CrissCut Fries	1 serv	410
Famous Star w/ Cheese	1	660
Fish & Chips	1 serv	630
French Fries	1 sm	290
Fried Zucchini	1 serv	320
Hamburger Big	1	470
Hamburger Kid's	1	460
Onion Rings	1 serv	430
Sandwich Bacon Swiss Crispy Chicken	1	720
Sandwich Carl's Catch Fish	1	660
Sandwich Charbroiled BBQ Chicken	1	360
Sandwich Charbroiled Chicken Club	1	550
Sandwich Charbroiled Santa Fe Chicken	1	610
Sandwich Spicy Chicken	1	560

FOOD	PORTION	CALS
Six Dollar Burger The Bacon Cheese	1	1070
Six Dollar Burger The Guacamole Bacon	1	1140
Six Dollar Burger The Jalapeno	1	1030
Six Dollar Burger The Low Carb	1	490
Six Dollar Burger The Original	1	1010
Six Dollar Burger The Western Bacon	1	1130
Super Star w/ Cheese	1	930
SALAD DRESSINGS		
Blue Cheese	1 serv (2 oz)	320
House	1 serv (2 oz)	220
Low Fat Balsamic	1 serv (2 oz)	35
Thousand Island	1 serv (2 oz)	240
SALADS		
Charbroiled Chicken	1	260
Side	1	50

CARVEL

FOOD	PORTION	CALS
Brown Bonnet	1	370
Cake Ice Cream	1 slice	270
Carvelanche Cake Mix	1 reg (16 oz)	720
Carvelanche Cookies & Cream	1 reg (16 oz)	550
Carvelanche Triple Fudge Cake Mix	1 reg (16 oz)	900
Chipsters	1	330
Cone Cake Chocolate	1 sm	260
Cone Cake Chocolate	1 lg	600
Cone Cake Vanilla	1 sm	280
Cone Cake Vanilla	1 lg	650
Cone Sugar Chocolate	1 sm	300
Cone Sugar Vanilla	1 sm	320
Cone Waffle Chocolate	1 sm	330
Cone Waffle Chocolate	1 lg	660
Cone Waffle Vanilla	1 sm	350
Cone Waffle Vanilla	1 lg	710
Dashers Banana Barge	1	940
Dashers Bananas Foster	1	600
Dashers Fudge Brownie	1	810
Dashers Mint Chocolate Chip	1	720
Dashers Peanut Butter Cup	1	1090
Dashers Strawberry Shortcake	1	590
Flying Saucer 98% Fat Free Chocolate	1	180
Flying Saucer 98% Fat Free Vanilla	1	180

FOOD	PORTION	CALS
Flying Saucer Chocolate	1	230
Flying Saucer Deluxe Sprinkles	1	330
Flying Saucer Vanilla	1	240
Ice Cream Chocolate	1 sm (4 oz)	250
Ice Cream Vanilla	1 sm (4 oz)	240
Ice Cream No Fat Chocolate	1 sm (4 oz)	160
Ice Cream No Fat Vanilla	1 sm (4 oz)	160
Sherbet All Flavors	1 sm (4 oz)	180
Sinful Love Bar	1	460
Sprinkle Cup	1	230
Sundae Bittersweet Fudge	1 reg	690
Sundae Caramel	1 reg	670
Sundae Hot Fudge	1 reg	670
Sundae Strawberry	1 reg	580
Sundae Mini Chocolate Syrup	1	200
Thick Shake Chocolate	1 reg (16 oz)	650
Thick Shake Vanilla	1 reg (16 oz)	610
Thinny Thin Classic Sundae No Fat Fudge	1 reg	380
Thinny Thin Classic Sundae No Fat Strawberry	1 reg	320
Thinny Thin Miniature Sundae No Fat	1	190
Thinny Thin Miniature Sundae No Sugar Added	1	200
Thinny Thin No Fat Carvelanche Strawberry	1 (16 oz)	430
Thinny Thin No Fat Chocolate	1 sm	160
Thinny Thin No Fat Vanilla	1 sm	160
Thinny Thin No Sugar Added Vanilla	1 sm	180
Thinny Thin Parfait No Fat	1	190
Thinny Thin Shake No Fat Chocolate	1 (16 oz)	440
Thinny Thin Shake No Fat Mocha	1 (16 oz)	440
Thinny Thin Shake No Fat Vanilla	1 (16 oz)	300

CHEVY'S

FOOD	PORTION	CALS
Black Beans	1 serv	59
Catch Of The Day w/ San Antonio Vegetables Salsa & Tomalito	1 serv	428
Chicken Fajitas w/ San Antonio Vegetables & Tomalito	1 serv	285
Fish Tacos w/ Taco Dressing Lettuce & Pico De Gallo	1 serv	483
Grilled Chicken Salad w/ Salsa Vinaigrette	1 serv	533
Guacamole	1 serv (2 oz)	103

FOOD	PORTION	CALS
Mexican Rice	1 serv	211
Mixed Green Salad w/ Salsa Vinaigrette	1 serv	358
Salsa	1 serv (5 oz)	40
Shrimp Fajitas w/ San Antonio Vegetables & Tomalito	1 serv	286
Sour Cream	1 serv	121
Tortilla Corn	1	80
Tortilla El Machino	1	167
Veggie Burrito w/ San Antonio Vegetables Pico De Gallo & Ranchero Sauce	1 serv	430
Veggie Fajitas w/ San Antonio Vegetables & Tomalito	1 serv	345

CHICKEN OUT ROTISSERIE
MAIN MENU SELECTIONS

FOOD	PORTION	CALS
Apple Cornbread Stuffing	1 serv (6 oz)	215
Baked Potato Wedges	1 serv (6 oz)	110
Biscuit	1	150
Chicken Burger w/o Cheese	1	285
Chunky Cinnamon Applesauce	1 serv (6 oz)	60
Creamed Spinach w/ Artichokes	1 serv (6 oz)	160
Farm Fresh Cole Slaw	1 serv (6 oz)	55
French Baguette	1	80
Fresh Fruit Salad	1 serv (6 oz)	77
Mandarin Walnut Cranberry Relish	1 serv (6 oz)	240
Mashed Sweet Potatoes	1 serv (6 oz)	120
Oriental Green Beans	1 serv (6 oz)	34
Real Cheese & Macaroni	1 serv (6 oz)	311
Red Skin Mashed Potatoes	1 serv (6 oz)	181
Rice Pilaf	1 serv (6 oz)	140
Roasted Peas Corn & Carrots	1 serv (6 oz)	120
Sandwich BBQ Pulled Chicken	1	406
Sandwich Grilled Chicken Breast	1	350
Sandwich Open Faced Pulled Chicken	1	682
Sandwich Pulled Chicken	1	320
Sandwich Signature Chicken Salad	1	370
Steamed Broccoli & Carrots	1 serv (6 oz)	30
Vegetarian Baked Beans	1 serv (6 oz)	150
Wrap Chinese Chicken Salad w/o Dressing	1	330
Wrap Fajita	1	360
Wrap Fresh Vegetable Salad w/o Dressing	1	170

FOOD	PORTION	CALS
Wrap Grilled Chicken Caesar	1	355
Wrap Pesto Chicken	1	405
Wrap Pulled Chicken	1	300
Wrap Skinless Grilled Chicken	1	330
SOUPS		
Chicken Noodle	1 serv (6 oz)	130
Vegetable Minestrone	1 serv (6 oz)	96

CHICK-FIL-A
BEVERAGES

FOOD	PORTION	CALS
Coca-Cola Classic	1 sm	110
Diet Coke	1 sm	0
Diet Lemonade	1 sm	25
Ice Tea Sweetened	1 sm	80
Iced Tea Unsweetened	1 sm	0
Lemonade	1 sm	170
BREAKFAST SELECTIONS		
Bagel Chicken Egg Cheese	1	500
Bagel Wheat	1	220
Biscuit Bacon	1	300
Biscuit Bacon Egg	1	390
Biscuit Bacon Egg Cheese	1	440
Biscuit Buttered	1	270
Biscuit Chicken	1	420
Biscuit Chicken w/ Cheese	1	470
Biscuit Egg	1	350
Biscuit Egg Cheese	1	400
Biscuit Sausage	1	410
Biscuit Sausage Egg	1	500
Biscuit Sausage Egg Cheese	1	550
Biscuit w/ Gravy	1	330
Burrito Chicken	1	420
Burrito Sausage	1	460
Chick-N-Minis	1 serv	270
Hashbrowns	1 serv	260
DESSERTS		
Cheesecake	1 slice	340
Fudge Nut Brownie	1	330
Icedream Cone	1 sm	160
Lemon Pie	1 slice	390

FOOD	PORTION	CALS
MAIN MENU SELECTIONS		
Chicken Filet	1	230
Chicken Filet Chargrilled	1	100
Chick-N-Strips	4	290
Cool Wrap Chargrilled Chicken	1	390
Cool Wrap Chicken Caesar	1	460
Cool Wrap Spicy Chicken	1	380
Fruit Cup	1 serv	60
Hearty Breast of Chicken Soup	1 cup	140
Nuggets	8	260
Polynesian Sauce	1 pkg	110
Sandwich Chargrilled Chicken	1	270
Sandwich Chicken	1	410
Sandwich Chicken Deluxe	1	420
Sandwich Chicken Salad On Wheat Bread	1	350
Waffle Potato Fries	1 sm	270
SALAD DRESSINGS AND SAUCES		
Barbecue Sauce	1 pkg	45
Blue Cheese	2 tbsp	150
Buffalo Sauce	1 pkg	15
Buttermilk Ranch	2 tbsp	160
Buttermilk Ranch Sauce	1 pkg	110
Caesar	2 tbsp	160
Fat Free Honey Mustard	2 tbsp	60
Honey Mustard	1 pkg	45
Honey Roasted BBQ Sauce	1 pkg	60
Light Italian	2 tbsp	15
Raspberry Vinaigrette Reduced Fat	2 tbsp	80
Spicy	2 tbsp	140
Thousand Island	2 tbsp	150
SALADS		
Carrot & Raisin Salad	1 sm	170
Chargrilled Chicken Garden Salad	1 serv	180
Chick-N-Strips Salad	1 serv	390
Cole Slaw	1 sm	260
Croutons Garlic & Butter	1 pkg	50
Honey Roasted Sunflower Kernels	1 pkg	80
Side Salad	1 serv	60
Southwest Chargrilled Salad	1 serv	240
Tortilla Strips	1 pkg	70

FOOD	PORTION	CALS
CHILI'S		
CHILDREN'S MENU SELECTIONS		
Corn Dog	1	250
Grilled Chicken Platter	1 serv	140
Little Chicken Crispers	1 serv	590
Little Mouth Burger	1 serv	280
Little Mouth Cheeseburger	1 serv	350
Macaroni & Cheese	1 serv	510
Pepper Pal Pasta w/ Alfredo	1 serv	410
Pepper Pal Pasta w/ Marinara	1 serv	290
Pizza	1 serv	570
Rib Basket	1 serv	370
Sandwich Grilled Cheese	1 serv	420
Sandwich Grilled Chicken	1 serv	140
DESSERTS		
Cheesecake	1 serv	760
Chocolate Chip Paradise Pie w/ Vanilla Ice Cream	1 serv	1600
Frosty Chocolate Shake w/ Chocolate Sprinkles	1 serv	850
Molten Chocolate Cake w/ Vanilla Ice Cream	1 serv	1270
MAIN MENU SELECTIONS		
Awesome Blossom	1 serv	2710
Baby Back Ribs & Chicken	1 serv	1460
Black Bean Burger	1 serv	650
Boneless Buffalo Wings	1 serv	1250
Boneless Shanghai Wings	1 serv	1260
Bottomless Tostada Chips	1 basket	400
Burger Bacon	1 serv	1080
Burger BBQ Ranch	1 serv	1110
Burger Chipotle Bleu Cheese Bacon	1 serv	1090
Burger Ground Peppercorn	1 serv	1050
Burger Mushroom Swiss	1 serv	1100
Burger Oldtimer	1 serv	800
Chicken Crispers	1 serv	1870
Chicken Tacos	1 serv	1200
Cinnamon Apples	1 serv	210
Citrus Fire Chicken & Shrimp	1 serv	760
Classic Nachos	1 serv	1570
Country Fried Steak	1 serv	1890

FOOD	PORTION	CALS
Fried Cheese w/ Marinara Sauce	1 serv	1210
Garlic Toast	1 piece	200
Grilled Baby Back Ribs	1 serv	1370
Grilled Salmon w/ Garlic & Herbs	1 serv	700
Guiltless Grill Chicken Pita	1 serv	550
Guiltless Grill Chicken Platter	1 serv	580
Guiltless Grill Chicken Sandwich	1 serv	490
Guiltless Grill Salmon	1 serv	480
Guiltless Grill Tomato Basil Pasta	1 serv	650
Homestyle Fries	1 serv	520
Kettle Black Beans	1 serv	140
Loaded Mashed Potatoes	1 serv	560
Margarita Grilled Chicken	1 serv	690
Monterey Chicken	1 serv	1170
Pasta Cajun Chicken	1 serv	1460
Pasta Grilled Shrimp Alfredo	1 serv	1340
Pasta Tomato Basil Chicken	1 serv	860
Pita Chicken Caesar	1 serv	650
Pita Chicken Fajita	1 serv	450
Pita Steak Fajita	1 serv	580
Quesadillas Fajita Chicken	1 serv	1720
Quesadillas Fajita Combo	1 serv	1840
Quesadillas Fajita Steak	1 serv	1970
Ribeye Cajun	1 serv	870
Ribeye Flame Grilled	1 serv	960
Rice	1 serv	210
Sandwich Cajun Chicken	1 serv	820
Sandwich Chicken Ranch	1 serv	1150
Sandwich Chili's Cheesesteak	1 serv	1010
Sandwich Grilled Chicken	1 serv	840
Sandwich Smoked Turkey	1 serv	930
Sauteed Mushrooms Onions & Bell Peppers	1 serv	120
Seasonal Grilled Veggies	1 serv	90
Seasonal Steamed Veggie w/ Parmesan Cheese	1 serv	60
Sirloin Chili's Classic	1 serv	530
Sirloin Honey BBQ	1 serv	800
Skillet Queso	1 serv	670
Southwestern Eggrolls	1 serv	810
Steamed Broccoli	1 serv	80

FOOD	PORTION	CALS
Sweet Corn On The Cob	1 serv	180
Triple Play	1 serv	2330
Wings Over Buffalo	1 serv	1140
SALAD DRESSINGS AND SAUCES		
Dressing Asian Sesame Ginger	1 serv (2 oz)	250
Dressing Avocado Ranch	1 serv (2 oz)	150
Dressing Bleu Cheese	1 serv (2 oz)	330
Dressing Caesar	1 serv (2 oz)	350
Dressing Chipotle Ranch	1 serv (2 oz)	170
Dressing Citrus Balsamic Vinaigrette	1 serv (2 oz)	350
Dressing Creamy Cilantro	1 serv (2 oz)	300
Dressing Honey Lime	1 serv (2 oz)	270
Dressing Honey Mustard	1 serv (2 oz)	260
Dressing Ranch	1 serv (2 oz)	240
Dressing Thousand Island	1 serv (2 oz)	270
Dressing Low Fat Ranch	1 serv (2 oz)	110
Dressing No Fat Balsamic Vinaigrette	1 serv (2 oz)	50
Dressing No Fat Honey Mustard	1 serv (2 oz)	90
Sauce Peanut Dipping	1 serv (2 oz)	190
Sauce Picante Salsa	1 serv (2 oz)	40
Sauce Sesame Dipping	1 serv (2 oz)	70
SALADS		
Boneless Buffalo Chicken	1 serv	870
Chicken Caesar w/ Dressing	1 serv	1010
Crispy Chicken	1 serv	810
Dinner Caesar w/ Dressing	1 serv	430
Dinner House	1 serv	140
Grilled Caribbean	1 serv	440
Lettuce Wraps	1 serv	330
Lime Grilled Shrimp Caesar w/ Dressing	1 serv	980
Quesadilla Explosion	1 serv	850
Southwestern Cobb	1 serv	650
SOUPS		
Broccoli Cheese	1 cup	160
Chicken Enchilada	1 cup	220
Chicken Noodle	1 cup	50
Chicken Tortilla	1 cup	140
Chili w/ Cheese	1 cup	500
New England Clam Chowder	1 cup	470
Potato	1 cup	220

FOOD	PORTION	CALS
Southwestern Vegetable	1 cup	110

CHIPOTLE
Barbacoa	1 serv (4 oz)	228
Black Beans	1 serv (4 oz)	130
Carnitas	1 serv (4 oz)	227
Cheese	1 serv (1 oz)	110
Chicken	1 serv (4 oz)	219
Chips	1 serv (4 oz)	490
Crispy Taco Shells	3	180
Fajita Vegetables	1 serv (3 oz)	100
Flour Tortilla	1 (6 inch)	300
Flour Tortilla	1 (13 inch)	330
Guacamole	1 serv (4 oz)	170
Lettuce	1 serv (1 oz)	5
Pinto Beans	1 serv (4 oz)	138
Rice	1 serv (3.5 oz)	168
Salsa Corn	1 serv (4 oz)	100
Salsa Tomato	1 serv (4 oz)	25
Sour Cream	1 serv (2 oz)	120
Steak	1 serv (4 oz)	230
Tomatillo Green	1 serv (2 oz)	15
Tomatillo Red	1 serv (2 oz)	28
Vinaigrette	1 serv (2 oz)	282

CHURCH'S CHICKEN
DESSERTS
Pie Apple	1 pie (3 oz)	280
Pie Edward's Double Lemon	1 pie (3 oz)	300
Pie Edward's Strawberry Cream Cheese	1 pie (2.8 oz)	280

MAIN MENU SELECTIONS
Biscuit Honey Butter	1	240
Cajun Rice	1 reg	130
Chicken Fried Steak w/ White Gravy	1 serv (7.5 oz)	610
Cole Slaw	1 reg	150
Corn On The Cob	1 ear	140
Country Fried Steak w/ White Gravy	1 serv (5.8 oz)	470
Crunchy Tenders	1 (2 oz)	120
French Fries	1 reg	290
Jalapeno Cheese Bombers	4 (4 oz)	240
Macaroni & Cheese	1 reg	210

FOOD	PORTION	CALS
Mashed Potatoes & Gravy	1 reg	70
Okra	1 reg	350
Original Breast	1	200
Original Leg	1	110
Original Thigh	1	330
Original Wing	1	300
Sandwich Bigger Better Chicken w/ Cheese	1	510
Sandwich Country Fried Steak	1	490
Sandwich Spicy Fish	1	320
Spicy Breast	1	320
Spicy Crunchy Tenders	1 (2 oz)	135
Spicy Fish Fillet	1 piece (2.3 oz)	160
Spicy Leg	1	180
Spicy Thigh	1	480
Spicy Wing	1	430
Sweet Corn Nuggets	1 reg	600
Whole Jalapeno Peppers	2	10
SAUCES		
BBQ	1 pkg	30
Creamy Jalapeno	1 pkg	100
Honey	1 pkg	27
Honey Mustard	1 pkg	110
Hot Sauce	1 pkg	0
Ketchup	1 pkg	18
Purple Pepper	1 pkg	45
Ranch	1 pkg	130
Sweet & Sour	1 pkg	30

CICI'S

FOOD	PORTION	CALS
EXTRAS		
Apple Pizza	1 slice	149
Brownie	1	143
Cinnamon Roll	1	139
Garlic Bread	1 slice	99
PIZZA		
Buffet 12 Inch Alfredo	1 slice	139
Buffet 12 Inch Bacon Cheddar	1 slice	145
Buffet 12 Inch Bar-B-Que	1 slice	172
Buffet 12 Inch Beef	1 slice	170
Buffet 12 Inch Cheese	1 slice	152
Buffet 12 Inch Ham & Pineapple	1 slice	141

FOOD	PORTION	CALS
Buffet 12 Inch Ole	1 slice	108
Buffet 12 Inch Pepperoni	1 slice	175
Buffet 12 Inch Pepperoni & Jalapeno	1 slice	163
Buffet 12 Inch Sausage	1 slice	197
Buffet 12 Inch Spinach Alfredo	1 slice	151
Buffet 12 Inch Zesty Ham & Cheese	1 slice	153
Buffet 12 Inch Zesty Pepperoni	1 slice	157
Buffet 12 Inch Zesty Tomato Alfredo	1 slice	136
Buffet 12 Inch Zesty Veggie	1 slice	124
To-Go 15 Inch Bar-B-Que	1 slice	289
To-Go 15 Inch Cheese	1 slice	223
To-Go 15 Inch Ham & Pineapple	1 slice	225
To-Go 15 Inch Ole	1 slice	169
To-Go 15 Inch Pepperoni	1 slice	240
To-Go 15 Inch Spinach Alfredo	1 slice	243
To-Go 15 Inch Zesty Pepperoni	1 slice	246
To-Go 15 Inch Zesty Veggie	1 slice	213

CINNABON
BAKED SELECTIONS

FOOD	PORTION	CALS
Caramel Pecanbon	1	1100
Cinnabon Bites	6	520
Cinnabon Classic	1	813
Cinnabon Stix	1	379
Cinnamon Filled Churro	1	281
Minibon	1	339

BEVERAGES

FOOD	PORTION	CALS
Caramelatta Chill	1 (16 oz)	520
Chillatta Cappuccino	1 (16 oz)	330
Chillatta Caramel	1 (16 oz)	480
Chillatta Chocolate Mocha	1 (16 oz)	460
Chillatta Mango	1 (16 oz)	340
Chillatta Strawberry	1 (16 oz)	330
Chillatta Strawberry Banana	1 (16 oz)	350
Chillatta Tropical Blast	1 (16 oz)	330
Mochalatta Chill	1 (16 oz)	450

COLD STONE CREAMERY

FOOD	PORTION	CALS
Waffle Cone Dipped	1	310
Waffle Cone Dipped w/ Candy	1	390
Waffle Cone Or Bowl	1	160

FOOD	PORTION	CALS
FROZEN YOGURT		
Cheesecake	1 serv (6 oz)	170
Low Fat Chocolate	1 serv (6 oz)	230
Nonfat Coffee	1 serv (6 oz)	220
Nonfat Sweet Cream	1 serv (6 oz)	220
ICE CREAM		
Amaretto	1 serv (6 oz)	390
Banana	1 serv (6 oz)	370
Black Cherry	1 serv (6 oz)	390
Butter Pecan	1 serv (6 oz)	390
Cake A Cheesecake Named Desire	1 slice (5 oz)	410
Cake Butterfinger Bonanza	1 slice (5 oz)	450
Cake Celebration Sensation	1 slice (4.5 oz)	350
Cake Chocolate Chipper	1 slice (4.6 oz)	450
Cake Coffeehouse Crunch	1 slice (5 oz)	530
Cake Cookie Dough Delirium	1 slice (4.8 oz)	420
Cake Cookies & Creamery	1 slice (4.5 oz)	390
Cake Midnight Delight	1 slice (5.3 oz)	510
Cake MMMMMM Chip	1 slice (4.5 oz)	380
Cake Peanut Butter Playground	1 slice (5 oz)	490
Cake Raspberry Truffle Temptation	1 slice (5 oz)	480
Cake Snicker's Supreme	1 slice (5 oz)	510
Cake Strawberry Passion	1 slice (5 oz)	380
Cake Zebra Stripes	1 slice (4.8 oz)	400
Candy Cane	1 serv (6 oz)	420
Caramel Latte	1 serv (6 oz)	400
Carrot Cake Batter	1 serv (6 oz)	450
Cheesecake	1 serv (6 oz)	390
Chocolate	1 serv (6 oz)	390
Cinnamon	1 serv (6 oz)	400
Coconut	1 serv (6 oz)	390
Coffee	1 serv (6 oz)	400
Cookie Batter	1 serv (6 oz)	450
Cotton Candy	1 serv (6 oz)	390
Dark Chocolate Peppermint	1 serv (6 oz)	410
Egg Nog	1 serv (6 oz)	400
Espresso	1 serv (6 oz)	350
French Vanilla	1 serv (6 oz)	400
Irish Cream	1 serv (6 oz)	390
Macadamia Nut	1 serv (6 oz)	390

FOOD	PORTION	CALS
Mango	1 serv (6 oz)	370
Mint	1 serv (6 oz)	400
Mocha	1 serv (6 oz)	390
Oatmeal Batter	1 serv (6 oz)	400
Orange Dreamsicle	1 serv (6 oz)	380
Peanut Butter	1 serv (6 oz)	440
Pecan Praline	1 serv (6 oz)	400
Pistachio	1 serv (6 oz)	390
Pumpkin	1 serv (6 oz)	390
Raspberry	1 serv (6 oz)	390
Sinless Sans Fat Sweet Cream	1 serv (6 oz)	160
Strawberry	1 serv (6 oz)	380
Sweet Cream	1 serv (6 oz)	390
Vanilla Bean	1 serv (6 oz)	400
White Chocolate	1 serv (6 oz)	390
MIX-INS AND TOPPINGS		
Almond Joy	1 piece	180
Apple Pie Filling	0.75 oz	60
Banana	½	60
Black Cherries	0.75 oz	80
Blackberries	0.75 oz	10
Blueberries	0.75 oz	10
Brownies	1 piece	180
Butterfinger	½ bar	140
Butterscotch Fat Free	1 oz	80
Caramel	1 oz	100
Caramel Topping Fat Free	1 oz	110
Cashews	1 oz	170
Chocolate Chips	1 oz	130
Cinnamon	⅛ tsp	15
Coconut	1 oz	80
Cookie Dough	1 piece	180
Fudge	1 oz	100
Fudge Topping Fat Free	1 oz	80
Granola	1 oz	120
Gumballs	1 oz	120
Gummi Bears	1 oz	120
Heath Candy	1 bar	110
Honey	1 oz	90
Kit Kat	½ bar	100

FOOD	PORTION	CALS
M&M's	1 oz	170
M&M's Peanut	1 oz	150
Macadamia Nuts	1 oz	180
Maraschino Cherry	1	5
Marshmallow Creme	1 oz	100
Marshmallows	1 oz	100
Nestle Crunch	½ bar	130
Nilla Wafers	3	70
Oreo Cookies	2	120
Peach Pie Filling	1 oz	60
Peanut Butter	0.75 oz	150
Peanuts	1 oz	200
Pecan Pralines	1 oz	210
Pecans	1 oz	140
Pie Crust Graham Cracker	1 oz	110
Pie Crust Oreo	1 oz	180
Pistachio Nuts	1 oz	210
Raisins	1 oz	80
Raspberries	0.75 oz	15
Reese's Peanut Butter Cup	1 piece	190
Reese's Pieces	1 oz	170
Roasted Almonds	1 oz	190
Sliced Almonds	1 oz	210
Snickers	½ bar	170
Sprinkles Chocolate	1 oz	25
Sprinkles Rainbow	1 oz	25
Strawberries	0.75 oz	20
Toasted Coconut	1 oz	180
Twix	1 cup	150
Walnuts	1 oz	130
Whip Topping	1 serv	45
White Chocolate Chips	1 oz	160
Whoppers	1 oz	100
Yellow Sponge Cake	1 piece	70
York Peppermint Patties	2 pieces	120
SORBET		
Sinless Lemon	1 serv (6 oz)	180
Sinless Raspberry	1 serv (6 oz)	200
Sinless Tangerine	1 serv (6 oz)	200

FOOD	PORTION	CALS
CORNER BAKERY		
BREAKFAST SELECTIONS		
Baked French Toast	1 serv	570
Buckhead Cheese Grits	1 serv	350
Fresh Berry Parfait	1 serv	330
Oatmeal	1 serv	280
Oatmeal Crunchy Honey Banana	1 serv	380
Oatmeal Swiss	1 serv	330
Panini Ham & Cheddar	1	720
Panini Smoked Bacon & Cheddar	1	680
Scrambler All American w/o Potatoes & Bread	1 serv	310
Scrambler Anaheim w/o Potatoes & Bread	1 serv	490
Scrambler Farmer's w/o Potatoes & Bread	1 serv	430
The Commuter Croissant	1	720
PASTA		
Chicken Carbonara	1 serv	740
Half Moon Cheese Ravioli	1 serv	550
Penne w/ Marinara	1 serv	550
Pesto Cavatappi	1 serv	930
SALAD DRESSINGS		
Caesar	1 serv	310
House	1 serv	280
Ranch	1 serv	160
Vinaigrette Balsamic	1 serv	300
SALADS		
Caesar	1 serv	520
Caesar w/ Roasted Chicken & Croutons	1 serv	640
Chopped w/o Bread	1 serv	810
Harvest	1 serv	860
Harvest w/ Roasted Chicken	1 serv	980
Santa Fe Ranch	1 serv	680
Santa Fe Ranch w/ Roasted Chicken	1 serv	800
Side Cucumber Tomato	1 (6 oz)	120
Side Egg	1 (6 oz)	570
Side Roasted Potato Bacon	1 (6 oz)	370
Side Seasonal Fruit Medley	1 (6 oz)	90
Side Tomato Mozzarella Pasta	1 (6 oz)	205
Side Tuna	1 (6 oz)	310
SANDWICHES		
Bavarian w/ Ham	1	720

FOOD	PORTION	CALS
Bavarian w/ Turkey	1	690
Chicken Pesto	1	840
Panini California Grille	1	700
Panini Chicken Pomodori	1	890
Panini Club	1	900
Panini Corned Beef Reuben	1	930
Panini Grilled Ham & Swiss	1	880
Southwest Roast Beef	1	840
Tomato Mozzarella	1	670
Tuna Salad On Olive Bread	1	450
Turkey Derby	1	650
Turkey Frisco	1	850
Uptown Turkey	1	660
SOUPS		
Big Al's Chili w/ Cheddar Cheese	1 (10 oz)	380
Bread Bowl	1	420
Cheddar	1 (10 oz)	310
Chicken Wild Mushroom Brie Stew	1 (10 oz)	260
Loaded Baked Potato w/ Garnish	1 (10 oz)	420
Mom's Chicken Noodle	1 (10 oz)	170
Old Fashioned Beef Stew	1 (10 oz)	260
Roasted Poblano Corn Chowder	1 (10 oz)	330
Roasted Tomato Basil w/o Garnish	1 (10 oz)	170
Zesty Chicken Tortilla w/ Tortilla Strips	1 (10 oz)	230

COSI
BEVERAGES

FOOD	PORTION	CALS
Arctic Double Chi	1 tall (12 oz)	621
Arctic Latte	1 tall (12 oz)	396
Arctic Mocha	1 tall (12 oz)	623
Arctic Raspberry Chai	1 tall (12 oz)	300
Arctic Thai as prep	1 tall (12 oz)	432
Caramel Mocha	1 tall (9 oz)	344
Chai Tea Latte	1 tall (8 oz)	109
Hot Chocolate	1 tall (12 oz)	436
Kefir Blueberry	1 (12 oz)	278
Lemonade	1 (15 oz)	112
Lemonade Strawberry	1 tall (12 oz)	290
Smoothie Mango Mania	1 tall (12 oz)	186
Smoothie Peach	1 tall (12 oz)	186
Smoothie Strawberry Banana	1 tall (12 oz)	186

FOOD	PORTION	CALS
Smores Latte	1 tall (11 oz)	401
Wildberry Blast	1 tall (12 oz)	186
BREAKFAST SELECTIONS		
Bagel Asiago Cheese	1 (6 oz)	327
Bagel Cinnamon Raisin	1 (6 oz)	438
Bagel Cranberry Orange	1 (6 oz)	372
Bagel Everything	1 (5.5 oz)	353
Bagel Plain	1 (5.5 oz)	326
Bagel Poppy Seed	1 (5.5 oz)	346
Cream Cheese Honey Pecan	1 serv (2 oz)	159
Cream Cheese Plain	1 serv (2 oz)	182
Cream Cheese Plain Low Fat	1 serv (2 oz)	121
Cream Cheese Veggie Low Fat	1 serv (2 oz)	113
Croissant Almond	1	340
Croissant Butter	1	330
Croissant Chocolate	1	370
Fruit Salad	1 serv	216
Granola Cereal	1 serv	564
Granola Parfait Peach	1 serv	389
Granola Parfait Strawberry	1 serv	426
Muffin Banana Nut	1	480
Muffin Blueberry	1	440
Muffin Carrot Raisin	1	470
Muffin Corn	1	450
Muffin Lowfat Bran	1	351
Scones Blueberry	1	410
DESSERTS		
Apple Tart	1 serv	396
Blondie Brownie	1	570
Cheesecake	1 serv	567
Cheesecake Brownie	1 serv	470
Cinnamon Apple Pie	1 serv	960
Cookie Chocolate Chunk	1	480
Cookie Oatmeal Raisin	1	440
Ice Cream Double Scoop	1 serv	225
Sundae	1 med	408
SALAD DRESSINGS		
Caesar	1 serv (2 oz)	301
Cosi Vinaigrette	1 serv (2 oz)	357
Fat Free Balsamic Vinaigrette	1 serv (2 oz)	45

FOOD	PORTION	CALS
Lowfat Ginger Soy	1 serv (2 oz)	74
Pepperanch	1 serv (2 oz)	262
Reduced Fat Roasted Shallot Sherry Vinaigrette	1 serv (2 oz)	85
Roasted Shallot Sherry Vinaigrette	1 serv (2 oz)	308
SALADS		
Bombay Chicken No Dressing	1 serv	176
Caesar No Dressing	1 serv	182
Caesar w/ Grilled Chicken No Dressing	1 serv	340
Cosi Cobb No Dressing	1 serv	419
Greek No Dressing	1 serv	236
Mixed Greens No Dressing	1 serv	46
Shanghai Chicken No Dressing	1 serv	221
Signature No Dressing	1 serv	375
SANDWICHES		
Buffalo Blue	1	649
Cosi Club	1	729
Green Market	1	555
Grilled Chicken T.B.M.	1	791
Hummus & Fresh Veggies	1	432
Italiano	1	834
Melts Bacon Turkey Cheddar	1	682
Melts Chicken TBM	1	926
Melts Grilled Chicken Parmesan	1	701
Melts Pesto Chicken	1	809
Melts Tomato Basil & Mozzarella	1	666
Melts Tuna	1	1012
Polpette Rustica	1	553
Roasted Turkey & Brie	1	772
Sesame Ginger Chicken	1	508
Shrimp Salad	1	471
Smoked Ham & Brie	1	639
T.B.M.	1	729
Tandoori Chicken	1	633
Tuna Cheddar	1	956
Turkey Light	1	476
Turkey Rustica	1	619
Tuscan Pesto Chicken	1	571
Vegi Muffaletta	1	824
Wasabi Roast Beef	1	626

FOOD	PORTION	CALS
SOUPS		
Cajun Gumbo	1 serv (10 oz)	251
Chicken Gumbo	1 serv (6 oz)	151
Chicken Noodle	1 serv (10 oz)	116
Grilled Chicken Corn Chowder	1 serv (10 oz)	305
Lentil	1 serv (10 oz)	199
Minestrone	1 serv (10 oz)	174
New England Clam Chowder	1 serv (10 oz)	440
Three Bean Chili	1 serv (10 oz)	162
DAIRY QUEEN		
FOOD SELECTIONS		
Chicken Strip Basket	4 pieces	520
Chili Cheese Dog	1	330
DQ Homestyle Bacon Double Cheeseburger	1	610
DQ Homestyle Burger	1	290
DQ Homestyle Cheeseburger	1	340
DQ Homestyle Double Cheeseburger	1	540
DQ Ultimate Burger	1	670
French Fries	1 sm	300
Grillburger ½ Lb	1	800
Grillburger ½ Lb w/ Cheese	1	930
Grillburger ¼ Lb FlameThrower	1	850
Grillburger Bacon Cheddar	1	710
Grillburger California	1	630
Grillburger Classic	1	540
Grillburger Classic w/ Cheese	1	610
Grillburger Mushroom Swiss	1	700
Hot Dog	1	240
Onion Rings	1 reg	470
Salad Crispy Chicken No Dressing	1 serv	350
Salad Grilled Chicken No Dressing	1 serv	240
Sandwich Crispy Chicken	1	590
Sandwich Gilled Chicken	1	340
Side Salad	1 serv	60
ICE CREAM		
Banana Split	1	510
Blizzard Banana Split	1 sm	460
Blizzard Chocolate Chip Cookie Dough	1 sm	720
Blizzard Oreo Cookies	1 sm	570
Blizzard Reese's Peanut Butter Cup	1 sm	600

FOOD	PORTION	CALS
Blizzard Strawberry Cheesecake	1 sm	530
Brownie Earthquake	1	740
Buster Bar	1	500
Cake 8 Inch Round	⅛ cake	370
Cake Blizzard Oreo Cookie	⅛ cake	490
Cake Blizzard Reese's Peanut Butter Cup	⅛ cake	490
Cone Chocolate	1 sm	240
Cone Dipped	1 sm	340
Cone Vanilla	1 sm	230
Dilly Bar Chocolate	1	220
DQ Fudge Bar No Sugar Added	1	50
DQ Sandwich	1	200
DQ Soft Serve Chocolate	½ cup	150
DQ Soft Serve Vanilla	½ cup	140
DQ Vanilla Orange Bar No Sugar Added	1	60
Malt Chocolate	1 sm	640
MooLatte Cappuccino	1 (16 oz)	490
MooLatte Caramel	1 (16 oz)	630
MooLatte French Vanilla	1 (16 oz)	570
MooLatte Mocha	1 (16 oz)	590
Peanut Buster Parfait	1	730
Shake Chocolate	1 sm	560
Slush Arctic Rush	1 sm	220
Starkiss	1	80
Sundae Chocolate	1 sm	280
Sundae Strawberry	1 sm	240
SALAD DRESSINGS		
Blue Cheese	1 serv (2 oz)	210
Honey Mustard	1 serv (2 oz)	260
Italian Fat Free	1 serv (2 oz)	10
Ranch	1 serv (2 oz)	310

D'ANGELO
CHILDREN'S MENU SELECTIONS

FOOD	PORTION	CALS
D'Lite Turkey	1	217
Sub Cheeseburger	1	294
Sub Ham & Cheese	1	227
Sub Kidz Tuna	1	438
Sub Meatball	1	330
SALAD DRESSINGS		
Bleu Cheese	1 serv	152

FOOD	PORTION	CALS
Caesar	1 serv	397
Caesar Fat Free	1 serv	57
Creamy Italian	1 serv	340
Greek w/ Feta Cheese	1 serv	227
Honey Mustard	1 serv	150
Olive Oil Vinaigrette	1 serv	170
Ranch Lite	1 serv	240
SALADS		
Antipasto	1 serv	284
Caesar w/ Dressing	1 serv	474
Chicken Caesar w/ Dressing	1 serv	533
Chicken Stir Fry w/o Dressing	1 serv	168
Cobb w/o Dressing	1 serv	292
Greek	1 serv	290
Lobster w/o Dressing	1 serv	376
Roast Beef w/o Dressing	1 serv	131
Steak Tip Caesar	1 serv	661
Tossed Garden w/o Dressing	1 serv	49
Turkey w/o Dressing	1 serv	157
SANDWICHES		
D'Lite Chicken Caesar Salad	1	374
D'Lite Chicken Stir Fry	1	426
D'Lite Classic Veggie	1	362
D'Lite Fresh Veggie	1	348
D'Lite Grilled Chicken Breast	1	388
D'Lite Roast Beef	1	338
D'Lite Turkey	1	347
D'Lite Turkey Cranberry	1	444
Pokket Big Papi	1	469
Pokket BLT & Cheese	1	397
Pokket Caesar Salad	1	616
Pokket Capicola & Cheese	1	362
Pokket Cheese	1	519
Pokket Cheeseburger	1	459
Pokket Chicken Caesar Salad	1	674
Pokket Chicken Club	1	526
Pokket Chicken Honey Dijon	1	508
Pokket Chicken Salad	1	623
Pokket Chicken Stir Fry	1	380
Pokket Classic Vegetable	1	368

FOOD	PORTION	CALS
Pokket Classic Veggie No Cheese	1	212
Pokket Greek	1	790
Pokket Grilled Chicken	1	303
Pokket Ham	1	229
Pokket Ham & Cheese	1	326
Pokket Ham & Salami	1	386
Pokket Hamburger	1	399
Pokket Italian	1	525
Pokket Lobster	1	530
Pokket Meatball	1	574
Pokket Mortadella & Cheese	1	410
Pokket Number 9	1	407
Pokket Pastrami	1	438
Pokket Pepperoni	1	407
Pokket Roast Beef	1	247
Pokket Salad	1	196
Pokket Salami & Cheese	1	509
Pokket Seafood Salad	1	449
Pokket Steak	1	305
Pokket Steak & Cheese	1	377
Pokket Steak Bomb	1	631
Pokket Steak Tip	1	452
Pokket Tuna	1	664
Pokket Turkey	1	256
Pokket Turkey Club	1	332
Sub Big Papi	1 sm	525
Sub BLT & Cheese	1 sm	463
Sub Capicola & Cheese	1 sm	408
Sub Cheese	1 sm	589
Sub Cheeseburger	1 sm	526
Sub Chicken Club	1	593
Sub Chicken Honey Dijon	1	575
Sub Chicken Salad	1 sm	692
Sub Chicken Stir Fry	1 sm	449
Sub Classic Veggie	1 sm	462
Sub Grilled Chicken	1 sm	369
Sub Ham	1 sm	302
Sub Ham & Cheese	1 sm	395
Sub Ham & Salami	1 sm	456
Sub Hamburger	1 sm	466

FOOD	PORTION	CALS
Sub Italian	1 sm	614
Sub Lobster	1 sm	598
Sub Meatball	1 sm	644
Sub Meatball & Cheese	1 sm	750
Sub Mortadella & Cheese	1 sm	479
Sub Number 9	1 sm	450
Sub Pastrami	1 sm	613
Sub Pepperoni	1 sm	603
Sub Roast Beef	1 sm	320
Sub Salad	1 sm	281
Sub Salami & Cheese	1 sm	579
Sub Seafood Salad	1 sm	498
Sub Steak	1 sm	373
Sub Steak & Cheese	1 sm	446
Sub Steak Bomb	1 sm	670
Sub Steak Tip	1 sm	545
Sub Tuna	1 sm	685
Sub Turkey Club	1 sm	401
Sub Toasted Italian Bistro	1 sm	585
Sub Toasted Pastrami Reuben	1 sm	750
Sub Toasted Roast Beef & Cheddar	1 sm	564
Sub Toasted Spicy Meatball	1 sm	933
Sub Toasted Tuna & Swiss	1 sm	796
Sub Toasted Turkey Thanksgiving	1 sm	705
Sub Toasted Turkey & Ham	1 sm	532
Wrap Big Papi	1	593
Wrap BLT & Cheese	1	544
Wrap Buffalo Chicken Salad	1	823
Wrap Caesar Salad	1	711
Wrap Capicola & Cheese	1	494
Wrap Cheese	1	675
Wrap Cheeseburger	1	609
Wrap Chicken Caesar Salad	1	830
Wrap Chicken Cobb	1	931
Wrap Chicken Filet & Bacon	1	639
Wrap Chicken Honey Dijon	1	672
Wrap Chicken Salad	1	782
Wrap Chicken Stir Fry	1	535
Wrap Classic Veggie	1	486
Wrap Greek	1	765

FOOD	PORTION	CALS
Wrap Grilled Chicken	1	422
Wrap Ham & Cheese	1	435
Wrap Ham & Salami	1	513
Wrap Hamburger	1	509
Wrap Italian	1	631
Wrap Lobster	1	749
Wrap Meatball	1	687
Wrap Mortadella & Cheese	1	522
Wrap Number 9	1	517
Wrap Pastrami	1	550
Wrap Peppercorn Steak	1	702
Wrap Pepperoni	1	519
Wrap Roast Beef	1	448
Wrap Salad	1	324
Wrap Salami & Cheese	1	605
Wrap Seafood Salad	1	541
Wrap Steak	1	392
Wrap Steak & Cheese	1	464
Wrap Steak Bomb	1	670
Wrap Steak Tip	1	432
Wrap Tuna	1	731
Wrap Turkey	1	369
Wrap Turkey Club	1	415
SOUPS		
Beef Stew	1 sm	220
Broccoli & Cheddar Cheese	1 sm	270
Chicken Noodle	1 sm	110
Hearty Vegetable	1 sm	40
Italian Wedding	1 sm	120
Lobster Bisque	1 sm	360
New England Clam Chowder	1 sm	320
Portuguese Kale	1 sm	130

DELTACO
BEVERAGES

Barq's Root Beer	1 sm	278
Classic Coke	1 sm	248
Diet Coke	1 sm	2
Iced Tea	1 sm	0
Light Lemonade Minute Maid	1 sm	13
Milk 2% Low Fat	1 serv	152

FOOD	PORTION	CALS
Orange Juice	1 serv	140
Pibb Xtra	1 sm	243
Shake Chocolate	1 (15 oz)	680
Shake Strawberry	1 (15 oz)	540
Shake Vanilla	1 (15 oz)	550
Sprite	1 sm	243
BREAKFAST SELECTIONS		
Burrito Breakfast	1	250
Burrito Egg & Cheese	1	450
Burrito Macho Bacon & Egg	1	1030
Burrito Steak & Egg	1	580
Hash Brown Sticks	5 pieces	250
Quesadilla Bacon & Egg	1	450
Side of Bacon	2 strips	50
MAIN MENU SELECTIONS		
Beans 'n Cheese Cup	1 serv	260
Bun Taco	1	440
Burrito Crispy Fish	1	497
Burrito Del Beef	1	550
Burrito Del Classic Chicken	1	560
Burrito Del Combo	1	530
Burrito Deluxe Combo	1	570
Burrito Deluxe Del Beef	1	590
Burrito Green Bean & Cheese	1	280
Burrito Green Half Pound	1	430
Burrito Macho Beef	1	1170
Burrito Macho Chicken	1	930
Burrito Macho Combo	1	1050
Burrito Red Bean & Cheese	1	270
Burrito Red Half Pound	1	430
Burrito Spicy Chicken	1	480
Burrito Works Chicken	1	520
Burrito Works Steak	1	590
Burrito Works Veggie	1	490
Cheeseburger	1	330
Cheeseburger Double Del	1	560
Cheeseburger Double Del Bacon	1	610
Chips & Salsa	1 sm	156
Del Cheeseburger	1	430
Fries	1 sm	350

FOOD	PORTION	CALS
Fries Chili Cheese	1 serv	670
Fries Deluxe Chili Cheese	1 serv	710
Hamburger	1	280
Nachos	1 serv	380
Nachos Macho	1 serv	1100
Quesadilla Cheddar	1	500
Quesadilla Chicken Cheddar	1	580
Quesadilla Spicy Jack	1	490
Quesadilla Spicy Jack Chicken	1	570
Rice Cup	1 serv	140
Taco	1	160
Taco Big Fat	1	320
Taco Big Fat Chicken	1	340
Taco Big Fat Steak	1	390
Taco Carne Asada	1	237
Taco Crispy Fish	1	290
Taco Del Carbon Chicken	1	170
Taco Del Carbon Steak	1	220
Taco Macho	1	504
Taco Soft	1	160
Taco Soft Chicken	1	210
SALADS		
Deluxe Chicken Salad	1 serv	740
Taco Salad	1 serv	350
Taco Salad Deluxe	1	780

DESERT MOON CAFE
CHILDREN'S MENU SELECTIONS

Burrito Bean & Cheese	1 serv	650
Kids Nachos	1 serv	500
Kids Taco w/ Chicken	1	280
Kids Taco w/ Steak	1	290
Kidsadilla	1 serv	630
MAIN MENU SELECTIONS		
Alamo Burger	1	810
Burrito Adobe Moon w/ Chicken	1	730
Burrito Adobe Moon w/ Steak	1	750
Burrito Black Bean w/ Chicken	1	770
Burrito Black Bean w/ Steak	1	790
Burrito Full Moon w/ Chicken	1	620
Burrito Full Moon w/ Steak	1	640

FOOD	PORTION	CALS
Burrito Get It Smothered	1	120
Burrito Harvest Wrap w/ Chicken	1	620
Burrito Harvest Wrap w/ Steak	1	300
Enchilada Mesa	1	710
Enchilada Queso	1	730
Enchilada Shrimp	1	830
Fajita Platter w/ Chicken	1 serv	1160
Fajita Platter w/ Shrimp	1 serv	1060
Fajita Platter w/ Steak	1	1190
Hell Canyon Chili	1 serv	260
Mucho Nachos	1 serv	800
Mucho Nachos w/ Chicken	1 serv	900
Mucho Nachos w/ Steak	1 serv	920
Pizza Texas BBQ	1	330
Quesadilla Baja Chicken	1	650
Quesadilla Coyote w/ Chicken	1	660
Quesadilla Coyote w/ Steak	1	680
Quesadilla Sonoran	1	660
Rice Bowl Black Bean w/ Chicken	1 serv	790
Rice Bowl Black Bean w/ Steak	1 serv	820
Rice Bowl Chili w/ Chicken	1 serv	760
Rice Bowl Chili w/ Steak	1 serv	790
Rice Bowl Shrimp Creole	1 serv	910
Shrimp Dippers	1 serv	430
Soup Black Bean	1 serv	360
Soup Tortilla	1 serv	330
Taco Acapulco Shrimp	1	230
Taco Classic w/ Chicken	1	190
Taco Classic w/ Steak	1	200
Taco Fajita w/ Chicken	1	200
Taco Fajita w/ Steak	1	210
SALAD DRESSINGS AND SAUCES		
BBQ Sauce	1 serv (1 oz)	50
Buffalo Wing Sauce	1 serv (1 oz)	45
Dressing Bleu Cheese	1 serv (2 oz)	300
Dressing Creamy Caesar	1 serv (2 oz)	320
Dressing Honey Dijon Fat Free	1 serv (2 oz)	80
Dressing Lite Ranch	1 serv (2 oz)	150
Dressing Lite Raspberry Vinaigrette	1 serv (2 oz)	150
Dressing Poblano	1 serv (1 oz)	150

FOOD	PORTION	CALS
Guacamole	1 serv (2 oz)	100
Pepper Cream Sauce	1 serv (2 oz)	100
Pico De Gallo	1 serv (2 oz)	15
Salsa Black Bean	1 serv (2 oz)	20
Salsa Fruit	1 serv (2 oz)	60
Salsa Mild Tomato	1 serv (2 oz)	15
Salsa Rattlesnake	1 serv (2 oz)	15
SALADS W/O TORTILLA BOWL		
Caesar	1 serv	530
Caesar w/ Chicken	1 serv	640
Caesar w/ Shrimp	1 serv	570
Chopped Chicken	1 serv	520
Taco w/ Chicken	1 serv	310
Taco w/ Steak	1 serv	340

DUNKIN' DONUTS
BAGELS AND CREAM CHEESE

FOOD	PORTION	CALS
Bagel Blueberry	1	330
Bagel Cinnamon Raisin	1	330
Bagel Everything	1	370
Bagel Harvest	1	350
Bagel Onion	1	320
Bagel Plain	1	320
Bagel Poppyseed	1	370
Bagel Reduced Carb w/ Cheese	1	380
Bagel Salsa	1	310
Bagel Salt	1	370
Bagel Sesame	1	380
Bagel Wheat	1	330
Cream Cheese Chive	2 oz	170
Cream Cheese Garden Vegetable	2 oz	170
Cream Cheese Lite	2 oz	110
Cream Cheese Plain	2 oz	190
Cream Cheese Salmon	2 oz	170
Cream Cheese Strawberry	2 oz	190
BAKED SELECTIONS		
Apple Fritter	1	300
Biscuit	1	250
Bismark Chocolate Iced	1	340
Coffee Roll	1	270
Coffee Roll Chocolate Frosted	1	290

FOOD	PORTION	CALS
Coffee Roll Maple Frosted	1	290
Coffee Roll Vanilla Frosted	1	290
Cookie Chocolate Chunk	2	220
Cookie Chocolate Chunk w/ Walnuts	2	230
Cookie Oatmeal Raisin Pecan	2	220
Cookie White Chocolate Chunk	2	230
Croissant Plain	1	330
Danish Apple	1	330
Danish Cheese	1	340
Danish Strawberry Cheese	1	320
Donut Apple Crumb	1	230
Donut Apple Crumb Cake	1	290
Donut Apple N' Spice	1	200
Donut Bavarian Kreme	1	210
Donut Black Raspberry	1	210
Donut Blueberry	1	290
Donut Blueberry Crumb	1	240
Donut Boston Kreme	1	240
Donut Bow Tie	1	300
Donut Chocolate Coconut	1	300
Donut Chocolate Frosted	1	360
Donut Chocolate Glazed	1	290
Donut Chocolate Kreme Filled	1	270
Donut Cinnamon	1	330
Donut Double Chocolate	1	310
Donut Frosted Lemon	1	240
Donut Glazed	1	180
Donut Glazed Gingerbread	1	260
Donut Glazed Lemon	1	240
Donut Jelly Filled	1	210
Donut Lemon Burst	1	300
Donut Maple Frosted	1	210
Donut Marble Frosted	1	200
Donut Old Fashioned	1	300
Donut Powdered	1	330
Donut Strawberry	1	210
Donut Strawberry Frosted	1	210
Donut Sugar Raised	1	170
Donut Vanilla Kreme Filled	1	270
Donut Whole Wheat Glazed	1	310

FOOD	PORTION	CALS
Eclair	1	270
English Muffin	1	160
French Cruller	1	150
Fritter Glazed	1	260
Muffin Banana Walnut	1	540
Muffin Blueberry	1	470
Muffin Chocolate Chip	1	630
Muffin Coffee Cake	1	580
Muffin Corn	1	510
Muffin Cranberry Orange	1	440
Muffin Honey Bran Raisin	1	480
Muffin Reduced Fat Blueberry	1	400
Munchkins Chocolate Glazed	3	200
Munchkins Cinnamon	4	270
Munchkins Glazed	3	280
Munchkins Jelly Filled	5	210
Munchkins Lemon Filled	4	170
Munchkins Plain	4	270
Munchkins Powdered	4	270
Munchkins Sugar Raised	7	220
Stick Cinnamon	1	450
Stick Glazed	1	490
Stick Glazed Chocolate	1	470
Stick Jelly	1	530
Stick Plain	1	420
Stick Powdered	1	450
BEVERAGES		
Cappuccino	1 (10 oz)	60
Cappuccino w/ Soy Milk	1 (10 oz)	70
Cappuccino w/ Soy Milk Sugar	1 (10 oz)	120
Cappuccino w/ Sugar	1 (10 oz)	130
Coffee Blueberry	1 (10 oz)	20
Coffee Caramel	1 (10 oz)	20
Coffee Chocolate	1 (10 oz)	20
Coffee Cinnamon	1 (10 oz)	20
Coffee Coconut	1 (10 oz)	20
Coffee French Vanilla	1 (10 oz)	20
Coffee Hazelnut	1 (10 oz)	20
Coffee Marshmallow	1 (10 oz)	20
Coffee Regular	1 (10 oz)	15

FOOD	PORTION	CALS
Coffee Toasted Almond	1 (10 oz)	20
Coffee w/ Cream	1 (10 oz)	70
Coffee w/ Cream Sugar	1 (10 oz)	120
Coffee w/ Milk	1 (10 oz)	35
Coffee w/ Milk Sugar	1 (10 oz)	80
Coffee w/ Skim Milk	1 (10 oz)	25
Coffee w/ Skim Milk Sugar	1 (10 oz)	70
Coffee w/ Sugar	1 (10 oz)	60
Coolatta Coffee w/ 2% Milk	1 (16 oz)	190
Coolatta Coffee w/ Cream	1 (16 oz)	350
Coolatta Coffee w/ Milk	1 (16 oz)	210
Coolatta Coffee w/ Skim Milk	1 (16 oz)	170
Coolatta Lemonade	1 (16 oz)	240
Coolatta Strawberry Fruit	1 (16 oz)	290
Coolatta Tropicana Orange	1 (16 oz)	370
Coolatta Vanilla Bean	1 (16 oz)	440
Dunkaccino	1 (10 oz)	230
Espresso	1 (2 oz)	0
Espresso w/ Sugar	1 (2 oz)	30
Hot Chocolate	1 (10 oz)	220
Iced Coffee	1 (16 oz)	15
Iced Coffee w/ Cream	1 (16 oz)	70
Iced Coffee w/ Cream Sugar	1 (16 oz)	120
Iced Coffee w/ Milk	1 (16 oz)	35
Iced Coffee w/ Milk Sugar	1 (16 oz)	80
Iced Coffee w/ Skim Milk	1 (16 oz)	25
Iced Coffee w/ Skim Milk Sugar	1 (16 oz)	70
Iced Coffee w/ Sugar	1 (16 oz)	60
Iced Latte	1 (16 oz)	120
Iced Latte w/ Skim Milk	1 (16 oz)	70
Iced Latte w/ Skim Milk Sugar	1 (16 oz)	120
Iced Latte w/ Sugar	1 (16 oz)	170
Iced Latte Caramel Creme	1 (16 oz)	260
Iced Latte Caramel Swirl	1 (16 oz)	240
Iced Latte Caramel Swirl w/ Skim Milk	1 (16 oz)	180
Iced Latte Lite	1 (16 oz)	80
Iced Latte Mocha Almond	1 (16 oz)	290
Iced Latte Mocha Swirl	1 (16 oz)	240
Iced Latte Mocha Swirl w/ Skim Milk	1 (16 oz)	180
Latte	1 (10 oz)	120

FOOD	PORTION	CALS
Latte w/ Soy Milk	1 (10 oz)	90
Latte w/ Soy Milk Sugar	1 (10 oz)	150
Latte w/ Sugar	1 (10 oz)	160
Latte Caramel Creme	1 (10 oz)	260
Latte Caramel Swirl	1 (10 oz)	230
Latte Caramel Swirl w/ Soy Milk	1 (10 oz)	210
Latte Lite	1 (10 oz)	70
Latte Mocha Almond	1 (10 oz)	290
Latte Mocha Swirl	1 (10 oz)	230
Latte Mocha Swirl w/ Soy Milk	1 (10 oz)	210
Smoothie Mango Passion Fruit	1 (16 oz)	360
Smoothie Reduced Calorie Berry	1 sm (16 oz)	250
Smoothie Strawberry Banana	1 (16 oz)	360
Smoothie Wildberry	1 (16 oz)	360
Tea Regular or Decaffeinated	1 (10 oz)	0
Tea w/ Milk	1 (10 oz)	25
Tea w/ Milk Sugar	1 (10 oz)	70
Tea w/ Skim Milk	1 (10 oz)	25
Tea w/ Skim Milk Sugar	1 (10 oz)	60
Tea w/ Sugar	1 (10 oz)	50
Turbo Ice	1 (16 oz)	120
Vanilla Chai	1 (10 oz)	230
SANDWICHES		
Bagel Bacon Egg Cheese	1	540
Bagel Egg Cheese	1	470
Bagel Ham Egg Cheese	1	510
Bagel Sausage Egg Cheese	1	660
Biscuit Egg Cheese	1	410
Biscuit Sausage Egg Cheese	1	610
Croissant Bacon Egg Cheese	1	520
Croissant Egg Cheese	1	550
Croissant Ham Egg Cheese	1	520
Croissant Sausage Egg Cheese	1	490
English Muffin Bacon Egg Cheese	1	360
English Muffin Egg Cheese	1	280
English Muffin Ham Egg Cheese	1	310
English Muffin Sausage Egg Cheese	1	530
Flatbread Egg White Turkey	1	280
Flatbread Egg White Veggie	1	290
Panini Meatball	1	480

FOOD	PORTION	CALS
Panini Southwestern Chicken	1	420
Panini Steak	1	450

EDDIE'S PIZZA
Bar Pie	1 pie	350
Bar Pie No Fat Cheese	1 pie	270

EL POLLO LOCO
DESSERTS
Caramel Flan	1 serv (5.5 oz)	290
Churros	2	300
Cone Vanilla	1	330
Soft Serve Vanilla	1 cup (5 oz)	300

MAIN MENU SELECTIONS
BBQ Black Beans	1 serv (6 oz)	200
Bowl The Original Pollo	1 serv	540
Burrito BRC	1 (7.5 oz)	390
Burrito Classic Chicken	1 (10.3 oz)	500
Burrito Twice Grilled	1 (15 oz)	830
Burrito Ultimate Grilled	1 (13.6 oz)	650
Chicken Breast	1 (4.3 oz)	220
Chicken Breast Skinless	1 (4 oz)	180
Chicken Leg	1 (1.8 oz)	90
Chicken Thigh	1 (3.1 oz)	220
Chicken Wing	1 (1.3 oz)	90
Cole Slaw	1 serv (6 oz)	120
Corn Cobbette	1 (5 oz)	90
French Fries	1 serv (5.5 oz)	440
Fresh Vegetables w/ Margarine	1 serv (4.1 oz)	60
Fresh Vegetables w/o Margarine	1 serv (4 oz)	35
Gravy	1 serv (1 oz)	10
Loco Nachos	1 serv	170
Macaroni & Cheese	1 serv (5.5 oz)	280
Mashed Potatoes	1 serv (5 oz)	100
Pinto Beans	1 serv (6 oz)	140
Quesadilla Cheese	1 (4.5 oz)	420
Refried Beans w/ Cheese	1 serv (6.3 oz)	270
Skinless Breast Meal	1 serv	310
Soup Chicken Tortilla w/o Tortilla Strips	1 serv (10 oz)	140
Spanish Rice	1 serv (4.5 oz)	160
Taco Al Carbon	1 (3.1 oz)	150

FOOD	PORTION	CALS
Taco Soft Chicken	1 (4.5 oz)	270
Taquito Chicken	1	190
Tortilla Chips	1 serv (1.5 oz)	210
Tortilla Corn 6 Inches	2	120
Tortilla Flour 6.5 Inches	2	210
SALAD DRESSINGS AND TOPPINGS		
Creamy Cilantro	1 serv (1.5 oz)	220
Creamy Cilantro Light	1 pkg	70
Guacamole	1 serv (1 oz)	45
Hot Sauce Jalapeno	1 pkg	5
Jack & Poblano Queso	1 serv (1.8 oz)	100
Ketchup	1 pkg	10
Light Italian	1 pkg	20
Pico De Gallo Medium	1 serv (1 oz)	10
Ranch	1 pkg	230
Salsa Avocado Hot	1 serv (1 oz)	30
Salsa Chipotle Hot	1 serv (1 oz)	5
Salsa House Mild	1 serv (1 oz)	5
Sour Cream	1 serv (1 oz)	60
Thousand Island	1 pkg	220
SALADS		
Caesar Pollo	1 (11.4 oz)	520
Ceasar Pollo w/o Dressing	1 (9.4 oz)	220
Garden	1 (4.8 oz)	120
Tostada Chicken	1 (17.3 oz)	840
Tostada Chicken w/o Shell	1 (14.7 oz)	410
EMERALD CITY SMOOTHIE		
Apple Andie	1 (11 oz)	230
Berry Berry	1 (13 oz)	350
Blueberry Blast	1 (13 oz)	380
Coconut Passion	1 (11 oz)	600
Cranberry Delight	1 (10 oz)	550
Energizer	1 (10 oz)	350
Fruity Supreme	1 (9 oz)	280
Grape Escape	1 (10 oz)	480
Guava Sunrise	1 (13 oz)	366
Kiwi Kic	1 (11 oz)	400
Lean Body	1 (11 oz)	330
Lean Out	1 (11 oz)	600
Low Carb	1 (10 oz)	350

FOOD	PORTION	CALS
Mango Mania	1 (8 oz)	370
Marionberry Fuel	1 (13 oz)	380
Mega Mass	1 (14 oz)	610
Mini Mass	1 (13 oz)	520
Mocha Bliss	1 (10 oz)	550
Nutty Banana	1 (11 oz)	720
Orange Twister	1 (10 oz)	140
Pacific Splash	1 (12 oz)	240
PB&J	1 (14 oz)	630
Peach Pleasure	1 (12 oz)	270
Peanut Passion	1 (11 oz)	580
Pineapple Bliss	1 (12 oz)	210
Power Fuel	1 (11 oz)	450
Quick Start	1 (10 oz)	280
Raspberry Dream	1 (13 oz)	410
Rejuvenator	1 (10 oz)	340
Sambazon	1 (15 oz)	410
Slim N Fit	1 (10 oz)	350
The Builder	1 (18 oz)	1270
Zesty Lemon	1 (14 oz)	430
Zip Zip	1 (10 oz)	240
Zone Zinger	1 (14 oz)	430

EVOS
BEVERAGES

FOOD	PORTION	CALS
Shake Mango Guava	1 reg (16 oz)	180
Shake Multi-Berry	1 reg (20 oz)	200
Shake Strawberry Banana	1 reg (16 oz)	190
Shake Organic Cappuccino	1 reg (16 oz)	230
Shake Organic Vanilla	1 reg (16 oz)	180

CHILDREN'S MENU SELECTIONS

FOOD	PORTION	CALS
Kids Champion Burger	1	400
Kids Chicken Strips	1 serv	130
Kids Freerange Steakburger	1	390
Kids Good Corn Dog	1	150

MAIN MENU SELECTIONS

FOOD	PORTION	CALS
Airbaked Chicken Strips	1 serv	260
Airfries	1 reg	230
American Champion	1	420
American DeLite	1	330
Burger Bun	1	190

FOOD	PORTION	CALS
Cheddar Cheese Slice	1	80
Crispy Mesquite Chicken	1 serv	330
Freerange Steakburger	1	400
Fresh Fruit Bowl	1 serv	200
Good Corn Dog	1	150
Herb Crusted Trout	1 serv	440
Honey Mesquite Chicken	1 serv	290
Spicy Chipotle Turkey	1 serv	370
Veggie Chili	1 reg	110
Veggie Garden Grill Italian	1	350
Wrap Honey Wheat	1	300
Wrap Spinach Herb	1	310
Wraps Avocado Turkey	1	480
Wraps Crispy Buffalo Chicken	1	440
Wraps Crispy Thai Trout	1	660
Wraps Freerange Beef Taco	1	600
Wraps Southwest Soy Taco	1	500
Wraps Spicy Thai Chicken	1	510
Wraps Tomato Basil Chicken	1	520
SALAD DRESSINGS AND TOPPINGS		
Balsamic Vinegar	1 serv (0.5 oz)	5
Crispy Noodles	1 serv (7 g)	35
Croutons Multi-Grain	1 serv (7 g)	30
Dressing Avocado	1 serv (3 oz)	190
Dressing Caesar	1 serv (1.7 oz)	300
Dressing Fat Free Vinaigrette	1 serv (1 oz)	5
Dressing Raspberry	1 serv (2 oz)	50
Dressing Spicy Thai	1 serv (1.4 oz)	150
Extra Virgin Olive Oil	1 serv (1 oz)	250
Herb Spread	1 serv (0.7 oz)	30
Ketchup Cayenne Firewalker	1 serv (1.2 oz)	35
Ketchup Garlic Gravity	1 serv (1.2 oz)	35
Ketchup Mesquite Magic	1 serv (1.2 oz)	35
Mesquite Honey Mustard	1 serv (0.7 oz)	80
Mustard	1 serv (0.5 oz)	10
Southwest Sour Cream	1 serv (1.4 oz)	60
Spicy Chipotle Mayo	1 serv (0.7 oz)	30
Tomato Basil Sauce	1 serv (1.4 oz)	150
SALADS		
Bordeaux Bistro w/o Dressing	1	260

FOOD	PORTION	CALS
For Salads Chicken Strips	1 serv (3 oz)	130
For Salads Grilled Chicken	1 serv (3 oz)	90
Mediterranean Summer w/o Dressing	1	200
Santa Ana Caesar w/o Dressing	1	20
Side Salad w/o Dressing	1	35
Spicy Thai w/o Dressing	1	35
SUPPLEMENTS		
Fat Burner	1 serv (5 g)	16
Go Energy	1 serv (5 g)	15
Mega Protein	1 serv (0.5 oz)	45
Multi-Vitamin	1 serv (5 g)	10

FAZOLI'S

FOOD	PORTION	CALS
BEVERAGES		
Lemon Ice All Flavors	1	360
Lemon Ice Original	1 reg	180
Lemon Ice Strawberry	1	320
CHILDREN'S MENU SELECTIONS		
Fettuccine Alfredo	1 serv	290
Meat Lasagna	1 serv	260
Ravioli w/ Marinara	1 serv	290
Spaghetti w/ Meat Sauce	1 serv	300
Spaghetti w/ Meatballs	1 serv	270
Ziti w/ Meat Sauce	1 serv	190
DESSERTS		
Cheesecake Original	1 slice	290
Cheesecake Turtle	1 slice	450
Cookie Chocolate Chunk	1	510
MAIN MENU SELECTIONS		
Breadstick	1	100
Breadstick Garlic	1	150
Fettuccine Alfredo	1 sm	520
Fettuccine w/ Marinara	1 serv	450
Fettuccine w/ Meat Sauce	1 serv	500
Oven Baked Chicken Parmesan	1 serv	960
Oven Baked Meat Lasagna	1 serv	510
Oven Baked Rigatoni Romano	1 serv	1090
Oven Baked Spaghetti	1 serv	680
Oven Baked Spaghetti w/ Meatballs	1 serv	940
Panini Four Cheese & Tomato	1	510
Panini Grilled Chicken	1	540

FOOD	PORTION	CALS
Panini Smoked Turkey	1	620
Penne w/ Alfredo	1 serv	520
Penne w/ Marinara	1 serv	450
Penne w/ Meat Sauce	1 serv	500
Pizza Slice Cheese	1	270
Pizza Slice Pepperoni	1	310
Platter Classic Sampler	1	810
Platter Ultimate Sampler	1	980
Ravioli w/ Marinara	1 serv	500
Ravioli w/ Meat Sauce	1 serv	550
Spaghetti w/ Alfredo	1 serv	520
Spaghetti w/ Marinara	1 sm	450
Spaghetti w/ Meat Sauce	1 sm	500
Submarinos Club	half	973
Submarinos Ham n' Swiss	1	680
Submarinos Italian Beef	half	660
Submarinos Original	half	940
Topping Broccoli	1 serv	25
Topping Broccoli & Tomatoes	1 serv	30
Topping Garlic Shrimp	1 serv	160
Topping Italian Sausage	1 serv	240
Topping Meatballs	1 serv	160
Topping Peppery Chicken	1 serv	70
Ziti w/ Meat Sauce	1 serv	480
SALAD DRESSINGS		
Caesar	1 serv	220
Fat Free Honey Mustard	1 serv	60
Fat Free Italian	1 serv	25
Honey French	1 serv	220
Italian	1 serv	160
Ranch	1 serv	220
Ranch Lite	1 serv	120
SALADS		
Chicken & Fruit	1	220
Chicken & Pasta Caesar	1	440
Chicken BLT Ranch	1	270
Parmesan Chicken	1	360
Side Caesar	1	40
Side Garden	1	25
Side Pasta	1 serv	320

FOOD	PORTION	CALS
FRESHENS		
PRETZELS		
Bites	1 serv (3 oz)	255
Gourmet	1 (6 oz)	510
SMOOTHIES		
Berry Berry	1 serv (21 oz)	280
Blueberry Breeze	1 serv (21 oz)	396
Caribbean Craze	1 serv (21 oz)	315
Cayman Cooler	1 serv (21 oz)	320
Club Trim	1 serv (21 oz)	291
Fitness Fuel	1 serv (21 oz)	521
Immune Support	1 serv (21 oz)	377
Jamaican Jammer	1 serv (21 oz)	378
Maui Mango	1 serv (21 oz)	354
Mocha Coffee	1 serv (21 oz)	385
Mystic Mango	1 serv (21 oz)	407
Orange Shooter	1 serv (21 oz)	330
Orange Sunrise	1 serv (21 oz)	367
Peach Sunset	1 serv (21 oz)	388
Peachy Pineapple	1 serv (21 oz)	415
Peanut Butter Chocolate	1 serv (21 oz)	312
Pina Colada	1 serv (21 oz)	451
Pineapple Passion	1 serv (21 oz)	389
Raspberry Royale	1 serv (21 oz)	346
Rockin' Raspberry	1 serv (21 oz)	332
Strawberry Shooter	1 serv (21 oz)	251
Strawberry Squeeze	1 serv (21 oz)	313
Vanilla Coffee	1 serv (21 oz)	438
Vanilla Fudge	1 serv (21 oz)	275
FRUITFULL		
BREADS		
Almond Cherry	½ slice	226
Apple Spice	½ slice	186
Banana	½ slice	165
Cappuccino Chocolate Chip	½ slice	229
Carrot	½ slice	190
Chocolate	½ slice	120
Lemon Blueberry	½ slice	120
Old Fashion Pound Cake	½ slice	227
Orange Cranberry	½ slice	130

FOOD	PORTION	CALS
Pumpkin	½ slice	150
Sweet Potato	½ slice	176
Zucchini	½ slice	190
DIPS		
Banana Cream	1 serv (4.5 oz)	250
Banana Split	1 serv (4.5 oz)	290
Cherry Cream	1 serv (4.5 oz)	280
Coconut Cream	1 serv (4.5 oz)	300
Mud Pie	1 serv (4.5 oz)	380
Strawberry Cream	1 serv (4.5 oz)	270
FROZEN BARS		
Cream Banana	1	110
Cream Coconut	1	130
Cream Peaches 'n' Cream	1	150
Cream Pina Colada	1	90
Cream Raspberry Cream	1	110
Cream Strawberry Cream	1	110
Happy Indulgence Berry Cobbler	1	200
Happy Indulgence Key Lime Pie	1	220
Happy Indulgence Peach Cobbler	1	170
Juice Fuzzy Navel	1	70
Juice Green Tea Melon	1	90
Juice Guava	1	70
Juice Lemon	1	90
Juice Lime	1	80
Juice Passionate Cherry	1	80
Juice Pineapple	1	80
Juice Raspberry	1	70
Juice Strawberry	1	70
Juice Tamarind	1	90
Juice Tropical Splash	1	80
Juice Watermelon	1	60
Yogurt Blueberry	1	120
Yogurt Chocolate	1	160
Yogurt Vanilla	1	140
SMOOTHIES		
Berry Berry Best	1 (4 oz)	160
Make Mine Mango	4 oz	160
Strawberry Ana Banana	4 oz	120

FOOD	PORTION	CALS
SNACKS		
All About Almonds	1 pkg (1 oz)	170
Buzzworthy Banana	1 pkg (1.1 oz)	140
Calypso Cashews	1 pkg (1.1 oz)	170
Chocolate Twisted Bliss	1 pkg (1.4 oz)	190
Debbie Loves Fruit	1 pkg (1 oz)	110
Got Nuts?	1 pkg (1.1 oz)	180
Hit The Road Jack	1 pkg (1.1 oz)	130
Honey I Ate The Peanuts	1 pkg (1 oz)	160
Jamaican Me Crazy Cranberry Mix	1 pkg (1.1 oz)	100
Judy's Apple Crisps	1 pkg (1 oz)	140
Nacho Chips They're Mine	1 pkg (1.1 oz)	120
Nature Lover's Choice	1 pkg (1.1 oz)	140
Power Pistachios	1 pkg (1.1 oz)	100
Reggae Rice Crackers	1 pkg (1.1 oz)	120
Rockin' Raisins	1 pkg (1.4 oz)	170
Rocky Mountain Munch	1 pkg (1.1 oz)	120
Sour Wiggle Giggle	1 pkg (1.5 oz)	150
Soy Glad You're Healthy	1 pkg (1.1 oz)	160
Survivor Snacks	1 pkg (1.1 oz)	140
Swinging Sesame Stix	1 pkg (1.1 oz)	180
Tammy's Flax Snacks	1 pkg (1.1 oz)	170
Whassup Wasabi!	1 pkg (1.1 oz)	150
Yogurt Twisted Bliss	1 pkg (1.4 oz)	190
You've Got Trail	1 pkg (1.1 oz)	150
Yummy Gummy In My Tummy	1 pkg (1.4 oz)	150
Zydeco Cajun Mix	1 pkg (1.1 oz)	108
GODFATHER'S PIZZA		
Breadstick	1	80
Golden All Meat Combo	1 med slice	300
Golden Apple Dessert	⅙ sm	202
Golden Bacon Cheeseburger	1 med slice	270
Golden Cheese	1 med slice	220
Golden Cherry Dessert	⅙ sm	206
Golden Cinnamon Streusel	⅙ sm	226
Golden Combo	1 med slice	290
Golden Hawaiian	1 med slice	240
Golden Hot Stuff	1 med slice	290
Golden Humble Pie	1 med slice	310
Golden M&M Streusel Dessert	⅙ sm	249

FOOD	PORTION	CALS
Golden Pepperoni	1 med slice	260
Golden Super Combo	1 med slice	320
Golden Super Hawaiian	1 med slice	250
Golden Super Taco	1 med slice	330
Golden Taco	1 med slice	300
Golden Veggie	1 med slice	230
Monkey Bread	⅙	120
Original All Meat Combo	1 med slice	370
Original Bacon Cheeseburger	1 med slice	330
Original Cheese	1 med slice	260
Original Combo	1 med slice	350
Original Hawaiian	1 med slice	280
Original Hot Stuff	1 med slice	360
Original Humble Pie	1 med slice	380
Original Pepperoni	1 med slice	290
Original Super Combo	1 med slice	390
Original Super Hawaiian	1 med slice	280
Original Super Taco	1 med slice	390
Original Taco	1 med slice	360
Original Veggie	1 med slice	270
Potato Wedges	1 serv (4 oz)	192
Thin All Meat Combo	1 med slice	280
Thin Bacon Cheeseburger	1 med slice	250
Thin Cheese	1 med slice	180
Thin Combo	1 med slice	250
Thin Hawaiian	1 med slice	200
Thin Hot Stuff	1 med slice	270
Thin Humble Pie	1 med slice	270
Thin Pepperoni	1 med slice	220
Thin Super Combo	1 med slice	300
Thin Super Hawaiian	1 med slice	230
Thin Super Taco	1 med slice	310
Thin Taco	1 med slice	260
Thin Veggie	1 med slice	190

HARDEE'S
BEVERAGES

Barq's Root Beer	1 sm (20 oz)	290
Cherry Coke	1 sm (20 oz)	260
Coca-Cola	1 sm (20 oz)	260
Coffee Black	1 sm (12 oz)	5

FOOD	PORTION	CALS
Diet Coke	1 sm (20 oz)	0
Dr Pepper	1 sm (20 oz)	260
Hi-C Fruit Punch	1 sm (20 oz)	260
Hi-C Orange	1 sm (20 oz)	280
Lemonade Minute Maid	1 sm (20 oz)	250
Mello Yellow	1 sm (20 oz)	265
Milk 2%	1 (10 oz)	150
Orange Juice	1 serv (10 oz)	150
Shake Chocolate	1 (16 oz)	700
Shake Strawberry	1 (16 oz)	700
Shake Vanilla	1 (16 oz)	710
Sprite	1 sm	260
BREAKFAST SELECTIONS		
Big Country Breakfast Platter Bacon	1 serv	980
Big Country Breakfast Platter Breaded Pork Chop	1 serv	1220
Big Country Breakfast Platter Chicken	1 serv	1140
Big Country Breakfast Platter Country Ham	1 serv	970
Big Country Breakfast Platter Country Steak	1 serv	1150
Big Country Breakfast Platter Grilled Pork Chop	1 serv	1130
Big Country Breakfast Platter Sausage	1 serv	1060
Biscuit Bacon	1 serv	430
Biscuit Bacon Egg Cheese	1	560
Biscuit Breaded Pork Chop	1 serv	690
Biscuit Chicken Fillet	1 serv	600
Biscuit Cinnamon 'N' Raisin	1	280
Biscuit Country Ham	1	440
Biscuit Country Steak	1 serv	620
Biscuit Country Steak & Egg	1 serv	690
Biscuit Egg	1 serv	450
Biscuit Ham Egg Cheese	1	560
Biscuit Loaded Omelet	1 serv	640
Biscuit Made From Scratch	1	370
Biscuit 'N' Gravy	1	530
Biscuit Sausage	1	530
Biscuit Sausage Egg	1	610
Breakfast Bowl Loaded Biscuit 'N' Gravy	1 serv	770
Breakfast Bowl Low Carb	1 serv	620
Burrito Loaded Breakfast	1	780

FOOD	PORTION	CALS
Burrito Steak 'N' Egg Breakfast	1	470
Folded Egg	1 serv	80
Frisco Breakfast Sandwich	1	410
Grits	1 serv	110
Hash Rounds	1 sm	260
Loaded Omelet	1	270
Pancake Platter	1 serv	300
Scrambled Egg	1 serv	160
Sunrise Croissant	1	210
Sunrise Croissant w/ Bacon	1	450
Sunrise Croissant w/ Ham	1	430
Sunrise Croissant w/ Sausage	1	550
CHILDREN'S MENU SELECTIONS		
French Fries	1 serv	250
Kids Meal Cheeseburger	1 serv	600
Kids Meal Chicken Strips	1 serv	500
Kids Meal Hamburger	1 serv	560
DESSERTS		
Apple Turnover	1	290
Cone Single Scoop	1	285
Cookie Chocolate Chip	1	290
Ice Cream Bowl Single Scoop	1 serv	235
Peach Cobbler	1 serv	280
MAIN MENU SELECTIONS		
Burger Six Dollar	1	1060
Cheeseburger	1	680
Cheeseburger Double	1	510
Chicken Strips	3 pieces	380
Cole Slaw	1 serv	170
Crispy Curls	1 sm	340
French Fries	1 sm	390
Fried Chicken Breast	1 piece	370
Fried Chicken Leg	1 piece	170
Fried Chicken Thigh	1 piece	330
Fried Chicken Wing	1 piece	200
Grilled Onions	1 serv	35
Hamburger	1	310
Hamburger Double	1	420
Hot Dog	1	420
Hot Ham 'N' Cheese	1	420

FOOD	PORTION	CALS
Hot Ham 'N' Cheese Big	1	520
Mashed Potatoes	1 sm	90
Roast Beef Big	1	470
Roast Beef Regular	1	330
Sandwich Big Chicken Fillet	1	850
Sandwich Charbroiled Chicken Club	1	560
Sandwich Fish Supreme	1	500
Thickburger	1	850
Thickburger Bacon Cheese	1	910
Thickburger Double	1	1240
Thickburger Double Bacon Cheese	1	1300
Thickburger Low Carb	1	420
Thickburger Monster	1	1410
Thickburger Mushroom 'N Swiss	1	720
SAUCES AND SPREADS		
Au Jus Sauce	1 serv (3 oz)	10
Chicken Gravy	1 serv (1.5 oz)	20
Dipping Sauce BBQ	1 serv (0.5 oz)	15
Dipping Sauce Honey Mustard	1 serv (1 oz)	110
Dipping Sauce Ranch Dressing	1 serv (1 oz)	160
Dipping Sauce Sweet N Sour	1 serv (1 oz)	45
Gravy Biscuit	1 serv (5 oz)	160
Horseradish Sauce	1 pkg	25
Hot Sauce	1 pkg	0
Jam Grape	1 serv	10
Jam Strawberry	1 serv	35
Ketchup	1 pkg	10
Mayonnaise	1 pkg	90
Pancake Syrup	1 serv (1 oz)	90

HUNGRY HOWIE'S PIZZA
OTHER MENU SELECTIONS

Cajun Bread	¼ bread	300
Chicken Tenders	2	140
Cinnamon Bread	¼ bread	313
Howie Bread	¼ bread	300
Howie Wings	5	180
Sub Deluxe Italian	½ sub	506
Sub Ham & Cheese	½ sub	475
Sub Pizza	½ sub	689
Sub Pizza Special	½ sub	606

FOOD	PORTION	CALS
Sub Steak & Cheese	½ sub	491
Sub Turkey	½ sub	466
Sub Turkey Club	½ sub	556
Sub Vegetarian	½ sub	530
Three Cheeser Bread	¼ bread	370
PIZZA		
Cheese Slice	1 sm	161
Cheese Slice	1 med	191
Cheese Slice	1 lg	208
Cheese Slice	1 extra lg	395
Cheese Slice Thin	1 med	111
Cheese Slice Thin	1 lg	124
Medium Topping Anchovies	1 serv	44
Medium Topping Bacon	1 serv	32
Medium Topping Banana Peppers	1 serv	6
Medium Topping Beef	1 serv	30
Medium Topping Black Olives	1 serv	7
Medium Topping Ham	1 serv	7
Medium Topping Mushrooms	1 serv	2
Medium Topping Pepperoni	1 serv	22
Medium Topping Pineapple	1 serv	5
Medium Topping Sausage	1 serv	27
SALAD DRESSINGS AND SAUCES		
Dressing Blue Cheese	1 serv (1 oz)	150
Dressing Creamy Italian	1 serv (1 oz)	120
Dressing Fat Free Italian	1 serv (1.5 oz)	25
Dressing Fat Free Ranch	1 serv (1.5 oz)	45
Dressing French Style	1 serv (1 oz)	30
Dressing Greek	1 serv (1 oz)	110
Dressing Italian	1 serv (1 oz)	80
Dressing Ranch	1 serv (1 oz)	180
Dressing Thousand Island	1 serv (1 oz)	140
Sauce Dipping	1 serv (3 oz)	45
SALADS		
Antipasto	1 sm	115
Chef	1 sm	114
Garden	1 sm	20
Greek	1 sm	126

FOOD	PORTION	CALS
IN-N-OUT BURGER		
BEVERAGES		
Coca-Cola	1 (16 oz)	198
Coffee Black	1 (10 oz)	5
Diet Coke	1 (16 oz)	0
Dr Pepper	1 (16 oz)	180
Iced Tea	1 (16 oz)	0
Lemonade	1 (16 oz)	180
Milk	1 (10 oz)	108
Root Beer	1 (16 oz)	222
Seven Up	1 (16 oz)	200
Shake Chocolate	1 (15 oz)	690
Shake Strawberry	1 (15 oz)	690
Shake Vanilla	1 (15 oz)	680
MAIN MENU SELECTIONS		
Cheeseburger w/ Onions	1	480
Cheeseburger w/ Onions Lettuce Bun	1	330
Cheeseburger w/ Onions Mustard Ketchup No Spread	1	400
French Fries	1 serv (4.4 oz)	400
Hamburger Double Double w/ Onions	1	670
Hamburger Double Double w/ Onions Lettuce Bun	1	520
Hamburger Double Double w/ Onions Mustard Ketchup No Spread	1	590
Hamburger w/ Onions	1	390
Hamburger w/ Onions Lettuce Bun	1	240
Hamburger w/ Onions Mustard Ketchup No Spread	1	310
IVAR'S SEAFOOD BARS		
Chicken	3 pieces (4.5 oz)	250
Chowder Salmon	1 cup	220
Chowder White	1 cup	330
Clams	1 serv (5 oz)	400
Cocktail Sauce	¼ cup	50
Fish	3 pieces	220
French Fries	1 serv (3.5 oz)	300
Oysters	5	290
Prawns	1 serv (5 oz)	290
Salmon Fried	3 pieces (4.5 oz)	210

FOOD	PORTION	CALS
Scallops	1 serv (5 oz)	240
Tartar Sauce	2 tbsp	140

JACK IN THE BOX
BEVERAGES

FOOD	PORTION	CALS
Barq's Root Beer	1 (20 oz)	180
Chocolate Milk Low Fat Chug	1 (3.5 oz)	200
Coca-Cola Classic	1 (20 oz)	170
Coffee Regular & Decaf	1 (11 oz)	5
Diet Coke	1 (20 oz)	0
Dr Pepper	1 (20 oz)	150
Fanta Orange	1 (20 oz)	150
Fanta Strawberry	1 (20 oz)	150
Iced Tea	1 (20 oz)	5
Lemonade	1 (20 oz)	160
Orange Juice	1 (10 oz)	140
Reduced Fat Milk Chug	1 (3.5 oz)	130
Shake Chocolate	1 (16 oz)	880
Shake Oreo	1 (16 oz)	910
Shake Strawberry	1 (16 oz)	880
Shake Vanilla	1 (16 oz)	790
Sprite	1 (20 oz)	160

BREAKFAST SELECTIONS

FOOD	PORTION	CALS
Biscuit Bacon Egg Cheese	1	430
Biscuit Chicken	1	450
Biscuit Sausage	1	440
Biscuit Sausage Egg Cheese	1	740
Biscuit Spicy Chicken	1	460
Breakfast Jack	1	290
Breakfast Jack Bacon	1	300
Breakfast Jack Sausage	1	450
Breakfast Sandwich Ciabatta	1	710
Breakfast Sandwich Ultimate	1	570
Burrito Hearty Breakfast	1	480
Burrito Sirloin Steak & Egg w/o Salsa	1	790
Croissant Sausage	1	580
Croissant Supreme	1	450
French Toast Sticks	4 (4.2 oz)	470
French Toast Sticks Blueberry	4	450
Hash Browns	1 serv	150
Sandwich Extreme Sausage	1	670

FOOD	PORTION	CALS
DESSERTS		
Cake Chocolate Overload	1 serv (3.2 oz)	300
Cheesecake	1 serv (3.6 oz)	310
MAIN MENU SELECTIONS		
Bacon Cheddar Potato Wedges	1 serv (9 oz)	720
Cheeseburger Bacon Ultimate	1	1090
Cheeseburger Junior Bacon	1	430
Cheeseburger Sourdough Ultimate	1	950
Cheeseburger Ultimate	1	1010
Chicken Fajita Pita	1	280
Chicken Sandwich	1	400
Chicken Strips Crispy	4	500
Chicken Strips Grilled	4 (5 oz)	180
Ciabatta Burger Bacon 'N Cheese	1	1120
Ciabatta Burger Single Bacon 'N' Cheese	1	870
Ciabatta Chipotle w/ Grilled Chicken	1	690
Ciabatta Chipotle w/ Spicy Crispy Chicken	1	750
Ciabatta Sirloin Steak 'N' Cheddar	1	770
Club Sourdough Grilled Chicken	1	530
Curly Fries Seasoned	1 sm (3 oz)	270
Dipping Sauce Barbeque	1 serv (1 oz)	45
Egg Rolls	1	130
Fish & Chips	1 serv (7.6 oz)	570
Fries Natural Cut	1 sm	340
Fruit Cup	1 serv	90
Hamburger	1	310
Hamburger Deluxe	1	370
Hamburger Deluxe w/ Cheese	1	460
Hamburger w/ Cheese	1	350
Jack's Spicy Chicken	1 serv	620
Jack's Spicy Chicken w/ Cheese	1	700
Jumbo Jack	1	600
Jumbo Jack w/ Cheese	1	690
Mozzarella Cheese Sticks	3	240
Onion Rings	8 (4.2 oz)	500
Sampler Trio	1 serv	750
Sandwich Bacon Chicken	1	440
Sirloin Burger w/ American Cheese & Red Onion	1	1120
Sirloin Burger w/ Swiss & Grilled Onions	1	1070

FOOD	PORTION	CALS
Sirloin Steak Melt	1	640
Sourdough Jack	1	710
Spicy Chicken Bites	1 serv	290
Stuffed Jalapeno	3 (2.5 oz)	230
Taco Monster Beef	1	240
Taco Regular Beef	1	160
SALAD DRESSINGS AND TOPPINGS		
Asian Sesame	1 serv (2.5 oz)	230
Dipping Sauce Buttermilk House	1 serv (0.9 oz)	130
Dipping Sauce Frank's Red Hot Buffalo	1 serv (1 oz)	10
Dipping Sauce Sweet & Sour	1 serv (1 oz)	45
Dipping Sauce Teriyaki	1 serv (1 oz)	60
Dipping Sauce Zesty Marinara	1 serv (0.8 oz)	15
Dressing Bacon Ranch	1 serv (2.5 oz)	320
Dressing Creamy Southwest	1 serv (2.5 oz)	270
Low Fat Balsamic	1 serv (2.5 oz)	40
Mayo Onion Sauce	1 serv (0.5 oz)	90
Ranch	1 serv (2.5 oz)	390
Ranch Lite	1 serv (2.5 oz)	190
Soy Sauce	1 serv (0.3 oz)	5
Syrup Log Cabin	1 serv (2 oz)	190
Taco Sauce	1 serv (0.3 oz)	0
Tartar Sauce	1 serv (1.5 oz)	210
SALADS		
Asian w/ Crispy Chicken w/o Dressing	1 (13.8 oz)	330
Asian w/ Grilled Chicken w/o Dressing	1 (12.8 oz)	160
Chicken Club w/ Crispy Chicken w/o Dressing	1 (14 oz)	480
Chicken Club w/ Grilled Chicken w/o Dressing	1 (13 oz)	320
Side w/o Dressing	1 (4.3 oz)	50
Southwest Chicken w/ Crispy Chicken w/o Dressing	1 (16 oz)	480
Southwest w/ Grilled Chicken w/o Dressing	1 (15 oz)	320
JAMBA JUICE		
Acai Supercharger Original	1 (24 oz)	420
Aloha Pineapple Original	1 (26 oz)	500
Banana Berry Original	1 (25 oz)	480
Berry Fulfilling Original	1 (24 oz)	290
Berry Lime Sublime Original	1 (26 oz)	460
Caribbean Passion Original	1 (26 oz)	440
Chocolate Moo'd Original	1 (24 oz)	680

FOOD	PORTION	CALS
Citrus Squeeze Original	1 (26 oz)	470
Coldbuster Original	1 (25 oz)	430
Grape Escape Original	1 (24 oz)	300
Mango Mantra Original	1 (25 oz)	310
Mango-A-Go-Go Original	1 (24 oz)	440
Matcha Green Tea Blast Original	1 (24 oz)	440
Matcha Green Tea Mist Original	1 (24 oz)	280
Mega Mango Original	1 (24 oz)	330
Mighty Cherry Charger Original	1 (24 oz)	490
Orange-A-Peel Original	1 (25 oz)	440
Orange Berry Blitz Original	1 (26 oz)	410
Orange Dream Machine Original	1 (24 oz)	540
Passion Berry Breeze Original	1 (24 oz)	270
Peach Pleasure Original	1 (25 oz)	460
Peanut Butter Moo'd Original	1 (24 oz)	840
Peenya Kowlada Original	1 (26 oz)	690
Protein Berry Pizazz Original	1 (24 oz)	440
Raspberry Rainbow Original	1 (24 oz)	300
Razzmatazz Original	1 (26 oz)	480
Strawberries Wild Original	1 (25 oz)	450
Strawberry Nirvana Original	1 (25 oz)	280
Strawberry Surf Rider Original	1 (25 oz)	490
Strawberry Whirl Original	1 (24 oz)	310

JIMMY JOHN'S
BEVERAGES

Coke	1 sm	248
Diet Coke	1 sm	0
Iced Tea	1 sm	3
Iced Tea Raspberry	1 sm	195
Lemonade	1 sm	243
Lemonade Light	1 sm	13
Sprite	1 sm	243

SANDWICHES

Giant Club Beach	1	798
Giant Club Billy	1	867
Giant Club Bootlegger	1	720
Giant Club Country	1	840
Giant Club Gourmet Smoked Ham	1	851
Giant Club Gourmet Veggie	1	856
Giant Club Hunter's	1	854

FOOD	PORTION	CALS
Giant Club Italian Night	1	975
Giant Club Lulu	1	790
Giant Club Tuna	1	719
Giant Club Ultimate Porker	1	843
Slim Double Provolone	1	588
Slim Ham & Cheese	1	534
Slim Salami Capicola Cheese	1	624
Slim Tuna Salad	1	577
Slim Turkey Breast	1	407
Sub Big John	1	564
Sub J.J.B.L.T.	1	662
Sub Pepe	1	684
Sub Totally Tuna	1	502
Sub Turkey Tom	1	555
Sub Vegetarian	1	640
Sub Vito	1	579
The J.J. Gargantuan	1	1008
Unwich Hunter's Club	1	520
Unwich The J.J. Gargantuan	1	769
SIDES		
Cookie Chocolate Chunk	1	421
Cookie Raisin Oatmeal	1	421
Jimmy Chips	1 pkg	160
Jimmy Chips BBQ	1 pkg	160
Jimmy Chips Jalapeno	1 pkg	150
Jimmy Chips Sea Salt & Vinegar	1 pkg	140
Pickle Spear	1	4
Pickle Whole	1	15

KENTUCKY FRIED CHICKEN
BEVERAGES

FOOD	PORTION	CALS
Diet Pepsi	1 med (14 oz)	0
Mt. Dew	1 med (14 oz)	190
Pepsi	1 med (14 oz)	180
DESSERTS		
Cake Double Chocolate Chip	1 slice	330
Cookie Sweet Life Chocolate Chip	1 (1.2 oz)	160
Cookie Sweet Life Oatmeal Raisin	1 (1.2 oz)	150
Cookie Sweet Life Sugar	1 (1.2 oz)	160
Little Bucket Chocolate Cream	1	280
Little Bucket Lemon Creme	1 serv	410

FOOD	PORTION	CALS
Little Bucket Strawberry Short Cake	1 serv	210
Pie Mini's Apple	3 (4 oz)	370
Teddy Graham Cinnamon Snacks	1 serv	90
MAIN MENU SELECTIONS		
Baked Beans	1 serv	220
Biscuit	1 (2 oz)	220
Bowl Chicken & Biscuit	1	870
Bowl Mashed Potato w/ Gravy	1	740
Bowl Rice w/ Gravy	1	620
Chicken Pot Pie	1 (15 oz)	770
Cole Slaw	1 serv	180
Corn On The Cob	1 ear (3 inch)	70
Crispy Strips	2 (3.5 oz)	240
Extra Crispy Breast	1 (5.7 oz)	440
Extra Crispy Drumstick	1 (2 oz)	160
Extra Crispy Thigh	1 (4 oz)	370
Extra Crispy Whole Wing	1 (1.8 oz)	170
Green Beans	1 serv	50
KFC Snacker	1	290
KFC Snacker Buffalo	1	260
KFC Snacker Fish	1	330
KFC Snacker Fish w/o Sauce	1	290
KFC Snacker Honey BBQ	1	210
KFC Snacker Ultimate Cheese	1	280
Macaroni & Cheese	1 serv	180
Mashed Potatoes w/ Gravy	1 serv	140
Mashed Potatoes w/o Gravy	1 serv	110
Original Breast	1 (5.6 oz)	360
Original Recipe Breast	1 (5.6 oz)	360
Original Recipe Breast w/o Skin or Breading	1 (3.8 oz)	140
Original Recipe Drumstick	1 (2 oz)	130
Original Recipe Thigh	1 (4.4 oz)	330
Original Recipe Whole Wing	1 (1.6 oz)	130
Popcorn Chicken	1 reg (4 oz)	400
Potato Salad	1 serv	180
Potato Wedges	1 serv	260
Sandwich Crispy Twister	1	550
Sandwich Double Crunch	1	470
Sandwich Honey BBQ	1	280
Sandwich Tender Roast	1	380

FOOD	PORTION	CALS
Sandwich Tender Roast w/o Sauce	1	300
Seasoned Rice	1 serv	180
Twister Oven Roasted	1	420
Twister Oven Roasted w/o Sauce	1	330
Wings Fiery Buffalo	5	380
Wings Honey BBQ	5	390
Wings Hot	5	350
Wings Hot & Spicy	5	400
Wings Teriyaki	5	480
Wings Boneless Fiery Buffalo	5	420
Wings Boneless Honey BBQ	5	450
Wings Boneless Sweet & Spicy	5	440
Wings Boneless Teriyaki	5	500
SALAD DRESSINGS		
Creamy Parmesan Caesar	1 serv (2 oz)	260
Golden Italian Light	1 serv (1.5 oz)	45
Ranch	1 serv (2 oz)	200
Ranch Fat Free	1 serv (1.5 oz)	35
SALADS		
Crispy BLT w/o Dressing	1 (12 oz)	330
Crispy Caesar w/o Dressing & Croutons	1 (11 oz)	350
Croutons Parmesan Garlic	1 pkg	60
Roasted BLT w/o Dressing	1 (12 oz)	200
Roasted Caesar w/o Dressing & Croutons	1 (11 oz)	220
Side Caesar w/o Dressing & Croutons	1 (3 oz)	50
Side House w/o Dressing	1 (3 oz)	15

KOO-KOO-ROO
MAIN MENU SELECTIONS

FOOD	PORTION	CALS
Baked Yam	1 serv (6 oz)	197
Black Beans	1 serv (6 oz)	125
Buffalo Wings	6	606
Burrito California Chicken	1	810
Burrito Fajita Chicken	1	750
Burrito Original Chicken	1	709
Butternut Squash	1 serv (6 oz)	66
Chicken Bowl Chargrilled w/o Sauce	1	569
Chicken Bowl Spicy Garlic Ginger w/o Sauce	1	485
Original Breast	1 (4.1 oz)	187
Original Chicken Dark	3 pieces (5 oz)	320
Rotisserie Chicken Breast & Wing	1 serv (6.5 oz)	355

FOOD	PORTION	CALS
Rotisserie Chicken Leg & Thigh	1 serv (4.8 oz)	300
Rotisserie Half Chicken	1 serv (11.3 oz)	655
Sandwich BBQ Chicken	1	562
Sandwich Chicken Caesar	1	781
Sandwich Original Chicken	1	661
Sandwich Turkey Hand Carved	1	599
Southwestern Bowl w/o Sauce	1	570
Tostada Bowl w/o Sauce w/o Shell	1	528
Traditional Turkey Dinner	1 serv	692
Turkey Breast Sliced	1 serv	182
Turkey Pot Pie	1	883
Wrap Caesar Chicken	1	757
Wrap Chipotle Chicken	1	924
SALADS		
BBQ Chicken w/o Dressing	1	365
Cantaloupe & Honeydew	1 serv (5 oz)	50
Chicken Caesar w/o Dressing	1	286
Chinese Chicken w/o Dressing	1	550
Creamy Coleslaw	1 serv (5 oz)	238
Cucumber	1 serv (4.5 oz)	41
House	1	113
Tangy Tomato	1 serv (4.5 oz)	60
Tossed w/ Dressing	1 serv (3 oz)	16
SOUPS		
Chicken Noodle	1 serv (5 oz)	71
Chicken Tortilla	1 serv (5 oz)	112
Ten Vegetable	1 serv (5 oz)	94

KRISPY KREME
BEVERAGES

FOOD	PORTION	CALS
Chillers Fruity Orange You Glad	1 (12 oz)	180
Chillers Fruity Very Berry	1 (12 oz)	170
Chillers Kremey Berries & Kreme	1 (12 oz)	620
Chillers Kremey Chocolate Chocolate	1 (12 oz)	970
Chillers Kremey Lemon Sherbert	1 (12 oz)	630
Chillers Kremey Lotta Latte	1 (12 oz)	670
Chillers Kremey Mocha Dream	1 (12 oz)	670
Chillers Kremey Oranges & Kreme	1 (12 oz)	630
DOUGHNUTS		
Apple Fritter	1	380
Caramel Kreme Crunch	1	380

FOOD	PORTION	CALS
Chocolate Iced w/ Sprinkles	1	270
Chocolate Iced Cake	1	280
Chocolate Iced Custard Filled	1	300
Chocolate Iced Glazed	1	250
Chocolate Iced Kreme Filled	1	350
Cinnamon Apple Filled	1	290
Cinnamon Bun	1	260
Cinnamon Twist	1	240
Dulce De Leche	1	300
Glazed Creme Filled	1	340
Glazed Lemon Filled	1	290
Glazed Raspberry Filled	1	300
Glazed Chocolate Cake	1	300
Glazed Cinnamon	1	210
Glazed Sour Cream	1	300
Glazed Cruller	1	240
Glazed Cruller Chocolate	1	290
Glazed Pumpkin Spice	1	300
Holes Glazed Blueberry	4	220
Holes Glazed Cake	4	210
Holes Glazed Chocolate Cake	4	210
Holes Glazed Original	4	200
Holes Glazed Pumpkin Spice	4	210
Maple Iced Glazed	1	240
New York Cheesecake	1	340
Original Glazed	1	200
Powdered Cake	1	290
Powdered Strawberry Filled	1	290
Sugar	1	200
Traditional Cake	1	230

KRYSTAL
BEVERAGES

Coca-Cola Classic	1 sm (16 oz)	129
Coco-Cola Classic frzn	1 (16 oz)	130
Diet Coke	1 sm (16 oz)	tr
Sprite	1 sm (16 oz)	126

BREAKFAST SELECTIONS

4 Carb Scrambler Bacon	1 serv	370
4 Carb Scrambler Sausage	1 serv	600
Biscuit Bacon Egg Cheese	1	390

FOOD	PORTION	CALS
Biscuit Chik	1	360
Biscuit Sausage	1	480
Biscuit & Gravy	1	280
Biscuit Plain	1	270
Country Breakfast	1 serv	660
Kryspers	1 serv	190
Krystal Sunriser	1	240
Scrambler	1 serv	440
DESSERTS		
Fried Apple Turnover	1	220
Lemon Icebox Pie	1 serv	260
MAIN MENU SELECTIONS		
BA Burger	1	470
BA Burger Cheese	1	530
BA Burger Double Bacon Cheese	1	800
Chik'n Bites	1 sm	310
Chik'n Bites Salad	1 serv	290
Fries	1 reg	470
Fries Chili Cheese	1 serv	540
Krystal	1	160
Krystal Bacon Cheese	1	190
Krystal Cheese	1	180
Krystal Chik	1	240
Krystal Chili	1 serv	200
Krystal Double	1	260
Krystal Double Cheese	1	310
Pup Chili Cheese	1	210
Pup Corn	1	260
Pup Plain	1	170

LONG JOHN SILVER'S
BEVERAGES

Coca-Cola	1 sm	150
Diet Coke	1 sm	0
Sprite	1 sm	140
DESSERTS		
Pie Chocolate Cream	1 pie	310
Pie Pecan	1 pie	370
Pie Pineapple Cream	1 pie	290
MAIN MENU SELECTIONS		
Baked Cod	1 piece	120

FOOD	PORTION	CALS
Battered Chicken	1 piece	140
Battered Fish	1 piece	230
Battered Shrimp	1 piece	45
Breaded Clams	1 serv	240
Cheesesticks	3 pieces	140
Clam Chowder	1 bowl	220
Corn Cobbette	1 piece	90
Crumblies	1 serv	170
Crunchy Shrimp	21 pieces	330
Fries	1 reg	230
Hushpuppy	1 piece	60
Rice	1 serv	180
Sandwich Chicken	1	360
Sandwich Fish	1	440
Sandwich Ultimate Fish	1	500
Slaw	1 serv	200

MARBLE SLAB CREAMERY

FOOD	PORTION	CALS
Cone Honey Wheat	1	130
Cone Sugar	1	130
Cone Vanilla Cinnamon	1	130
Frozen Yogurt Nonfat	½ cup	100
Frozen Yogurt Nonfat No Sugar Added	½ cup	90
Ice Cream Reduced Fat	1 serv (6.75 oz)	390
Ice Cream Superpremium	1 serv (6.75 oz)	450
Sorbet	½ cup	90

MAUI WOWI
SMOOTHIES

FOOD	PORTION	CALS
Fresh Fruit Banana Banana	1 (12 oz)	210
Fresh Fruit Black Raspberry	1 (12 oz)	240
Fresh Fruit Kiwi Lemon Lime	1 (12 oz)	180
Fresh Fruit Lemon Wave	1 (12 oz)	415
Fresh Fruit Mango Orange Banana	1 (12 oz)	240
Fresh Fruit Passion Papaya	1 (12 oz)	220
Fresh Fruit Pina Colada	1 (12 oz)	240

MAX & ERMA'S

FOOD	PORTION	CALS
Black Bean Roll Up	1 serv	577
Caribbean Chicken Lunch Portion	1 serv	536
Fruit Smoothie	1	124
Garlic Breadstick	1	156

FOOD	PORTION	CALS
Hula Bowl w/ Fat Free Honey Mustard Dressing w/o Breadsticks	1 serv	823
Salad Baby Greens w/o Breadstick	1 serv	119
Salad Shrimp Stack	1 serv	322
Salad Dressing Bleu Cheese	2 tbsp	201
Salad Dressing French Fat Free	2 tbsp	126
Salad Dressing Honey Mustard Fat Free	2 tbsp	60
Salad Dressing Italian	2 tbsp	110
Salad Dressing Ranch	2 tbsp	120
Salad Dressing Tex Mex Low Fat	2 tbsp	23

MCALISTER'S DELI
CHILDREN'S MENU SELECTIONS

FOOD	PORTION	CALS
Kid's Nacho	1 serv	734
Mac's Dog	1	307
Pita Pizza	1	503
Sandwich Ham & Cheese	1	455
Sandwich PB&J	1	714
Sandwich Toasted Cheese	1	620
Sandwich Turkey & Cheese	1	451

DESSERTS

FOOD	PORTION	CALS
Brownie Chocolate	1 (3.5 oz)	424
Brownie Delight	1 (11 oz)	917
Chocolate Loving Spoon Cake	1 (4 oz)	538
Ice Cream Vanilla Bean	1 scoop (5 oz)	160
Kentucky Pie	1 slice (12 oz)	807
New York Cheesecake	1 slice (5 oz)	505
Sundae Topping Caramel	2 tbsp	100
Sundae Topping Chocolate	1 tbsp	110

MAIN MENU SELECTIONS

FOOD	PORTION	CALS
Appetizers Chips & Salsa	1 serv (5 oz)	87
Appetizers Dip Cheese & Chili	1 serv (5 oz)	572
Appetizers Dip Cheese & Veggie Chili	1 serv (5 oz)	552
Appetizers Nacho Basket	1 serv (6 oz)	579
Appetizers Nacho Chili	1 serv (6 oz)	564
Appetizers Nacho Veggie Chili	1 serv (6 oz)	537
Chicken Cordon Bleu	1 serv	810
Chili Vegetarian	1 serv (8 oz)	133
Cole Slaw	1 serv (4 oz)	190
Fruit Cup	1 serv (4 oz)	98
Giant Spud Cheese	1 (27 oz)	930

FOOD	PORTION	CALS
Giant Spud Grilled Chicken	1 (27 oz)	839
Giant Spud Just A Spud	1 (26 oz)	604
Giant Spud Ole	1 (30 oz)	1252
Giant Spud Ole w/ Chili	1 (33 oz)	1512
Giant Spud Ole w/ Veggie Chili	1 (33 oz)	1457
Giant Spud Veggie	1 (28 oz)	668
Macaroni & Cheese	1 serv (4 oz)	200
Mashed Potatoes	1 serv (4 oz)	136
Meatloaf w/ Gravy	1 serv	340
Open-Faced Roast Beef	1 serv	751
Pot Roast Spud	1 serv	906
Potato Salad	1 serv (4 oz)	200
Salmon Filet	1 serv	235
Steamed Vegetables	1 serv (4 oz)	43
SALAD DRESSINGS AND SAUCES		
Au Jus	1 serv (4 oz)	10
Comeback Gravy	1 serv (4 oz)	37
Dressing Bleu Cheese	2 tbsp	140
Dressing Greek	2 tbsp	90
Dressing Parmesan Peppercorn	2 tbsp	150
Dressing Ranch	2 tbsp	100
Dressing Tomato Basil	2 tbsp	30
Dressing Lite Olive Oil Vinaigrette	2 tbsp	60
Dressing Lite Ranch	2 tbsp	100
Dressing Low Calorie Italian	2 tbsp	25
SALADS		
Caesar w/ Salmon	1 (17 oz)	800
Chicken Fiesta	1 (20 oz)	493
Chicken Grill	1 (21 oz)	840
Garden	1 (15 oz)	264
Garden w/ Chicken Salad	1 (18 oz)	537
Garden w/ Salmon	1 (17 oz)	315
Garden w/ Tuna Salad	1 (18 oz)	373
Greek Chicken	1 (19 oz)	584
Side Caesar	1 (6 oz)	328
Side Garden	1 (8 oz)	138
Taco	1 (26 oz)	641
Taco w/ Veggie Chili	1 (26 oz)	641
SANDWICHES		
BLT	1	654

FOOD	PORTION	CALS
Chicken Salad	1	677
Deli Corned Beef On Wheat	1	369
Deli Ham On Wheat	1	350
Deli Pastrami On Wheat	1	371
Deli Roast Beef On Wheat	1	398
Deli Salami On Wheat	1	565
Deli Turkey On Wheat	1	342
French Dip	1	676
Grilled Chicken Breast	1	751
Grilled Chicken Club	1	1234
Ham Melt	1	700
McAlister's Club	1	1225
Meatloaf Parmesan	1	708
Memphian	1	585
Muffuletta	¼ (8 oz)	615
New Yorker	1	628
Orange Cranberry Club	1	954
Reuben On Rye	1	492
Roast Beef Melt	1	635
Salmon	1	608
Submarine	1	833
Sweetberry Chicken On Wheatberry	1	701
Tuna Salad On Wheat	1	452
Turkey Melt	1	700
Veggie On Pita	1	522
Wrap Greek Chicken	1	630
Wrap Grill Chicken Caesar	1	533
SOUPS		
Asiago Cheese Bisque	1 (8 oz)	240
Broccoli Cheddar	1 (8 oz)	213
Cheddar Potato	1 (8 oz)	213
Cheesy Chicken Tortilla	1 (8 oz)	150
Chicken & Sausage Gumbo	1 (8 oz)	150
Clam Chowder	1 (8 oz)	200
Country Potato	1 (8 oz)	173
Country Vegetable	1 (8 oz)	93
French Onion	1 (8 oz)	80
Red Beans & Rice	1 (8 oz)	107
Southwest Roasted Corn	1 (8 oz)	90

FOOD	PORTION	CALS
MCDONALD'S		
BEVERAGES		
Apple Juice	1 box (6.8 oz)	90
Chocolate Milk 1% Low Fat	8 oz	170
Coca-Cola Classic	1 sm (16 oz)	150
Coffee	1 sm (12 oz)	0
Diet Coke	1 sm (16 oz)	0
Half & Half Creamer	1 pkg	20
Hi-C Orange Lavaburst	1 sm (16 oz)	160
Iced Coffee Caramel	1 sm (16 oz)	130
Iced Coffee Hazelnut	1 sm (16 oz)	130
Iced Coffee Regular	1 sm (16 oz)	140
Iced Coffee Vanilla	1 sm (16 oz)	130
Iced Tea	1 sm (16 oz)	0
Milk 1% Low Fat	1 pkg	100
Orange Juice	1 sm (12 oz)	140
Powerade Mountain Blast	1 sm (16 oz)	100
Shake Triple Thick Chocolate	1 sm (12 oz)	440
Shake Triple Thick Strawberry	1 sm (12 oz)	420
Shake Triple Thick Vanilla	1 sm (16 oz)	420
Sprite	1 sm (16 oz)	150
BREAKFAST SELECTIONS		
Big Breakfast Regular Biscuit	1 serv	720
Biscuit	1 reg	250
Biscuit Regular Bacon Egg Cheese	1	450
Biscuit Regular Sausage	1	410
Biscuit Regular Sausage w/ Egg	1	500
Burrito Sausage	1	300
Deluxe Breakfast Regular Biscuit w/o Syrup & Margarine	1 serv	1070
English Muffin	1	160
Hash Browns	1 serv	140
Hotcake Syrup	1 pkg (2 oz)	180
Hotcakes & Sausage w/o Syrup & Margarine	1 serv	520
Hotcakes w/o Syrup & Margarine	1 serv	350
McGriddles Bacon Egg Cheese	1	460
McGriddles Sausage	1	420
McGriddles Sausage Egg Cheese	1	560
McMuffin Sausage	1	370
McMuffin Sausage w/ Egg	1	250

FOOD	PORTION	CALS
McSkillet Burrito w/ Sausage	1	610
McSkillet Burrito w/ Steak	1	570
Sausage Patty	1	170
Scrambled Eggs	2	170
DESSERTS		
Apple Dippers	1 pkg	35
Apple Pie Baked	1	270
Caramel Dip Low Fat	1 pkg	70
Cinnamon Melts	1 serv	460
Cookie Chocolate Chip	1	180
Cookie Oatmeal	1 (1.1 oz)	150
Cookie Sugar	1 (1.1 oz)	150
Cookies McDonaldland	1 pkg (2 oz)	250
Cookies McDonaldland Chocolate Chip	1 pkg	270
Fruit 'n Yogurt Parfait	1 serv	160
Ice Cream Cone Reduced Fat Vanilla	1	150
Kiddie Cone	1	45
McFlurry Oreo	1 (12 oz)	560
McFlurry w/ M&M's	1 (12 oz)	620
Peanuts For Sundae	1 serv	45
Sundae Hot Caramel	1	340
Sundae Hot Fudge	1	330
Sundae Strawberry	1	280
MAIN MENU SELECTIONS		
Apple Sauce Strawberry	1 serv	90
Big Mac	1	540
Big N' Tasty	1	460
Big N' Tasty w/ Cheese	1	510
Cheeseburger	1	300
Cheeseburger Double	1	440
Cheesy Tots	6 pieces	210
Chicken McNuggets	4 pieces	170
Chicken Selects	3 pieces	380
Filet-O-Fish	1	380
French Fries	1 sm	250
French Fries	1 lg	570
Hamburger	1	250
McChicken	1	360
McRib	1	500
Onion Rings	1 sm	140

FOOD	PORTION	CALS
Quarter Pounder	1	410
Quarter Pounder Double w/ Cheese	1	740
Quarter Pounder w/ Cheese	1	510
Sandwich Chicken Classic Crispy	1	500
Sandwich Chicken Classic Grilled	1	420
Sandwich Club Chicken Crispy	1	660
Sandwich Club Chicken Grilled	1	570
Sandwich Ranch BLT Chicken Crispy	1	600
Sandwich Ranch BLT Chicken Grilled	1	520
Snack Wrap Grilled w/ Chipotle BBQ	1	260
Snack Wrap Grilled w/ Honey Mustard	1	260
Snack Wrap Grilled w/ Ranch	1	270
Snack Wrap w/ Chipotle BBQ	1	320
Snack Wrap w/ Honey Mustard	1	320
Snack Wrap w/ Ranch	1	140
SALAD DRESSINGS AND SAUCES		
Dipping Sauce Buffalo	1 serv (1 oz)	80
Dipping Sauce Zesty Onion Ring	1 serv (1 oz)	150
Dressing Ken's Light Italian	1 pkg (2 oz)	120
Dressing Newman's Own Creamy Caesar	1 pkg (2 oz)	170
Dressing Newman's Own Creamy Southwest	1 pkg (1.5 oz)	100
Dressing Newman's Own Low Fat Balsamic Vinaigrette	1 pkg (1.5 oz)	40
Dressing Newman's Own Low Fat Family Recipe Italian	1 pkg (1.5 oz)	60
Dressing Newman's Own Low Fat Sesame Ginger	1 pkg (1.5 oz)	90
Dressing Newman's Own Ranch	1 pkg (2 oz)	170
Honey	1 pkg (0.5 oz)	50
Ketchup	1 pkg	15
Sauce Barbecue	1 pkg (1 oz)	50
Sauce Creamy Ranch	1 pkg (1.5 oz)	200
Sauce Hot Mustard	1 pkg (1 oz)	60
Sauce Southwestern Chipotle Barbeque	1 pkg (1.5 oz)	70
Sauce Spicy Buffalo	1 pkg (1.5 oz)	60
Sauce Sweet'N Sour	1 pkg (1 oz)	50
Sauce Tangy Honey Mustard	1 pkg (1.5 oz)	70
SALADS		
Asian w/ Crispy Chicken w/o Dressing	1 serv	380
Asian w/ Grilled Chicken w/o Dressing	1 serv	300

FOOD	PORTION	CALS
Asian w/o Chicken & Dressing	1 serv	150
Bacon Ranch w/ Crispy Chicken	1 serv	350
Bacon Ranch w/ Grilled Chicken w/o Dressing	1 serv	260
Bacon Ranch w/o Chicken	1 serv	140
Caesar w/ Crispy Chicken	1 serv	300
Caesar w/ Grilled Chicken	1 serv	220
Caesar w/o Chicken	1 serv	90
Croutons Butter Garlic	1 pkg	60
Fruit & Walnut Snack Size	1 serv	210
Side Salad	1 serv	20
Southwest w/ Crispy Chicken w/o Dressing	1 serv	400
Southwest w/ Grilled Chicken	1 serv	320
Southwest w/o Chicken & Dressing	1 serv	140

MIMIS CAFE
BEVERAGES

Cappuccino	1 serv	86
Cappuccino Iced	1 serv	86
Espresso	1 serv	8
Hot Chocolate w/ Whipped Cream	1 serv	986
Mocha Iced	1 serv	376
Mocha Latte	1 serv	376

CHILDREN'S MENU SELECTIONS

Chicken Fingers	1 serv	408
Grilled Cheese	1 serv	273
Macaroni & Cheese	1 serv	353
Mini Burger	1 serv	554
Mini Corn Dogs	1 serv	460
Pancakes Chocolate Chip	1 serv	563
Pancakes Mimi Mouse	1 serv	477
PB&J Soldiers	1 serv	730
Pepperoni Pizzadillas	1 serv	617
Scrambled Eggs & Bacon	1 serv	216
Spaghetti	1 serv	343
Turkey Dinner	1 serv	337

DESSERTS

Apple Crisp Cinnamon	1 serv	898
Bread Pudding	1 serv	819
Brownie Triple Chocolate	1 serv	1950
Cheesecake New York Style	1 serv	1075
Pie Banana Foster Mud	1 serv	1245

FOOD	PORTION	CALS
Pie Pecan Chocolate Chip	1 serv	1879
MAIN MENU SELECTIONS		
Appetizer Dip Spinach & Artichoke	1 serv	2459
Appetizer Fried Chicken Tenders	1 serv	800
Appetizer Fried Dill Pickles	1 serv	972
Appetizer Jazz Fest	1 serv	1252
Appetizer Zucchini Parmesan	1 serv	626
Blackened Soul w/ Shrimp Creole	1 serv	852
Broiled Flat Iron Steak	1 serv	1026
Burger Half Pound	1	684
Cafe Fish & Chips	1 serv	1290
Cajun Blackened Salmon	1 serv	919
Cheeseburger BBQ Ranch	1	999
Cheeseburger Half Pound	1	855
Chicken Cordon Bleu	1 serv	1360
Chicken Feta Penne	1 serv	1879
Ciabatta Chicken	1	1251
Ciabatta Meatloaf	1	1036
Ciabatta Turkey Pesto	1	1248
Club Cafe	1	1132
Country Fried Steak	1 serv	1061
Crab Cake Dinner	1 serv	1662
Diablo Center Cut Pork Chops	1 serv	1094
Dip Classic Beef	1	521
Fillet Of Soul	1 serv	636
French Quarter	1	1480
Garlic Shrimp Spaghettini	1 serv	860
Grilled Beef Liver	1 serv	1003
Grilled Chicken Tuscan Style	1 serv	880
Habachi Salmon	1 serv	846
Mimi's Meatloaf	1 serv	910
Mimi's Pot Roast	1 serv	1291
Original Patty Melt	1	976
Parmesan Crusted Chicken Breast	1 serv	1820
Pasta Jambalaya	1 serv	1223
Pot Pie Chicken	1 serv	1403
Reuben West Coast	1	2015
Sandwich 5 Way Grilled Cheese	1	703
Sandwich Albacore & Avocado	1	993
Sandwich Bacon Lettuce & Tomato	1	586

FOOD	PORTION	CALS
Sandwich Fresh Roasted Turkey Breast	1	532
Sandwich Turkey Walnut Salad On Raisin Bread	1	549
Sandwich Veggie Stack	1	836
Slow Roasted Turkey Breast	1 serv	851
Small Bites Black & Blue Quesadilla	1 serv	1241
Small Bites Chicken & Fruit	1 serv	460
Small Bites Citrus Salmon	1 serv	699
Small Bites Crab Cakes	1 serv	412
Small Bites Smoky Chicken Enchiladas	1 serv	1154
Small Bites Sweet & Sour Coconut Shrimp	1 serv	608
Small Bites Thai Chicken Wrap	1 serv	1004
Top Sirloin 12 oz	1 serv	947
SALAD DRESSINGS		
Balsamic Vinaigrette	1 serv	316
Bleu Cheese	1 serv	298
Caesar	1 serv	273
Chinese Sesame	1 serv	263
Dijon Vinaigrette	1 serv	296
Honey Mustard	1 serv	243
Non Fat French	1 serv	65
Ranch	1 serv	194
Thousand Island	1 serv	232
SALADS		
Asian Chopped	1 serv	751
Bleu Cheese & Walnut	1 serv	728
Caesar Blackened Chicken	1 serv	570
Chopped Cobb	1 serv	524
Fried Chicken	1 serv	764
Zesty Chicken Tostada	1 serv	1046
SOUPS		
Broccoli Cheddar	1 serv	270
Chicken Gumbo	1 serv	235
Clam Chowder	1 serv	240
Corn Chowder	1 serv	196
Cream Of Chicken	1 serv	337
French Market Onion	1 serv	207
Red Bean & Andouille Sausage	1 serv	256
Split Pea	1 serv	194
Vegetarian Vegetable	1 serv	60

FOOD	PORTION	CALS
NEWPORT CREAMERY		
Ice Cream Chocolate No Sugar Added	½ cup	110
Ice Cream Vanilla No Sugar Added	½ cup	100
Vanilla Yogurt	½ cup	120
Vanilla Yogurt Nonfat	½ cup	100
NOAH'S BAGELS		
BAGELS AND BREADS		
Bagel Asiago Cheese Topped	1 (4.2 oz)	330
Bagel Blueberry	1 (3.7 oz)	270
Bagel Candy Cane	1 (3.7 oz)	270
Bagel Cheddar Shtick	1 (4.2 oz)	330
Bagel Chocolate Chip	1 (3.7 oz)	290
Bagel Chopped Garlic	1 (3.9 oz)	290
Bagel Cinnamon Raisin	1 (3.7 oz)	270
Bagel Cinnamon Sugar	1 (4.1 oz)	310
Bagel Cracked Pepper	1 (3.7 oz)	280
Bagel Cranberry Orange	1 (3.5 oz)	250
Bagel Dutch Apple	1 (5 oz)	340
Bagel Egg	1 (3.7 oz)	290
Bagel Everything	1 (3.9 oz)	280
Bagel Good Grains	1 (3.9 oz)	280
Bagel Jalapeno Cheddar	1 (4.9 oz)	350
Bagel Onion	1 (3.7 oz)	270
Bagel Plain	1 (3.7 oz)	270
Bagel Poppyseed	1 (3.9 oz)	290
Bagel Power	1 (4 oz)	310
Bagel Pumpernickel	1 (3.7 oz)	260
Bagel Sesame Seed	1 (3.9 oz)	290
Bagel Six Cheese	1 (4.5 oz)	340
Bagel Spinach Florentine	1 (4.9 oz)	350
Bagel Sun Dried Tomato	1 (3.7 oz)	270
Bagel Whole Wheat	1 (3.7 oz)	260
Bagel Whole Wheat Sesame & Sunflower Seeds	1 (4.4 oz)	370
Bialy	1 (5.3 oz)	380
Bread Ciabatta	1 serv (4.25 oz)	290
Bread Corn Meal Rye	1 slice (2 oz)	150
Bread Harvest Grain	1 slice (2.3 oz)	180
Bread Marble Rye	1 slice (1.7 oz)	160
Bread Potato	1 slice (1.7 oz)	140

FOOD	PORTION	CALS
Challah Braided	1 serv (2 oz)	160
Challah Roll	1 (3 oz)	230
Pizza Bagel Artichoke Tomato & Red Onion	1 (11.1 oz)	550
Pizza Bagel Artichoke & Spinach	1 (12 oz)	670
Pizza Bagel Cheese	1 (6.2 oz)	420
Pizza Bagel Cheesy Garlic & Herb	1 (6.2 oz)	500
Pizza Bagel Pepperoni	1 (6.8 oz)	500
Pizza Bagel Spinach & Mushroom	1 (9.5 oz)	580
Pizza Bagel Tomato & Rosemary	1 (8.7 oz)	540
BEVERAGES AND EXTRAS		
Cafe Latte Low Fat	1 reg (12 oz)	160
Cafe Latte Nonfat	1 reg (12 oz)	110
Cafe Latte Whole	1 reg (12 oz)	200
Cappuccino Low Fat	1 reg (12 oz)	120
Cappuccino Nonfat	1 reg (12 oz)	90
Cappuccino Whole	1 reg (12 oz)	150
Chai Tea Low Fat Milk	1 reg (12 oz)	220
Chai Tea Non Fat Milk	1 reg (12 oz)	210
Chai Tea Whole Milk	1 reg (12 oz)	230
Coca-Cola	8 oz	99
Coca-Cola Cherry	8 oz	104
Coffee Iced Americano	8 oz	0
Coffee Regular or Decaf	1 (12 oz)	0
Diet Coke	8 oz	1
Espresso	1 reg (2 oz)	0
Fanta Orange	8 oz	106
Frozen Drinks Cafe Caramel	1 (18 oz)	620
Frozen Drinks Cafe Mocha	1 (18 oz)	510
Frozen Drinks Strawberry Cream	1 (18 oz)	450
Frozen Drinks Wild Berry Fat Free	1 (18 oz)	270
Half & Half Creamer	1 oz	40
Hi-C Fruit Punch	8 oz	104
Hot Chocolate Nonfat	1 reg (12 oz)	220
Hot Chocolate Whole	1 reg (12 oz)	290
Iced Cappuccino Nonfat	1 reg (12 oz)	90
Iced Mocha Low Fat	1 reg (12 oz)	230
Iced Tea Raspberry	8 oz	78
Iced Tea Unsweetened	8 oz	1
Lemonade	8 oz	97
Lemonade	1 (16 oz)	200

FOOD	PORTION	CALS
Lemonade Blackberry	1 (16 oz)	310
Macchiato Nonfat	1 reg (12 oz)	230
Macchiato Whole	1 reg (12 oz)	290
Macha Nonfat	1 reg (12 oz)	190
Milk Low Fat	8 oz	120
Milk Skim	8 oz	80
Milk Whole	8 oz	150
Mocha Low Fat	1 reg (12 oz)	230
Mocha Whole	1 reg (12 oz)	270
Mr. Pibb	8 oz	97
On Top Reduced Fat Topping	2 tbsp (0.3 oz)	20
Orange Juice	1 (10 oz)	143
Sprite	8 oz	97
Syrup Blackberry	2 tbsp (1 oz)	100
Syrup Caramel	2 tbsp (1 oz)	70
Syrup Hazelnut	2 tbsp (1 oz)	100
Syrup Vanilla	2 tbsp (1 oz)	100
Syrup Vanilla Sugar Free	2 tbsp (1 oz)	116
Tea Hamey & Sons All Flavors	8 oz	0
Whipped Cream Light	2 tbsp (1 oz)	36
CREAM CHEESE AND SPREADS		
Butter	1 tbsp (0.5 oz)	110
Cream Cheese Whipped Onion & Chive	2 tbsp (0.7 oz)	70
Cream Cheese Whipped Plain	2 tbsp (0.7 oz)	70
Cream Cheese Whipped Reduced Fat Blueberry	2 tbsp (0.7 oz)	70
Cream Cheese Whipped Reduced Fat Garden Vegetable	2 tbsp (0.7 oz)	60
Cream Cheese Whipped Reduced Fat Garlic Herb	2 tbsp (0.7 oz)	60
Cream Cheese Whipped Reduced Fat Honey Almond	2 tbsp (0.7 oz)	70
Cream Cheese Whipped Reduced Fat Jalapeno Salsa	2 tbsp (0.7 oz)	60
Cream Cheese Whipped Reduced Fat Plain	2 tbsp (0.7 oz)	60
Cream Cheese Whipped Reduced Fat Strawberry	2 tbsp (0.7 oz)	60
Cream Cheese Whipped Reduced Fat Sun Dried Tomato & Basil	2 tbsp (0.7 oz)	60
Cream Cheese Whipped Smoked Salmon	2 tbsp (0.7 oz)	60

FOOD	PORTION	CALS
Deli Mustard	1 tsp (5 g)	0
Garlic Mayo	1 serv (1.5 oz)	270
Grape Jam	1 serv (1 oz)	110
Honey	1 serv (1 oz)	90
Hummus	1 serv (2 oz)	90
Mayo	1 tbsp (0.5 oz)	110
DESSERTS		
Cinnamon Twists	1 serv (3.8 oz)	370
Coffee Cake Apple Cinnamon	1 serv (6.6 oz)	700
Coffee Cake Chocolate Chip	1 serv (6.1 oz)	760
Coffee Cake Mixed Berry	1 serv (6.9 oz)	710
Cookie Chocolate Chip	1 (2.8 oz)	360
Cookie Chocolate Mudslide	1 (2.75 oz)	320
Cookie Iced Sugar	1 (3.7 oz)	480
Cookie Oatmeal Raisin	1 (2.8 oz)	320
Cookie Snickerdoodle	1 (2.8 oz)	400
Cookie Mini Chocolate Mudslide	1 (1.38 oz)	160
Cookie Mini Chocolate Chip	1 (1.38 oz)	180
Cookie Mini Iced Sugar	1 (1.87 oz)	230
Cookie Mini Oatmeal Raisin	1 (1.38 oz)	160
Marshmallow Crispy Treat	1 (3.9 oz)	410
Muffin Blueberry	1 (5 oz)	480
Muffin Cranberry Orange	1 (4.6 oz)	460
Muffin Strawberry White Chocolate	1 (5.5 oz)	550
Strudel Cinnamon Walnut	1 serv (5.4 oz)	630
SALAD DRESSINGS		
Caesar	2 tbsp (1 oz)	150
Harvest Chicken Salad	2 tbsp (1 oz)	90
Raspberry Vinaigrette	2 tbsp	160
SALADS		
Caesar	1 (10.5 oz)	600
Caesar Side	1 (4.5 oz)	280
Caesar Chicken	1 (14 oz)	720
City	1 (11.5 oz)	830
City w/ Chicken	1 (15 oz)	950
Southwestern Chicken	1 (15.2 oz)	710
SANDWICHES		
Bagel & Lox	1 (11.2 oz)	520
Bagel Dog Asiago	1 (7.1 oz)	510
Bagel Dog Everything	1 (7.1 oz)	510

FOOD	PORTION	CALS
Bagel Dog Original	1 (6.9 oz)	490
Bagel Plain w/ Peanut Butter & Jelly	1 (6.2 oz)	550
Breakfast Wrap Santa Fe	1 (14.5 oz)	750
Breakfast Wrap Veggie	1 (15.6 oz)	810
California Chicken	1 (9.9 oz)	360
Club Blackened Chicken	1 (10.4 oz)	630
Club Deli Pesto Turkey	1 (10.9 oz)	670
Deli Chicken Salad	1 (11 oz)	1150
Deli Corned Beef	1 (14 oz)	740
Deli Egg Salad Kosher	1 (11.5 oz)	650
Deli Pastrami	1 (14 oz)	750
Deli Roast Beef	1 (14 oz)	730
Deli Tuna Salad	1 (13 oz)	740
Deli Turkey	1 (14.5 oz)	720
Deli Melts Hummus	1 (10.2 oz)	570
Deli Melts Pastrami	1 (9.6 oz)	530
Deli Melts Roast Beef	1 (9.6 oz)	530
Deli Melts Tuna	1 (11.6 oz)	700
Deli Melts Turkey	1 (9.6 oz)	500
Deli Melts Veggie	1 (12.3 oz)	590
Deli Whitefish	1 (12.2 oz)	850
Egg Mit Artichoke & Tomato	1 (12 oz)	620
Egg Mit Bacon & Cheddar	1 (9.2 oz)	620
Egg Mit Cheese	1 (8.5 oz)	520
Egg Mit Cheese & Tomato	1 (10 oz)	530
Egg Mit Lox & Chives	1 (8.8 oz)	490
Egg Mit Plain	1 (7.9 oz)	450
Egg Mit Spinach Mushroom & Swiss	1 (9.8 oz)	530
Egg Mit Turkey Sausage	1 (9.9 oz)	590
Kosher Vegetarian On Plain Bagel	1 (13.9 oz)	860
Panini Albacore Tuna	1 (13.6 oz)	750
Panini Egg Spinach Bacon	1 (11.8 oz)	790
Panini Egg Vegetarian Omelete	1 (13.8 oz)	670
Panini Italian Chicken	1 (12.5 oz)	810
Panini Mediterranean	1 (10.6 oz)	550
Panini Tomato Mozzarella	1 (7.9 oz)	440
Panini Turkey Club	1 (12.3 oz)	610
Sandwich Rachel	1 (13.9 oz)	1030
Sandwich Reuben	1 (13.9 oz)	770
Sandwich Veg Out	1 (10.1 oz)	490

FOOD	PORTION	CALS
Wrap Albacore Tuna	1 (12.3 oz)	600
Wrap Chicken Caesar	1 (12.6 oz)	790
Wrap Southwestern Turkey	1 (13.5 oz)	750
Wrap Veggie	1 (9.8 oz)	460
SIDES		
Cole Slaw	1 serv (3 oz)	120
Egg Salad	1 serv (5 oz)	330
Fresh Fruit Cup	1 (11 oz)	140
Fruit & Yogurt Parfait	1 (12 oz)	220
Kosher Pickle	1	5
Redskin Potato Salad	1 serv (3 oz)	160
Tuna Salad	1 serv (5 oz)	280
SOUPS		
Broccoli Cheese	1 cup (8.7 oz)	290
Chicken Noodle	1 cup (8.7 oz)	110
Italian Wedding	1 cup (8.7 oz)	160
Tortilla	1 cup (8.7 oz)	300
Turkey Chili	1 cup (8.7 oz)	220

NOODLES & COMPANY
MAIN MENU SELECTIONS

FOOD	PORTION	CALS
Bangkok Curry	1 sm	250
Bangkok Curry	1 reg	490
Beef Braised	1 serv	190
Beef Sauteed	1 serv	210
Buttered Noodles	1 sm	310
Buttered Noodles	1 reg	620
Chicken Breast Seasoned	1 serv	130
Chicken Parmesan Crusted	1 serv	190
Ciabatta Roll	1	160
Flatbread	1 serv	210
House Marinara	1 reg	650
House Marinara	1 sm	330
Mushroom Stroganoff	1 sm	390
Mushroom Stroganoff	1 reg	780
Organic Tofu	1 serv	180
Pad Thai	1 sm	350
Pad Thai	1 reg	700
Pasta Fresca	1 sm	420
Pasta Fresca	1 reg	780
Penne Rosa	1 sm	420

FOOD	PORTION	CALS
Penne Rosa	1 reg	810
Pesto Cavatappi	1 sm	510
Pesto Cavatappi	1 reg	910
Potstickers	3	200
Shrimp Sauteed	1 serv	35
Whole Grain Tuscan Linguine	1 sm	450
Whole Grain Tuscan Linguine	1 reg	770
Wisconsin Mac & Cheese	1 sm	450
Wisconsin Mac & Cheese	1 reg	900
SALADS		
Caesar	1 sm	160
Caesar	1 reg	320
Chinese Chopped	1 sm	150
Chinese Chopped	1 reg	310
Cucumber Tomato Side Salad	1	80
The Med	1 sm	150
The Med	1 reg	310
Tossed Green	1	60
SOUPS		
Chicken Noodle	1 sm	150
Chicken Noodle	1 reg	300
Thai Curry	1 sm	240
Thai Curry	1 reg	480
Tomato Basil	1 sm	210
Tomato Basil	1 reg	420

OLD SPAGHETTI FACTORY
CHILDREN'S MENU SELECTIONS

Grilled Cheese Sandwich	1 serv	360
Macaroni & Cheese	1 serv	350
Spaghetti w/ Tomato Sauce	1 serv	300
Spaghetti w/ Tomato Sauce & Meatballs	1 serv	440
DESSERTS		
Caramel Turtle Pie	1 serv	660
Mud Pie	1 serv	680
New York Cheese Cake w/ Strawberry Topping	1 serv	690
MAIN MENU SELECTIONS		
Baked Chicken	1 dinner serv	880
Chicken Marsala	1 dinner serv	960
Fettuccine Alfredo	1 dinner serv	1130
Fettuccine Chicken	1 dinner serv	960

FOOD	PORTION	CALS
Lasagne	1 dinner serv	630
Parmigiana Chicken	1 dinner serv	840
Parmigiana Eggplant	1 dinner serv	670
Pot Pourri	1 dinner serv	710
Ravioli Spinach & Cheese	1 dinner serv	480
Salmon Tuscany	1 dinner serv	680
Sandwich Meatball	1	860
Sandwich Sausage	1	730
Sandwich Tuscan Chicken	1	1060
Seafood Cheddar Melt	1 serv	790
Spaghetti w/ Clam Sauce	1 dinner serv	690
Spaghetti w/ Clam Sauce & Mizithra	1 dinner serv	960
Spaghetti w/ Meat & Clam Sauces	1 dinner serv	980
Spaghetti w/ Meat Sauce	1 dinner serv	470
Spaghetti w/ Meat Sauce & Mizithra	1 dinner serv	850
Spaghetti w/ Meat Sauce & Sausage	1 dinner serv	830
Spaghetti w/ Meatballs	1 dinner serv	840
Spaghetti w/ Mizithra	1 dinner serv	1010
Spaghetti w/ Mushroom & Clam Sauces	1 dinner serv	830
Spaghetti w/ Mushroom & Meat Sauces	1 dinner serv	460
Spaghetti w/ Mushroom Sauce	1 dinner serv	460
Spaghetti w/ Mushroom Sauce & Mizithra	1 dinner serv	850
Spaghetti w/ Tomato & Mizithra	1 dinner serv	840
Spaghetti w/ Tomato & Meat Sauces	1 dinner serv	460
Spaghetti w/ Tomato Sauce	1 dinner serv	440
Spaghetti w/ Tomato Sauce & Clam Sauce	1 dinner serv	560
Starter Tortellini	1 serv	930
Tortellini Mortadella & Chicken	1 dinner serv	930

ON THE BORDER
CHILDREN'S MENU SELECTIONS

Border Chicken Strips	1 serv	570
Corn Dog	1	320
Crispy Taco Mexican Dinner Beef	1 serv	740
Crispy Taco Mexican Dinner Chicken	1 serv	740
Hamburger	1	390
Nachos Bean & Cheese	1 serv	980
Nachos Cheese	1 serv	670
Quesadillas Chicken	1 serv	720
Sandwich Grilled Chicken	1	630
Soft Taco Mexican Dinner Beef	1 serv	840

FOOD	PORTION	CALS
Soft Taco Mexican Dinner Chicken	1 serv	750
Sundae w/ Chocolate Syrup	1 serv	300
Sundae w/ Strawberry Puree	1 serv	340
DESSERTS		
Border Brownie Sundae	1	440
Chocolate Turtle Empanadas	1 serv	1280
Dulce De Leche Cheesecake	1 serv	1160
Kahlua Ice Cream Pie	1 serv	850
Sizzling Apple Crisp	1 serv	960
Sopapillas	1 serv	1230
Vanilla Ice Cream	1 scoop	180
MAIN MENU SELECTIONS		
Bacon Wrapped Shrimp	1 serv	730
Baja Chicken	1 serv	610
Bandera Sirloin	1 serv	640
Beans Black	1 serv	180
Beans Refried	1 serv	290
Black Bean & Corn Relish	1 serv	80
Border Chimichanga Fajita Chicken w/ Onions & Mushrooms	1 serv	1230
Border Chimichanga Ground Beef	1 serv	1310
Border Chimichanga Spicy Chicken	1 serv	1160
Border Sampler	1 serv	1940
Bordurrito Big Beef w/ Side Salad	1 serv	1600
Bordurrito Big Chicken w/ Side Salad	1 serv	1420
Burrito Beef	1 serv	1080
Burrito Chicken	1 serv	880
Burrito Three Sauce Fajita Chicken	1 serv	870
Burrito Three Sauce Fajita Steak	1 serv	1050
Carne Asada & Shrimp	1 serv	1040
Cheese Chile Relleno	1	880
Cheesy Pepper Jack Mashed Potatoes	1 serv	380
Chicken Flautas Appetizer	1 serv	970
Chile Con Queso	1 cup	250
Chile Con Queso	1 bowl	390
Corona Extra Dinner	1 serv	2040
Crispy Taco Beef	1	330
Crispy Taco Chicken	1	240
Crispy Taco Veggie	1	250
Dos XX Fish Tacos	1 serv	1590

FOOD	PORTION	CALS
Empanadas Beef	1	440
Empanadas Chicken	1 serv	1090
Empanadas Chicken	1	390
Empanadas Ground Beef	1 serv	1150
Enchilada Beef	1	340
Enchilada Cheese & Onion	1	410
Enchilada Chicken	1	350
Fajitas 7 Pepper Steak	1 serv	910
Fajitas Blackened Chicken w/ Portobello Mushrooms	1 serv	640
Fajitas Carnitas	1 serv	830
Fajitas Chicken Con Queso	1 skillet	1130
Fajitas Grilled Vegetables w/ Portobello Mushrooms	1 serv	390
Fajitas Jalapeno BBQ Chicken	1 serv	760
Fajitas Mesquite Grilled Chicken	1 serv	440
Fajitas Mesquite Grilled Steak	1 serv	620
Fajitas Monterey Ranch Chicken	1 serv	840
Fajitas Shrimp	1 serv	750
Fajitas Ultimate	1 serv	1230
Firecracker Stuffed Jalapenos	1 serv	980
French Fries	1 serv	390
Grande Fajita Nachos Beef	1 serv	1970
Grande Fajita Nachos Chicken	1 serv	1890
Grande Fajita Nachos Combo	1 serv	1940
Guacamole	1 serv	130
Guacamole Live	1 serv	570
Margarita Chicken	1 serv	290
Mexican Rice	1 serv	220
Mexican Shrimp Scampi	1 serv	740
Pico Chicken & Shrimp	1 serv	730
Quesadillas Combo Fajita	1 serv	1450
Quesadillas Double Stacked Club	1 serv	1860
Quesadillas Fajita Chicken	1 serv	1430
Quesadillas Fajita Steak	1 serv	1530
Quesadillas Spinach & Mushroom	1 serv	1420
Ranchiladas	1 serv	1360
Red Chili Ribeye	1 serv	900
Salmon Mexican	1 serv	650
Sandwich Chicken Blackened w/ French Fries	1 serv	1510

FOOD	PORTION	CALS
Sandwich Chicken Grilled w/ French Fries	1 serv	1430
Sauteed Shrimp	4	170
Shaken Margarita Shrimp Cocktail	1 serv	280
Shaken Margarita Shrimp Cocktail w/ Tortilla Chips	1 serv	780
Soft Taco Beef	1	340
Soft Taco Chicken	1	250
Soft Taco Veggie	1	210
Superior Dinner	1 serv	1350
Tamale	1	310
Tortilla Soup	1 bowl	350
Tortillas Corn	3	230
Tortillas Flour	3	300
Tres Enchilada Dinner Beef	1 serv	1010
Tres Enchilada Dinner Cheese	1 serv	1210
Tres Enchilada Dinner Chicken	1 serv	1040
Ultimate Loaded Queso	1 serv	900
Vegetables Grilled	1 serv	50
Vegetables Sauteed	1 serv	70
SALAD DRESSINGS AND SAUCES		
Chili Con Carne Sauce	1 serv (2 oz)	70
Chipotle Mayonnaise	1 serv (1 oz)	190
Dressing Chipotle Honey Mustard	1 serv (2 oz)	310
Dressing Ranch	1 serv (2 oz)	220
Dressing Smoked Jalapeno Vinaigrette	1 serv (2 oz)	230
Dressing Sweet Pepper Vinaigrette	1 serv (2 oz)	270
Dressing Fat Free Balsamic Vinaigrette	1 serv (2 oz)	50
Dressing Lo Fat Ranch	1 serv (2 oz)	110
Parrila Butter	1 serv (1 oz)	120
Pico De Gallo	1 scoop	20
Ranchero Sauce	1 serv (2 oz)	18
Salsa	1 serv (2 oz)	25
Sour Cream	1 serv (2 oz)	140
SALADS		
Chopped Chicken w/ Dressing	1 serv	1330
Fiesta Blackened Chicken w/ Dressing	1 serv	1150
Fiesta Chicken w/ Dressing	1 serv	1140
Grande Taco Beef	1 serv	1450
Grande Taco Chicken	1 serv	1280
House	1 serv	170

FOOD	PORTION	CALS
Sizzling Fajita Chicken	1 serv	760
Sizzling Fajita Steak	1 serv	910

P.F. CHANG'S CHINA BISTRO
DESSERTS
Banana Spring Rolls	1 serv	814
Cake The Great Wall Of Chocolate	1 serv	2237
Flourless Chocolate Dome Gluten Free	1 serv	572
Ice Cream Pineapple Coconut	1 serv	111
Mini Dessert Apple Pie	1	170
Mini Dessert Banana Split	1	167
Mini Dessert Carrot Cake	1	295
Mini Dessert Creamy Strawberry Cheesecake	1	239
Mini Dessert Great Wall Of Chocolate	1	336
Mini Dessert S'mores	1	323
Mini Dessert Tiramisu	1	202
Mini Dessert Tres Leche Lemon Dream	1	216

MAIN MENU SELECTIONS
Almond & Cashew Chicken	1 serv	815
Asian Marinated New York Strip	1 serv	1432
Asian Slaw	1 serv	585
Beef A La Sichuan	1 serv	1172
Beef w/ Broccoli	1 serv	1118
Buddha's Feast Steamed	1 serv	137
Buddha's Feast Stir Fried	1 serv	367
Calamari Salt & Pepper	1 serv	720
Cantonese Chow Fun w/ Beef	1 serv	1212
Cantonese Chow Fun w/ Chicken	1 serv	1045
Cantonese Scallops	1 serv	408
Cantonese Shrimp	1 serv	330
Chang's Spicy Chicken	1 serv	923
Chengdu Spiced Lamb	1 serv	1056
Chicken w/ Black Bean Sauce	1 serv	678
Chow Fun Vegetable	1 serv	878
Chow Mein Combo	1 serv	912
Chow Mein w/ Beef	1 serv	793
Chow Mein w/ Chicken	1 serv	689
Chow Mein w/ Pork	1 serv	898
Chow Mein w/ Shrimp	1 serv	625
Citrus Soy Salmon w/ Brown Rice	1 serv	1000
Citrus Soy Salmon w/ White Rice	1 serv	1025

FOOD	PORTION	CALS
Coconut Curry Vegetables	1 serv	686
Crispy Green Beans	1 serv	507
Crispy Honey Chicken	1 serv	867
Crispy Honey Shrimp	1 serv	1061
Dali Chicken	1 serv	1091
Double Pan Fried Noodles Combo	1 serv	1384
Double Pan Fried Noodles w/ Beef	1 serv	1186
Double Pan Fried Noodles w/ Chicken	1 serv	1072
Double Pan Fried Noodles w/ Pork	1 serv	1208
Double Pan Fried Noodles w/ Shrimp	1 serv	1031
Dumplings Peking Pan Fried	1 serv	367
Dumplings Peking Steamed	1 serv	327
Dumplings Shrimp Pan Fried	1 serv	305
Dumplings Shrimp Steamed	1 serv	265
Dumplings Vegetable Pan Fried	1 serv	307
Dumplings Vegetable Steamed	1 serv	267
Eggplant Stir Fried	1 serv	590
Fried Rice Combo	1 serv	1539
Fried Rice w/ Beef	1 serv	1228
Fried Rice w/ Chicken	1 serv	1208
Fried Rice w/ Pork	1 serv	1360
Fried Rice w/ Shrimp	1 serv	1154
Garlic Noodles	1 serv	612
Garlic Snap Peas	1 sm	129
Ginger Chicken w/ Broccoli	1 serv	656
Ginger Chicken w/ Broccoli Gluten Free	1 serv	677
Ground Chicken & Eggplant	1 serv	792
Harvest Spring Rolls	1 serv	287
Hot Fish	1 serv	1338
Kung Pao Chicken	1 serv	1228
Kung Pao Scallops	1 serv	1136
Kung Pao Shrimp	1 serv	977
Lemon Pepper Shrimp	1 serv	701
Lemon Scallops	1 serv	952
Lemongrass Prawns	1 serv	907
Lettuce Wraps Chicken	1 serv	377
Lettuce Wraps Gluten Free Chicken	1 serv	477
Lettuce Wraps Vegetarian	1 serv	281
Lo Mein Combo	1 serv	1409
Lo Mein w/ Beef	1 serv	1374

FOOD	PORTION	CALS
Lo Mein w/ Chicken	1 serv	1198
Lo Mein w/ Pork	1 serv	1400
Lo Mein w/ Shrimp	1 serv	1134
Lunch Bowl Almond & Cashew Chicken w/ White Rice	1	955
Lunch Bowl Beef w/ Broccoli w/ Brown Rice	1	844
Lunch Bowl Beef w/ Broccoli w/ White Rice	1	890
Lunch Bowl Buddha's Feast w/ Brown Rice	1	541
Lunch Bowl Buddha's Feast w/ White Rice	1	587
Lunch Bowl Citrus Soy Salmon w/ Brown Rice	1	1047
Lunch Bowl Citrus Soy Salmon w/ White Rice	1	1093
Lunch Bowl Crispy Honey Chicken w/ Brown Rice	1	943
Lunch Bowl Crispy Honey Chicken w/ White Rice	1	989
Lunch Bowl Moo Goo Gai Pan w/ Brown Rice	1	545
Lunch Bowl Moo Goo Gai Pan w/ White Rice	1	591
Lunch Bowl Pepper Steak w/ Brown Rice	1	820
Lunch Bowl Pepper Steak w/ White Rice	1 serv	968
Lunch Bowl Shrimp w/ Lobster Sauce w/ Brown Rice	1	686
Lunch Bowl Shrimp w/ Lobster Sauce w/ White Rice	1	732
Mongolian Beef	1 serv	1178
Moo Goo Gai Pan	1 serv	661
Mu Shu Chicken	1 serv	715
Mu Shu Pork	1 serv	871
Noodles Dan Dan	1 serv	1087
Noodles Tam's	1 serv	1678
Oolong Marinated Sea Bass	1 serv	521
Orange Peel Beef	1 serv	1568
Orange Peel Chicken	1 serv	1151
Orange Peel Shrimp	1 serv	1010
Pepper Steak	1 serv	971
Philip's Better Lemon Chicken	1 serv	1051
Rice Brown	1 cup	254
Rice Sticks	1 serv	135
Rice White	1 cup	295
Salt & Pepper Prawns	1 serv	844
Seared Ahi Tuna	1 serv	210

FOOD	PORTION	CALS
Shanghai Cucumbers	1 serv	124
Shrimp w/ Candied Walnuts	1 serv	1225
Shrimp w/ Lobster Sauce	1 serv	480
Sichuan Asparagus	1 sm	97
Sichuan Chicken Flatbread	1 serv	1160
Sichuan From The Sea Calamari	1 serv	1078
Sichuan From The Sea Scallops	1 serv	1030
Sichuan From The Sea Shrimp	1 serv	728
Singapore Street Noodles	1 serv	572
Singapore Street Noodles Gluten Free	1 serv	566
Spare Ribs Chang's	1 serv	1356
Spare Ribs Northern Style	1 serv	720
Spicy Green Beans	1 sm	234
Spinach w/ Garlic Stir Fried	1 sm	77
Sweet & Sour Chicken	1 serv	764
Sweet & Sour Pork	1 serv	1095
Vegetarian Ma Po Tofu	1 serv	537
Wild Alaskan Sockeye Salmon Steamed w/ Ginger	1 serv	646
Wild Alaskan Sockeye Salmon Steamed w/ Ginger Gluten Free	1 serv	672
Wok Charred Beef	1 serv	941
Wok Seared Lamb	1 serv	1081
Wontons Crab	1 serv	440
SALAD DRESSINGS AND SAUCES		
Dressing Creamy Wedge	1 serv	443
Dressing Signature Ginger	1 serv	483
Sauce Chili Bean	1 serv	81
Sauce Crispy Green Bean	1 serv	451
Sauce Potsticker	1 serv	36
Sauce Shrimp Dumpling	1 serv	24
Sauce Special	1 serv	55
Sauce Spicy Plum	1 serv	110
Sauce Sweet & Sour	1 serv	57
Vinaigrette Mustard	1 serv	66
Vinaigrette Watermelon Citrus	1 serv	240
SALADS		
Bikini Shrimp w/o Dressing	1 serv	192
Chang's Wedge w/ Chicken w/o Dressing	1 serv	595
Chang's Wedge w/o Dressing	1 serv	244

FOOD	PORTION	CALS
Chopped Chicken w/o Dressing	1 serv	401
SOUPS		
Chicken Noodle	1 bowl	512
Egg Drop	1 cup	48
Hot & Sour	1 cup	85
Wonton	1 bowl	354
PACIUGO GELATO		
Milk Base Amarena Black Cherry Swirl	1 scoop (3.5 oz)	160
Milk Base Banana Creme Pie	1 scoop (3.5 oz)	80
Milk Base Cheesecake	1 scoop (3.5 oz)	90
Milk Base Chocolate	1 scoop (3.5 oz)	80
Milk Base Chocolate Cookies'N Milk	1 scoop (3.5 oz)	90
Milk Base Coconut	1 scoop (3.5 oz)	80
Milk Base Coffee	1 scoop (3.5 oz)	75
Milk Base Fiordilatte	1 scoop (3.5 oz)	75
Milk Base French Vanilla Bean	1 scoop (3.5 oz)	80
Milk Base Green Tea	1 scoop (3.5 oz)	70
Milk Base Hazelnut	1 scoop (3.5 oz)	85
Milk Base Lemon Custard	1 scoop (3.5 oz)	75
Milk Base Mascarpone Chocolate Rum	1 scoop (3.5 oz)	95
Milk Base Pannacotta	1 scoop (3.5 oz)	75
Milk Base Peppermint	1 scoop (3.5 oz)	75
Milk Base Rose	1 scoop (3.5 oz)	70
Milk Base Tiramisu	1 scoop (3.5 oz)	80
Milk Base Zabajone	1 scoop (3.5 oz)	80
No Sugar Added Chocolate	1 scoop (3.5 oz)	28
No Sugar Added Mint	1 scoop (3.5 oz)	25
No Sugar Added Mocha	1 scoop (3.5 oz)	28
No Sugar Added Strawberry Milk	1 scoop (3.5 oz)	23
Soy Banana	1 scoop (3.5 oz)	40
Soy Blueberry	1 scoop (3.5 oz)	40
Soy Chocolate	1 scoop (3.5 oz)	38
Soy Coffee	1 scoop (3.5 oz)	35
Soy Hazelnut	1 scoop (3.5 oz)	35
Soy Strawberry	1 scoop (3.5 oz)	38
Soy Wild Berries	1 scoop (3.5 oz)	40
Water Base Blackberry	1 scoop (3.5 oz)	28
Water Base Ginger Lemon	1 scoop (3.5 oz)	25
Water Base Green Apple	1 scoop (3.5 oz)	28
Water Base Lemon Sage	1 scoop (3.5 oz)	25

FOOD	PORTION	CALS
Water Base Lychee	1 scoop (3.5 oz)	25
Water Base Orange Vidalia	1 scoop (3.5 oz)	25
Water Base Passion Fruit	1 scoop (3.5 oz)	23
Water Base Pineapple	1 scoop (3.5 oz)	28
Water Base Strawberry Port	1 scoop (3.5 oz)	25
Water Base Watermelon	1 scoop (3.5 oz)	25

PANDA EXPRESS
MAIN MENU SELECTIONS

FOOD	PORTION	CALS
BBQ Pork	1 serv	350
Beef & Broccoli	1 serv	150
Beef w/ String Beans	1 serv	170
Black Pepper Chicken	1 serv	180
Chicken w/ Mushrooms	1 serv	130
Chicken w/ Potato	1 serv	220
Chicken w/ String Beans	1 serv	170
Egg Roll Chicken	1 (3 oz)	190
Fried Shrimp	6 pieces	260
Mandarin Chicken	1 serv	250
Mixed Vegetables	1 serv	70
Orange Chicken	1 serv	480
Spicy Chicken w/ Peanuts	1 serv	200
Spring Roll Veggie	1 (1.7 oz)	80
Steamed Rice	1 serv	330
String Beans w/ Fried Tofu	1 serv	180
Sweet & Sour Chicken	1 serv	310
Sweet & Sour Pork	1 serv	410
Vegetable Chow Mein	1 serv	330
Vegetable Fried Rice	1 serv	390

SAUCES

FOOD	PORTION	CALS
Hot	2 tsp	10
Hot Mustard	1 serv	18
Mandarin	1 serv	70
Soy	1 tbsp	16
Sweet & Sour	1 serv	60

PEI WEI ASIAN DINER
CHILDREN'S MENU SELECTIONS

FOOD	PORTION	CALS
Kid's Wei Honey Seared Chicken w/o Noodles or Rice	1 serv	290

FOOD	PORTION	CALS
Kid's Wei Lo Mein Chicken w/o Noodles or Rice	1 serv	180
Kid's Wei Teriyaki Chicken w/o Noodles or Rice	1 serv	240
DESSERTS		
Cookie Chocolate Chip	1	342
Cookie Fortune	1	30
MAIN MENU SELECTIONS		
Bowl w/ Brown Rice Japanese Teriyaki Beef	1 serv	580
Bowl w/ Brown Rice Japanese Teriyaki Chicken	1 serv	460
Bowl w/ Brown Rice Japanese Teriyaki Shrimp	1 serv	410
Bowl w/ Brown Rice Japanese Teriyaki Vegetables & Tofu	1 serv	410
Bowl w/ White Rice Japanese Teriyaki Beef	1 serv	560
Bowl w/ White Rice Japanese Teriyaki Chicken	1 serv	440
Bowl w/ White Rice Japanese Teriyaki Shrimp	1 serv	390
Bowl w/ White Rice Japanese Teriyaki Vegetables & Tofu	1 serv	390
Crispy Potstickers	4	130
Edamame	1 serv	156
Fried Rice Beef	1 serv	630
Fried Rice Chicken	1 serv	525
Fried Rice Shrimp	1 serv	475
Fried Rice Vegetable & Tofu	1 serv	440
Ginger Broccoli Beef	1 serv	450
Ginger Broccoli Chicken	1 serv	300
Ginger Broccoli Shrimp	1 serv	230
Ginger Broccoli Vegetables & Tofu	1 serv	170
Honey Seared Chicken	1 serv	420
Honey Seared Shrimp	1 serv	370
Hot & Sour Soup	1 cup	150
Lemon Pepper Beef	1 serv	550
Lemon Pepper Chicken	1 serv	440
Lemon Pepper Shrimp	1 serv	380
Lemon Pepper Vegetables & Tofu	1 serv	230
Mandarin Kung Pao Beef	1 serv	610
Mandarin Kung Pao Chicken	1 serv	450
Mandarin Kung Pao Shrimp	1 serv	400
Mandarin Kung Pao Vegetables & Tofu	1 serv	290

FOOD	PORTION	CALS
Minced Chicken w/ Cool Lettuce Wraps w/o Rice Sticks	1 serv	250
Mongolian Beef	1 serv	420
Mongolian Chicken	1 serv	280
Mongolian Shrimp	2 serv	210
Mongolian Vegetables & Tofu	2 serv	180
Noodles Dan Dan Chicken	1 serv	390
Noodles Lo Mein Beef	1 serv	570
Noodles Lo Mein Chicken	1 serv	460
Noodles Lo Mein Shrimp	1 serv	400
Noodles Lo Mein Vegetables & Tofu	1 serv	400
Noodles Thai Blazing Beef	1 serv	630
Noodles Thai Blazing Chicken	1 serv	520
Noodles Thai Blazing Shrimp	1 serv	482
Noodles Thai Blazing Vegetables & Tofu	1 serv	430
Noodles Egg	1 serv	210
Noodles Rice	1 serv	130
Orange Peel Beef	1 serv	660
Orange Peel Chicken	1 serv	520
Orange Peel Shrimp	1 serv	460
Orange Peel Vegetables & Tofu	1 serv	330
Pad Thai Beef	1 serv	670
Pad Thai Chicken	1 serv	560
Pad Thai Shrimp	1 serv	490
Pei Wei Spicy Beef	1 serv	480
Pei Wei Spicy Chicken	1 serv	330
Pei Wei Spicy Shrimp	1 serv	300
Rice Brown	1 serv	170
Rice Fried	1 serv	260
Rice Sticks	1 cup	130
Rice White	1 serv	200
Spicy Korean Beef	1 serv	490
Spicy Korean Chicken	1 serv	350
Spicy Korean Shrimp	1 serv	280
Spicy Korean Vegetables & Tofu	1 serv	240
Spring Rolls	2	90
Sweet & Sour Chicken	1 serv	440
Sweet & Sour Shrimp	1 serv	390
Thai Coconut Curry Beef	1 serv	550
Thai Coconut Curry Chicken	1 serv	380

FOOD	PORTION	CALS
Thai Coconut Curry Shrimp	1 serv	300
Thai Coconut Curry Vegetables & Tofu	1 serv	220
Thai Dynamite Chicken	1 serv	390
Thai Dynamite Shrimp	1 serv	280
Thai Dynamite Vegetables & Tofu	1 serv	220
Wontons Crab	4	190
SALAD DRESSINGS AND SAUCES		
Dressing Sesame Ginger	1 serv (2 oz)	170
Lime Vinaigrette	1 serv (2 oz)	230
Sauce Lettuce Wrap	1 serv (2 oz)	70
Sauce Sweet Chili	1 serv (2 oz)	140
Sauce Thai Peanut	1 serv (2 oz)	168
SALADS		
Asian Chopped Chicken w/ Dressing	1 serv	280
Asian Chopped Chicken w/o Dressing	1 serv	200
Pei Wei Spicy Chicken w/ Dressing	1 serv	350
Pei Wei Spicy Chicken w/o Dressing	1 serv	210
Vietnamese Chicken Salad Rolls	3	53

PINKBERRY

FOOD	PORTION	CALS
Frozen Yogurt Coffee	½ cup	90
Frozen Yogurt Green Tea	½ cup	50
Frozen Yogurt Original	½ cup	70

PIZZA HUT

FOOD	PORTION	CALS
APPETIZERS		
Breadstick	1	150
Breadstick Cheese	1	200
Hot Wings	2 pieces	110
Mild Wings	2 pieces	110
BEVERAGES		
Diet Pepsi	1 med (14 oz)	0
Mt. Dew	1 med (14 oz)	190
Pepsi	1 med (14 oz)	180
DESSERTS		
Apple Pizza	1 slice	260
Cherry Pizza	1 slice	240
Cinnamon Sticks	2	170
PIZZA		
Fit 'N Delicious Diced Chicken Mushroom Jalapeno	1 med slice	170

FOOD	PORTION	CALS
Fit 'N Delicious Diced Chicken Red Onion Green Pepper	1 med slice	170
Fit 'N Delicious Diced Red Tomato Mushroom Jalapeno	1 med slice	150
Fit 'N Delicious Green Pepper Red Onion Diced Red Tomato	1 med slice	150
Fit 'N Delicious Ham Pineapple Diced Red Tomato	1 med slice	160
Fit 'N Delicious Ham Red Onion Mushroom	1 med slice	160
Hand Tossed Cheese	1 med slice	240
Hand Tossed Chicken Supreme	1 med slice	230
Hand Tossed Ham	1 med slice	220
Hand Tossed Meat Lover's	1 med slice	300
Hand Tossed Pepperoni	1 med slice	250
Hand Tossed Pepperoni Lover's	1 med slice	300
Hand Tossed Super Supreme	1 med slice	300
Hand Tossed Supreme	1 med slice	270
Hand Tossed Veggie Lover's	1 med slice	220
Pan Cheese	1 med slice	280
Pan Chicken Supreme	1 med slice	280
Pan Ham	1 med slice	260
Pan Meat Lover's	1 med slice	340
Pan Pepperoni	1 med slice	290
Pan Pepperoni Lover's	1 med slice	340
Pan Super Supreme	1 med slice	340
Pan Supreme	1 med slice	320
Pan Veggie Lover's	1 med slice	260
Personal Pan Cheese	1 pie	630
Personal Pan Chicken Supreme	1 pie	620
Personal Pan Meat Lover's	1 pie	800
Personal Pan Pepperoni	1 pie	660
Personal Pan Pepperoni Lover's	1 pie	800
Personal Pan Super Supreme	1 pie	790
Personal Pan Supreme	1 pie	750
Personal Pan Veggie Lover's	1 pie	580
Stuffed Crust Cheese	1 lg slice	360
Stuffed Crust Chicken Supreme	1 lg slice	380
Stuffed Crust Ham	1 lg slice	
Stuffed Crust Meat Lover's	1 lg slice	
Stuffed Crust Pepperoni	1 lg	

FOOD	PORTION	CALS
Stuffed Crust Pepperoni Lover's	1 lg slice	420
Stuffed Crust Super Supreme	1 lg slice	440
Stuffed Crust Supreme	1 lg slice	400
Stuffed Crust Veggie Lover's	1 lg slice	360
Thin'N Crispy Cheese	1 med slice	200
Thin'N Crispy Chicken Supreme	1 med slice	200
Thin'N Crispy Ham	1 med slice	180
Thin'N Crispy Meat Lover's	1 med slice	270
Thin'N Crispy Pepperoni	1 med slice	210
Thin'N Crispy Pepperoni Lover's	1 med slice	260
Thin'N Crispy Super Supreme	1 med slice	260
Thin'N Crispy Veggie Lover's	1 med slice	180
XL Full House Cheese	1 slice	280
XL Full House Chicken Supreme	1 slice	270
XL Full House Ham	1 slice	260
XL Full House Meat Lover's	1 slice	380
XL Full House Pepperoni	1 slice	290
XL Full House Pepperoni Lover's	1 slice	310
XL Full House Super Supreme	1 slice	330
XL Full House Supreme	1 slice	310
XL Full House Veggie Lover's	1 slice	280
SALAD DRESSINGS AND SAUCES		
Dipping Cup White Icing	1 serv	170
Dipping Sauce Breadstick	1 serv	45
Dipping Sauce Wing Blue Cheese	1 serv	230
Dipping Sauce Wing Ranch	1 serv	210
Dressing Caesar	2 tbsp	150
Dressing French	2 tbsp	140
Dressing Italian	2 tbsp	140
Dressing Ranch	2 tbsp	100
Dressing Thousand Island	2 tbsp	110
Dressing Lite Italian	2 tbsp	60
Dressing Lite Ranch	1 tbsp	70

POLLO TROPICAL
DESSERTS

Flan	1 serv (4 oz)	390
Key Lime	1 serv (3.9 oz)	210
Tres Leches	1 serv (5.4 oz)	410
MAIN MENU SELECTIONS		
Balsamic Tomato	1 combo	88

FOOD	PORTION	CALS
Balsamic Tomato	1 sm	176
Bananas Tropical	1 serv	437
Beef Skewers	1 (1 oz)	77
Black Beans	1 combo	90
Black Beans	1 sm	203
Boiled Yuca	1 combo	188
Boiled Yuca	1 sm	251
Caesar Salad	1 combo	130
Caesar Salad	1 sm	207
Chicken Boneless Breast	2 pieces	240
Chicken ¼ Dark Meat	1 serv	291
Chicken ¼ Dark Meat No Skin	1 serv	191
Chicken ¼ White Meat	1 serv	323
Chicken ¼ White Meat No Skin	1 serv	204
Chicken Caesar Salad	1 serv	669
Corn	1 combo	121
French Fries	1 sm	311
Ribs	¼ rack (2 oz)	200
Ribs	½ rack (4 oz)	400
Roast Pork	1 serv	392
Sandwich Chicken Caesar	1	881
Sandwich Grilled Chicken	1	827
Sandwich Roast Pork	1	773
Steak & Chicken Dark Meat	1 serv	437
TropiChop Chicken w/ Yellow Rice & Vegetables	1 serv	341
TropiChop Chicken w/ White Rice & Black Beans	1 serv	564
TropiChop Grilled Chicken Deluxe	1 serv	409
TropiChop Pork w/ White Rice & Black Beans	1 serv	714
TropiChop Pork w/ Yellow Rice & Vegetables	1 serv	480
TropiChop Ropa Vieja	1 serv	618
TropiChop Shrimp Creole	1 serv	506
TropiChop Vegetarian	1 serv	580
TropiChop Max Chicken w/ Yellow Rice & Vegetables	1 serv	864
TropiChop Max Chicken w/ White Rice & Black Beans	1 serv	1117
TropiChop Max Grilled Chicken Deluxe	1 serv	753

FOOD	PORTION	CALS
TropiChop Max Pork w/ White Rice & Black Beans	1 serv	1273
TropiChop Max Pork w/ Yellow Rice & Vegetables	1 serv	1020
TropiChop Max Ropa Vieja	1 serv	1160
TropiChop Max Shrimp Creole	1 serv	102
TropiChop Max Vegetarian	1 serv	950
White Rice	1 combo	203
White Rice	1 sm	339
Wrap Chicken Caesar	1	901
Wrap Chicken Classic	1	694
Wrap Curry Chicken	1	930
Wrap Steak	1	993
Yellow Rice w/ Vegetables	1 sm	245
Yellow Rice w/ Vegetables	1 combo	163
Yucatan Fries	1 serv	497
SALAD DRESSINGS AND SAUCES		
BBQ Sauce	1 serv (1.8 oz)	83
BBQ Sauce Guava	1 serv (1.8 oz)	83
Dressing Caesar	1 serv (1 oz)	161
Guacamole Sauce	1 serv (1.8 oz)	75
Mojo Sauce	1 serv (0.9 oz)	97
Mustard Curry Sauce	1 serv (1.8 oz)	265
Salsa	1 serv (1.8 oz)	8
SOUPS		
Caribbean Chicken	1 sm (8 oz)	121
Tropical Shrimp	1 sm (8 oz)	134
POPEYE'S		
Buttermilk Biscuit	1	240
Cajun Rice	1 reg	180
Coleslaw	1 serv	230
Collard Greens	1 serv	50
Corn On The Cob	1	220
Etouffee Chicken	1 serv	223
Etouffee Crawfish	1 serv	200
French Fries	1 serv	261
Fried Catfish	1 serv	300
Fried Crawfish	1 serv	370
Green Beans	1 serv	40
Jambalaya Chicken Sausage	1 serv	257

FOOD	PORTION	CALS
Mashed Potatoes & Gravy	1 serv	120
Mashed Potatoes w/o Gravy	1 serv	100
Mild Breast	1	510
Mild Breast Skinless	1	280
Mild Leg	1	200
Mild Leg Skinless	1	110
Mild Strips	2	280
Mild Strips w/o Breading	2	200
Mild Thigh	1	390
Mild Thigh Skinless	1	210
Mild Wing	1	220
Mild Wing Skinless	1	130
Naked Chicken Strips	3	170
Popcorn Shrimp	1 serv	280
Red Beans & Rice	1 reg	340
Sandwich Catfish Fully Dressed	1	640
Sandwich Deluxe Tame w/ Mayo	1	728
Sandwich Deluxe Tame w/o Mayo	1	530
Sandwich Shrimp Fully Dressed	1	740
Smothered Chicken	1 serv	210
Spicy Breast	1	530
Spicy Breast Skinless	1	290
Spicy Leg	1	190
Spicy Leg Skinless	1	120
Spicy Strips	2	310
Spicy Strips w/o Breading	2	190
Spicy Thigh	1	390
Spicy Thigh Skinless	1	200
Spicy Wing	1	220
Spicy Wing Skinless	1	140
Turnover Cinnamon Apple	1	250

PRETZELMAKER

Bites	1 sm (5.3 oz)	450
Bites	1 med (7.4 oz)	640
Bites Cinnamon Sugar	1 serv (5.8 oz)	520
Breezer Coffee	1 (20 oz)	640
Breezer Mocha	1 (20 oz)	620
Breezer Peach	1 (20 oz)	650
Breezer Raspberry	1 (20 oz)	650
Breezer Strawberry Banana	1 (20 oz)	650

FOOD	PORTION	CALS
Carmel Nut	1 (4.5 oz)	390
Cinnamon Sugar	1 (4.3 oz)	370
Cream Cheese	1 serv (1.5 oz)	200
Diet Coke	1 sm (20 oz)	0
Garlic	1 (4.1 oz)	350
Icing Cream Cheese	1 serv (1.5 oz)	180
Ketchup	2 pkg (0.6 oz)	20
Lemonade	1 sm (20 oz)	160
Mustard	2 pkg (0.4 oz)	5
Original	1 (4 oz)	340
Parmesan	1 (4.2 oz)	360
Plain	1 (4 oz)	209
PT Pretzel Dog	1 (6 oz)	440
Ranch	1 (4.1 oz)	240
Sauce Caramel	1 serv (1.5 oz)	140
Sauce Cheddar Cheese	1 serv (1.5 oz)	70
Sauce Nacho Cheese	1 serv (1.5 oz)	80
Sauce Pizza	1 serv (1.5 oz)	30

QUIZNO'S
COOKIES
Dark Chocolate Chunk	1	380
Double Chocolate Chip	1	370
Oatmeal Raisin	1	340
Snickerdoodle	1	400

SANDWICHES
Breakfast Bacon Egg Cheddar	1	380
Breakfast Black Angus Steak & Cheddar	1 sm	330
Breakfast Egg & Cheddar	1	240
Breakfast Garden Vegetable Cheddar	1	250
Breakfast Ham Egg Cheddar	1	290
Deli Honey Ham & Swiss	1	260
Deli Oven Roasted Turkey & Cheese	1	250
Deli Roast Beef & Cheddar	1	230
Deli Tuna Melt	1	500
Sammie Alpine Chicken	1	200
Sammie Balsamic Chicken	1	170
Sammie Bistro Steak Melt	1	180
Sammie Black Angus Steak	1	180
Sammie Italiano	1	240
Sammie Sonoma Turkey	1	160

FOOD	PORTION	CALS
Sub Baja Chicken w/ Bacon	1 sm	320
Sub Black Angus Steak On Rosemary Parmesan	1 sm	380
Sub Chicken Carbonara w/ Bacon	1 sm	360
Sub Classic Club w/ Bacon	1 sm	320
Sub Classic Italian	1 sm	360
Sub Honey Bacon Club	1 sm	320
Sub Honey Bourbon Chicken	1 sm	260
Sub Honey Mustard Chicken w/ Bacon	1 sm	330
Sub Mesquite Chicken w/ Bacon	1 sm	330
Sub Prime Rib Cheesesteak	1 sm	360
Sub Prime Rib & Peppercorn	1 sm	380
Sub Steakhouse Beef Dip	1 sm	260
Sub The Traditional	1 sm	260
Sub Turkey Bacon Guacamole	1 sm	360
Sub Turkey Ranch & Swiss	1 sm	250
Sub Tuscan Turkey On Rosemary Parmesan	1 sm	300
Sub Veggie	1 sm	270
SOUPS		
Bread Bowl Chili	1 serv	730
Bread Bowl Country French	1 serv	720
Broccoli Cheese	1 cup	150
Chicken Noodle	1 cup	130
Chili	1 cup	140

RANCH 1
BEVERAGES

FOOD	PORTION	CALS
Barq's Root Beer	1 sm (16 oz)	167
Coca-Cola	1 sm (16 oz)	150
Diet Coke	1 sm (16 oz)	2
Sprite	1 sm (16 oz)	150
CHILDREN'S MENU SELECTIONS		
Kids Meal Chicken Tenders	1 (2 oz)	111
Kids Meal Fries	1 serv (4 oz)	279
Kids Meal Popcorn Chicken	1 (2 oz)	112
MAIN MENU SELECTIONS		
Bowl Chicken Teriyaki	1 (19.3 oz)	504
Chicken Crispy	1 serv (5 oz)	326
Chicken Grilled	1 serv (3.9 oz)	146
Chicken On Mixed Greens	1 serv (21 oz)	340
Chicken Popcorn	1 serv (5.5 oz)	325

FOOD	PORTION	CALS
Chicken Tenders	1 serv (5.6 oz)	387
Fajita Mix Tomtoes Onion & Carrot	1 serv (3.2 oz)	20
Fajitas Chicken	1 serv (10 oz)	540
Fries	1 med	381
Fries Cheese	1 reg	493
Green Mix For Sandwiches	1 serv (2.5 oz)	31
Peppers & Onions	1 serv (1.6 oz)	27
Platter Chicken Rice	1 (10.9 oz)	273
Popcorn Chicken	1 sm	325
Rice	1 serv (4 oz)	97
Sandwich Chicken & Cheese	1 (11.2 oz)	389
Sandwich Chicken Philly	1 (9.2 oz)	410
Sandwich Crispy Chicken	1 (11.4 oz)	711
Sandwich Crispy Spicy Chicken	1 (11.4 oz)	543
Sandwich Grilled Spicy Chicken	1 (10.3 oz)	363
Sandwich Ranch 1 Classic	1 (9.4 oz)	683
Streamed Vegetables	1 serv (3 oz)	27
Wrap Grilled Chicken Caesar	1 (13.2 oz)	746
SALAD DRESSINGS AND SAUCES		
Dressing Balsamic Vinaigrette	1 oz	71
Dressing Classic Caesar	1 oz	103
Dressing Salad	1 oz	201
Sauce Ancho Chili Pepper	1 oz	134
Sauce BBQ	1 oz	84
Sauce Honey Mustard	1 oz	110
Sauce Pepper & Onion Saute	1 oz	143
Sauce Roasted Red Pepper	1 oz	232
Sauce Teriyaki	1 oz	24
SALADS		
Caesar	1 (7 oz)	34
Caesar Grilled Chicken	1 (11.3 oz)	223
Crispy Chicken Club	1 (13.6 oz)	495
Mandarin Chicken	1 (14.5 oz)	553
Mixed Greens w/o Cheese	1 (17 oz)	194
Salad Blend	1 serv (10.3 oz)	45
Southwest Chicken Chop	1 (17.6 oz)	681
RED MANGO		
Blenders Blueberry Moon	1 cup	150
Blenders Captain Berry	1 cup	140
Blenders Green Tea Blueberry	1 cup	130

FOOD	PORTION	CALS
Blenders Green Tea Honeydew	1 cup	130
Blenders Mango Island	1 cup	150
Blenders Pina Colada	1 cup	160
Blenders Tri-Berry	1 cup	130
Blenders Watermelon Breeze	1 cup	130
Frozen Yogurt All Flavors	½ cup	90

RITA'S

FOOD	PORTION	CALS
Cream Ice	1 reg	312
Cream Ice Kids	1 serv	193
Custard	1 reg	385
Custard Kids	1 serv	285
Gelati w/ Chocolate Custard	1 reg	351
Gelati w/ Cream Ice w/ Chocolate Custard	1 reg	368
Gelati w/ Cream Ice w/ Vanilla Custard	1 reg	392
Gelati w/ Vanilla Custard	1 reg	120
Ice	1 reg	263
Ice Kids	1 serv	165
Misto w/ Chocolate Custard	1 reg	409
Misto w/ Cream Ice w/ Chocolate Custard	1 reg	463
Misto w/ Cream Ice w/ Vanilla Custard	1 reg	473
Misto w/ Vanilla Custard	1 reg	420
Sugar Free Gelati w/ Chocolate Custard	1 reg	268
Sugar Free Gelati w/ Vanilla Custard	1 reg	288
Sugar Free Ice	1 reg	160
Sugar Free Ice Kids	1 serv	63
Sugar Free Misto w/ Chocolate Custard	1 reg	233
Sugar Free Misto w/ Vanilla Custard	1 reg	245

ROBEKS
FREEZES AND SHAKES

FOOD	PORTION	CALS
800 Lb Gorilla	12 oz	375
Freeze Lemon	12 oz	279
Freeze Orange	12 oz	242
Shake Bananasplit	12 oz	302
Shake P-Nut Power	12 oz	422

SMOOTHIES

FOOD	PORTION	CALS
Acai Energizer	12 oz	167
Awesome Acai	12 oz	183
Banzai Blueberry	12 oz	175
Berry Brilliance	12 oz	194

FOOD	PORTION	CALS
Big Wednesday	12 oz	172
Cardio Cooler	12 oz	215
Citrus Stinger	12 oz	194
Cranberry Quest	12 oz	173
Dr. Robeks	12 oz	181
Guava Lava	12 oz	180
Hummingbird	12 oz	185
Infinite Orange	12 oz	181
Mahalo Mango	12 oz	174
Malibu Peach	12 oz	153
Outrageous Raspberry	12 oz	174
Passionfruit Cove	12 oz	168
Pina Koolada	12 oz	261
Polar Pineapple	12 oz	164
Pomegranate Passion	12 oz	196
Pomegranate Power	12 oz	211
Pro Arobek	12 oz	265
Raspberry Romance	12 oz	172
Robeks MuscleMax	12 oz	202
Robeks Rejuvenator	12 oz	193
South Pacific Squeeze	12 oz	188
Strawnana Berry	12 oz	179
Venice Burner	12 oz	231
Zen Berry	12 oz	190

SALADWORKS
SALAD DRESSINGS

FOOD	PORTION	CALS
Balsamic Vinaigrette	1 serv (2 oz)	192
Blue Cheese	1 serv (2 oz)	192
Creamy Italian	1 serv (2 oz)	232
Dijon Honey	1 serv	272
Fat Free Balsamic w/ Sundried Tomatoes	1 serv (2 oz)	28
French	1 serv (2 oz)	266
Herbal Ranch	1 serv (2 oz)	198
Italian Vinaigrette	1 serv (2 oz)	255
Lowfat Ranch	1 serv (2 oz)	34
Oriental Sesame	1 serv (2 oz)	147
Royal Caesar	1 serv (2 oz)	266
Russian	1 serv (2 oz)	221

SALADS

FOOD	PORTION	CALS
B.L.T.	1 serv	262

FOOD	PORTION	CALS
Bently	1 serv	340
Caesar	1 serv	283
Caesar Chicken	1 serv	423
Caesar Shrimp	1 serv	350
Fiesta	1 serv	460
Garden	1 serv	58
Mandarin Chicken	1 serv	589
Newport	1 serv	184
Nicoise	1 serv	407
Spinach	1 serv	433
Tivoli	1 serv	563
Turkey Club	1 serv	720

SAMURAI SAM'S
BOWLS

FOOD	PORTION	CALS
Low Carb	1 reg	230
Spicy Beef 'N Broccoli	1 reg	620
Spicy Beef 'N Broccoli Brown Rice	1 reg	580
Sumo Brown Rice	1	1022
Sumo White Rice	1	1083
Sweet & Sour Dark Chicken	1 reg	610
Sweet & Sour Dark Chicken Brown Rice	1 reg	570
Sweet & Sour White Chicken	1 reg	580
Sweet & Sour White Chicken Brown Rice	1 reg	540
Teriyaki Dark Chicken	1 reg	540
Teriyaki Dark Chicken Brown Rice	1 reg	500
Teriyaki Dark Chicken & Shrimp	1 reg	492
Teriyaki Dark Chicken & Shrimp Brown Rice	1 reg	451
Teriyaki Dark Chicken & Steak	1 reg	540
Teriyaki Dark Chicken & Steak Brown Rice	1 reg	490
Teriyaki Salmon	1	643
Teriyaki Shrimp Brown Rice	1 reg	407
Teriyaki Steak	1 reg	530
Teriyaki Steak & Shrimp	1 reg	483
Teriyaki Steak & Shrimp Brown Rice	1 reg	442
Teriyaki Steak Brown Rice	1 reg	490
Teriyaki Veggie	1 reg	363
Teriyaki Veggie Brown Rice	1 reg	323
Teriyaki White Chicken	1 reg	520
Teriyaki White Chicken Brown Rice	1 reg	470
Teriyaki White Chicken & Shrimp	1 reg	478

FOOD	PORTION	CALS
Teriyaki White Chicken & Shrimp Brown Rice	1 reg	437
Teriyaki White Chicken & Steak	1 reg	520
Teriyaki White Chicken & Steak Brown Rice	1 reg	480
Yakisoba Dark Chicken	1	842
Yakisoba Dark Chicken & Steak	1	825
Yakisoba Shrimp	1	677
Yakisoba Steak	1	809
Yakisoba Veggie	1	509
Yakisoba White Chicken	1	794
Yakisoba White Chicken & Steak	1	801
SALADS AND SIDES		
Crab Rangoon	1 serv	210
Dressing Chinese	1 serv (3.5 oz)	230
Dressing Chinese Ginger	1 serv (1 oz)	85
Dressing Oriental	1 serv (1 oz)	70
Egg Roll Grilled Chicken	1	150
Salad Oriental Chicken	1 serv	220
Salad Side	1	10
Salad Toss Sesame Chicken	1	490
Soup Asian Noodle	1 serv	89
Teriyaki Sauce	1 serv (1 oz)	40
WRAPS		
Teriyaki Dark Chicken	1	670
Teriyaki Dark Chicken Brown Rice	1	650
Teriyaki Steak	1	650
Teriyaki Steak Brown Rice	1	630
Teriyaki Veggie	1	510
Teriyaki Veggie Brown Rice	1	490
Teriyaki White Chicken	1	640
Teriyaki White Chicken Brown Rice	1	620
Teriyaki White Chicken & Steak	1	649
Teriyaki White Chicken & Steak Brown Rice	1	628

SBARRO
DESSERTS

Black Forest Cake	1 serv (4.6 oz)	480
Deluxe Carrot Cake	1 serv (5 oz)	540
Deluxe Cheese Cake	1 serv (5.7 oz)	560
Deluxe Milk Chocolate Cake	1 serv (4.3 oz)	490
MAIN MENU SELECTIONS		
Baked Ziti w/ Sauce	1 serv (14 oz)	700

FOOD	PORTION	CALS
Calzone Cheese	1 (12 oz)	770
Chicken Francese	1 serv (11 oz)	640
Chicken Parmigiana	1 serv (11 oz)	520
Chicken Portofino	1 serv (12 oz)	730
Chicken Vesuvio	1 serv (11 oz)	690
Eggplant Rollatini w/ Cheese	1 serv (11 oz)	580
Garlic Roll	1 (2.2 oz)	170
Meat Lasagna	1 serv (13 oz)	650
Meatballs	1 serv (3.7 oz)	140
Mixed Vegetables	1 serv (7 oz)	190
Pasta Milano	1 serv (20 oz)	640
Pasta Rustica	1 serv (14 oz)	600
Penne Alla Vodka	1 serv (14 oz)	640
Penne w/ Sausage & Peppers	1 serv (14 oz)	710
Pizza Cheese	1 slice	460
Pizza Chicken Vegetable	1 slice	530
Pizza Fresh Tomato	1 slice	450
Pizza Mushroom	1 slice	460
Pizza Pepperoni	1 slice	730
Pizza Sausage	1 slice	670
Pizza Sauteed Spinach & Yellow Pepper	1 slice	670
Pizza Supreme	1 slice	630
Pizza White	1 slice	570
Pizza Gourmet Broccoli & Spinach	1 slice	720
Pizza Gourmet Cheese	1 slice	660
Pizza Gourmet Ham Pineapple & Bacon	1 slice	680
Pizza Gourmet Meat Delight	1 slice	780
Pizza Gourmet Mushroom	1 slice	610
Pizza Gourmet Mushroom & Spinach	1 slice	710
Pizza Gourmet Tomato & Basil	1 slice	700
Pizza Low Carb Cheese	1 slice	310
Pizza Low Carb Pepperoni	1 slice	420
Pizza Low Carb Sausage Pepperoni	1 slice	560
Pizza Stuffed Pepperoni	1 slice	960
Pizza Stuffed Philly Cheesesteak	1 slice	830
Pizza Stuffed Spinach & Broccoli	1 slice	790
Sausage & Peppers	1 serv (10 oz)	410
Spaghetti w/ Chicken Francese	1 serv (15 oz)	800
Spaghetti w/ Chicken Parmigiana	1 serv (15 oz)	930
Spaghetti w/ Chicken Vesuvio	1 serv (15 oz)	850

FOOD	PORTION	CALS
Spaghetti w/ Meatballs	1 serv (18 oz)	680
Spaghetti w/ Sauce	1 serv (20 oz)	820
Stromboli Pepperoni	1 (10 oz)	890
Stromboli Spinach Tomato Broccoli	1 (10 oz)	680
SALADS		
Caesar	1 serv (8 oz)	80
Cucumber & Tomato	1 serv (8 oz)	130
Fruit Salad	1 serv (12 oz)	130
Greek	1 serv (8 oz)	60
Mixed Garden	1 serv (8 oz)	35
Pasta Primavera	1 serv (8 oz)	190
Stringbean & Tomato	1 serv (8 oz)	100

SEASON 52

FOOD	PORTION	CALS
CHILDREN'S MENU SELECTIONS		
Children's Chicken	1 serv	344
Children's Flatbread	1	468
Children's Pasta	1 serv	177
DESSERTS		
Boston Cream Pie	1 serv	188
Carrot Cake	1 serv	320
Chocolate & Peanut Butter Harlequin	1 serv	330
Fresh Spring Fruit	1 serv	35
Key Lime Pie	1 serv	283
Pecan Pie	1 serv	263
Sorbet w/ Fruit	1 serv	213
Strawberry Mango Cheesecake	1 serv	226
Strawberry Shortcake	1 serv	154
Toasted Almond Amaretto	1 serv	324
FLATBREADS		
Artichoke & Goat Cheese	1	469
Garlic Chicken	1	474
Parmesan Crispbread	1	363
Spicy Shrimp	1	474
Steak & Mushroom	1	474
Tomato	1	460
MAIN MENU SELECTIONS		
Appetizer Goat Cheese Ravioli	1 serv	473
Appetizer Grilled Artichokes	1 serv	185
Appetizer Grilled Asparagus	1 serv	186
Appetizer Roasted Potato Wedges	1 serv	333

FOOD	PORTION	CALS
Appetizer Shrimp Cocktail	1 serv	221
Appetizer Shrimp Stuffed Mushrooms	1 serv	302
Appetizer Steak Skewers w/ Thai Salad	1 serv	438
Appetizer Steamed Mussels	1 serv	472
Cedar Salmon	1 serv	472
Chicken Boccone Pasta	1 serv	434
Chicken Breast	1 serv	403
Filet Mignon	1 serv	473
Grilled Rainbow Trout	1 serv	410
Grilled Scallops	1 serv	471
Pork Tenderloin	1 serv	392
Sandwich Chicken Breast	1	472
Sandwich Fresh Fish	1	437
Sandwich Grilled Steak	1	463
Sandwich Vegetable Stack	1	461
Shrimp Stuffed w/ Crab	1 serv	470
Soup Chicken Tortilla	1 serv (8 oz)	181
Soup Vegetable	1 serv (8 oz)	153
Spring Vegetable Plate	1 serv	465
Tuna w/o Soy Sauce	1 serv	175
Turkey Skewer	1 serv	404
Yellowfin Tuna	1 serv	466
SALADS		
Chicken Cobb	1 entree	474
Greek	1 entree	478
Mesclun Greens	1 side	315
Portobello & Romaine	1 entree	270
Salmon	1 entree	470
Spinach	1 side	272
Spring Greens	1 side	240
Tabbouleh	1 side	417
Tomato & Blue Cheese Stack	1 side	352
SIZZLER		
Grilled Salmon w/ Broccoli	1 serv	393
Hibachi Chicken w/ Broccoli	1 serv	290
Petite Steak w/ Broccoli	1 serv	520
SOUPER SALAD		
BEVERAGES		
Lemonade	1 (24 oz)	190

FOOD	PORTION	CALS
Lemonade Mango	1 (24 oz)	220
Lemonade Raspberry	1 (24 oz)	220
Lemonade Strawberry	1 (24 oz)	220
Smoothie Mango	1 tall	250
Smoothie Peach	1 tall	230
Smoothie Raspberry	1 tall	230
Smoothie Strawberry	1 tall	230
DESSERTS		
Blueberry Bread	1 piece	150
Brownies	2 pieces	120
Cornbread	1 piece	170
Cottage Cheese	½ cup	90
Gingerbread	1 piece	180
Peaches	½ cup	70
Pineapple Tidbits	¼ cup	60
Pudding Banana	½ cup	160
Pudding Chocolate	½ cup	170
Soft Serve Cone Chocolate	1	120
Soft Serve Cone Vanilla	1	120
Sponge Cake	4 pieces	80
Strawberry Parfait	½ cup	100
Vanilla Wafers	4	70
Whipped Topping	½ cup	100
PASTA AND PIZZA		
Chicken Alfredo	1 cup	320
Macaroni & Cheese	1 cup	380
Pizza Slice Cheese	1	70
Pizza Slice Garden	1	80
Pizza Slice Pepperoni	1	90
Pizza Slice Sausage	1	80
Spaghetti & Meatballs	1 cup	280
SALAD DRESSINGS AND SAUCES		
Balsamic Vinegar	1 oz	60
Bleu Cheese	2 oz	220
Caesar	2 oz	280
Chipotle Ranch	2 oz	280
Fat Free French	2 oz	60
Fat Free Italian w/ Cheese	2 oz	30
Green Goddess	2 oz	260
Honey Mustard	2 oz	240

FOOD	PORTION	CALS
Mayonnaise	2 tbsp	200
Olive Oil	1 oz	240
Peppercorn Ranch	2 oz	220
Pesto Basil	1 tbsp	45
Ranch	2 oz	220
Reduced Calorie Ranch	2 oz	120
Sauce Alfredo	1½ tbsp	45
Sauce Chipotle Pepper	¼ tsp	0
Sauce Cholula Hot	¼ tsp	0
Sauce Jalapeno Cheese	1 serv (2 oz)	35
Sauce Marinara	1½ tbsp	10
Sauce Meaty Marinara	1½ tbsp	40
Sauce Sriracha Hot	¼ tsp	0
Sour Cream Light	2 tbsp	40
Tangy Oriental	2 oz	160
Thousand Island	1 oz	300
Vinaigrette Cranberry	2 oz	100
Vinaigrette House	2 oz	220
SALADS		
Apple Walnut	1 cup	130
Asian Chicken	1 cup	80
Asian Shrimp	1 cup	100
Buffalo Chicken	1 cup	70
Caesar Shrimp	1 cup	90
Caesar Chicken	1 cup	90
Caesar Chicken Salsa	1 cup	80
California Chicken Salad	⅓ cup	80
Capri	1 cup	50
Chicago Chopped	1 cup	120
Chickpea	⅓ cup	110
Cobb	1 cup	100
Coleslaw Broccoli	⅓ cup	80
Edamame	⅓ cup	70
Fisherman's Kettle Shrimp & Crab	⅓ cup	120
Gazpacho	⅓ cup	30
Green Goddess Crab	1 cup	70
Italian Antipasto	1 cup	70
Mango Berry	1 cup	110
Marinated Mushrooms	⅓ cup	60
Marinated Oriental Cucumber	⅓ cup	10

FOOD	PORTION	CALS
Marinated Tomato	1 cup	60
Melon Couscous	⅓ cup	50
Mustard Potato	⅓ cup	80
Paco's Taco	⅓ cup	100
Pasta De Garden	⅓ cup	80
Pasta Fettuccine	⅓ cup	100
Pasta Primavera	⅓ cup	45
Pasta Thai Chicken	⅓ cup	100
Pasta Tuna Skroodle	⅓ cup	130
Red Potato	⅓ cup	50
Rice Florentine	⅓ cup	90
Roasted Mushrooms & Artichokes w/ Feta Cheese	⅓ cup	40
Roasted Vegetables	⅓ cup	20
Salad Of The Sea	⅓ cup	50
Salmon Medley	1 cup	70
Santa Fe Corn	⅓ cup	100
Shrimp & Crab Louie	1 cup	130
Southwest Chicken Chipotle	1 cup	90
Sweet Garden Slaw	⅓ cup	35
Tropical Tuxedo	⅓ cup	60
Tuna Fish	⅓ cup	70
SOUPS		
Adobe Rice & Chicken	1 (5 oz)	100
Alaskan Salmon Chowder	1 (5 oz)	70
Beef Mushroom Barley	1 (5 oz)	80
Beef Noodle	1 (5 oz)	80
Beef Shellini	1 (5 oz)	90
Beef Stroganoff	1 (5 oz)	120
Black Bean	1 (5 oz)	80
Broccoli Cheese	1 (5 oz)	70
Cajun Gumbo	1 (5 oz)	110
Cauliflower Cheese	1 (5 oz)	70
Cheddar Chicken Broccoli Stew	1 (5 oz)	140
Cherokee Joe Cornbread	1 (5 oz)	70
Chicken Creole	1 (5 oz)	100
Chicken Enchilada	1 (5 oz)	180
Chicken Gumbo	1 (5 oz)	90
Chicken Mushroom Barley	1 (5 oz)	80
Chicken Noodle	1 (5 oz)	80

FOOD	PORTION	CALS
Chicken Tetrazini	1 (5 oz)	120
Chicken Tortilla	1 (5 oz)	60
Cream Of Asparagus	1 (5 oz)	140
Cream Of Broccoli	1 (5 oz)	60
Cream Of Cauliflower	1 (5 oz)	60
Cream Of Chicken	1 (5 oz)	100
Cream Of Mushroom	1 (5 oz)	80
Holiday Harvest	1 (5 oz)	90
Vegan Split Pea	1 (5 oz)	90
Vegetable Beef	1 (5 oz)	80
Vegetable Cheese	1 (5 oz)	80
Vegetable Lentil	1 (5 oz)	70
Vegetarian Butter Bean	1 (5 oz)	70
Vegetarian Vegetable	1 (5 oz)	50

SOUTHERN TSUNAMI SUSHI BAR

SALADS

Calamari	1 serv (4 oz)	148
Edamame	1 serv (4 oz)	124
Harusame	1 serv (5 oz)	148
Seabreeze	1 serv (4 oz)	113

SUSHI

California Roll	1 (0.8 oz)	31
Cream Cheese Roll w/ Salmon	1 piece (0.8 oz)	43
Crunchy Shrimp Roll	1 piece (0.9 oz)	42
Dragon Roll	1 piece (0.8 oz)	42
Freshwater Eel Roll	1 piece (0.8 oz)	41
Green Horseradish	1 tsp	7
Inari	1 piece (1.9 oz)	105
Nigiri Cuttlefish	1 piece (1 oz)	42
Nigiri Egg Cake	1 piece (1.4 oz)	73
Nigiri Fish Roe	1 piece (1.4 oz)	61
Nigiri Fresh Salmon	1 piece (1.3 oz)	68
Nigiri Fresh Water Eel	1 piece (1.6 oz)	108
Nigiri Octopus	1 piece (1.1 oz)	57
Nigiri Sea Eel	1 piece (1.6 oz)	90
Nigiri Shrimp	1 piece (1.1 oz)	44
Nigiri Smoked Salmon	1 piece (1.3 oz)	68
Nigiri Tilapia	1 piece (1.2 oz)	49
Nigiri Tuna	1 piece (1.3 oz)	60
Nigiri Yellowtail	1 piece (1.2 oz)	54

FOOD	PORTION	CALS
Ocean Crab Roll	1 piece (0.8 oz)	33
Orange Roll	1 piece (0.8 oz)	32
Pickled Ginger	1 tbsp	9
Rainbow Roll	1 piece (1 oz)	41
Sea Eel Roll	1 piece (0.8 oz)	36
Soy Sauce	1 pkg	16
Spicy Roll Salmon	1 piece (0.8 oz)	40
Spicy Roll Shrimp	1 piece (0.8 oz)	31
Spicy Roll Tuna	1 piece (0.8 oz)	37
Tempura Roll	1 piece (0.9 oz)	44
Tofu Roll	1 piece (0.8 oz)	27
Tsunami Roll Crab & Fish Roe	1 piece (0.8 oz)	39

STARBUCKS
BAKED SELECTIONS

FOOD	PORTION	CALS
Apple Fritter	1	480
Bagel French Toast	1	280
Bagel Multigrain	1	280
Bagel Plain	1	280
Bar Cranberry Bliss	1	320
Bar Toffee Almond	1	400
Brownie Espresso	1	340
Cinnamon Roll	1	470
Cocoa Crispy Square	1	420
Cookie Chocolate Chunk	1	420
Cookie Coffee Ginger	1	470
Cookie Penguin	1	370
Cookie Rainbow	1	420
Cookies Mini Black & White	2	240
Croissant Butter	1	370
Dougnut Glazed	1	490
Loaf Banana Nut	1 serv	470
Loaf Iced Lemon	1 serv	500
Loaf Marble	1 serv	410
Loaf Pumpkin	1 serv	380
Mallorca Sweet Bread	1	420
Muffin Blueberry	1	310
Muffin Pumpkin Cream Cheese	1	490
Muffin Reduced Fat Chocolate	1	290
Muffin Walnut Bran	1	430

FOOD	PORTION	CALS
Reduced Fat Coffee Cake Banana Chocolate Chip	1	390
Reduced Fat Coffee Cake Blueberry	1 serv	320
Reduced Fat Coffee Cake Cinnamon Swirl	1 serv	290
Reduced Fat Coffee Cake Pumpkin Chocolate Chip	1	300
Rustic Apple Tart	1	190
Scone Blueberry	1	480
Scone Cran Apple Crumb	1	490
Scone Raspberry	1	470
BEVERAGES		
Apple Juice	1 grande	250
Cafe Americano	1 grande	15
Cafe Au Lait Nonfat Milk	1 grande	70
Caffe Mocha No Whip Nonfat Milk	1 grande	220
Caffe Mocha Whip Nonfat Milk	1 grande	290
Cappuccino Nonfat Milk	1 grande	80
Caramel Apple Cider Whip	1 grande	380
Caramel Apple Spice No Whip	1 grande	310
Caramel Macchiato Nonfat Milk	1 grande	190
Chocolate Milk Nonfat	1 grande	280
Cinnamon Dolce Creme No Whip Nonfat Milk	1 grande	220
Cinnamon Dolce Whip Nonfat Milk	1 grande	290
Coffee Of The Week	1 grande	5
Coffee Of The Week Decafe	1 grande	5
Frappuccino Blended Coffee Cafe Vanilla Whip Nonfat Milk	1 grande	430
Frappuccino Blended Coffee Cafe Vanilla No Whip Soy	1 grande	310
Frappuccino Blended Coffee Cafe Vanilla Whip Soy	1 grande	430
Frappuccino Blended Coffee Cafe Vanilla No Whip Nonfat Milk	1 grande	310
Frappuccino Blended Coffee Caramel No Whip Nonfat Milk	1 grande	270
Frappuccino Blended Coffee Caramel No Whip Soy	1 grande	270
Frappuccino Blended Coffee Caramel Whip Soy	1 grande	380

FOOD	PORTION	CALS
Frappuccino Blended Coffee Cinnamon Dolce No Whip Nonfat Milk	1 grande	260
Frappuccino Blended Coffee Cinnamon Dolce No Whip Soy	1 grande	260
Frappuccino Blended Coffee Cinnamon Dolce Whip Soy	1 grande	370
Frappuccino Blended Coffee Coffee Whip Nonfat Milk	1 grande	380
Frappuccino Blended Coffee Espresso Nonfat Milk	1 grande	190
Frappuccino Blended Coffee Java Chip No Whip Nonfat Milk	1 grande	340
Frappuccino Blended Coffee Java Chip No Whip Soy	1 grande	190
Frappuccino Blended Coffee Java Chip Whip Nonfat Milk	1 grande	460
Frappuccino Blended Coffee Java Chip Whip Soy	1 grande	460
Frappuccino Blended Coffee Mocha No Whip Nonfat Milk	1 grande	260
Frappuccino Blended Coffee Mocha No Whip Soy	1 grande	260
Frappuccino Blended Coffee Mocha Whip Nonfat Milk	1 grande	380
Frappuccino Blended Coffee Pumpkin Spice No Whip Nonfat Milk	1 grande	290
Frappuccino Blended Coffee Pumpkin Spice No Whip Soy	1 grande	290
Frappuccino Blended Coffee Pumpkin Spice Whip Nonfat Milk	1 grande	400
Frappuccino Blended Coffee Pumpkin Spice Whip Soy	1 grande	400
Frappuccino Blended Coffee Whip Nonfat Milk	1 grande	370
Frappuccino Blended Coffee White Chocolate Mocha No Whip Nonfat Milk	1 grande	300
Frappuccino Blended Coffee White Chocolate Mocha No Whip Soy	1 grande	300
Frappuccino Blended Coffee White Chocolate Mocha Whip Nonfat Milk	1 grande	410

FOOD	PORTION	CALS
Frappuccino Blended Coffee White Chocolate Mocha Whip Soy	1 grande	410
Frappuccino Blended Creme Tazo Chai No Whip Nonfat Milk	1 grande	330
Frappuccino Blended Creme Tazo Chai Whip Nonfat Milk	1 grande	570
Frappuccino Blended Creme Vanilla Bean No Whip Nonfat Milk	1 grande	350
Frappuccino Blended Creme Vanilla Bean Whip Nonfat Milk	1 grande	470
Frappuccino Light Blended Coffee Cafe Vanilla Nonfat Milk	1 grande	190
Frappuccino Light Blended Coffee Caramel	1 grande	160
Frappuccino Light Blended Coffee Cinnamon Dolce Nonfat Milk	1 grande	140
Frappuccino Light Blended Coffee Java Chip Nonfat Milk	1 grande	200
Frappuccino Light Blended Coffee Mocha Nonfat Milk	1 grande	140
Frappuccino Light Blended Coffee Nonfat Milk	1 grande	130
Frappuccino Light Blended Coffee Pumpkin Spice Nonfat Milk	1 grande	150
Frappuccino Light Blended Creme Double Chocolaty Chip Whip Nonfat Milk	1 grande	510
Frappuccino Light Blended Creme Pumpkin Spice No Whip Nonfat Milk	1 grande	360
Frappuccino Light Blended Creme Pumpkin Spice Whip Nonfat Milk	1 grande	470
Frappuccino Light Blended Creme Tazo Green Tea No Whip Nonfat Milk	1 grande	380
Frappuccino Light Blended Creme Tazo Green Tea Whip Nonfat Milk	1 grande	490
Frappuccino Light Blended Creme White Chocolate No Whip Nonfat Milk	1 grande	480
Frappuccino Light Blended Creme White Chocolate Whip Nonfat Milk	1 grande	610
Frappuccino Light Espresso Nonfat Milk	1 grande	110
Hot Chocolate No Whip Nonfat Milk	1 grande	240
Hot Chocolate Whip Nonfat Milk	1 grande	320

FOOD	PORTION	CALS
Iced Brewed Coffee	1 grande	90
Iced Cafe Mocha Whip Nonfat Milk	1 grande	290
Iced Caffe Americano	1 grande	15
Iced Caffe Latte Nonfat Milk	1 grande	90
Iced Caffe Mocha No Whip Nonfat Milk	1 grande	170
Iced Caramel Macchiato Nonfat Milk	1 grande	190
Iced Latte Pumpkin Spice No Whip Nonfat Milk	1 grande	220
Iced Latte Pumpkin Spice Whip Nonfat Milk	1 grande	330
Iced Latte Skinny Cinnamon Dolce No Whip Nonfat Milk	1 grande	80
Iced Latte Sugar Free Flavored Syrup Nonfat Milk	1 grande	80
Iced Latte Syrup Flavored Nonfat Milk	1 grande	160
Iced Latte Vanilla Nonfat Milk	1 grande	160
Iced Peppermint White Chocolate Mocha No Whip Nonfat Milk	1 grande	370
Iced Peppermint White Chocolate Mocha Whip Nonfat Milk	1 grande	490
Iced Tazo Latte Black Tea Nonfat Milk	1 grande	170
Iced Tazo Latte Black Tea Soy	1 grande	200
Iced Tazo Latte Chai Nonfat Milk	1 grande	200
Iced Tazo Latte Green Tea Nonfat Milk	1 grande	220
Iced Tazo Latte Green Tea Soy	1 grande	260
Iced Tazo Latte Red Tea	1 grande	200
Iced Tazo Latte Red Tea Nonfat Milk	1 grande	170
Iced White Chocolate Mocha No Whip Nonfat Milk	1 grande	310
Iced White Chocolate Mocha Whip Nonfat Milk	1 grande	430
Latte Caffe Nonfat Milk	1 grande	130
Latte Cinnamon Dolce No Whip Nonfat Milk	1 grande	210
Latte Cinnamon Dolce w/ Sugar Free Syrup Nonfat Milk	1 grande	130
Latte Cinnamon Dolce Whip Nonfat Milk	1 grande	280
Latte Pumpkin Spice No Whip Nonfat Milk	1 grande	260
Latte Pumpkin Spice Whip Nonfat Milk	1 grande	330
Latte Skinny Caramel No Whip Nonfat Milk	1 grande	130
Latte Skinny Cinnamon Dolce No Whip Nonfat Milk	1 grande	130

FOOD	PORTION	CALS
Latte Skinny Hazelnut No Whip Nonfat Milk	1 grande	130
Latte Skinny Vanilla No Whip Nonfat Milk	1 grande	130
Latte Syrup Flavored Nonfat Milk	1 grande	200
Milk Nonfat	1 grande	180
Peppermint White Chocolate Mocha No Whip Nonfat Milk	1 grande	420
Peppermint White Chocolate Mocha Whip Nonfat Milk	1 grande	490
Pumpkin Spice Creme No Whip Nonfat Milk	1 grande	270
Pumpkin Spice Creme Whip Nonfat Milk	1 grande	340
Shaken Black Iced Tea & Lemonade	1 grande	130
Shaken White Iced Tea Blueberry	1 grande	80
Steamed Apple Juice	1 grande	230
Tazo Black Shaken Iced Tea & Lemonade	1 grande	130
Tazo Chai Latte Iced Tea Soy	1 grande	230
Tazo Chai Latte Nonfat Milk	1 grande	200
Tazo Chai Latte Soy	1 grande	230
Tazo Latte Black Tea Nonfat Milk	1 grande	170
Tazo Latte Black Tea Soy	1 grande	190
Tazo Latte Green Tea Nonfat Milk	1 grande	200
Tazo Latte Green Tea Soy	1 grande	220
Tazo Latte Red Tea Nonfat Milk	1 grande	170
Tazo Latte Red Tea Soy	1 grande	190
Tazo Shaken Iced Tea Green	1 grande	80
Tazo Shaken Iced Tea Green & Lemonade	1 grande	130
Tazo Shaken Iced Tea Orange Passion	1 grande	70
Tazo Shaken Iced Tea Passion	1 grande	80
Tazo Shaken Iced Tea Passion & Lemonade	1 grande	130
Tazo Tea	1 grande	0
Vanilla Creme No Whip Nonfat Milk	1 grande	200
Vanilla Creme Whip Nonfat Milk	1 grande	270
Vivanno Blend Banana Chocolate	1 grande (20 oz)	85
Vivanno Blend Organe Mango Banana	1 grande (20 oz)	250
White Chocolate Mocha No Whip Nonfat Milk	1 grande	360
White Chocolate Mocha Whip Nonfat Milk	1 grande	430
SALADS		
Fiesta	1 (9.4 oz)	320
Fruit & Cheese Plate	1 (8.6 oz)	400
Vegetable Vinaigrette	1 (10.7 oz)	310

FOOD	PORTION	CALS
SANDWICHES		
Club Chicken Cheddar Bacon w/ Mayo	1	480
Club Turkey & Avocado	1	390
Egg Salad On Multigrain	1	470
Turkey & Swiss w/ Mayo	1	310
TOPPINGS		
Caramel	1 tbsp	15
Chocolate	1 tsp	5
Flavored Sugar Free Syrup	1 pump	0
Flavored Syrup	1 pump	20
Mocha Syrup	1 pump	25
Sprinkles	1 serv	0
SUBWAY		
ADD-ONS AND SALAD DRESSINGS		
American Cheese	1 serv (0.4 oz)	40
Bacon Strips	2	45
Banana Pepper Slices	3	0
Cheddar	1 serv (0.5 oz)	60
Fat Free Italian	1 serv (2 oz)	35
Fat Free Red Wine Vinaigrette	1 serv (0.7 oz)	30
Jalapeno Pepper Slices	3	<5
Mayonnaise	1 tbsp	110
Mayonnaise Light	1 tbsp	50
Monterey Cheddar Shredded	1 serv (0.5 oz)	50
Mustard Yellow or Deli	2 tsp	5
Olive Oil Blend	1 tsp	45
Pepperjack Cheese	1 serv (0.5 oz)	50
Provolone	1 serv (0.5 oz)	50
Ranch	1.5 tbsp	120
Ranch	1 serv (2 oz)	320
Red Wine Vinaigrette	1 serv (2 oz)	80
Sauce Chipotle Southwest	1.5 tbsp	100
Sauce Fat Free Honey Mustard	1.5 tbsp	30
Sauce Fat Free Sweet Onion	1.5 tbsp	40
Swiss	1 serv (0.5 oz)	50
Vinegar	1 tsp	0
BREADS		
Hearty Italian	6 inch	220
Honey Oat	6 inch	250
Italian	6 inch	200

FOOD	PORTION	CALS
Italian Herb & Cheese	6 inch	250
Italian White	1 mini	140
Monterey Cheddar	6 inch	240
Parmesan Oregano	6 inch	220
Wheat	1 mini	140
Wheat	6 inch	200
Wrap	1	190
DESSERTS		
Apple Slices	1 pkg	35
Cookie Chocolate Chip	1	210
Cookie Chocolate Chip w/ M&M's	1 (1.6 oz)	210
Cookie Chocolate Chunk	1	220
Cookie Double Chocolate Chip	1 (1.6 oz)	210
Cookie Oatmeal Raisin	1	200
Cookie Peanut Butter	1	220
Cookie Sugar	1	220
Cookie White Chip Macadamia Nut	1	220
Raisins	1 pkg	150
SALADS		
Ham w/o Dressing & Croutons	1 serv	120
Oven Roasted Chicken Breast w/o Dressing & Croutons	1 serv	140
Roast Beef w/o Dressing & Croutons	1 serv	120
Subway Club w/o Dressing & Croutons	1 serv	150
Sweet Onion Chicken Teriyaki w/o Dressing & Croutons	1 serv	210
Turkey Breast	1 serv	110
Turkey Breast & Ham w/o Dressing & Croutons	1 serv	120
Veggie Delight w/o Dressing & Croutons	1 serv	60
SANDWICHES		
6 Inch Chicken & Bacon Ranch	1	580
6 Inch Cold Cut Combo	1	410
6 Inch Double Stacked Cold Cut Combo	1	550
6 Inch Double Stacked Italian BMT	1	630
6 Inch Double Stacked Steak & Cheese	1	540
6 Inch Double Stacked Subway Club	1	420
6 Inch Double Stacked Sweet Onion Chicken Teriyaki	1	480
6 Inch Double Stacked Turkey Breast	1	330
6 Inch Ham	1	290

FOOD	PORTION	CALS
6 Inch Italian BMT	1	450
6 Inch Meatball Marinara	1	560
6 Inch Oven Roasted Chicken Breast	1	310
6 Inch Roast Beef	1	290
6 Inch Spicy Italian	1	480
6 Inch Steak & Cheese	1	400
6 Inch Subway Club	1	320
6 Inch Subway Melt	1	380
6 Inch Sweet Onion Chicken Teriyaki	1	370
6 Inch Tuna	1	530
6 Inch Turkey Breast	1	280
6 Inch Turkey Breast & Ham	1	290
6 Inch Veggie Delite	1	230
Mini Sub Ham	1	180
Mini Sub Roast Beef	1	190
Mini Sub Tuna w/ Cheese	1	320
Mini Sub Turkey Breast	1	190
Softwich Santa Fe Turkey	1	520

TACO BELL

FOOD	PORTION	CALS
Border Bowl Southwest Steak	1 serv	600
Border Bowl Zesty Chicken	1 serv	640
Border Bowl Zesty Chicken w/o Dressing	1 serv	440
Burrito 7 Layer	1	490
Burrito Bean	1	350
Burrito Chili Cheese	1	370
Burrito Grilled Stuft Chicken	1	640
Burrito Supreme Beef	1	420
Burrito ½ Lb Beef & Potato	1	530
Burrito ½ Lb Combo Beef	1	440
Burrito Fiesta Chicken	1	360
Burrito Fiesta Steak	1	370
Burrito Stuft Grilled Steak	1	630
Burrito Supreme Chicken	1	400
Burrito Supreme Steak	1	390
Chalupa Baja Beef	1	410
Chalupa Baja Chicken	1	390
Chalupa Baja Steak	1	390
Chalupa Nacho Cheese Beef	1	370
Chalupa Nacho Cheese Chicken	1	360
Chalupa Nacho Cheese Steak	1	340

FOOD	PORTION	CALS
Chalupa Supreme Beef	1	380
Chalupa Supreme Chicken	1	360
Chalupa Supreme Steak	1	360
Cheesy Fiesta Potatoes	1 serv	290
Cinnamon Twists	1 serv	170
Crunchwrap Supreme	1	560
Crunchwrap Supreme Spicy Chicken	1	540
Crunchy Taco	1	170
Crunchy Taco Supreme	1	210
Empanada Caramel Apple	1	290
Enchirito Beef	1	360
Enchirito Chicken	1	340
Fresco Border Bowl Zesty Chicken w/o Dressing	1 serv	350
Fresco Burrito Bean	1	330
Fresco Burrito Fiesta Chicken	1	330
Fresco Burrito Supreme Chicken	1	330
Fresco Burrito Supreme Steak	1	330
Fresco Crunchy Taco	1	150
Fresco Soft Taco Beef	1	180
Fresco Soft Taco Grilled Steak	1	160
Fresco Soft Taco Ranchero Chicken	1	170
Gordita Baja Beef	1	340
Gordita Baja Chicken	1	320
Gordita Baja Steak	1	320
Gordita Nacho Cheese Beef	1	300
Gordita Nacho Cheese Chicken	1	280
Gordita Nacho Cheese Steak	1	270
Gordita Supreme Beef	1	310
Gordita Supreme Chicken	1	290
Gordita Supreme Steak	1	290
Guacamole Side	1 serv	70
Mexican Pizza	1	530
Mexican Rice	1 serv	180
MexiMelt	1 serv	260
Nacho Supreme	1 serv	440
Nachos	1 serv	330
Nachos Bellgrande	1 serv	770
Pintos 'n Cheese	1 serv	160
Quesadilla Cheese	1	470

FOOD	PORTION	CALS
Quesadilla Chicken	1	520
Quesadilla Steak	1	520
Salsa Side	1 serv	15
Soft Taco Grande	1	430
Soft Taco Grilled Steak	1	270
Soft Taco Ranchero Chicken	1	270
Soft Taco Supreme Beef	1	250
Sour Cream Side	1 serv	80
Taco Double Decker	1	320
Taco Double Decker Supreme	1	370
Taco Spicy Chicken	1	170
Taco Salad Express	1	610
Taco Salad Fiesta	1	840
Taco Salad Fiesta Chicken	1	790
Taco Salad Fiesta Chicken w/o Shell	1	430
Taco Salad Fiesta w/o Shell	1	470
Taquitos Grilled Chicken	1 serv	310
Taquitos Grilled Steak	1 serv	310
Tostada	1	240

TACO BUENO
MAIN MENU SELECTIONS

FOOD	PORTION	CALS
Bueno Chilada Beef	1 (7.9 oz)	523
Bueno Chilada Beef w/o Chili	1 (5.5 oz)	412
Bueno Chilada Beef w/o Queso	1 (5.6 oz)	337
Bueno Chilada Chicken	1 (7.4 oz)	477
Bueno Chilada Chicken w/o Chili	1 (5 oz)	366
Bueno Chilada Chicken w/o Queso	1 (5.1 oz)	290
Burrito Bean	1 (6.4 oz)	490
Burrito Bean w/o Cheddar Cheese	1 (5.9 oz)	412
Burrito Bean w/o Chili	1 (5.2 oz)	434
Burrito Beef	1 (6.9 oz)	510
Burrito Beef w/o Cheddar Cheese	1 (6.4 oz)	432
Burrito Beef w/o Chili	1 (5.7 oz)	455
Burrito Beef Potato	1 (4.8 oz)	350
Burrito Beef Potato w/o Queso	1 (4.1 oz)	305
Burrito Beef Potato w/o Sour Cream	1 (4.3 oz)	330
Burrito Big Ol' Beef	1 (10.6 oz)	772
Burrito Big Ol' Beef w/o Cheddar Cheese	1 (9.6 oz)	615
Burrito Big Ol' Beef w/o Chili	1 (9.4 oz)	716
Burrito Big Ol' Beef w/o Sour Cream	1 (9.6 oz)	715

FOOD	PORTION	CALS
Burrito Big Ol' Chicken	1 (8.4 oz)	607
Burrito Big Ol' Chicken w/o Cheddar Cheese	1 (7.4 oz)	450
Burrito Big Ol' Chicken w/o Sour Cream	1 (7.4 oz)	551
Burrito Chicken Potato	1 (4.5 oz)	327
Burrito Chicken Potato w/o Queso	1 (3.8 oz)	274
Burrito Chicken Potato w/o Sour Cream	1 (4 oz)	299
Burrito Combination	1 (6.8 oz)	507
Burrito Combination w/o Cheddar Cheese	1 (6.3 oz)	429
Burrito Combination w/o Chili	1 (5.6 oz)	452
Burrito Combination w/o Refried Beans	1 (5.7 oz)	440
Burrito Party	1 (4 oz)	298
Burrito Party w/o Cheddar Cheese	1 (3.8 oz)	259
Cheese Nachos	1 serv (5.5 oz)	572
Cheesecake Chimichanga	1 (2 oz)	210
Cinnamon Chips	1 serv (4.5 oz)	676
Corn Tortilla Chips	1 serv (1.5 oz)	219
Guacamole	1 serv (0.9 oz)	55
Jalapenos	1 serv (0.7 oz)	3
Mexican Rice	1 serv (4.2 oz)	469
Muchaco Beef	1 (5.2 oz)	449
Muchaco Beef w/o Cheddar Cheese	1 (4.9 oz)	410
Muchaco Beef w/o Refried Beans	1 (4.2 oz)	392
Muchaco Chicken	1 (4.6 oz)	387
Muchaco Chicken w/o Cheddar Cheese	1 (4.4 oz)	348
Quesadilla Beef	1 (8.5 oz)	823
Quesadilla Cheese	1 (6.5 oz)	709
Quesadilla Chicken	1 (7.9 oz)	761
Quesadilla Kids Cheese	1 (2.2 oz)	219
Quesadilla Mini Cheese	1 (2.7)	274
Refried Beans Powdered	1 serv (6.3 oz)	406
Refried Beans w/o Cheddar Cheese	1 serv (5.8 oz)	327
Refried Beans w/o Chili	1 serv (5.1 oz)	360
Salsa Red	1 serv (2 oz)	14
Soup Tortilla	1 bowl	237
Soup Tortilla w/o Tortilla Strips & Cheese	1 bowl	148
Sour Cream	1 serv (1 oz)	57
Taco w/o Cheddar Cheese	1 (1.5 oz)	104
Taco Crispy Beef	1 (2.6 oz)	200
Taco Crispy Chicken	1 (1.9 oz)	140
Taco Crispy Chicken w/o Cheddar Cheese	1 (1.7 oz)	100

FOOD	PORTION	CALS
Taco Crispy w/o Cheddar Cheese	1 (2.4 oz)	161
Taco Party	1 (1.9 oz)	143
Taco Soft Beef	1 (3.5 oz)	245
Taco Soft Beef w/o Cheddar Cheese	1 (3.2 oz)	206
Taco Soft Chicken	1 (2.9 oz)	184
Taco Soft Chicken w/o Cheddar Cheese	1 (2.5 oz)	145
Tostada	1 (4.1 oz)	324
Tostada w/o Cheddar Cheese	1 (3.3 oz)	207
Tostada w/o Chili	1 (2.9 oz)	269
Tostada w/o Refried Beans	1 (2.5 oz)	234
SALADS		
Nacho Beef	1 (9.3 oz)	759
Nacho Beef w/o Cheddar Cheese	1 (8.8 oz)	681
Nacho Beef w/o Chili	1 (6.9 oz)	648
Nacho Chicken	1 (8.9 oz)	713
Nacho Chicken w/o Cheddar Cheese	1 (8.4 oz)	634
Nacho Chicken w/o Chili	1 (6.5 oz)	601
Taco Beef	1 (12.7 oz)	1043
Taco Beef w/o Cheddar Cheese	1 (11.7 oz)	886
Taco Beef w/o Chili	1 (11.5 oz)	987
Taco Beef w/o Guacamole	1 (11.7 oz)	988
Taco Beef w/o Sour Cream	1 (11.7 oz)	986
Taco Beef w/o Tortilla Bowl	1 (9.7 oz)	564
Taco Chicken	1 (9.6 oz)	838
Taco Chicken w/o Cheddar Cheese	1 (8.6 oz)	680
Taco Chicken w/o Guacamole	1 (8.6 oz)	783
Taco Chicken w/o Sour Cream	1 (8.6 oz)	781
Taco Chicken w/o Tortilla Bowl	1 (6.6 oz)	359
TACOTIME		
DESSERTS		
Churro Plain	1 (1.5 oz)	205
Churro w/ Cinnamon & Sugar	1 (2 oz)	245
Crustos	1 serv	294
Empanada Apple	1 (4 oz)	234
Empanada Cherry	1 (4 oz)	240
Empanada Pumpkin	1 (4 oz)	256
MAIN MENU SELECTIONS		
Burrito Big Juan Seasoned Ground Beef	1 (13 oz)	651
Burrito Big Juan Shredded Beef	1 (13 oz)	633
Burrito Big Juan Chicken	1 (13 oz)	594

FOOD	PORTION	CALS
Burrito Casita Chicken	1 (12 oz)	494
Burrito Casita Seasoned Ground Beef	1 (12 oz)	552
Burrito Casita Shredded Beef	1 (12 oz)	533
Burrito Chicken & Black Bean	1 (10 oz)	478
Burrito Chicken BLT	1 (10 oz)	721
Burrito Chicken Ranchero	1 (10.8 oz)	654
Burrito Crisp Chicken	1 (5.5 oz)	336
Burrito Crisp Meat	1 (5.8 oz)	450
Burrito Crisp Pinto Bean	1 (6 oz)	394
Burrito Soft Meat	1 (6.7 oz)	426
Burrito Soft Pinto Bean	1 (6.7 oz)	377
Burrito Veggie	1 (11 oz)	534
Cheddar Fries	1 sm (6 oz)	374
Cheddar Melt	1 (2.8 oz)	250
Mexi-Fries	1 sm (5 oz)	290
Mexi-Rice	1 serv (4 oz)	87
Nachos Grande	1 serv (16.5 oz)	1132
Refritos w/ Chips	1 serv (7 oz)	304
Refritos w/o Chips	1 serv (6.7 oz)	285
Stuffed Fries	1 sm (5 oz)	321
Taco ½ Lb Shredded Beef	1 (9 oz)	440
Taco ½ Lb Soft Chicken	1 (9 oz)	401
Taco ½ Lb Soft Seasoned Ground Beef	1 (9 oz)	459
Taco Chips	1 serv (2 oz)	150
Taco Crisp Seasoned Ground Beef	1 (4.3 oz)	225
Taco Super Soft Chicken	1 (11 oz)	540
Taco Super Soft Seasoned Ground Beef	1 (11 oz)	598
Taco Super Soft Shredded Beef	1 (11 oz)	579
Taco Value Soft	1 (5.3 oz)	314
SALAD DRESSINGS AND TOPPINGS		
Cheddar Cheese	1 serv (2 oz)	223
Dressing Chipotle Ranch	1 serv (1 oz)	165
Dressing Ranch	1 serv (1 oz)	181
Dressing Thousand Island	1 serv (1 oz)	132
Guacamole	1 serv (1 oz)	50
Salsa Nuevo	1 serv (1 oz)	8
Salsa Verde	1 serv (1 oz)	6
Sour Cream	1 serv (1.5 oz)	85
SALADS		
Taco Chicken	1 reg (9.2 oz)	351

FOOD	PORTION	CALS
Taco Seasoned Ground Beef	1 reg (7.8 oz)	396
Taco Shredded Beef	1 reg (7.8 oz)	377
Tostada Delight Chicken	1 (10.5 oz)	565
Tostada Delight Seasoned Ground Beef	1 (10.5 oz)	623
Tostada Delight Shredded Beef	1 (10.5 oz)	604

TASTI D-LITE
Vanilla	1 sm (4 oz)	40

TCBY
FROZEN YOGURT AND SORBET
Hand Scooped Butter Pecan Perfection	½ cup	110
Hand Scooped Chocolate Chocolate Swirl	½ cup	120
Hand Scooped Chocolate Chunk Cookie Dough	½ cup	160
Hand Scooped Cookies & Cream	½ cup	140
Hand Scooped Cotton Candy	½ cup	120
Hand Scooped Mint Chocolate Chunk	½ cup	140
Hand Scooped Mocha Almond	½ cup	150
Hand Scooped No Sugar Added Chocolate Chocolate Swirl	½ cup	90
Hand Scooped No Sugar Added Vanilla	½ cup	80
Hand Scooped No Sugar Added Vanilla Fudge Brownie	½ cup	100
Hand Scooped Pralines & Cream	½ cup	140
Hand Scooped Psychedelic Sorbet	½ cup	290
Hand Scooped Rainbow Cream	½ cup	120
Hand Scooped Rocky Road	½ cup	220
Hand Scooped Strawberries & Cream	½ cup	120
Hand Scooped Vanilla Bean	½ cup	120
Hand Scooped Vanilla Chocolate Chunk	½ cup	140
Soft Serve Frozen Yogurt All Flavors 96% Fat Free	½ cup	140
Soft Serve Frozen Yogurt All Flavors Nonfat	½ cup	110
Soft Serve Frozen Yogurt All Flavors Nonfat No Sugar Added	½ cup	90
Soft Serve Frozen Yogurt All Flavors Low Carb	½ cup	110
Soft Serve Sorbet All Flavors Nonfat Nondairy	½ cup	100

SMOOTHIES
Berrylicious	1 (16 oz)	290
Black 'N Blueberry	1 (16 oz)	280

FOOD	PORTION	CALS
Mango Tango	1 (16 oz)	330
Mangolada	1 (16 oz)	340
Mondo Mango	1 (16 oz)	310
Pina Paradise	1 (16 oz)	350
Pink Pineapple	1 (16 oz)	340
Straight Up Strawberry	1 (16 oz)	280
Strawberry Bonanza	1 (16 oz)	320
Strawberry Fling	1 (16 oz)	340

TIM HORTONS
BAKED SELECTIONS

FOOD	PORTION	CALS
Bagel Blueberry	1	270
Bagel Cinnamon Raisin	1	270
Bagel Everything	1	280
Bagel Flax Seed	1	290
Bagel Onion	1	260
Bagel Plain	1	260
Bagel Poppy Seed	1	270
Bagel Sesame Seed	1	270
Bagel Sun Dried Tomato	1	310
Bagel Twelve Grain	1	330
Cinnamon Roll Frosted	1	470
Cinnamon Roll Glazed	1	420
Cookie Caramel Chocolate Pecan	1	230
Cookie Chocolate Chip	1	230
Cookie Oatmeal Raisin Spice	1	220
Cookie Peanut Butter Chocolate Chunk	1	260
Cookie Triple Chocolate	1	250
Cookie White Chocolate Macadamia Nut	1	240
Croissant Butter	1	340
Croissant Cheese	1	370
Danish Cherry Cheese	1	330
Danish Chocolate	1	430
Danish Maple Pecan	1	380
Donut Apple Fritter	1	300
Donut Chocolate Dip	1	210
Donut Chocolate Glazed	1	260
Donut Honey Dip	1	210
Donut Maple Dip	1	210
Donut Old Fashion Glazed	1	320
Donut Old Fashion Plain	1	260

FOOD	PORTION	CALS
Donut Sour Cream Plain	1	270
Donut Walnut Crunch	1	360
Donut Filled Angel Cream	1	310
Donut Filled Blueberry	1	230
Donut Filled Boston Cream	1	250
Donut Filled Canadian Maple	1	260
Donut Filled Strawberry	1	230
Honey Cruller	1	320
Muffin Blueberry	1	330
Muffin Blueberry Bran	1	300
Muffin Carrot Wheat	1	400
Muffin Chocolate Chip	1	430
Muffin Cranberry Blueberry Bran	1	290
Muffin Cranberry Fruit	1	350
Muffin Fruit Explosion	1	360
Muffin Raisin Bran	1	360
Muffin Strawberry Sensation	1	350
Muffin Low Fat Blueberry	1	290
Muffin Low Fat Cranberry	1	290
Tea Biscuit Plain	1	250
Tea Biscuit Raisin	1	290
Timbits Apple Fritter	1	50
Timbits Chocolate Glazed	1	70
Timbits Honey Dip	1	60
Timbits Old Fashion Plain	1	70
Timbits Filled Banana Cream	1	60
Timbits Filled Lemon	1	60
Timbits Filled Strawberry	1	60
BEVERAGES		
Cafe Mocha	1 (10 oz)	160
Cappuccino Iced	1 (12 oz)	300
Coffee Decaffeinated + Sugar & Cream	1 (10 oz)	75
Coffee + Sugar & Cream	1 (10 oz)	75
English Toffee	1 (10 oz)	220
Flavor Shot	1 serv	5
French Vanilla	1 (10 oz)	240
Hot Chocolate	1 (10 oz)	240
Hot Smoothie	1 (10 oz)	260
Iced Cappuccino w/ Milk	1 (12 oz)	180
Tea + Sugar & Milk	1 (10 oz)	50

FOOD	PORTION	CALS
CREAM CHEESE		
Garden Vegetable	1.5 oz	120
Light Plain	1.5 oz	60
Plain	1.5 oz	130
Strawberry	1.5 oz	120
SANDWICHES		
B.L.T.	1	450
Breakfast Bacon Egg Cheese	1	410
Breakfast Egg Cheese	1	360
Breakfast Sausage Egg Cheese	1	520
Chicken Salad	1	380
Egg Salad	1	390
Ham & Swiss	1	440
Toasted Chicken Club	1	460
Turkey Breast	1	390
SOUPS		
Beef Stew	1 serv (10 oz)	236
Chicken Noodle	1 serv (10 oz)	120
Chili	1 serv (10 oz)	300
Country Field Mushroom	1 serv (10 oz)	150
Cream Of Broccoli	1 serv (10 oz)	160
Hearty Vegetable	1 serv (10 oz)	70
Minestrone	1 serv (10 oz)	120
Potato Bacon	1 serv (10 oz)	180
Split Pea w/ Ham	1 serv (10 oz)	150
Turkey Rice	1 serv (10 oz)	120
Vegetable Beef Barley	1 serv (10 oz)	110
YOGURT		
Low Fat Creamy Vanilla w/ Berries	1 (6 oz)	160
Low Fat Strawberry w/ Berries	1 (6 oz)	150
TJ CINNAMONS		
Chocolate Twist	1	250
Cinnamon Twist	1	280
Mocha Chill w/ Whipped Cream	1 (12.5 oz)	306
Mocha Chill w/o Whipped Cream	1 (12.5 oz)	264
Original Roll w/o Icing	1	507
Pecan Sticky Bun	1	688
TJ Icing	1 serv (1 oz)	117

FOOD	PORTION	CALS
WENDY'S		
BEVERAGES		
Chocolate Milk 1%	8 oz	170
Coca-Cola	1 med (12 oz)	140
Dasani Water	1 bottle	0
Diet Coke	1 med (11 oz)	0
Frosty	1 sm (8 oz)	330
Milk 2%	8 oz	120
Sprite	1 med (12 oz)	130
CHILDREN'S MENU SELECTIONS		
French Fries	1 serv (3.2 oz)	280
Kid's Meal Cheeseburger	1	320
Kid's Meal Chicken Nuggets	4 pieces	180
Kid's Meal Ham & Cheese	1 serv	240
Kid's Meal Hamburger	1	270
Kid's Meal Turkey & Cheese	1 serv	250
SALAD DRESSINGS AND TOPPINGS		
Ancho Chipotle Ranch	1 pkg	110
Blue Cheese	1 pkg	260
Buttery Best Spread	1 pkg	50
Caesar	1 pkg	120
Cheddar Cheese Shredded	2 tbsp	70
Creamy Ranch	1 pkg	230
Creamy Ranch Reduced Fat	1 pkg	100
Crispy Noodles	1 pkg	60
Croutons Homestyle Garlic	1 pkg	70
Dipping Sauce Deli Honey Mustard	1 pkg	170
Dipping Sauce Heartland Ranch	1 pkg	200
Dipping Sauce Spicy Southwest Chipotle	1 pkg	150
Dipping Sauce Sweet & Sour Hawaiian	1 pkg	70
Dipping Sauce Wild Buffalo Ranch	1 pkg	180
French Fat Free	1 pkg	80
Granola Topping	1 pkg	110
Honey Mustard	1 pkg	280
Honey Mustard Low Fat	1 pkg	110
Hot Chili Seasoning	1 pkg	5
Italian Vinaigrette	1 pkg	140
Ketchup	1 tsp	7
Mayonnaise	1 tsp	30
Mustard	½ tsp	5

FOOD	PORTION	CALS
Nuggets Sauce Barbeque	1 pkg	45
Nuggets Sauce Honey Mustard	1 pkg	130
Nuggets Sauce Sweet & Sour	1 pkg	50
Oriental Sesame	1 pkg	190
Roasted Almonds	1 pkg	130
Saltines	2	25
Sour Cream Reduced Fat	1 pkg	45
Thousand Island	1 pkg	260
Tortilla Strips	1 pkg	110
SALADS		
Caesar Chicken w/o Dressing & Croutons	1 serv	180
Ceasar Side Salad w/o Dressing & Croutons	1 serv	70
Chicken BLT w/o Dressing & Croutons	1 serv	340
Mandarin Chicken w/o Dressing	1 serv	170
Side Salad w/o Dressing	1	35
Southwest Taco w/o Dressing Tortilla Strip & Sour Cream	1 serv	440
SANDWICHES AND SIDES		
Baked Potato Plain	1	270
Baked Potato w/ Sour Cream & Chives	1 serv	320
Big Bacon Classic	1	580
Chicken Nuggets	5 pieces	220
Chili	1 sm (8 oz)	220
Classic Single w/ Everything	1	420
French Fries	1 med (5 oz)	440
Frescata Black Forest Ham & Swiss	1	480
Frescata Club	1	440
Frescata Roasted Turkey & Basil Pesto	1	420
Frescata Roasted Turkey & Swiss	1	490
Hamburger	1	280
Homestyle Chicken Strips	3 pieces	410
Jr. Bacon Cheeseburger	1	370
Jr. BBQ Cheeseburger	1	330
Jr. Cheeseburger	1	320
Jr. Cheeseburger Deluxe	1	360
Mandarin Orange Cup	1 serv	80
Sandwich Crispy Chicken	1	380
Sandwich Spicy Chicken Fillet	1	510
Sandwich Ultimate Chicken Grill	1	360
Yogurt Low Fat Strawberry	1 pkg	140

FOOD	PORTION	CALS
WETZEL'S PRETZELS		
Original w/ Butter	1	320
Original w/o Butter	1	280
WHATABURGER		
BEVERAGES		
Barq's Root Beet	1 sm (16 oz)	220
Cherry Coke	1 sm (16 oz)	210
Coca-Cola	1 sm (16 oz)	207
Coffee	1 sm (8 oz)	5
Coffee Decaf	1 sm (8 oz)	5
Diet Coke	1 sm (16 oz)	0
Dr Pepper	1 sm (16 oz)	190
Fanta Orange	1 sm (16 oz)	210
Fanta Strawberry	1 sm (16 oz)	230
Iced Tea Sweetened	1 (34 oz)	430
Iced Tea Unsweetened	1 sm (19 oz)	0
Lemonade Hi-C Poppin' Pink	1 sm (16 oz)	200
Malt Chocolate	1 sm (16 oz)	670
Malt Strawberry	1 sm (16 oz)	670
Malt Vanilla	1 sm (16 oz)	600
Milk Reduced Fat	8 oz	120
Orange Juice Tropicana	1 (10 oz)	140
Powerade Fruit Punch	1 sm (16 oz)	130
Shake Chocolate	1 sm (16 oz)	630
Shake Strawberry	1 sm (16 oz)	630
Shake Vanilla	1 sm (16 oz)	560
Sprite	1 sm (16 oz)	200
CHILDREN'S MENU SELECTIONS		
Kid's Meal Chicken Strips	1 serv	770
Kid's Meal Justaburger	1 serv	570
DESSERTS		
Apple Pie A La Mode	1 serv	520
Apple Pie Hot	1	230
Cinnamon Roll	1	400
Cookie Chocolate Chunk	1 (2 oz)	230
Cookie White Chocolate Chunk Macadamia	1 (2 oz)	250
Peach Pie Al La Mode	1 serv	570
MAIN MENU SELECTIONS		
Biscuit	1	300
Biscuit Honey Butter Chicken	1	610

FOOD	PORTION	CALS
Biscuit Sandwich Bacon Egg & Cheese	1	500
Biscuit Sandwich Egg & Cheese	1	450
Biscuit Sandwich Sausage Egg & Cheese	1	690
Biscuit w/ Bacon	1	355
Biscuit w/ Gravy	1	530
Biscuit w/ Sausage	1	540
Breakfast Platter w/ Bacon	1 serv	730
Breakfast Platter w/ Sausage	1 serv	930
Breakfast On A Bun w/ Bacon	1	380
Breakfast On A Bun w/ Sausage	1	570
Chicken Strips	1	200
Chicken Strips w/ Gravy	4	840
French Fries	1 sm	260
Gravy White Peppered	1 serv	60
Hashbrown Sticks	4	200
Justaburger	1	329
Onion Rings	1 med	420
Pancakes Plain	1 serv	580
Pancakes w/ Bacon	1 serv	630
Pancakes w/ Sausage	1 serv	820
Sandwich Chicken Strip Honey BBQ	1	1110
Sandwich Chicken Strip Junior Honey BBQ	1	720
Sandwich Egg	1	330
Sandwich Grilled Chicken	1	450
Taquito Sausage & Egg	1	410
Taquito w/ Bacon & Egg	1	370
Taquito w/ Bacon Egg & Cheese	1	420
Taquito w/ Potato & Egg	1	430
Taquito w/ Potato Egg & Cheese	1	470
Taquito w/ Sausage Egg & Cheese	1	450
Texas Toast	1 slice	180
Whataburger	1	640
Whataburger Double Meat	1	890
Whataburger Jr.	1	330
Whataburger Triple Meat	1	1140
Whataburger w/ Bacon & Cheese	1	800
Whatacatch	1	480
Whatacatch Dinner	1 serv	1095
Whatachick'n	1	530

FOOD	PORTION	CALS
SALADS		
Chicken Strips	1 serv	570
Garden Salad	1	60
Grilled Chicken	1 serv	230
WHITE CASTLE		
BEVERAGES		
Barq's Red Cream Soda	1 sm (21 oz)	260
Barq's Root Beer	1 sm (21 oz)	250
Coca-Cola	1 sm (21 oz)	220
Coffee Black	1 sm (12 oz)	<5
Crave Cooler Coke	1 sm (21 oz)	150
Diet Coke	1 sm (21 oz)	0
Fanta Orange	1 sm (21 oz)	240
Hi-C Flashing Fruit Punch	1 sm (21 oz)	240
Hot Chocolate	1 sm (12 oz)	220
Hot Tea	1 sm (12 oz)	0
Iced Tea Sweetened w/ Lemon	1 sm (21 oz)	170
Iced Tea Unsweetened	1 sm (21 oz)	0
Lemonade Raspberry	1 sm (21 oz)	290
Pibb Xtra	1 sm (21 oz)	220
Powerade Mountain Blast	1 sm (21 oz)	140
Sprite	1 sm (21 oz)	220
MAIN MENU SELECTIONS		
Cheeseburger	1	170
Cheeseburger Bacon	1	200
Cheeseburger Bacon Double	1	370
Cheeseburger Double	1	300
Cheeseburger Jalapeno	1	180
Cheeseburger Jalapeno Double	1	320
Chicken Rings	6	210
Clam Strips	1 reg	250
Fish Nibblers	1 reg	280
French Fries	1 reg	310
Mozzarella Cheese Sticks	3	250
Onion Chips	1 reg	480
Sandwich Chicken Breast w/ Cheese	1	200
Sandwich Chicken Ring	1	180
Sandwich Chicken Ring w/ Cheese	1	200
Sandwich Fish w/ Cheese	1	180
White Castle	1	140

FOOD	PORTION	CALS
White Castle Double	1	250
SAUCES AND SPREADS		
Dressing Ranch	1 serv (1 oz)	150
Ketchup	1 pkg	10
Lemon Juice	1 pkg	0
Mayonnaise	1 pkg	60
Sauce BBQ	1 serv (1 oz)	35
Sauce Hot	1 pkg	0
Sauce Marinara	1 serv (1 oz)	15
Sauce Seafood	1 serv (1 oz)	30
Sauce Tartar	1 pkg	30
Sauce Zesty Zing	1 serv (1 oz)	110
Sauce Fat Free Honey Mustard	1 serv (1 oz)	50

WINCHELL'S DONUTS

FOOD	PORTION	CALS
Chocolate Bar	1	240
Chocolate Round	1	240
Chocolate Twist	1	240
Croissant	1	260
Glazed Round	1	230
Glazed Twist	1	230
Iced Chocolate	1	230
Traditional	1	215

WORLD WRAPPS

FOOD	PORTION	CALS
CHILDREN'S MENU SELECTIONS		
Kid's Bean & Cheese	1	332
Kid's Chicken & Cheese	1	229
Kids' Quesadilla	1	410
Kid's Teriyaki Chicken	1	407
SALADS		
BBQ Ranch Chicken	1 serv	633
Caesar Blackened Salmon	1 serv	612
Caesar Classic	1 serv	417
California Cobb	1 serv	636
Garden Veggie	1 serv	492
Thai Asian Chicken	1 serv	613
SIDES AND SOUPS		
Chips & Mango Salsa	1 serv	224
Chips & Tomato Corn Salsa	1 serv	184
Potstickers	3	170

FOOD	PORTION	CALS
Soup Thai Lemongrass	1 cup	256
Soup Tortilla	1 cup	191
Yogurt Parfait	1 serv	281
SMOOTHIES		
Black & Blue	1 (16 oz)	319
Blue Mango Boost	1 (16 oz)	295
Caribbean C	1 (16 oz)	276
Georgia Peach	1 (16 oz)	343
Peanut Butter Banana	1 (16 oz)	502
Strawberry Orange Banana	1 (16 oz)	268
Triathlete	1 (16 oz)	341
Tropical Storm	1 (16 oz)	309
WRAPS		
Baja Veggie w/ Cheese Sour Cream Avocados	1 sm	541
Barcelona	1 sm	460
Bean & Cheese	1 sm	452
Bombay Curry Veggie	1 sm	495
Buffalo w/ Shrimp	1 sm	422
Burrito w/ Chicken Cheese Sour Cream Avocado	1 sm	576
Burrito w/ Steak Cheese Sour Cream Avocado	1 sm	573
Caribbean Sole	1 sm	523
Chicken Caesar	1 sm	547
Chicken Parmesan	1 sm	495
Portabello & Goat Cheese	1 sm	391
Samurai Salmon	1 sm	543
Spicy Southwest Shrimp	1 sm	460
Tequila Lime Shrimp	1 sm	422
Teriyaki Chicken	1 sm	482
Teriyaki Steak	1 sm	497
Teriyaki Tofu & Mushroom	1 sm	387
Texas Roadhouse BBQ Chicken	1 sm	512
Texas Roadhouse BBQ Steak	1 sm	569
Thai Chicken	1 sm	508
YOGURTLAND		
Arctic Vanilla	½ cup (3 oz)	108
Blueberry Tart	½ cup (3 oz)	127
Cafe Con Leche	½ cup (3 oz)	108

FOOD	PORTION	CALS
Chocolate Mint	½ cup (3 oz)	100
Double Cookies & Cream	½ cup (3 oz)	121
Dutch Chocolate	½ cup (3 oz)	118
Fresh Strawberry	½ cup (3 oz)	108
Green Tea	½ cup (3 oz)	107
Heath Bar	½ cup (3 oz)	132
Mango	½ cup (3 oz)	96
Mango Tart	½ cup (3 oz)	127
No Sugar Added French Vanilla	½ cup (3 oz)	89
NY Cheesecake	½ cup (3 oz)	100
Peach	½ cup (3 oz)	100
Peach Tart	½ cup (3 oz)	127
Peanut Butter	½ cup (3 oz)	119
Pineapple Tart	½ cup (3 oz)	127
Pistachio	½ cup (3 oz)	100
Plain Tart	½ cup (3 oz)	108
Strawberry Tart	½ cup (3 oz)	127
Taro	½ cup (3 oz)	102

ZOUP!
DESSERTS

FOOD	PORTION	CALS
Cookie Chocolate Chunk	1	410
Cookie Peanut Butter	1	420

SANDWICHES

FOOD	PORTION	CALS
Grilled Turkey Club	½	470
Panini Italian Chicken	½	370
Pesto Three Cheese	1	720
Tuna Melt	1	600
Wrap American Farm	½	435
Wrap Asian	½	615
Wrap Chicken Caesar w/o Dressing	½	505
Wrap Greek w/o Dressing	½	485
Wrap Sonoma	½	595
Wrap Tuna	½	365
Zesty Southwest Turkey	½	310

SOUPS

FOOD	PORTION	CALS
Chicken & Dumplings	1 (8 oz)	130
Chicken Potpie	1 (8 oz)	200
Italian Wedding w/ Turkey Meatballs	1 (8 oz)	120
Jamaican Bay Gumbo	1 (8 oz)	140
Lobster Bisque	1 (8 oz)	260

FOOD	PORTION	CALS
Pepper Steak	1 (8 oz)	160
Potato Cheddar	1 (8 oz)	210
Sesame Noodle Bowl	1 (8 oz)	80
Shrimp & Crawfish Etouffee	1 (8 oz)	130
Sicilian Pizza	1 (8 oz)	150
Spicy Crab & Rice	1 (8 oz)	110
Turkey Chili	1 (8 oz)	120
Wild Mushroom Barley	1 (8 oz)	108